THE OLYMPIC BOOK OF

SPORTS MEDICINE

THE ENC

AN INTE

IN COLL

INTERNA

EDITED

A. DIRI

...JBLICATION

...DICINE

OXFORD

BLACKWELL SCIENTIFIC PUBLICATIONS

LONDON EDINBURGH BOSTON

MELBOURNE PARIS BERLIN VIENNA

© 1988 International Olympic Committee

Published by Blackwell Scientific Publications
Editorial Offices:
Osney Mead, Oxford OX2 0EL
25 John Street, London WC1N 2BL
23 Ainslie Place, Edinburgh EH3 6AJ
3 Cambridge Center, Cambridge
  Massachusetts 02142, USA
54 University Street, Carlton
  Victoria 3053, Australia

Other Editorial Offices:
Arnette SA, 2 rue Casimir-Delavigne
  75006 Paris, France
Blackwell Wissenschaft, Meinekestrasse 4
  D-1000 Berlin 15, Germany
Blackwell MZV, Feldgasse 13
  A-1238 Wien, Austria

First published 1988
Paperback reissue 1991

Set by Oxprint Ltd, Oxford
Printed and bound by Mohndruck Ltd, Germany

Part title illustrations by Grahame Baker

DISTRIBUTORS

Marston Book Services Ltd
PO Box 87
Oxford OX2 0DT
Orders:
Tel: 0865 791155
Fax: 0865 791927
Telex: 837515

USA
  Mosby-Year Book, Inc.
  11830 Westline Industrial Drive
  St Louis, Missouri 63146
  Orders: Tel: 800 633-6699

Canada
  Mosby-Year Book, Inc.
  5240 Finch Avenue East
  Scarborough, Ontario
  Orders: Tel: 416 298-1588

Australia
  Blackwell Scientific Publications
  (Australia) Pty Ltd
  54 University Street
  Carlton, Victoria 3053
  Orders: Tel: 03 347-0300

British Library Cataloguing in Publication Data

The Olympic book of sports medicine.
1. Sports. Performance. Medical aspects
I. Dirix, A.   II. Knuttgen, H.G.
III. Tittel, K.   IV. International Sports Committee
612'.044
ISBN 0-632-03084-4

Contents

Preface

H. E. Juan Antonio Samaranch
President of the International Olympic Committee

It is a fact of life nowadays, that as soon as one deals with competition sport, and particularly top level sport, the doctor, scientist and coach are involved straight away. Everywhere multidisciplinary teams spring up around training sites, seeking to isolate and identify the ingredients of success, to improve performances by changing this movement, that method of preparation, one piece of equipment or another, etc.

Sport has in fact become a vast realm of experiments, experimentation and discoveries, the significance of which, going far beyond the world of sport, often has implications which may affect the whole of mankind. In sport, as elsewhere, the uses to which science is put depend on the integrity and honesty of those whose job it is to delve into its secrets. One of the major difficulties in this respect lies in the extraordinary isolation of the practitioner, sometimes submerged beneath a never-ending flood of information without a free moment to sift through it, sometimes, at the other extreme, cut off from access to any worthwhile source of new ideas.

This difference is even more marked when one compares the situation in the industrialized countries with that which exists in developing countries. But all are faced with the same dilemma: finding the right information, quickly, and in a usable form.

In an attempt to remedy this problem, at least in part, the International Olympic Committee, through the intermediary of its Medical Commission, decided to undertake an ambitious project in collaboration with the International Federation of Sports Medicine to produce *The Encyclopaedia of Sports Medicine*. This first volume, *The Olympic Book of Sports Medicine*, is the result. Thanks to the joint efforts of over 50 contributing authors from two dozen countries, all recognized authorities in their respective fields, this first part of the project has been completed. We look forward to the development of additional volumes on specialized topics in the near future.

Our goal was simple: to offer all those working in the field, sometimes in far from ideal conditions, a general reference work which would bring them up to date, and enable them to find the vital information they lacked, that indispensable reference, the idea needed to complete the job in hand in the best possible conditions. We do not pretend to offer here, in a single volume, the source of all knowledge about sports medicine. We wanted more simply just to provide an approach, a key which could be used by everyone and permit those who have the time, the inclination or the opportunity to go further without the risk of losing their bearings.

We very much hope we will be able to complete this work by adding a series of much more specialized volumes which will attempt to cover, each within a particular field, the most recent discoveries and most sophisticated techniques.

Some may find it surprising to see the International Olympic Committee involving itself in a field which would, at first sight, appear to be totally foreign to it. However, serious reasons have led us to adopt this position—reasons which the Chairman of our Medical Commission, Prince Alexandre de Merode, put forward so brilliantly during the first European Symposium on Doping, held in Paris on 24 and 25 January 1988. It is indeed time, I feel, for serious reflection concerning worrying recent developments in top level sports, and to consider whether these current trends might not in fact contain the seeds of their own destruction.

I see here two kinds of danger. The danger of division between the industrialized countries and the others; between those who have the resources to carry out highly specialized—and very costly—research, and those who strive simply to spread and instil a few simple principles of hygiene and nutrition, for want of anything better; thus the danger of creating a sporting élite restricted to a few countries, which goes totally against the universality of our movement and our ideals. But also the danger of 'manufacturing' a programmed athlete, medically prepared to attain the highest performances at the very real risk of endangering health, and sometimes even his or her life.

Apart from the abandonment of the ethical and moral principles which have been the cornerstone of the Olympic Movement's success for nearly a century, I see in such an attitude a refusal—even a denial—of the profoundly 'human' and educative character of sport. I would put the same vigour and conviction into fighting such a concept of 'sport' that I now employ in defending our ideals.

How then to ward off these dangers, compensate for the regrettable deficiencies of our modern society, and put all our strength into defending those principles which we hold dear? Such was the question we had to ask ourselves, and so the idea of *The Encyclopaedia of Sports Medicine*, put forward by Prince de Merode, immediately struck us as being one of the best answers to this question. It will be up to you, the people who use the work, to tell us whether we have succeeded.

Before I let you go on to discover this work, however, I would like to appeal to you in my capacity as President of the International Olympic Committee. Since ancient times, sport has always been synonymous with joy, relaxation, health, balance and perfection. Whilst it is perfectly legitimate to strive to reach one's own limits, it is a totally different matter to go beyond these limits, be it with the help, complicity or at the behest of anyone else. It is the duty of all of us, athletes, leaders, doctors, coaches, researchers, etc. to be self-critical if necessary, to see to it that these limits are respected, and to ensure that sport remains the sphere where one can witness the miracle of a transient perfection resulting solely from the abilities and willpower of the individual athlete.

That, then, is the essence of our mission, and this book will have already served a useful purpose if it in any way contributes towards this necessary awareness.

List of contributors

Editors

A. Dirix Prof MD, *St Niklaas, Belgium; Secretary IOC Medical Commission*

H. G. Knuttgen Prof PhD, *Boston University, Boston, USA; Co-chairman FIMS Scientific Commission*

K. Tittel Prof MD, *German University for Physical Culture and Sports, Leipzig, GDR; Co-chairman FIMS Scientific Commission*

Authors

C. Abouker MD, *St Roch Hospital, Nice, France*

C. Argenson Prof MD, *St Roch Hospital, Nice, France*

O. Bar-Or Prof MD, *McMaster University, Hamilton, Canada*

A. Beckett Prof PhD, *London University, London, UK*

P. Berteau MD, *Institute of Sports Medicine, Rouen, France*

A. Bouzayen MD, *National Centre of Sports Medicine, Tunis, Tunisia*

G. Caldarone Prof MD, *Institute of Sports Science, Rome, Italy*

G. Caselli MD, *Institute of Sports Science, Rome, Italy*

A. Chouchane MD, *St Roch Hospital, Nice, France*

F. A. Commandré MD, *University of Marseilles, Marseilles, France*

D. L. Costill Prof PhD, *Ball State University, Muncie, USA*

W. Crasselt PhD, *German University for Physical Culture and Sports, Leipzig, GDR*

A. Dal Monte Prof MD, *Institute of Sports Science, Rome, Italy*

Prince Alex. de Merode, *Vice President IOC; Chairman IOC Medical Commission, Lausanne, Switzerland*

E. H. De Rose Prof MD, *Federal University Rio Grande do Sul, Port Alegre, Brazil*

F. Denis MD, *St Roch Hospital, Nice, France*

I. Diop Mar Prof MD, *National Olympic Committee of Senegal, Dakar, Senegal*

M. Donike Prof MD, *German University of Sports, Cologne, FRG*

I. Drăgan Prof MD PhD, *University Policlinic 'Vitan', Bucharest, Romania*

B. Drinkwater Prof PhD, *Pacific Medical Center, Seattle, USA*

K. D. Fitch MD, *Mount Hospital Medical Centre, Perth, Australia*

R. Frenkl Prof MD, *Hungarian University of Physical Education, Budapest, Hungary*

G. Grimby Prof MD, *Sahlgren Hospital, Gothenburg, Sweden*

K. Häkkinen MD, *University of Jyväskylä, Jyväskylä, Finland*

D. Hannemann MD, *Sports Medical Service, Berlin, GDR*

Y. Hayashi MD, *Tokyo Metropolitan Geriatric Hospital, Tokyo, Japan*

M. Hebbelinck Prof PhD, *Vrije University, Brussels, Belgium*

G. P. H. Hermans MD, *R. C. Hospital, Hilversum, The Netherlands*

W. Hollman Prof MD, *German University of Sports, Cologne, FRG; President FIMS*

R. S. Hutton Prof PhD, *University of Washington, Seattle, USA*

S. Israel Prof MD PhD, *German University for Physical Culture and Sports, Leipzig, GDR*

L. Komadel Prof MD DSc, *Comenius University, Bratislava, Czechoslovakia*

P. V. Komi Prof PhD, *University of Jyväskylä, Jyväskylä, Finland*

Y. Kuroda Prof MD PhD, *University of Juntendo, Tokyo, Japan*

R. Leach Prof MD, *Boston University Medical Center, Boston, USA*

H. Liesen Prof MD, *German University of Sports, Cologne, FRG*

R. Lorentzon Prof MD, *University of Umeå, Sweden*

M. Máček Prof MD, *Charles University, Prague, Czechoslovakia*

A. Mader Prof, *German University of Sports, Cologne, FRG*

S. Mironov Prof MD, *Central Institute of Traumatology and Orthopaedics, Moscow, USSR*

A. R. Morton Prof, *University of Western Australia, Perth, Australia*

G. Neumann Prof MD, *German University for Physical Culture and Sports, Leipzig, GDR*

ix

B. Nigg Prof Dr sc nat, *University of Calgary, Calgary, Canada*

M. O'Brien Prof MD, *Trinity College, Dublin, Ireland*

A. Pelliccia MD, *Institute of Sports Science, Rome, Italy*

P. Renström Prof MD, *Sahlgren Hospital, Gothenburg, Sweden*

A. Rogopoulous MD, *St Roch Hospital, Nice, France*

W. D. Ross Prof PhD, *Simon Fraser University, Burnaby BC, Canada*

R. Rost Prof MD, *German University of Sports, Cologne, FRG*

C. Roux Prof MD, *University Hospital Center of Cocody, Abidjan, Ivory Coast*

R. J. Shephard Prof MD, *University of Toronto, Toronto, Canada*

P. N. Sperryn MD, *Hillingdon Hospital, New Malden, UK*

R. H. Strauss Prof MD, *Ohio State University, Colombus, USA*

R. Thomée BDPC, *Gothenburg University, Gothenburg, Sweden*

A. Thorstensson PhD, *Karolinska Institute, Stockholm, Sweden*

P. Vanuxem Prof MD, *University of Marseilles, Marseilles, France*

A. Venerando Prof MD, *Institute of Sports Science, Rome, Italy*

R. O. Voy MD, *US Olympic Committee, Colorado Springs, USA*

R. Ward MD, *Simon Fraser University, Burnaby BC, Canada*

H. Weicker Prof MD, *University of Heidelburg, Heidelburg, FRG*

H. Zakarian MD, *University of Marseilles, Marseilles, France*

P. Zeppilli Prof MD, *Institute of Sports Science, Rome, Italy*

The definition and scope of sports medicine

W. HOLLMANN
President of the International Federation of Sports Medicine

Carrying out everyday tasks requires a basic level of physical fitness. For this reason, the treatment of reduced physical capacity due to illness or age has always been a part of medicine. Seen from this point of view, sports medicine is as old as medicine itself.

Precise methods of physical measurement are a precondition of scientifically-based medicine. In 1883, the German physician Speck developed the first ergometer. That year, therefore, can perhaps be regarded as the birth of sports medicine based on precise physical measurement data. At the end of the 19th century, the physiologist Zuntz expanded these beginnings of ergometry with the development of the first motor-driven treadmill.

The term 'sports medicine' is a traditional name which no longer corresponds to the special field of sports medicine as we see it today. The first modern definition was made in 1958 on the occasion of the foundation of the Institute for Cardiology and Sports Medicine, Cologne: 'Sports medicine includes those theoretical and practical branches of medicine which investigate the influence of exercise, training, and sport on healthy and ill people, as well as the effects of lack of exercise, to produce useful results for prevention, therapy, rehabilitation, and the athlete.' This definition was adopted by the FIMS Scientific Commission in 1977.

Accordingly, prevention stands firmly in the foreground of today's sports medicine. There are two main aspects:

1 Due to the increased technology and automation in our lives, there is an almost compulsory lack of physical activity, with negative effects on health. In this situation, physical training and sport mean a restoration of physiological conditions to a certain extent.

2 Appropriate quantitative and qualitative training produces a large number of biochemical and biophysical adaptations in the human body. They can prevent a whole range of illnesses and diseases, and act against age-induced loss of physical capacity.

Performance diagnosis and rehabilitation are also important aspects of sports medicine. Physical training is the precondition for improvement in physical performance capacity during rehabilitation after operations or illness. Sometimes the ability to work can only be recovered by such measures. In various medical fields, performance diagnosis is the prerequisite for prompt diagnosis of early-stage damage or functional impairment. It also has many other functions, including assessment of the effect of therapy, the influence of medication on physical capacity, and a training effect for scientifically-controlled training.

Many classic medical disciplines have been able to profit from sports medicine research in the past few decades. This holds good from the technical-equipment point of view, as well as in the detection of physiological and pathophysiological regulations, and their consequences in diagnosis, therapy and rehabilitation. Internal medicine (especially cardiology and pulmonology), paediatrics, geriatrics, orthopaedics, gynaecology, neurology, clinical pharmacology and environmental medicine have all particularly profited from sports medicine.

The main aspects of sports medicine can be summarized as:

1 Medical treatment of injuries and illnesses.
2 Medical examination before starting a sport to detect any damage which could be worsened by the sport.
3 Medical performance investigation to assess the performance capacity of heart, circulation, respiration, metabolism and the skeletal musculature.
4 Performance diagnosis specific to the type of sport.
5 Medical advice on life-style and nutrition.
6 Medical assistance in developing optimal training methods.
7 Scientifically-based control of training.

Sport, in its individual categories of popular sport, sport for health, and performance and high performance sport, has been an important part of our lives for a long time. Partly for this reason, sports medicine has become an important branch of medicine, particularly over the past 20 years. It is recognized in many countries as an independent branch in research, teaching and practice. Today, in 1988, 82 nations belong to the International Federation of Sports Medicine (FIMS), which was founded in 1928; it is one of the largest medical societies in the world.

This publication has the task of putting over a basic knowledge of sports medicine in a short, clear form. For further education, reference must be made to the appropriate textbooks.

We thank the International Olympic Committee (President: H. E. Juan Antonio Samaranch) and its medical commission (Chairman: Prince Alexandre de Merode) for their generous support. This thanks is also extended to the publisher.

PART 1

INTRODUCTION

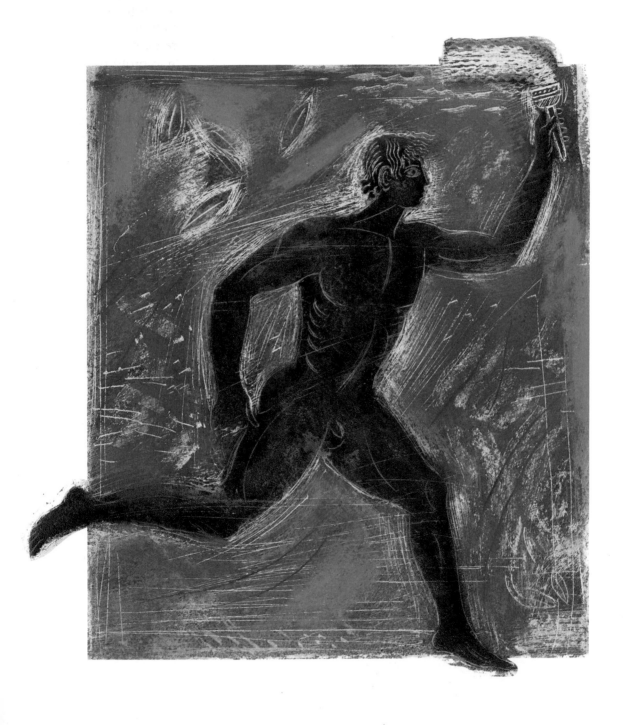

1.1 The development, objectives and activities of the IOC Medical Commission

PRINCE A. DE MERODE
Vice President of IOC
Chairman of IOC Medical Commission

The International Olympic Committee (IOC) Medical Commission was created in 1966 when measures to counter doping were still practically non-existent. After the 1960 Games when two athletes fell victim to an overdose of amphetamines, and further scandals at the 1964 Games which were overcome only with difficulty, the IOC resolved to lead the way. It took up a position firmly against the trend of 'winning at all costs' which was on the increase throughout the sporting world. Our action is founded on three basic principles:

1 The defence of ethics.
2 The protection of the health of athletes.
3 Ensuring an equal chance for everyone.

Harking back to the purest notions of the Olympic ideal, these three fundamental points still answer a need which has become one of the burning issues of our time. Originally the Medical Commission had set itself the urgent task of combating doping which, through a social phenomenon, was finding its way into sport. During the 20 years which have followed, the sophistication of methods used, the multiplicity of interests at stake and the appearance of alarming new factors have led the Commission to widen the scope of its activities.

As a result, in 1981 it was decided to restructure the Commission by dividing it into four subcommissions whose individual objectives are united by a common concern.

Subcommission 'Doping and biochemistry'

Its role, as its name suggests, is to fight against a form of cheating which involves doctoring human beings as if they were articles of sports equipment. It has thus:

1 Established a system of guidelines for procedure and sanctions which

will only be fully effective when it is totally standardized and universally adopted by all the governing bodies in sport.

2   Created a system of accreditation for laboratories in order to guarantee that an acceptable minimum of analyses is carried out and to avoid any unfairness resulting from differences in competence. Today there are 21 accredited laboratories worldwide, and it is hoped that six more will be added to that total by the end of 1988.

3   Created a system of 2-yearly re-accreditation with the aim of ensuring that necessary standards are maintained both in terms of qualifications of the staff and the quality of the equipment used.

4   Ensured coordination between accredited laboratories in the scientific research they carry out.

5   Set up a bank of vital reference substances for research carried out by the laboratories, with the collaboration of the Narcotics Control Board in Vienna.

6   Studied with the other subcommissions possibilities for educative measures which provide an indispensable additional element in the fight against doping.

Subcommission 'Biomechanics and physiology of sport'

The negative aspect of the fight against doping, namely bans and threats, has naturally led the Medical Commission towards seeking positive measures. Cheating and the obvious dangers involved in doping could by no means by considered to be an acceptable way of improving sporting performances. We therefore thought it imperative to show top level athletes a reliable way of improving performance, and one which does not contravene the basic principles that we are defending.

Moreover, with the level of results obtained going up all the time, the increasing number of competitions organized all over the world and the demands made by increasingly rigorous training, we were forced to ask some essential questions: 'What will happen to that vital asset of a top level athlete—his/her health—during and after his/her sporting career?' 'Little by little, by progressing from compromise to unconscious sacrifice, are we not going to go beyond the fundamental limits of what human beings are capable of achieving?' 'Would sport not then risk becoming a bringer of disease?' 'Would the old axiom, sport = health, then be invalidated by this example?'

In response to these questions and to provide a serious alternative to doping, the Medical Commission has recommended a modern scientific training method. Based on the biomechanics and physiology of sport, it allows, by means of regular checks, the peak of unrivalled physical form to be attained, in conjunction with perfection of movement and of equipment. These techniques manage, without in any way damaging health, to bring about a spectacular improvement in performance while at the same time avoiding the dangers of an empirical training programme often backed up by reprehensible practices.

The subcommission has launched a huge campaign of scientific studies by:

1 Making biomechanics films measuring forces during the Olympic Games and several world championships and intended for use in universities and research institutes.
2 Making biomechanics films for coaches during these same competitions, enabling them to compare the movements of different athletes.
3 Publishing the results of this research in the *International Journal of Sport Biomechanics*.
4 Setting up a biomechanics film library for general use.
5 Producing simpler programmes for developing countries.

Subcommission 'Sports medicine and orthopaedics'

This subcommission has a more traditional character, but one which is extremely important. It forms an indispensable complement to the biochemistry and doping subcommission, although it is linked to the biomechanics subcommission. In actual fact, the studies it carries out enable athletes to avoid the harmful movements which bring on microtrauma and which, if repeated regularly, can lead to irreversible traumas.

This subcommission undertakes the following:

1 It takes part in the fight against doping.
2 Together with the International Amateur Boxing Federation it has carried out a study which has brought about a complete revision of the rules in order to provide greater protection for boxers.
3 It has the task of studying and eliminating the dangers relating to certain sports.
4 It works closely with the subcommission on coordination with the NOCs.

Subcommission 'Coordination with the NOCs'

This subcommission came about as a result of the lack of communication that the Medical Commission felt existed with the National Olympic Committees (NOCs). Consequently, the NOC Continental Associations were asked to set up a medical commission whose president would be a member of our subcommission. At the same time, each NOC was asked to appoint a medical representative to enable the IOC Medical Commission to discover the needs, strong points and weak points of each continent and each NOC. This facility for finding out information has enabled requirements to be met and everyone's point of view to be known. It has carried out important work:

1 In setting up and directing, with the help of a budget financed by Olympic Solidarity, a programme of courses in sports medicine across the five continents.

2 In producing a document entitled *Minimum guidelines for medical facilities at the Olympic Village*, which is included with the contract sent to each candidate city to hold the Olympic Games.

3 By elaborating together with the other subcommissions on the 16 points which constitute a true code of ethics in the field of medical care. This document is essential in that we have discovered that when medical staff are living with athletes and are anxious to help them to the best of their ability, certain members may forget the fundamental principles which should govern how they act.

4 By producing with the help of a group of Canadian specialists and doctors a simple manual which will enable those attending courses in sports medicine to keep a tangible reminder and to enable them to find out straightaway what action they need to take or what medical care is required in whatever circumstances may arise.

Finally, *The Encyclopaedia of Sports Medicine*, of which this is the first volume, is the product of joint work by the different subcommissions of the IOC Medical Commission together with the International Federation of Sports Medicine. Its aim is to create a source of information in which any doctor wishing to treat a top level athlete or someone practising sport in general, can find an answer to the questions which may arise.

The IOC Medical Commission wishes, by taking practical action, to provide effective help to athletes; it is serving sport and the Olympic ideal. I should like to thank all those who have contributed in whatever way towards achieving its objectives, and whose unstinting devotion has as its only reward the satisfaction of seeing the work accomplished.

1.2 The development, objectives and activities of the International Federation of Sports Medicine (FIMS)

K. TITTEL & H. G. KNUTTGEN
Co-chairmen of FIMS Scientific Commission

Immediately following the annual meeting of the Deutscher Ärztebund zur Förderung der Leibesübungen held in Berlin, October 1927, physicians interested in sports medicine from 12 countries were invited to meet for informal discussion of the possibilities for international cooperation. The invitation was based on the desire to share knowledge and experience regarding the relationship of the physiological processes to regular physical exercise, to improve and standardize methods of medical examination for sports performance, and to cooperate with the International Olympic Committee in providing the best possible medical care for athletes taking part in the Olympic Summer and Winter Games. General agreement was reached that the time had come to establish an international organization of sports medicine.

During the IInd Olympic Winter Games held in St Moritz, 50 physicians from 11 countries participated in an official meeting held on 14 February 1928. Professor W. Knoll (Switzerland) outlined the aims and objectives of an international sports medicine association and, following discussion, the Association Internationale Médico-Sportive (AIMS) was founded. The objectives of the organization were seen as cooperation with, and support of, international sports federations, provision of support for the further development of national sports medical associations, and the organization on a regular basis of the exchange of information and experiences about the basic science and practical aspects of sports medicine. Professor Knoll was elected President, Dr A. Mallwitz (Germany) was elected Secretary General, and Professor A. Latarjet (France), Professor F. J. J. Buytendijk (Netherlands) and Dr W. Dybowski (Poland) were elected members of the Executive Committee.

Subsequently, Professor Buytendijk was requested to organize the First International AIMS Congress to be held during the IXth Olympic Summer Games, held in Amsterdam in August 1928. The Congress was highly successful and attracted 280 physicians from 20 countries. It

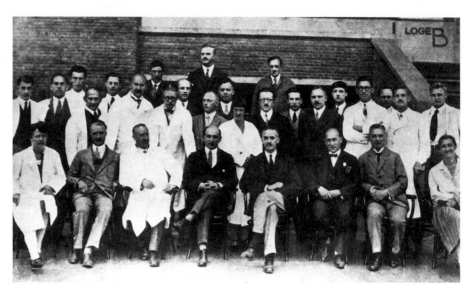

Fig. 1.2.1 Team of physicians and scientists who examined athletes during the IXth Olympic Summer Games in Amsterdam 1928. Professor Buytendijk is sitting in the first row (fourth from the left).

served as an excellent stimulus for further development of sports medicine in many countries. In connection with the Congress, a large team of physicians and scientists (Fig. 1.2.1) examined many of the participating athletes and collected anthropometric, cardiovascular, X-ray and metabolic information.

The IInd AIMS Congress was held in September 1933 at Torino, Italy. It was at this meeting that the General Assembly made the decision to change the name of the organization to Fédération Internationale Médico-Sportive et Scientifique. At the IIIrd International Congress held in Chamonix, France, in September 1934, the name of the organization was further changed to Fédération Internationale de Médecine Sportive (FIMS) and the organization has retained this name since that time.

Further development of sports medicine on both national and international levels was greatly aided by the succeeding three international congresses of FIMS, held in 1936 at Berlin, in 1937 at Paris and in 1939 at Bruxelles. Further development of international sports medicine was then interrupted by World War II and international activity was suspended for many years.

On 16 May 1946, a meeting was organized for a small group by Professor A. Govaerts (Belgium) and Professor J. Kral (Czechoslovakia) for the purpose of renewing activity and reorganizing FIMS. Other participants in this meeting, held in Bruxelles, were Professor P. Chailley-Bert (France), Dr L. Merklen (France), and Dr H. Brandt (Switzerland). The group also organized a meeting of the General Assembly which took place on 21 June 1947, in Bruxelles. New statutes were developed and approved and the following persons were elected to office: Professor

Govaerts as President, Professor Kral as Secretary General, and Dr Merklen, Dr Brandt and Professor Chailley-Bert as members of the Executive Committee. The rejuvenation of FIMS had an immediate and stimulating effect on the development of many national sports medicine organizations, although progress was slow because of the lingering effects of the war on the economy of many nations.

The VIIth World Congress of Sports Medicine constituted the first such meeting held after the war. The meeting was held in July 1948, in Prague, and attracted 135 physicians from 22 countries. The VIIIth World Congress was held in May 1958 at Firenze and Monte Catini, Italy, and it was at this meeting that the FIMS Executive Committee initiated a concerted effort to cooperate and collaborate with the International Olympic Committee and other international organizations. The results of these efforts were announced at the IXth World Congress of Sports Medicine (May/June 1952, in Paris) in that the International Olympic Committee recognized FIMS as the designated competent international organization for biological and medical research related to medicine and sport and the medical care of athletes. This recognition was of great importance and resulted in the establishment of medical commissions within the various international sports federations, the organization of sports medicine meetings on the occasion of each of the Olympic Games as well as other international sports competitions, and the increasing support given to sports medicine by the various national sports organizations.

In 1960, FIMS was officially recognized by the World Health Organization and the International Council of Sport and Physical Education of UNESCO. Since this time FIMS has expanded the list of international organizations with which it has established an official relationship and activities of cooperation, including the General Assembly of International Federations (GAIF), and the International Committee for Physical Fitness Research.

A major challenge for FIMS through the years has been the provision of support for the growth and development of national sports medical associations and the promotion of the exchange of information on an international level. FIMS continued to organize international meetings on a regular basis in various parts of the world and, on the occasion of the XIIth FIMS World Congress of Sports Medicine held in May/June 1958, at Moscow, participants from over 33 countries celebrated the 30th anniversary of the organization. FIMS published the proceedings of each international meeting as well as books and monographs on various topics in sports medicine. In 1961, the FIMS Executive Committee made the decision to produce its own publication, *Journal of Sports Medicine and Physical Fitness*, for the purpose of disseminating information about the various activities of FIMS, to report news from the various national sports medicine associations, and to summarize and report information from other sports medicine publications. The journal was edited by Professor G. La Cava (Italy) and was published for 15 years. It was decided by the FIMS Executive Committee in 1983 to terminate its relationship with the journal, and a bulletin, *The World of Sports Medicine*, was subsequently initiated and edited by Dr A. J. Ryan (USA).

At its meeting in January 1964, in Torino, the FIMS Executive Committee expanded the organization's structure and established a technical and scientific commission which eventually came to be designated the FIMS Scientific Commission. The original charge of the Scientific Commission was to enhance the exchange of information among sports medicine professionals, stimulate research in both basic and practical aspects of sports medicine, support the organization of international meetings, and establish relationships with cognate international organizations.

Through the years, a number of activities have been initiated and maintained by FIMS with the direct leadership or the cooperation and support of the Scientific Commission. An Olympic Medical Archive was proposed by Dr J. B. Wolffe (USA) in 1961 to collect clinical and scientific data from international élite athletes around the world. The long-term objective is to study the effects of prolonged intensive conditioning on health and longevity. This FIMS project has been supported by the International Olympic Committee, the World Health Organization and 22 national sports medical associations.

At the FIMS Executive Committee meeting in November 1962 in Luxembourg, Professor L. Prokop (Austria) proposed the organization of international FIMS courses to be held in various parts of the world. The first FIMS course was held in München-Grünwald in March 1965 and served as the prototype for subsequent courses held all over the world, with special consideration for developing nations. Financial support was obtained from Olympic Solidarity. As an adjunct to the courses, the *Basic Book of Sports Medicine* was prepared for the physicians and other professionals who enrolled in the FIMS courses. This text was prepared by the collaborative efforts of over 40 international authorities and submitted to the International Olympic Committee on the occasion of the XXIst Olympic Summer Games of 1976 in Montreal. The project constituted the contribution of FIMS to the spirit of Olympic Solidarity and the development of sports medicine programmes throughout the world.

By the early 1960s, the field of sports medicine experienced rapid growth and development in various parts of the world, partly because of the interest generated within individual nations and partly attributable to FIMS projects and initiatives. At the FIMS Executive Committee meeting in January 1964 in Torino, steps were taken to encourage the formation of sports medicine groupings based on geographical and linguistic criteria. As a result, the following organizations came into being: Confederación Panamericana de Medicina del Deporte, Confederación Centroamericana de Medicina del Deporte, Northwest European Chapter of Sports Medicine, Groupement Latin de Médecine du Sport, Union Balkanique de FIMS, Asian Confederation of Sports Medicine, Arab Federation of Sports Medicine, Union Africaine de Médecine du Sport, and Société Méditerranéene de Médecine du Sport. Each federation has engaged in cooperative activities with FIMS and has organized meetings, symposia, courses and congresses for their particular region.

As presently described in the statutes of FIMS, the Scientific Commission has several purposes or responsibilities:

1 The promotion of scientific research.
2 The documentation and publication of position statements regarding specific problems in sports medicine.
3 The maintenance of contact with other international scientific organizations, institutions and individual professionals.
4 Cooperation with organizers of international sports medicine meetings and events regarding programme planning and the publication of proceedings.
5 Cooperation with the editors of the official FIMS publication regarding scientific content of the journal.

The Scientific Commission maintains that international sports medicine must concern itself with all of the various phases and aspects of the sports experience. Authoritative information regarding the preparation of the athlete for participation and competition must be provided for the athletes, as well as for the various personnel who work with, and are responsible for, the athlete: physicians, trainers, coaches and therapists. Preparation includes conditioning of the athlete as related to both competitive success and injury prevention.

Sports medicine must work for advancement in the treatment of injuries in terms of immediate treatment, long-term care and rehabilitation. Careful attention must be given to the role of sports and exercise in health conservation and promotion for the general population. Education is necessary for all concerned with sport and sports medicine, and this must be considered in the planning of the activities of FIMS and all national sports medicine organizations.

Professional personnel in sports medicine must consider an extensive range of competitions and exercise participation. They must consider the responses, adaptations and health aspects of all persons engaged in sport and exercise. The élite athlete can be a marvel to observe in action and a fascinating person with whom to work. However, serious attention must also be given to the athletes competing on lower levels of competition, including those who participate in school sports programmes and in club competitions. Sports medicine also serves recreational athletes who enjoy both informal competition and the benefits to functional fitness and health enhancement.

In summary, it is possible to divide the development of FIMS into three periods. The first period consists of the organization of FIMS and the involvement of European professionals and national sports medicine organizations. The period lasted from 1928 until 1939 and the advent of World War II. The second period began in 1946 with the restructuring of the federation and a major expansion in membership. During this period, FIMS was recognized by the International Olympic Committee and the World Health Organization as the international organization for clinical and scientific aspects of sports participation. The third period began in 1964 on the occasion of the XVth FIMS World Congress and a return to the Olympic traditions of the development of the physical and moral qualities which are the basis of sport and the education of young people, in a spirit of better understanding and friendship through sports participation. Since 1964, sports medicine has experienced a tremendous growth in knowledge, service to athletes and international cooperation and collaboration.

FIMS can now look back on 60 productive years in which its original objectives have been attained as a result of the dedication and efforts of thousands of sports medicine professionals from all over the world. At the present time, FIMS represents a federation of over 80 national sports medical associations that have a combined membership of approximately 50 000 sports physicians and sports scientists.

The participation of the FIMS Scientific Commission with the Medical Commission of the International Olympic Committee to produce *The Olympic Book of Sports Medicine* constitutes a major effort of collaboration that should serve to herald an era of cooperative effort. Successful development of such projects helps both organizations to realize the objectives of the welfare of athletes and the benefits of a world community.

PART 2

THE IMPACT OF REGULAR TRAINING ON HUMAN BIOLOGICAL SYSTEMS

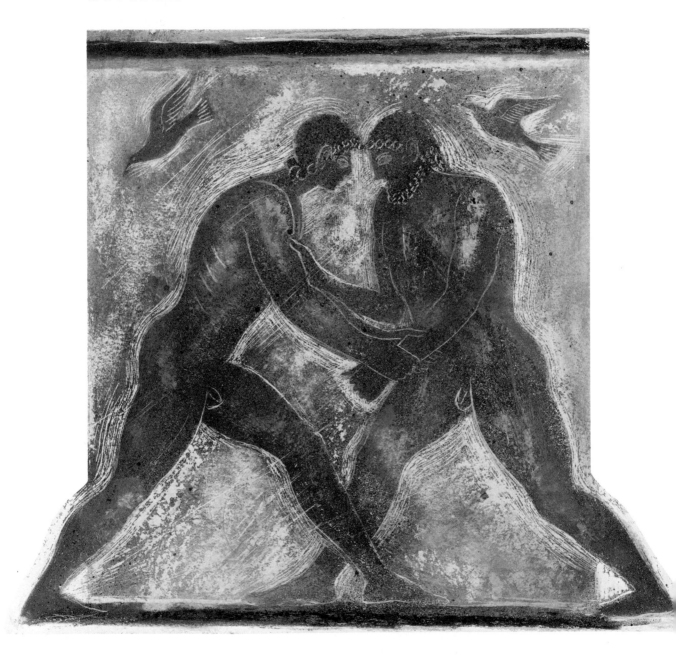

2.1 The musculoskeletal system

P. V. KOMI

Introduction

Initiation and maintenance of movement of the human body involves several structural and functional components. The central nervous system plays a major role in activating and coordinating the final action, together with the information coming from the various receptors residing in skeletal muscles, joints, eyes, ears, etc. The various skeletal muscles (Fig. 2.1.1) have a specific role in the execution of movement. They

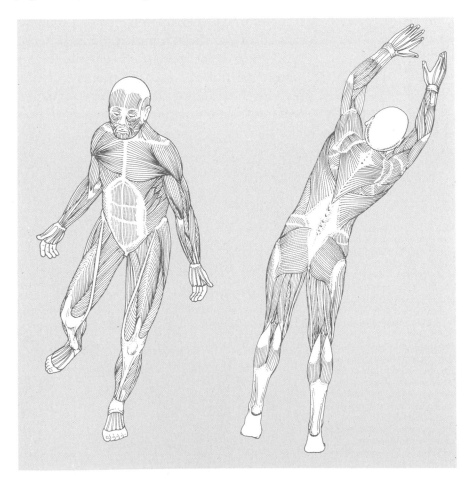

Fig. 2.1.1 Large superficial skeletal muscles are responsible for major locomotry action in the human body. For details of specific muscles see any functional anatomy textbook. Redrawn from McNaught & Callander (1970).

15

possess an ability to contract either by shortening (concentric action) or resisting external loads (lengthening contraction or eccentric action). The final direction, rate and magnitude of the action is controlled by complex interactive processes between the following three components: nervous system, skeletal muscle and external load characteristics. This chapter explains some of these processes by taking into consideration both structural and functional aspects in the neuromuscular system.

The motor unit and its relation to physical performance

In human skeletal muscle, muscle fibres are innervated by only one motor neuron branch; but this branch may be one from between 10 to 1000 similar branches all having the same axon. All the muscle fibres which are innervated by the same α-motoneuron compose a functional unit. A motor unit is therefore defined as a combination of an α-motoneuron and all of the skeletal muscle fibres innervated by that neuron (Fig. 2.1.2). Size of the motor unit (muscle fibres per α-motoneuron) varies within the muscle, and the number of motor units varies between muscles. In addition to these major structural differences the motor units within a specific muscle differ in regard to: (a) rate of force development;

Fig. 2.1.2 Schematic presentation of the basic components in skeletal muscle which are responsible for movement. Activation of the muscle begins either directly from the motor cortex and via the lower (α) motoneurons, or indirectly via reflex pathways. Muscle spindle and the corresponding afferent route is an example of the latter system. Despite the selection of the commanding pathway the muscle always receives its activation through the axonal branches of the α-motoneuron, which is an essential part of the motor unit.

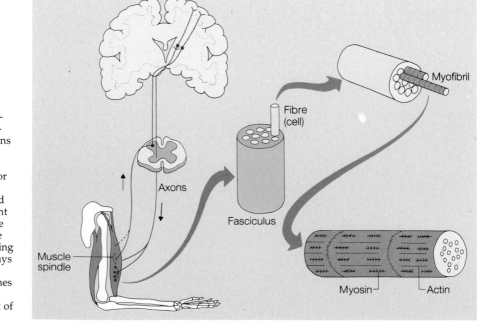

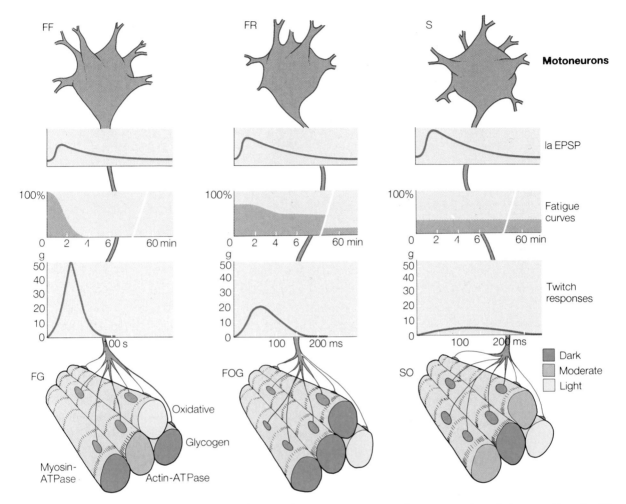

Fig. 2.1.3 An illustrative example to show the functional interrelationship between a motoneuron and its muscle fibres within different types of motor units. Motoneurons may be phasic (fire rapidly but with short bursts) or tonic (slow and continuous). Axon diameter size is directly related to conduction velocity. The muscle fibres have been stained to show: myosin-ATPase, acid-ATPase, succinate dehydro-genase (an oxidative enzyme), and glycogen. Note the differences in twitch tension for each motor unit: FF, fast, fatigable; FR, fast, fatigue resistant; S, slow; Ia EPSP, sensory excitatory, post-synaptic potentiation; FG, fast twitch glycolytic; FOG, fast twitch high-oxidative glycolytic; SO, slow twitch oxidative muscle fibres. From Edington & Edgerton (1976).

(b) peak force production; and (c) maintenance of force level without loss of tension. As is presented in Fig. 2.1.3, the FF unit develops tension fast, but it is also very fatigable. The SO unit, on the other hand, has a slow rate of force production, but it can produce the same tension repeatedly for longer periods of time without signs of fatigue. It is therefore also a fatigue-resistant-type motor unit. Figure 2.1.4 illustrates further the differences in response of the two extreme types of motor units. The units were first stimulated to tetany with the fast motor unit needing a

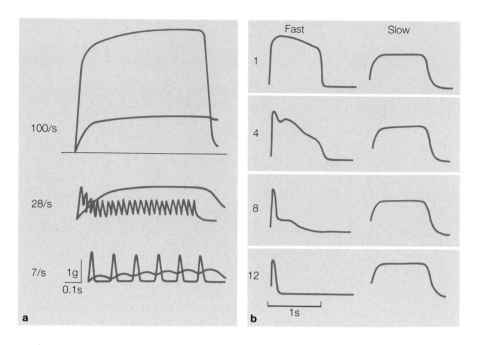

Fig. 2.1.4 Mechanical responses of the two different type motor units of the same muscle. (a) A slow-type unit reaches tetany at a stimulus frequency of 28 Hz, compared to 100 Hz for a faster unit. (b) The same motor units were stimulated with a tetanic frequency of 100 Hz for 1 s, with 2 s intervals. The response to the first, fourth, eighth and 12th tetanic stimulations are shown. Note that the fast motor unit already shows signs of fatigue during the fourth response, whereas the force record of the slow unit is similar in all examples. From Steg (1964).

much higher fusion frequency than the slow unit. They were then subjected to repetitive tetanic stimulation, and the difference in response between the two types is remarkable. The fast motor unit shows clear signs of fatigue (loss of force) after the fourth successive tetanic stimulation, whereas the slow unit has a similar tension response even after the 12th tetanic stimulation.

It is a common agreement that the stimulus which the muscle fibres receive, and thus the type of α-motoneurons, determines the histochemical structure and biochemical performance of the individual muscle fibres in a motor unit. All the fibres in the same unit, therefore, have similar chemical profiles (Fig. 2.1.3). The classification of the muscle fibre types is not uniform in the literature. In addition to the ones presented in Fig. 2.1.3 as FF, FOG and SO, the respective types have been classified, e.g. as IIB, IIA and I (Brooke & Kaiser, 1974), or simply as fast twitch white, fast twitch red and slow twitch intermediate (Henneman & Olson, 1965). It seems, however, that any scheme of classifying muscle fibres is an over-simplification. Depending on the pre-incubation media in the histochemical staining of muscle samples one can identify also a type IIC fibre (Billeter et al., 1981a, 1981b). For further details of fibre classification and metabolic potentials and adaptation of the different fibre types the reader is referred to an excellent review of Saltin and Gollnick (1983).

Since needle biopsy technique was introduced to investigate human

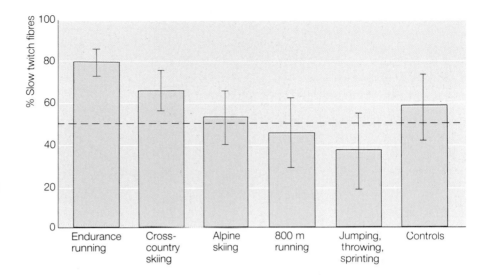

Fig. 2.1.5 Mean ± s.d. of the percent distribution of the slow twitch (type I) fibre distribution in the vastus lateralis muscles of different athlete groups. From Komi (1983).

skeletal muscle function (Bergström, 1962), numerous reports have appeared to demonstrate that long-distance runners, cyclists, rowers and cross-country skiers have relatively more slow (type I) fibres in vastus lateralis, gastrocnemius or deltoideus muscle. The sprinters, jumpers and general-power athletes usually have a greater proportion of fast (type II) fibres in, for example, vastus lateralis muscle. Figure 2.1.5 shows an example of muscle fibre distribution among various athletic groups. Differences in muscle fibre composition observed among athletes have raised the question whether the muscle structure of an individual athlete is an acquired phenomenon or is due to a genetically determined code. There is naturally no direct answer to this problem. Studies in monozygotic twins have demonstrated almost complete identity within twin pairs (Komi *et al.*, 1977), and this finding could be used to emphasize the strength of the genetic factor in influencing muscle fibre composition. There is, however, strong evidence that both the ultrastructure and metabolic capacity of the individual muscle fibres can adapt specifically to different athletic training (e.g. Howald, 1985). With regard to conversion from one fibre type to another, it is probably easier to demonstrate changes between populations of the different fast twitch fibres (IIA, IIB and IIC) rather than a complete conversion to, or from, the slow twitch (type 1) fibres. It is, however, clear that the muscle fibre profile during the peak performance of an Olympic athlete is determined both by genetic and environmental (training) factors.

In a biological system one should expect that structure and function have a close relationship. In isolated muscle fibre, motor unit or even whole muscle preparations, this relationship has demonstrated that

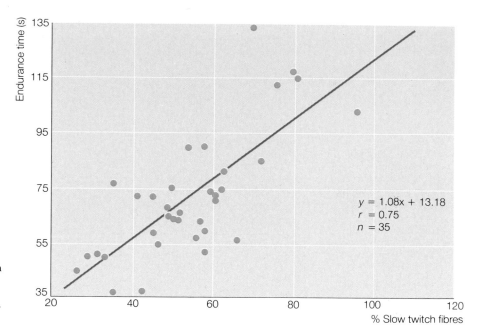

Fig. 2.1.6 Relationship between the percentage of slow twitch fibres in the vastus lateralis muscle and the time needed to maintain 60% maximal isometric leg extension force until exhaustion. From Komi *et al.* (1982).

such important mechanical parameters as rate of force development, force rise time, ½ relaxation time, force–velocity response, etc. are quite different between the various types (fast or slow) of preparations. And, as already discussed earlier, resistance to fatigue varies between different fibre, motor unit or muscle types. If this is the case in closed systems of isolated preparations, one should ask the question whether similar relationships could be demonstrated in human skeletal muscle. As mentioned earlier (see also Fig. 2.1.5) the athletic populations have different slow twitch fibre (STF) composition, which reflect differences in endurance capacity. Laboratory experiments have confirmed this by showing that a close relationship exists between relative amounts of slow twitch fibres (vastus lateralis muscle) and time to maintain a 60% isometric force level (Fig. 2.1.6). Thus, people who possess a greater proportion of slow twitch (or type I) muscle fibres can sustain the same relative fatigue loading longer than people whose muscles are richer in fast twitch (or type II) fibres. Rate of force development and rate of relaxation should—according to isolated preparation models—take place faster in people who have primarily fast twitch fibres (FTF) in their muscles. Similarly, in force–velocity measurements, the velocity end of the curve should be at much higher levels in people with primarily fast-type muscles.

It must be admitted, however, that existing experimental evidence using the measurement of muscle mechanical performance does not

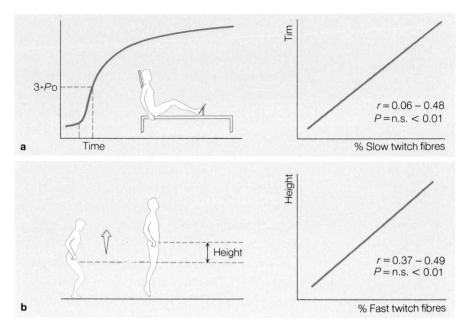

Fig. 2.1.7 The measurement of a maximum isometric force–time curve (a) or an explosive squatting jump (b) does not always demonstrate a significant interrelationship between muscle structure and performance. The correlation coefficients shown for the two regression lines indicate the ranges obtained in the various studies. From Viitasalo *et al.* (1984).

always support the interrelationships (structure vs. function) found in isolated muscle preparations. For example, some studies (Viitasalo & Komi, 1978; Viitasalo *et al.*, 1982) have demonstrated a significant relationship between structure and function in the case of isometric force production, while others (Viitasalo & Komi, 1981) have failed to do so. Similar inconsistencies have been observed for the vertical jump (Fig. 2.1.7). Thus force–time characteristics of either isometric or dynamic origin seem to be under strong environmental influence. Specific strength and power training (see Chapter 5.1) has influence on the force–time curve. Effects of training are probably of greater importance than the muscle structure itself (Viitasalo *et al.*, 1982). Voluntary explosive-type force production requires a well-controlled, synchronized activation process, and thus the experimental situation is very different from those of isolated preparations, which utilize electrical stimulation either on the muscle or its nerve. Great sex differences in force–time characteristics (Komi *et al.*, 1977) and electromechanical delays (Bell & Jacobs, 1986) gives an additional problem to this question.

Force–velocity relationships in human skeletal muscle is another biomechanical attribute which has not always demonstrated similar results as those found in isolated preparations. With the exception of the report of Tihanyi *et al.* (1982), the demonstration of interdependence between muscle fibre composition and the force–velocity curve has been much less than would have been expected from animal experiments. The primary reason for the small amount of valid research in this area is probably due to the lack of available dynamometers that can load the muscles through the entire physiological range of contraction speeds. The maximum speed of most of the commercially-available instruments can cover only 20–30% of the different physiological maxima. As Goldspink (1978) has demonstrated, the peak efficiencies of isolated fast and slow twitch fibres occur at completely different contraction speeds. Therefore, it is possible that in measurements of the force–velocity curve, when the maximum angular velocity reaches the value of 3–4 rad/s, only the efficient contraction speed of STF will be reached. The peak power of fast twitch-type muscle may occur at angular velocities more than three times greater than our present measurement systems allow (Fig. 2.1.8).

Human locomotion is dependent on a non-systematic relationship between structure and function in physical performance, and will probably, therefore, vary substantially from results based on studies of isolated preparations or using force/speed-measuring instruments. Our

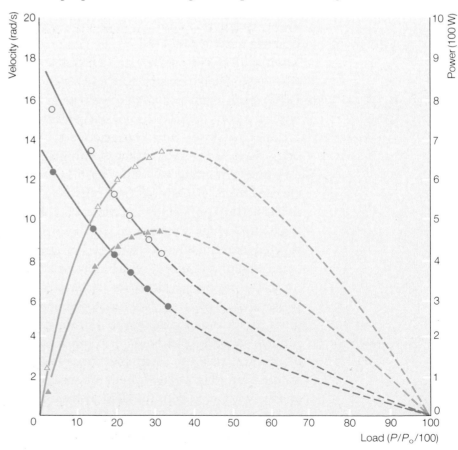

Fig. 2.1.8 Load–velocity (circles) and load–power (triangles) relationships in concentric leg extension movement for two groups of subjects who differed in fast twitch fibre composition of the vastus lateralis muscle. Open symbols, % FT 61 ± 3.2%; solid symbols, % FT 41.2 ± 1.7%. From Tihanyi *et al.* (1982).

muscles have perhaps been designed to function quite differently—and in a more elaborate way—than those exercise and loading modes currently used in many muscle-testing laboratories.

Types of muscle action

The term contraction may be thought of as the state of muscle when tension is generated across a number of actin and myosin filaments. Depending on the external load, direction and magnitude of action (Table 2.1.1), contraction may be: (a) concentric, in which the muscle shortens (i.e. the net muscle moment is in the same direction as the change in joint angle, and mechanical work is positive); (b) eccentric, in which the muscle is lengthened (i.e. net muscle moment is in the opposite direction to the change in joint angle, and mechanical work is negative); or (c) isometric, in which neither muscle length nor joint angle changes and mechanical work is zero. The use of the term 'muscle contraction' is therefore sometimes confusing, and a suggestion has been made to replace it with the term 'muscle action' (Cavanagh, 1988).

Table 2.1.1 Classification of muscle action or exercise types.

Type of action	Function	External mechanical work*
Concentric	Acceleration	Positive ($W = F\,(+D)$)
Isometric	Fixation	Zero (no change in length)
Eccentric	Deceleration	Negative ($W = F\,(-D)$)

* W = work; F = force; D = distance.

The force production in all three types of muscle action is seen through the internal rearrangements in length between the contractile and elastic components. In Fig. 2.1.9 these rearrangements are sketched according to Braunwald *et al.* (1967) to show the simplest possible mechanical model of muscle, where there is a contractile component (CC) and, with it, an elastic component in series (SEC). In isometric contraction the force is generated through the action of CC on SEC, which is stretched. Concentric action, where the load is attached to the end of the muscle, is always preceded by an isometric-type of contraction with rearrangements of the lengths of CC and SEC. The final movement begins when the pulling force of CC on the SEC equals, or slightly exceeds, that of the load. In eccentric action some external force, e.g. gravity and antagonist muscles, forces the muscle to lengthen.

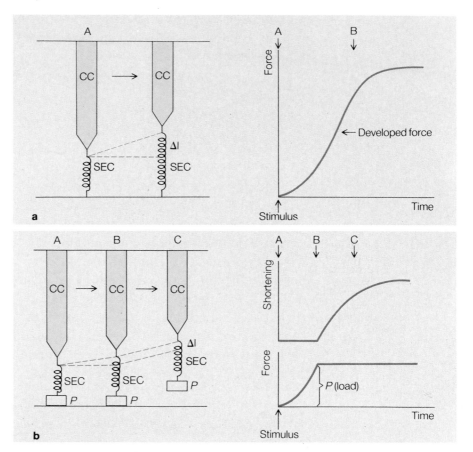

Fig. 2.1.9 Models of isometric (a) and concentric (b) muscle action. In isometric contraction the total length of the muscle does not change, but activation (A → B) causes the contractile component (CC) to shorten and stretch the series elastic component (SEC). Concentric action begins with an isometric phase, where CC first shortens and stretches SEC (A → B). Actual movement occurs when the pulling force of CC on SEC equals or slightly exceeds that of the load P (B → C). From Braunwald *et al.* (1967).

It is in the eccentric mode that the force and power capacities of the skeletal muscle are greatest. According to the force–velocity curve, the maximum force decreases (concentric action) or increases (eccentric action) as a function of the shortening or stretching velocities, respectively (Fig. 2.1.10). The increase in force output in eccentric contraction is primarily of chemomechanical origin. This was demonstrated by Edman *et al.* (1978), who showed that the force of an isolated sarcomere increases beyond P_o when the fibril is being stretched after the isometric maximum is reached with a constant tetanic stimulation. Principally, the same explanation should also apply to the human skeletal muscle, and Fig. 2.1.11 demonstrates this schematically.

This 'mechanical' origin of the high force in eccentric action was also emphasized in studies with human forearm flexors (Komi, 1973b), when the maximum integrated EMG (IEMG) was similar in both eccentric and concentric actions at relatively slow velocities. On the other hand, it has been suggested that when human skeletal muscle is stretched after the

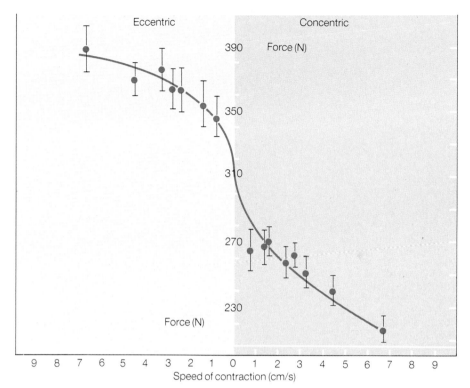

Fig. 2.1.10 Force–velocity relationship in eccentric and concentric muscle action for elbow flexor muscles. The measurements were performed with an electro-mechanical dynamometer, which was designed to arrange a constant velocity of shortening or lengthening for the biceps brachii muscle. From Komi (1973b).

maximum isometric force has been reached, EMG activity is also increased, perhaps through increased activation of Ia afferents (Bührle *et al.*, 1983). Although the contribution of this additional motor unit activation to the eccentric force is probably a small part of the entire force enhancement, it emphasizes the important role of the nervous system in influencing the force and stiffness characteristics of the contracting muscle. As will become evident, this role is also important in the stretch-shortening cycle (SSC).

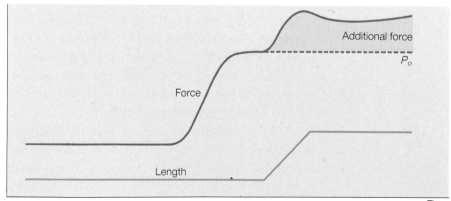

Fig. 2.1.11 A schematic presentation to show that if the human skeletal muscle is stretched (eccentric action) after maximal isometric force (P_o) has been attained, the force increases considerably. Similar phenomenon takes place in isolated sarcomeres (see text).

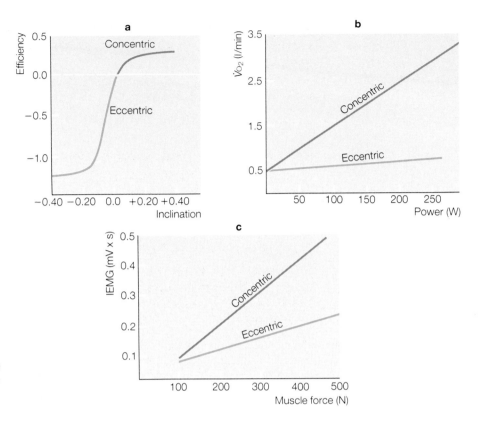

Fig. 2.1.12 (a) Mechanical efficiency of negative (eccentric) and positive (concentric) work during treadmill walking at different downhill and uphill inclinations, respectively (Margaria, 1938). (b) Relationship between oxygen uptake ($\dot{V}_{O_2}$) and work rate during positive (concentric) and negative (eccentric) work (Asmussen, 1952). (c) Relationship between integrated electromyographic (IEMG) activity of the biceps brachii muscle and the elbow flexor force under concentric and eccentric contraction performed with comparable velocities of shortening and stretching, respectively (Komi, 1973a).

Two additional differences between eccentric and concentric actions need to be mentioned. First, it is well documented that the slopes representing IEMG and force relationships are different in these two types of exercise (Bigland & Lippold, 1954; Komi, 1973a) (Fig. 2.1.12). To attain a certain force level requires much less motor unit activation in eccentric than concentric action. Second, oxygen consumption is much lower during eccentric exercise than in comparable concentric exercise (Asmussen, 1952; Knuttgen, 1986) (Fig. 2.1.12b). These findings indicate quite clearly that input/output relationships of the two exercises may be several times higher than that of pure concentric exercise. This can also be seen from Fig. 2.1.12a, which shows Margaria's (1938) findings that in higher stretch–velocity conditions the mechanical efficiency of eccentric exercise (negative work) may reach values higher than 100%.

The great force and power production capacity of the eccentric muscle action should also be seen as beneficial for specific purposes of muscle training. Despite the fact that repeated eccentric exercise causes soreness in muscles which have not been accustomed to such exercise loads, the strength training possibilities of high-tension eccentric muscle action are obvious (Komi & Buskirk, 1972). As will be explained in more detail in

Chapter 5.1 the recommendation is usually given to use high-force eccentric loads progressively, as a part of the regular strength training routine.

Stretch-shortening cycle

The discussion on muscle contraction above, outlines the restricted conditions applying to various contraction modes. The types of muscle action listed in Table 2.1.1 do not take place as isolated forms during normal locomotion. This is because the body segments are periodically subjected to impact forces (Fig. 2.1.13), as in running or jumping, or because some external force such as gravity lengthens the muscle. In these phases the muscles are acting eccentrically, and concentric action follows. This combination of eccentric and concentric actions forms a natural type of muscle function called the stretch-shortening cycle (SSC)

Fig. 2.1.13 Human walking and running do not resemble the movement of a rotating wheel, where the centre of gravity is always directly above the point of contact and perpendicular to the line of progression. Instead they resemble the action of a 'rolling' cubic box and have considerable impact loads when contact takes place with the ground. Before contact the muscles are preactivated (A) and ready to resist the impact, during which they are stretched (B). The stretch phase is followed by shortening (concentric) action (C). The lower part of the figure demonstrates the SSC, which is the natural form of muscle function. From Komi (1984).

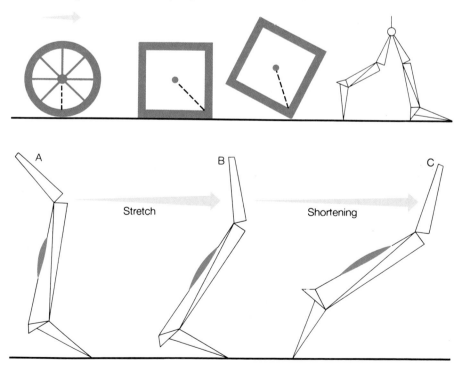

(Norman & Komi, 1979; Komi, 1984). The purpose of SSC behaviour is to make the final action (concentric phase) more powerful than that resulting from concentric action alone. SSC action is also very important in protecting the muscle from unnecessary slack periods. An isolated concentric action (see Fig. 2.1.9) requires considerable time before any movement occurs. In SSC the muscle has developed a high-level tension by the beginning of concentric action. Depending on the stretch velocity, this tension can be even higher than the final force is during isolated concentric action.

The final mechanism for performance potentiation during SSC is unclear. It has, however, been well demonstrated that both the mechanical and metabolic behaviour of the skeletal muscle is modified in concentric action during SSC. Experimental evidence has come from studies performed both on isolated muscle preparations and human experiments. For example, Edman *et al.* (1978) demonstrated that, especially at higher sarcomere lengths, the sarcomere force–velocity curve is shifted to the right where the shortening follows an active stretch. Experiments of Cavagna *et al.* (1965) with isolated frog sartorius muscle can, however, be used as a model to demonstrate how the performance of muscle in concentric action is potentiated when this contraction is preceded by an active stretch. A similar phenomenon has been demonstrated in human leg extensor muscles (Komi, 1983). It is important for this potentiation that the coupling between stretch and shortening phases is as short as possible (Bosco *et al.*, 1981).

Force–length and force–velocity curves have been regarded as basic attributes to demonstrate the mechanical behaviour of skeletal muscle. Cavagna *et al.* (1968) have shown that SSC action both in isolated muscle preparations and in human forearm flexors modifies the concentric phase so that its force is increased at a given muscle length or shortening velocity. When the force–velocity ($F-V$) curve is measured during a complex movement involving several joints (vertical jumps) preparatory countermovement shifts the $F-V$ curve to the right, and thus causes the leg extensor muscles to exert much higher forces at any knee angular velocity of concentric phase (Bosco & Komi, 1979) (Fig. 2.1.14).

The nervous system is thought to play an important role in performance potentiation in the SSC. However, the original study of Cavagna *et al.* (1965) was performed with isolated frog sartorius muscle, and therefore it is possible that the performance potentiation in the SSC was due solely to the effects of elastic potentiation. Later, Cavagna *et al.* (1968) were able to obtain similar results with intact human elbow flexor muscles. The experiments of Edman *et al.* (1982) with isolated fibrils also support pure

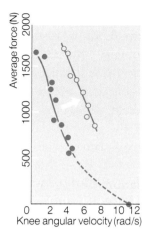

Fig. 2.1.14 Average force and average knee angular velocity relationship in vertical jumps performed with weights on the shoulders. The upper and lower curves are for the situations with and without preliminary countermovement, respectively. Note the great potentiation of performance (the curve shifts to the right and up) when the performance begins with countermovement. The potentiation may be explained partly, but not totally, by the efficient use of elastic energy. From Bosco & Komi (1979).

elastic (chemomechanical) potentiation. However, because the stretching of muscles in the eccentric phase must activate muscle spindles, some potentiation via the reflex loops could be expected as well. Evidence has been presented that the myoelectrical activity of the leg extensor muscles could be potentiated during the contact phase of the running cycle (Dietz *et al.*, 1979). Thus, it is likely that when the nervous connections are intact, the enhancement of performance in the SSC can be attributed to the combined effects of restitution of elastic energy and stretch reflex potentiation of muscle.

The reflex influence on performance potentiation is perhaps more complex than one would expect from the possible behaviour of the muscle spindle receptors. When an active muscle is put under stretch, both the spindles and the Golgi tendon organs become activated. The magnitude of the potentiation will depend on which one of these reflexes—facilitatory or inhibitory—dominates.

Muscle stiffness is very much influenced by the presence of stretch reflexes. A high degree of stiffness is also characteristic of the eccentric phase in SSC. As Hoffer and Andreassen (1981) have demonstrated in animal experiments, muscle stiffness in the normal muscle is larger with the same operating force than in an areflexive muscle (Fig. 2.1.15). Thus the stretch reflex plays a role in causing additional (reflex) contribution to stiffness during the stretch (eccentric) phase of SSC. However, it is very difficult to correctly isolate in normal SSC the potentiation effects of pure elasticity from those of reflex influences. Any increase in reflex activation should lead to enhancement of elastic influences. It must also be emphasized that all the components which contribute to enhanced performance in SSC are adaptive and their relative roles may change depending on the training/detraining status of the various parts of the neuromuscular system (see also Chapter 5.1).

Fig. 2.1.15 Presence of (stretch) reflex has considerable influence in increasing muscle stiffness. The figure shows the dependence of incremental stiffness on operating force, for 1 mm × 500 ms triangular perturbations in conditions with reflex present and with intrinsic muscle stiffness (reflex absent). From Hoffer & Andreassen (1981).

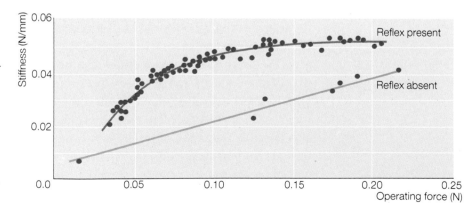

Mechanics of the human skeletal muscle during SSC

In isotonic contraction of an isolated muscle the speed of contraction depends on the force. Thus the smaller the force, the faster the contraction speed is. This relationship between force and velocity can be described by Hill's characteristics equation for the shortening contraction:

$$V (P + a) = b (P_o - P)$$

in which P is the force, P_o the developed isometric tension, V the velocity of shortening, and a and b are constants, whose values vary from muscle to muscle. Successful attempts have been made to demonstrate that this equation also fits the specific conditions of human muscle action (Wilkie, 1950).

Because the force–velocity relationship as described by Hill is a steady-state relationship, it could be expected that the form of the curve may not be applicable to situations where the load on the muscle is changing. Similarly, the eccentric part of the force–velocity curve shown in Fig. 2.1.10 may not be representative for a normal locomotory action, especially that of SSC.

In order to get an understanding of the true force–velocity relationship in natural SSC, one must be able to either: (a) estimate, mathematically with the help of film analysis and external force measurements, the muscular forces around a specific joint; or (b) approach the problem by directly measuring *in vivo* forces on the tendon. The *in vivo* registration has been applied primarily in animal experiments and it has produced considerable information on the mechanical behaviour of AT (Achilles tendon), e.g. in cat locomotion (Walmsley *et al.*, 1978). A method which directly records forces on human AT with an implanted transducer is described by Komi *et al.* (1987). This *in vivo* technique utilizes either an E-form or a buckle-type transducer, of which the latter has proven to be more convenient. The transducer is implanted under local anaesthesia around the AT of adult male volunteers. After appropriate calibration procedures the subjects can perform normal unrestricted locomotion including walking, running at different speeds, hopping, jumping and bicycling. In some cases even maximal efforts were performed without any discomfort. All movements were performed either on a long force platform or on a bicycle which had special force transducers on the pedals. EMG activities were registered from the major leg muscles. AT force (ATF) and EMGs were telemetered, and all the signals were stored on magnetic tape. The entire measurement lasted 2–3 h, after which the transducer was removed.

Each performance was also filmed at 100 frames/s for estimation of the percent change of the lengths of the gastrocnemius and soleus muscles

(Grieve *et al.*, 1977). This estimation was then used to calculate the force–length and force–velocity curves for the two muscles. It must be emphasized that in this analysis the force values represent the two muscles simultaneously because AT is a common tendon for both of them.

Figure 2.1.16 presents an example of ATF response during foot contact, together with F_z and F_y ground reaction forces and EMG activities of the selected muscle groups. The peak tendon force occurred approximately at the time when the F_y force crossed to the positive side. This peak force was dependent on running velocity so that it first increased when running velocity increased to 6 m/s. Thereafter, there was a decreasing trend in the peak ATF (Fig. 2.1.17a). However, the peak rate of the tendon force development increased continuously with increase in running speed (Fig. 2.1.17b).

Applying the technique of estimating muscle length changes (Grieve *et al.*, 1978) for the ground contact phase, the force–length and force–velocity curves shown in Fig. 2.1.18 can be obtained. As the figure demonstrates, the shape of the force–length curves show potentiation of the force response during the concentric phase (which is marked with a descending arrow). When the ball running was performed at medium

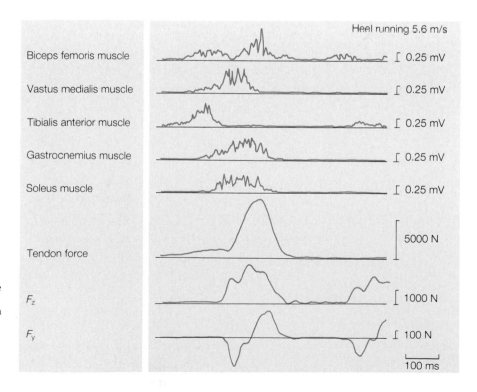

Fig. 2.1.16 A representative record of Achilles tendon force response together with F_z and F_y ground reaction forces and selected EMG activities when the subject was running with ball contact.

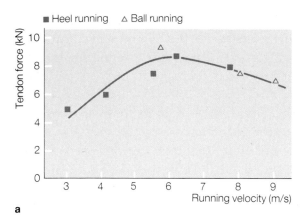

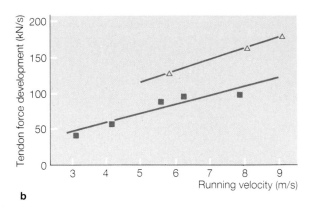

a

b

Fig. 2.1.17 Peak tendon forces (a) and peak rates of the tendon force development (b) at different running velocities.

(5.78 m/s) and high (9.02 m/s) velocities, the loop in the force–length curve was smaller at the higher velocity running. However, the rate of force development during the eccentric part (ascending arrow) was very high and it took place with a very small change in length of the muscle. This suggests that the gastrocnemius muscle demonstrates a characteristic short-range stiffness phenomenon in the stretching phase (e.g. Flitney & Hirst, 1978). The results were similar for the soleus muscle.

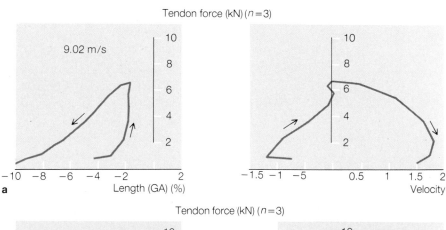

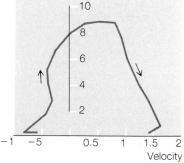

Fig. 2.1.18 Force–length and force–velocity curves of the gastrocnemius (GA) muscle for the ground contact phase when the subject ran with ball contact at two different velocities: (a) 9.02 m/s; (b) 5.78 m/s.

The force–length analysis gives a basis for estimation of the force–velocity curve for the ground contact phase. The right-hand curves in Fig. 2.1.18 are very different from the classic-type force–velocity curve. (see also Fig. 2.1.10). The concentric part of the curves particularly demonstrates performance potentiation. Much of this potentiation takes place as a recoil phenomenon, because the two muscles become inactive before the end of the concentric phase (see Fig. 2.1.16). Thus, the suggestion can be made that in running, where SSC is typical for the triceps surae muscle, the stretching phase is characterized by a small change in length and a high level of stiffness. This enables the muscles to resist high impact loads and to modify the conditions for subsequent concentric action, with corresponding shifts in the force–velocity response. This phenomenon has considerable practical consequences as explained in more detail in Chapter 5.1.

The direct *in vivo* technique of ATF measurements, however, has limitations. First, the Achilles tendon is common for both gastrocnemius and soleus muscles and therefore the force recordings are not for a single muscle only. Second, estimation of the length changes are representative for the entire muscle, but not specifically for the tendon or for the muscle tissue component. Despite these limitations it can be concluded that the change in muscle length during the stretching phase of SSC is very small and in all probability represents the phenomenon of short-range stiffness. It seems that the importance of the short-range stiffness, e.g. in various sports activities, has been ignored in the past. Considering the fact that efficient SSC action is characterized by a fast stretch and short coupling between eccentric and concentric actions, then the true meaning of the short-range stiffness becomes more relevant. An actiomyosin cross-bridge theory for the short-range component of muscle stiffness has

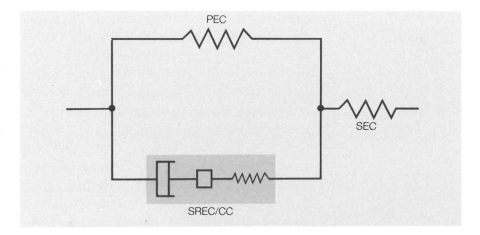

Fig. 2.1.19 The concept of short-range stiffness and its likely dependence on sarcomere cross-bridge function has introduced modifications of the mechanical model of the skeletal muscle. Short-range elastic component (SREC) resides in this model inside the contractile component (CC). PEC = parallel elastic component; SEC = series elastic component. From Haugen & Sten-Knudsen (1981).

been developed (Rack & Westbury, 1974; Flitney & Hirst, 1978). This then resulted in the development of a new mechanical model of an isolated muscle, which shows a short-range elastic component residing within the contractile component (Fig. 2.1.19). The present available evidence favours the use of this model in human skeletal muscle function as well.

Mechanical efficiency

There is still some confliction in our understanding of how efficient human locomotion is, primarily due to problems in correct calculation or estimation of mechanical efficiency (ME). Another important reason is that different forms of muscle action have different ME, and the situation becomes even more complicated when ME is measured under conditions of SSC exercises.

Conventionally, mechanical efficiency of work (ME) is the ratio of external work performed to the extra energy production:

$$\text{ME} = \frac{W \times 100}{E - e}$$

where E is the gross energy output, e is the resting metabolic rate, and W is the external work performed.

In the following discussion some new experimental findings are presented to emphasize that human locomotion and muscle action may indeed have a variety of ME values.

Mechanical efficiency of isolated concentric and eccentric exercises

To examine the ME values of either isolated eccentric or concentric exercises, or their combination, the sledge apparatus (Fig. 2.1.20) was constructed. The apparatus consists of: (a) a sledge ($m = 33$ kg) to which the subject is fixed in a sitting position; (b) a 'slide' on which the sledge runs along the slow-friction aluminium track; and (c) the force-plate placed perpendicularly with the sliding surface (for details of the method see Kaneko *et al.*, 1984; Aura & Komi 1986a, 1986b; Komi *et al.*, 1987). The relationship between energy expenditure and mechanical work was shown to be linear in a small range of shortening velocities of the concentric exercise (Kaneko *et al.*, 1984), but when the contraction velocity was increased (Aura & Komi, 1986b) this linearity was no longer true. For this reason ME of concentric exercise was not constant, but decreased with increasing shortening velocities (Fig. 2.1.21). In eccentric exercise ME increased in all subjects when mechanical work was increased,

Fig. 2.1.20 The sledge apparatus and other necessary equipment used to investigate the mechanical efficiency of isolated concentric and eccentric exercises and SSC exercise. A, sledge; B, ankle support; C, aluminic slide-bars; D, force-plate; E, electric goniometer; F, EMG-telemetry transmitters; G, audio signal; H, amplifier, force; I, amplifier, 'Elgon'; J–M, EMG-telemetry receiving units; N, FM recorder Racal 7 DS; O, oxygen-4 analyser. For details see Aura & Komi (1986b).

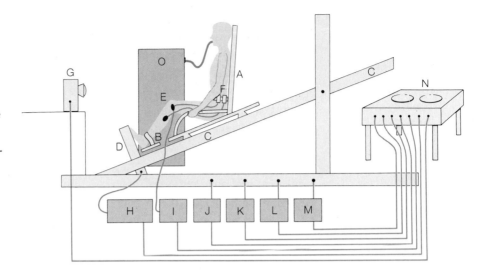

and in some individuals it reached values which exceeded −1.5 (150%). The evidence suggests that the mechanical efficiency of eccentric exercise is very high but not constant. Great variation between individuals is characteristic of eccentric exercise ME. The high efficiency can be improved by increasing stretch velocity, and efficiencies above 100% can be obtained with low motor unit activation. However, in concentric exercise EMG, energy expenditure and mechanical work change in parallel in slow contractions, but increasing shortening velocities will modify these relationships.

Fig. 2.1.21 The relative IEMG (open circles) related to the work intensity: (a) rel W_{neg}; (b) rel W_{pos}. Corresponding efficiency values are marked by dots. In (a) the relative IEMG during a 100 ms preactivation phase are marked by open triangles. The IEMG values are averages of the three muscles studied (vastus lateralis, vastus medialis and gastrocnemius). From Aura & Komi (1986a).

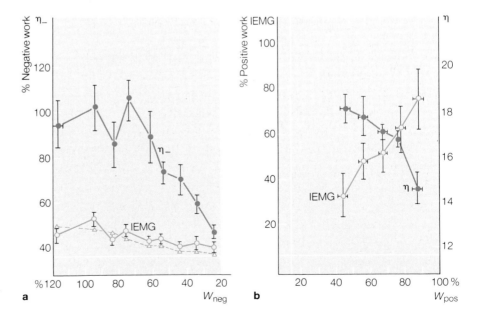

Mechanical efficiencies in SSC exercises

Prestretching of an active muscle during SSC exercise probably also influences the mechanical efficiency of the positive work phase (concentric action) of the cycle. Accepting that negative work does not have a constant efficiency value, then investigation of the ME of SSC exercise must be preceded by first defining that the ME of pure eccentric exercise is exactly the same in stretching velocity and amplitude as the one to be used in SSC exercise. This method was applied in the sledge apparatus described above by Aura and Komi (1986a). Maximum concentric exercise (W_{max}) was defined as the energy level which the subject is able to exert in one pure concentric action. For each subject the positive work intensity was always kept at 60% of W_{max}, and the preceding eccentric contraction was varied from day to day. SSC contractions were repeated 80 times in each situation at a rate of one every 3 s.

At the beginning of each exercise cycle, the sledge was released from a certain distance corresponding to the specific energy level. The height of dropping varied the potential energy of the sledge–subject system and subsequently varied the negative (kinetic) work done during the breakdown. Within each exercise the dropping height was constant, but was varied between exercises, being 20–120% of W_{max}. During contact with the force-plate, the subject resisted the downward movement (negative work), and immediately after stopping the sledge (knee angle 90°) the legs were extended to perform positive work. The effort in positive work was controlled so that the change in the potential energy of the sledge–subject system corresponded to 60% of W_{max}. When the sledge had

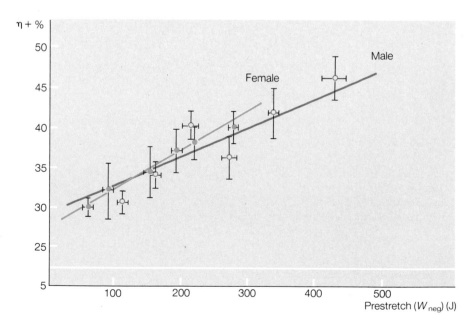

Fig. 2.1.22 The mechanical efficiency of the positive work ($\eta+$) in SSC exercise, related to the prestretch intensity (W_{neg}) in both sexes. From Aura & Komi (1986b).

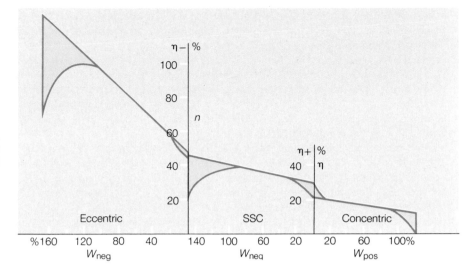

Fig. 2.1.23 Net mechanical efficiencies of pure eccentric (left), pure concentric (right) and SSC (middle) exercises. The shaded areas represent those parts of the curves which need more exact experimentation and in which the adaptational response may vary greatly. From Aura & Komi (1987).

reached its highest position, two assistants checked the starting position corresponded to the specific energy level of the negative work. The mechanical efficiencies of the pure negative and pure positive work were measured individually for all of the subjects 1 or 2 days prior to the actual SSC exercises. Exact formulae for calculating mechanical efficiency during SSC exercises are given elsewhere (Aura & Komi, 1986a).

Figure 2.1.22 shows how the efficiency of positive work increases in SSC exercise when the prestretch load (negative work) is increased. The results therefore suggest that the efficiency of the constant concentric exercise can be changed considerably by modifying the preceding eccentric stretch load. Figure 2.1.23, on the other hand, summarizes recent results by showing the efficiency values for the differing isolated eccentric (left) and concentric (right) actions and also for the SSC (middle) exercise (Aura & Komi, 1987).

References

Asmussen, E. (1952) Positive and negative muscular work. *Acta Physiol. Scand.* **28**, 364.

Aura, O. & Komi, P. V. (1986a) Mechanical efficiency of pure positive and pure negative work with special reference to the work intensity. *Int. J. Sports Med.* **7**, 44.

Aura, O. & Komi, P. V. (1986b) Effects of prestretch intensity on mechanical efficiency of positive work and on elastic behavior of skeletal muscle in stretch-shortening cycle exercise. *Int. J. Sports Med.* **7**, 137.

Aura, O. & Komi, P. V. (1987) The mechanical efficiency of human locomotion in different work intensity levels. (Submitted for publication in the *Proceedings of XI International Congress of Biomechanics, Amsterdam.*)

Bell, D. G. & Jacobs, I. (1986) Electromechanical response times and rate of force development in males and females. *Med. Sci. Sports Exerc.* **18(1)**, 31.

Bergström, J. (1962) Muscle electrolytes in man. *Scand. J. Clin. Lab. Invest.* (Suppl.) **68**, 11.

Bigland, B. & Lippold, O. C. J. (1954) The relation between force, velocity and integrated electrical activity in human muscles. *J. Physiol.* **123**, 214.

Billeter, R., Heizmann, C. W. & Howald, H. (1981a) Analysis of myosin light and heavy chain types in single human skeletal muscle fibers. *Eur. J. Biochem.* **116**, 389.

Billeter, R., Heizmann, C. W., Reist, U., Howald, H. & Jenny, E. (1981b) α- and β-tropomyosin in typed single fibers of human skeletal muscle. *FEBS Lett.* **132**, 133.

Bosco, C. & Komi, P. V. (1979) Mechanical characteristics and fiber composition of human leg extensor muscles. *Eur. J. Appl. Physiol.* **41**, 275.

Bosco, C., Komi, P. V. & Ito, A. (1981) Prestretch potentiation of human skeletal muscle during ballistic movement. *Acta Physiol. Scand.* **111**, 135.

Braunwald, E., Ross jr, J. & Sonnenblick, E. H. (1967) Mechanisms of contraction of the normal and failing heart. *New Engl. J. Med.* **227(15)**, 794.

Brooke, M. H. & Kaiser, K. K. (1974) The use and abuse of muscle histochemistry. *Ann. NY Acad. Sci.* **228**, 121.

Bührle, M., Schmidtbleicher, D. & Ressel, H. (1983) Die spezielle Diagnose der einzelnen Kraftkomponenten im Hochleistungssport. *Leistungssport* **13**, 11.

Cavanagh, P. R. (1988) On 'muscle action' vs. 'muscle contraction'. *J. Biomech.* **22(1)**, 69.

Cavagna, G. A., Dusman, B. & Margaria, R. (1968) Positive work done by the previously stretched muscle. *J. Appl. Physiol.* **24**, 21.

Cavagna, G. A., Saibene, F. P. & Margaria, R. (1965) Effect of negative work on the amount of positive work performed by an isolated muscle. *J. Appl. Physiol.* **20**, 157.

Dietz, V., Schmidtbleicher, D. & Noth, J. (1979) Neuronal mechanisms of human locomotion. *J. Neurophysiol.* **42**, 1212.

Edington, D. W. & Edgerton, V. R. (1976) *The Biology of Physical Activity*. Houghton Mifflin Co., Boston.

Edman, K. A. P., Elzinga, G. & Noble, M. I. M. (1978) Enhancement of mechanical performance by stretch during tetanic contractions of vertebrate skeletal muscle fibres. *J. Physiol. (Lond.)* **281**, 139.

Edman, K. A. P., Elzinga, G. & Noble, M. I. M. (1982) Residual force enhancement after stretch of contracting frog single muscle fibers. *J. Gen. Physiol.* **80**, 769.

Flitney, F. W. & Hirst, D. G. (1978) Cross-bridge detachment and sarcomere give during stretch of active frog's muscle. *J. Physiol. (Lond.)* **276**, 449.

Goldspink, G. (1978) Energy turnover during contraction of different types of muscles. In E. Asmussen & K. Jørgensen (eds) *Biomechanics VI-A*, pp. 27–39. University Park Press, Baltimore.

Grieve, D. W., Pheasant, S. & Cavanagh, P. R. (1978) Prediction of gastrocnemius length from knee and ankle joint posture. In E. Asmussen & K. Jørgensen (eds) *Biomechanics VI-A*, pp. 405–412. University Park Press, Baltimore.

Haugen, P. & Sten-Knudsen, O. (1981) The effect of a small stretch in the latency relaxation and the short-range elastic stiffness in isolated frog muscle fibres. *Acta Physiol. Scand.* **112**, 121.

Henneman, E. & Olson, C. B. (1965) Relations between structure and function in the design of skeletal muscles. *J. Neurophysiol.* **28**, 581.

Hoffer, J. A. & Andreassen, S. (1981) Regulation of soleus muscle stiffness in premammillary cats: intrinsic and reflex components. *J. Neurophysiol.* **45(2)**, 267.

Howald, H. (1985) Morphologische und funktionelle Veränderungen der Muskelflasern durch Training. In M. Bührle (ed) *Grundlagen der Maximal- und Schnellkrafttrainings*, pp. 35–52. Verlag Karl Hofmann, Schorndorf.

Kaneko, M., Komi, P. V. & Aura, O. (1984) Mechanical efficiency of concentric and eccentric exercises performed with medium to fast contraction rates. *Scand. J. Sports Sci.* **6(1)**, 15.

Knuttgen, H. G. (1986) Human performance in high-intensity exercise with concentric and eccentric muscle contractions. *Int. J. Sports Med.* (Suppl.) **7**, 6.

Komi, P. V. (1973a) Relationship between muscle tension, EMG and velocity of contraction under concentric and eccentric work. In J. E. Desmedt (ed) *New Developments in Electromyography and Clinical Neurophysiology*, Vol. 1, pp. 596–606. Karger, Basel.

Komi, P. V. (1973b) Measurement of the force–velocity relationship in human muscle under concentric and eccentric contractions. In *Medicine and Sport, Vol. 8: Biomechanics III*, pp. 224–229. Karger, Basel.

Komi, P. V. (1983) Elastic potentiation of muscles and its influence on sport performance. In W. Baumann (ed) *Biomechanik und Sportliche Leistung*, pp. 59–70. Verlag Karl Hofmann, Schorndorf.

Komi, P. V. (1984) Physiological and biomechanical correlates of muscle function: effects of muscle structure and stretch-shortening cycle on force and speed. In R. L. Terjung (ed) *Exercise and Sport Sciences Reviews*, Vol. 12, pp. 81–121. The Collamore Press, Lexington, Mass.

Komi, P. V. & Buskirk, E. R. (1972) Effect of eccentric

and concentric muscle conditioning on tension and electrical activity of human muscle. *Ergonomics* **15(4)**, 417.

Komi, P. V., Kankeko, M. & Aura, O. (1987) EMG activity of the leg extensor muscles with special reference to mechanical efficiency in concentric and eccentric exercises. *Int. J. Sports Med.* (Suppl.) **8**, 22.

Komi, P. V., Karlsson, J., Tesch, P., Suominen, H. & Heikkinen, E. (1982) Effects of heavy resistance and explosive-type strength training methods on mechanical, functional, and metabolic aspects of performance. In P. V. Komi (ed) *Exercise and Sport Biology*, pp. 90–102. Human Kinetics, Champaign.

Komi, P. V., Viitasalo, J. H. T., Havu, M., Thorstensson, B., Sjödin, B. & Karlsson, J. (1977) Skeletal muscle fibers and muscle enzyme activities in monozygous and dizygous twins of both sexes. *Acta Physiol. Scand.* **100**, 335.

McNaught, A. B. & Callander, R. (1970) *Illustrated Physiology*. E. & S. Livingstone, Edinburgh, London.

Margaria, R. (1938) Sulla fisiologia e specialmente il consumo energitico della marcia e della corca a varia velocita ed inclinazione del terrano. *Atti R. Acc. Naz. Lincei (Rendiconti)* **7**, 299.

Norman, R. W. & Komi, P. V. (1979) Electromyographic delay in skeletal muscle under normal movement conditions. *Acta Physiol. Scand.* **106**, 241.

Rack, P. M. H. & Westbury, D. R. (1974) The short range stiffness of active mammalian muscle and its effect on mechanical properties. *J. Physiol. (Lond.)* **240**, 331.

Saltin, B. & Gollnick, P. D. (1983) Skeletal muscle adaptability: significance for metabolism and performance. In L. D. Peachy, R. H. Adrian & S. R. Geiger (eds) *Handbook of Physiology*, Section 10, pp. 555–631. Williams & Wilkins, Baltimore.

Steg, G. (1964) Efferent muscle innervation and rigidity. *Acta Physiol. Scand.* **61(225)**, 5.

Tihanyi, J., Apor, P. & Fekete, G. (1982) Force–velocity-power characteristics and fiber composition in human leg extensor muscles. *Eur. J. Appl. Physiol.* **48**, 331.

Viitasalo, J. T., Häkkinen, K. & Komi, P. V. (1982) Isometric and dynamic force production and muscle fibre composition in man. *J. Human Mov. Studies* **7**, 199.

Viitasalo, J. & Komi, P. V. (1978) Force–time characteristics and fiber composition in human leg extensor muscles. *Eur. J. Appl. Physiol.* **40**, 7.

Viitasalo, J. & Komi, P. V. (1981) Interrelationships between electromyographic, mechanical, muscle structure and reflex time measurements in man. *Acta Physiol. Scand.* **111**, 97.

Viitasalo, J. T., Komi, P. V. & Bosco, C. (1984) Muscle structure, a determinant of explosive force production? In M. Kumamoto (ed) *Neural and Mechanical Control of Movement*.

Walmsley, B., Hodgson, J. A. & Burke, R. E. (1978) Forces produced by medial gastrocnemius and soleus muscles during locomotion in freely moving cats. *J. Neurophysiol.* **41**, 1203.

Wilkie, D. R. (1950) The relation between force and velocity in human muscle. *J. Physiol.* **110**, 249.

2.2 The cardiovascular system

W. HOLLMANN, R. FRENKL, P. BERTEAU & R. ROST

Introduction

Physiological and pathological considerations of the heart have pre-occupied thinking in sports medicine more than any other organ. The beginnings of this interest date back to 1899 when Henschen declared that the heart's performance and size could be improved by endurance training as a physiological process. This theory was particularly relevant in a damaged or diseased heart, where the question of its existing or desirable workload was of great importance. Most of the pathological and physiological aspects of the heart are now understood, but the discovery of the heart as a hormone-producing gland (natriuretic hormone) is awakening further medical interest.

The vital processes are characterized by metabolism, genetic reproduction and the ability to adapt. The human organism functions on the basis of about 65 billion body cells. About 25 to 50% of these are muscle cells. The supply of nutrients and the removal of waste products are preconditions for the metabolic process, which continues even when the

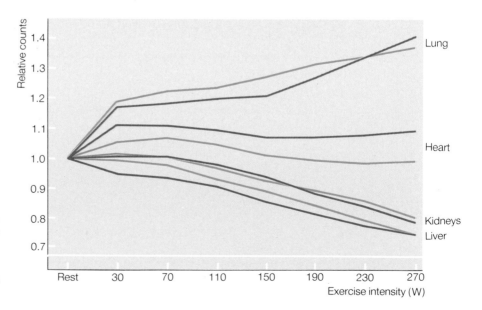

Fig. 2.2.1 Relative impulse rates of lung, heart, kidneys and liver at increasing power-production during cycle ergometer exercise while breathing oxygen (——) and air (——).

body is at rest. The cardiopulmonary system is decisive for this function. Muscular exercise requires a higher energy output. The corresponding increased need for oxygen and nutrients is covered by increased demands on the cardiopulmonary system. At the same time the blood distribution changes; more blood is transported to the exercising muscles, less to some internal organs (Fig. 2.2.1). Systematic repetition of large muscular demands over enough time leads to biochemical and biophysical adaptation. This appears to be an economic achievement by the body, and to result in an increase in maximal performance capacity.

The amount of oxygen to be taken up in the lungs and transported by the cardiovascular system depends on the cardiac output, a product of the heart rate and stroke volume, and on the arteriovenous oxygen difference (peripheral utilization). The performance limit of the heart is given by the maximal cardiac output (stroke volume × heart rate), while the capacity for endurance exercise in man depends on the oxygen uptake over given periods of time.

Performance limits of the normal heart

The deciding factor for the selective cardiac performance limit is the maximal cardiac output. It is reached by progressively increasing dynamic exercise with the largest possible muscle groups. With progressive loading, an increase in oxygen uptake corresponds to an

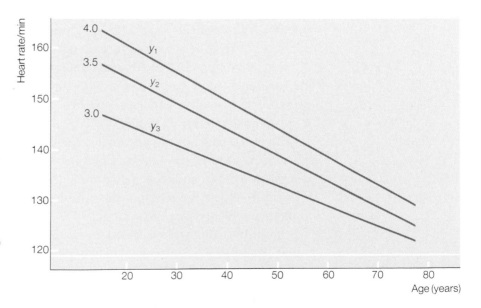

Fig. 2.2.2 Regression lines between age (abscissa) and heart rate related to arterial lactate levels of 3.0, 3.5 and 4.0 mmol/1. The equations are:
$y_1 = 172.4 - 0.57\,x$;
$n = 110$; $r = 0.47$ ($P < 0.001$)
$y_2 = 164.4 - 0.52\,x$; $n = 110$;
$r = 0.43$ ($P < 0.001$)
$y_3 = 152.7 - 0.40\,x$; $n = 110$;
$r = 0.33$ ($P < 0.001$).

increase in cardiac output. In sitting cycle ergometry with a rising intensity of exercise, the stroke volume can increase by between 30 and 50% of the resting value. The maximum stroke volume of the heart is reached with a heart rate of 130 to 150/min. In contrast to this, the heart rate increases linearly up to a performance capacity of about 90% of the maximal oxygen uptake, and then moves more and more horizontally with increases in the load intensity.

The maximal heart rate is reached in puberty, and lies between 205 and 220/min. With increasing age, it regresses. A 25-year-old has average values of 195 ± 10/min, and a 70-year-old average values of 165 ± 10/min. As a rule of thumb, one can say that the maximal attainable heart rate as one ages is 235 minus the age in years. Attention must, however, be paid to the large variations between individuals (Fig. 2.2.2).

Increases in the stroke volume are a result of increased contractility through increased sympathetic tone brought about by muscular exercise and an increase in left ventricular filling with elevation of the end diastolic volume (EDV). In man, this is on average $70 ± 20$ ml/m^2 body surface area (BSA). The highest possible EDV is achieved while lying; sitting up or standing up leads to a reduction. During the systolic emptying phase, the shortening of the heart muscle fibres brings about an increase in stroke volume (SV). This amounts to 45–55 ml/m^2 BSA. The blood remaining in the ventricles at the end of systole is described as the end systolic volume (ESV). It represents the blood left in the ventricle. On average, 67% of the EDV is expelled during systole (normal range between 60 and 75%). The SV/EDV relationship is designated the ejection fraction. With a mean heart rate of 72/min, the mean cardiac output is about 6.5 litre. The maximal cardiac output is ~20 l/min in men, and 13 l/min in women. The end diastolic pressure increases very little during increasing physical exercise, and with high-intensity exercise the mean pressure in the lung capillary bed lies under 22 mmHg, and in the A. pulmonalis under 30 mmHg.

With increasing age the maximal cardiac output is reduced. The cause is: (a) reduction of the maximal attainable heart rate frequency in the process of ageing; and (b) a reduction in the stroke volume. At the same time, there is less reduction of the peripheral resistance during exercise in older people than in the young.

Systolically, the arterial blood pressure increases linearly with dynamic exercise, while the diastolic pressure increases slightly, depending on the type of exercise (intra-arterial measurement). Training under physiological conditions does not bring about significant alterations.

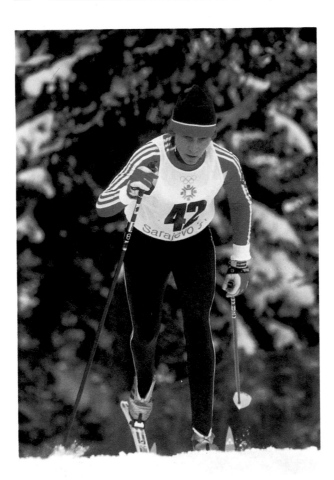

Fig. 2.2.3 Cross-country skiing typifies those sports events that depend on aerobic endurance training and cardiovascular performance. Courtesy of the IOC archives.

Endurance training and heart performance capacity

Of the five main forms of motor demand in the body, coordination, flexibility, strength, speed and endurance, only one is suitable for increasing the performance of the heart: general dynamic aerobic endurance. It is brought about only through an increase in the stroke volume. The maximal attainable heart rates remain generally uninfluenced and even become lower in athletes whose hearts are especially large. Increases in stroke volume are observed both during exercise and at rest as a result of aerobic exercise conditioning. It is made possible by a larger EDV with a comparable or increased ejection fraction, in comparison to the untrained state. While the normal heart size in man is 700 to 800 ml in the lying position, athletes' hearts can be over 1400 ml. The biggest athletes' hearts reported in the literature were found in

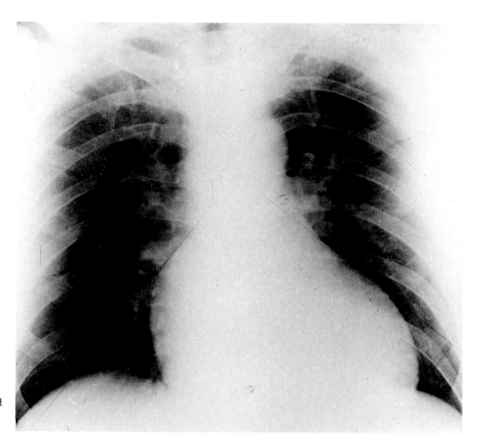

Fig. 2.2.4 Healthy heart of a world champion in road cycling, heart volume 1700 ml.

leading international professional cyclists, with values of 1700 and 1600 ml (Fig. 2.2.4). At the time of the investigations (1964 and 1976), both athletes were reigning world champions. In the course of time, both hearts have returned to values of 958 and 1180 ml, respectively. When they were in a state of high endurance training, there was a resting bradycardia of 32–36/min. A negative T-wave stood out in the ECG in one of the two subjects in the chest leads up to, and including, V4. Twelve years later this finding had returned to normal.

The linear relationship between cardiac output and oxygen uptake with increasing dynamic exercise until submaximal load intensities is retained even under extreme endurance training conditions. The maximal values of the cardiac output are more than 40 l/min. Echocardiographic and other investigations have shown that all heart chambers are enlarged in endurance athletes. At the same time, there is an increase in the absolute thickness of the septum wall and the posterior wall. This explains the increase in heart weight in athletes, which, even so, does not exceed the so-called critical heart weight of 500 g.

Table 2.2.1 Comparison of cardiovascular characteristics of endurance-trained male and female athletes (not world class) and physically inactive people. The spiro-ergometrical data was attained during cycle ergometer exercise (standardized testing method according to Hollmann & Venrath). It is noteworthy that trained people have a greater blood volume/kg bodyweight at unchanged relative haemoglobin contents (g%). Data from the Institute for Cardiology and Sports Medicine, German Sports University, Cologne (Hollmann & Hettinger, 1980).

	Male	Female	Inactive males
Age (years)	25.8 ± 10.7, $n = 216$	20.6 ± 4.6, $n = 55$	43.3 ± 13.0, $n = 69$
Height (cm)	179.6 ± 6.2, $n = 224$	169.1 ± 5.2, $n = 55$	174.9 ± 6.3, $n = 73$
Bodyweight (kg)	75.1 ± 8.8, $n = 224$	60.4 ± 6.5, $n = 55$	76.8 ± 9.8, $n = 73$
Vital capacity (litre)	5.47 ± 0.83, $n = 222$	3.69 ± 0.62, $n = 54$	4.55 ± 0.77, $n = 72$
Maximal ventilatory volume (litre)	183.0 ± 37.1, $n = 222$	119.9 ± 25.4, $n = 54$	155.5 ± 36.7, $n = 71$
Heart volume (ml)	892.9 ± 121.2, $n = 213$	610.0 ± 90.3, $n = 53$	788.5 ± 122.0, $n = 69$
Heart volume/kg (ml)	11.88 ± 1.56, $n = 212$	10.12 ± 1.01, $n = 53$	10.29 ± 1.34, $n = 69$
Blood volume (ml)	6143.0 ± 712.5, $n = 224$	4474.0 ± 615.5, $n = 55$	5650.0 ± 667.9, $n = 73$
Blood volume/kg (ml)	81.92 ± 6.88, $n = 223$	74.06 ± 6.73, $n = 55$	74.16 ± 8.92, $n = 73$
Haemoglobin (g%)	15.9 ± 1.06, $n = 202$	14.3 ± 1.17, $n = 52$	16.0 ± 1.01, $n = 68$
Total haemoglobin (g)	979.9 ± 137.0, $n = 191$	639.7 ± 119.2, $n = 52$	913.7 ± 122.9, $n = 64$
Total haemoglobin (g/kg)	13.03 ± 1.31, $n = 191$	10.62 ± 1.46, $n = 52$	11.93 ± 1.52, $n = 64$
Maximal oxygen uptake (ml/min)	3663.0 ± 570.7, $n = 224$	2389.0 ± 397.0, $n = 55$	2718.0 ± 568.1, $n = 73$
Maximal oxygen uptake/ kg (ml/min)	48.95 ± 6.84, $n = 224$	39.54 ± 5.44, $n = 55$	35.81 ± 8.2, $n = 73$
Maximal oxygen pulse (ml)	20.55 ± 3.08, $n = 223$	13.23 ± 2.34, $n = 55$	16.59 ± 2.48, $n = 73$

With improvement of endurance, the arteriovenous oxygen difference increases during exercise to the limit of physical performance capacity. When this is considered in connection with the larger stroke volume, the large maximal oxygen uptake of those who are trained is understandable.

In principle, the above statements apply to women as well as men. The mean female heart size is 500–600 ml. The biggest female athlete's heart reported in the literature was 1100 ml (Medved et al., 1975). Table 2.2.1 compares cardiovascular characteristics of male and female athletes and physically inactive people (Hollmann & Hettinger, 1980).

Effect of training on peripheral adaptation

The peripheral adaptation has a major significance in both the physiological and pathological fields. From the cardiological point of view it is often underestimated. The haemodynamic and metabolic processes in exercising muscle are decisive for the end performance capacity achieved, provided there is an intact cardiopulmonary system and normal oxygen transport in the blood. Local blood supply and oxygen utilization

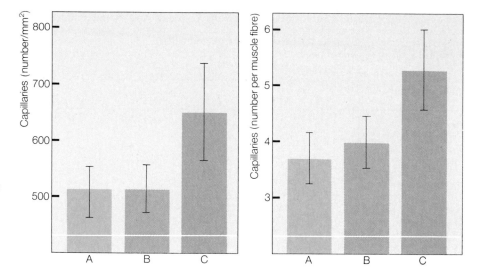

Fig. 2.2.5 Capillarization within the vastus lateralis muscle of physically inactive people (left bars, A), physically active people not performing endurance sports (middle bars, B) and endurance-trained athletes (right bars, C).

(oxidation capacity) correspond directly with total distribution of blood in the organism in limiting performance.

The influence of endurance training on peripheral haemodynamics can, in theory, have three effects:

1   Improved capillarization (Fig. 2.2.5). There is still controversy over whether this effect is achieved through the enlargement of existing capillaries or through the opening up of reserve capillaries. Muscle biopsy studies have shown a mean increase in capillary area of 36% due to endurance training (Schön *et al.*, 1978).
2   Collateral improvement.
3   A more efficient intramuscular blood distribution.

Providing evidence for the last two points is difficult for technical reasons. However, it has been shown that blood flow characteristics are improved by endurance training, with an improvement in the elasticity of the erythrocyte membrane, which increases the ability of the erythrocytes to change their shape in the capillaries.

The peripheral metabolic adaptations are:

1   Increase of number and size of mitochondria.
2   Enlargement of the activity of some aerobic and anaerobic enzymes.
3   Augmentation of myoglobin.
4   Increase of the intramuscular glycogen content.

The sum of the peripheral adaptations causes a reduction of the sympathetic drive of the heart.

Training effects with preventive cardiological significance

The functional basis of all degenerative cardiovascular diseases is the appearance of an imbalance between oxygen requirement and available oxygen in a circumscribed tissue area. Endurance training can counteract this in a variety of ways.

1 In the heart itself, through:
(a) Reduction of the heart rate at rest and in given submaximal exercise intensities in connection with an enlarged stroke volume.
(b) Prolongation of diastole.
(c) Reduced contractility.
(d) Reduction of catecholamine release.
(e) Stabilization of electrical stability.
These factors cause a decrease in the myocardial oxygen requirement, and prolong the phase of intramyocardial blood supply. The occurrence of heart rhythm disturbances is counteracted.
2 With the above mentioned improvements in the properties of blood flow there is a reduction in thrombocyte aggregation and adhesion, with less danger of thrombosis.
3 Levels of high-density lipoprotein (HDL), a protective factor against the occurrence of arteriosclerosis, are increased. This applies especially to the HDL_2 fraction, which is of special anti-arteriosclerotic significance. At the same time, low-density lipoprotein (LDL) and triglycerides may be reduced, again having an anti-arteriosclerotic effect.

Prevention of loss of cardiopulmonary performance due to ageing

Endurance training is the only scientifically-based method to counteract performance loss due to ageing. This is especially true for the cardiopulmonary system. The training adaptations mentioned can be brought about in men and women until at least an age of 70 years, if the people concerned are able to accept the exercise load. In experiments on individuals, aged 55 to 70 years, who had been untrained for decades, it was established that the same training adaptations take place at this age as in young subjects. There are only quantitative differences in comparison to young people. It is thus possible for a healthy person of 60 to have a cardiopulmonary capacity roughly equal to that of a 30- to 40-year-old.

In this sense, the 'senile heart' does not exist. The muscle cells in a healthy 100-year-old are no different than those of a young person; there is just more deposition of connective tissue. Investigations on subjects aged between 100 and 110 years showed that in general they have an LDL/HDL quotient which is well below the average, as well as lower blood pressure.

References

Henschen, S. W. (1899) Skilauf und Skiwettlauf. Eine medizinische Sportstudie. *Mitt. Med. Klin. Uppsala* **2**, 15.

Hollmann, W. & Hettinger, Th. (1980) *Sportmedizin— Arbeits- und Trainingsgrundlagen.* Schattauer-Verlag, Stuttgart.

Medved, R., Pavisie, V. & Stuka, K. (1975) Das größte gesund Sportherz bei Frauen. *Sportarzt Sportmed.* **26**, 174.

Schön, F. A., Hollmann, W., Liesen, H. & Waterloh, E. (1980) Elektronen-mikroskopische Befunde am M. vastus lat. von Untrainierten und Marathon-läufern sowie ihre Beziehung zur relativen maximalen Sauerstoffaufnahme und Laktatproduktion. *Dtsch. Z. Sportmed.* **31(12)**, 343.

Further reading

Bevegard, B. S. (1962) Studies on the regulation of the circulation in man. *Acta Physiol. Scand.* (Suppl.) **57**, 200.

Broustet, J. B., Boisseau, M., Bouloumie, J., Emerian, J. P., Series, E. & Bricaud, H. (1978) The effects of acute exercise and physical training on platelet function in patients with coronary artery disease. *Cardiac Rehabil.* **9(2)**, 28.

Heck, H., Rost, R. & Hollmann, W. (1984) Normwerte des Blutdrucks bei der Fahrradergometrie. *Dtsch. Z. Sportmed.* **35(7)**, 243.

Hollmann, W., Rost, R., Dufaux, B. & Liesen, H. (1983) *Prävention und Rehabilitation von Herz-Kreislaufkrankheiten durch körperliches Training.* Hippokrates-Verlag, Stuttgart.

Reindell, H., König, K. & Roskamm, H. (1967) *Funktionsdiagnostik des Gesunden und Kranken Herzens.* Thieme-Verlag, Stuttgart.

Reindell, H. & Roskamm, H. (1977) *Herz-Krankheiten.* Springer-Verlag, Berlin, Heidelberg.

Rost, R. (1984) *Herz und Sport.* Perimed-Verlag, Erlangen.

2.3 The respiratory system

W. HOLLMANN & A. MADER

Introduction

Pulmonary respiration transforms venous blood into arterial blood by exposing it to oxygen, and allowing the removal of carbon dioxide. In addition, respiration plays an important role in maintaining a constant pH value in the blood. In man, the part played by the lung in temperature regulation and water loss is of lesser importance. The driving forces of gaseous exchange are the partial pressure gradients of oxygen and carbon dioxide. The gas exchange between lung and blood takes place in the alveoli via the alveolocapillary membrane. The anatomical dead space allows the cleansing and humidifying of the air and adjusting it to body temperature.

The challenge to the muscles of pulmonary ventilation consists of producing a pressure difference between the intrathoracic space and the external air. It has to be performed against the resistance in the airway and the chest. Only about 20% of lung resistance is due to tissue resistance; 80% comes from resistance in the airway. During intense physical exercise, the speed of air movement increases, and with it the turbulence in the trachea and large bronchi. On the other hand, the increase in sympathetic tone due to exercise causes a relaxation of the bronchial musculature, with an expansion of the bronchi that results in a lowering of respiratory resistance.

Elastic resistance increases with increased respiratory depth. The measure of lung flexibility is the 'compliance'. It depends on the properties of the lung tissue and the size of the lung volume. The smaller the expiratory volume, the smaller the compliance.

At rest, the cost expenditure for respiration amounts to an oxygen uptake of 0.5–1.0 ml/l ventilation. In intense physical exercise, it increases significantly and can amount to 10–12% of the total oxygen uptake. As the air resistance in nasal breathing is two to three times greater than in mouth breathing, this factor also influences the oxygen requirement.

Lung volume

The maximal lung volume represents the air content of the lungs in maximal inspiration. The volume remaining after normal expiration is the functional residual capacity (FRC). After maximal deep expiration, the residual volume (RV) remains. The maximal amount of air that can be expired after maximal inspiration is the maximal respiratory volume (vital capacity, VC). The total lung capacity (TLC), is the volume of air that is in the lungs after maximal inspiration (VC + RV = TLC). In a healthy person, the VC is about 74%, and the RV about 26% of the total capacity.

The individual volumes are in general dependent on sex, age, body surface and state of training. In addition, the body position plays a role. For example, the standing VC is about 10%, and the sitting VC about 5%, greater than the lying VC. The total capacity remains similar, as the RV is independent of body position. The respiratory reserve volume increases by about 60% on sitting and by about 70% on standing, when compared to the lying position. The lung volume in women is more than 10% smaller than in men of the same age and size; training, however, can increase the pulmonary volume.

After the third decade of life, the RV increases and the VC decreases. Between the age of 25 and 60 years the share of the RV in the TLC rises by up to 30–35% of the TLC. The causes are increasing thoracic rigidity and a loss of elasticity in the lung tissues.

In pulmonary function diagnosis, 'dynamic' lung volumes are measured as well as the 'static' volumes mentioned above. The forced expiratory volume (FEV_1) is the volume that can be forced out through the mouth under maximum exertion in the first second after maximal inspiration. Its considerable clinical significance lies in the possibility of diagnosing and differentiating disturbances of ventilation in this way.

Obstructive ventilation disturbances with increased bronchial resistance permit the movement of only a reduced amount of air in the first second of expiration. A restrictive ventilation disturbance gives, however, a broadly normal value in terms of percentage of VC; because although the VC is reduced, a normal bronchial flow resistance is present. The normal value for a healthy person in the third decade of life is above 80%. A dependence of this value on the body length and VC has been observed. VC values of over 5 litre let the forced expiratory volume sink physiologically to about 75% in many cases. In people with a VC of more than 7 litre this can be nearer 70%. These values were established in studies of national basketball players, where the VC was 7–9 litre (Hollmann & Hettinger, 1980).

The maximal voluntary ventilation is used to determine the lung ventilatory reserve. To obtain this value, the subject breathes in and out as rapidly and deeply as possible through the open mouth. The duration of registration is 10 s; the product of the breathing rate and depth is multiplied by six to give the value/min. The normal range for healthy males in the third decade of life is between 100 and 180 l/min, and for women, 70–120 l/min. The maximal ventilatory capacity is never reached in maximal dynamic exercise.

The respiratory flow rate represents the first derivation of volume according to time, measured in l/s or ml/s. The flow rate in forced expiration increases from 0.1 to a maximum of 10–15 l/s.

Lung ventilation

By ventilation one understands the movement of air in and out of the lungs. The amount of ventilation is given by the product of respiratory rate and tidal volume, giving the minute volume of pulmonary ventilation ($\dot{V}_E$). It is controlled so that the oxygen and carbon dioxide partial pressures in the alveolar air and arterial blood remain at an optimal level. At rest, the respiratory rate is 8–14/min and the tidal volume 400–600 ml. With the start of physical exercise, the oxygen needs of the organism rise, and ventilation increases. The respiratory rate and tidal volume increase almost at the moment of starting the activity. Endurance-trained people adjust themselves to a greater tidal volume faster than the untrained.

In the case of submaximal dynamic work of constant intensity, with the use of larger muscle groups, the $\dot{V}_E$ reaches a steady state value after 3–6 min. Up to an exercise intensity of 30–50% of the $\dot{V}_{O_2\ max}$, the $\dot{V}_E$ increases in proportion to the oxygen uptake, and then as the exercise intensity increases, rises increasingly out of proportion. This switch from a linear to an exponential rise of $\dot{V}_E$, associated with the stage of increasing power production and oxygen uptake, is called the point of most effective respiration (Hollmann, 1961) or the anaerobic threshold (Wasserman & McIlroy, 1964). Figure 2.3.1 shows some of the metabolic changes occurring during an increasing exercise intensity. At the same time, there is a significant difference in the lactate content of the arterial and venous blood, as resting musculature, which is not taking part in the acute exercise, metabolizes part of the lactate (Hollmann, 1961). This connection between the amount of ventilation and the arterial lactate level will be discussed later.

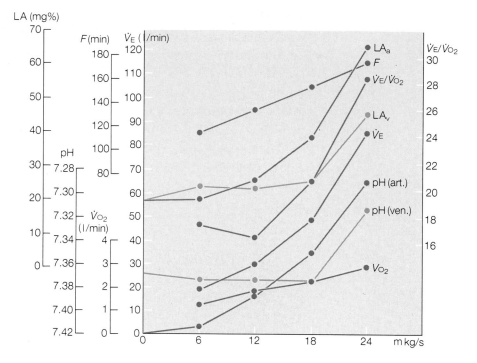

Fig. 2.3.1 Ventilation ($\dot{V}_E$), oxygen uptake ($\dot{V}_{O_2}$), pulse rate (F), respiratory equivalent ($\dot{V}_E/\dot{V}_{O_2}$), arterial lactate level (LA_a), venous lactate level (LA_v), arterial and venous pH value during increasing exercise on the cycle ergometer. Mean values of 12 males (third decade of life) at the end of the third minute of exercise at every level of power production.

If the tidal volume exceeds about 50% of the VC with an increasing workload, there is, above all, an increase in respiratory rate. At the borders of performance capacity, the tidal volume becomes significantly less. After the exercise has ended, the $\dot{V}_E$ reverts at first quickly, and then increasingly slowly, to the initial resting value.

During physical exercise, the state of training, age and sex have an influence on the minute volume. Methodological conditions (crank-turning exercise standing, cycle ergometer exercise, pedalling exercise lying, step-test exercise, treadmill exercise) influence the size of the minute volume to a great extent.

If 100 vol% oxygen is used instead of air (21 vol% oxygen), the $\dot{V}_E$ rises in an almost straight line. If gas mixtures with less oxygen content than 21 vol% are used, the curved increase in $\dot{V}_E$ takes place at correspondingly lower levels of exercise intensity (altitude conditions).

The relationship between the amount of oxygen uptake and the $\dot{V}_E$ can be defined as the respiratory equivalent value. This is a quotient obtained from the $\dot{V}_E$ (ml) divided by the oxygen uptake (ml) in the same minute. The smaller the value, the better the respiratory economics, due to the higher oxygen utilization of the ventilated air. In the uppermost steady state area of $\dot{V}_E$ during exercise, the respiratory equivalent value of an untrained male in the third decade of life is 25–30, depending on the type

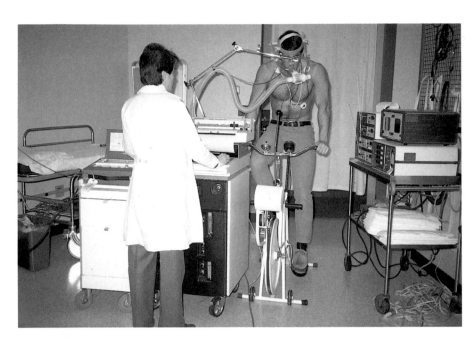

Fig. 2.3.2 Circulatory and pulmonary function can be assessed through monitored exercise testing in the clinical or research laboratory. Courtesy of L. H. Hartley.

of power production demanded. An improvement of the endurance-training state, and with it the aerobic capacity, permits a reduction in ventilation effort. At the same time, there is a reduction in the lactate level and an increase of the pH value of the arterial blood at submaximal exercise loads. A similar effect can be obtained by increasing the amount of oxygen in the inspired air.

Similarly to the $\dot{V}_E$, the carbon dioxide elimination increases with rising exercise intensity. At low levels of power production, the respiratory quotient (CO_2 in ml/O_2 in ml) falls to a lower level than at physical rest, as does the respiratory equivalent value. So the lung function in light to moderate physical exercise is more efficient than in a state of physical rest.

The uppermost level of exercise intensity attainable without a further rise in arterial lactate, and thus without an increase of $\dot{V}_E$ in longer-lasting exercise, has been called the 'Sauerstoff-Dauerleistungsgrenze' (aerobic border for long-lasting exercise) (Hollmann, 1961). The value is identical to the point of optimal respiratory efficiency (Hollmann, 1961) and to the anaerobic threshold of Wasserman and McIlroy (1964).

Rhythmic movements, especially in sports like swimming, influence the respiratory rate, and without exception lead to a reduction in frequency. A compensatory increase in the tidal volume takes place. Healthy people basically choose the respiratory rate and tidal volume which is optimal for the most effective respiration. Each artificial alteration thus leads to a reduction in efficiency.

Breathing through the nose is not sufficient for a ventilation expenditure greater than 50 l/min. At this point, or earlier, the mouth must also be used.

Diffusion in the lungs

The diffusion capacity of the lungs is the gas diffusion in unit of time per mmHg partial pressure difference between alveolar air and erythrocyte content. At physical rest, the value for oxygen is 20–50 ml/min/mmHg. As a consequence of the good diffusion conditions for carbon dioxide, the partial pressure in alveolar air is practically identical to that found in arterial blood. The oxygen partial pressure is, however, 105 mmHg in the alveoli and 100 mmHg in arterial blood. The level of gas pressure at the capillary end thus depends on the level of gas pressure in venous mixed blood and alveolar air, on the ventilation/perfusion pressure, on the gas-binding capacity of the blood, and on the solubility coefficients of the gases. Oxygen undersaturation in normal alveolar air conditions can be traced to the following factors:

1   Incomplete compensation between alveolar air and lung capillary blood (membrane gradient).
2   Disproportion of distribution of ventilation and perfusion (distribution gradient).
3   Admixture of venous mixed blood with capillary blood (venous mixing gradient).

The diffusion pressure increases with physical effort because additional vessel areas are opened; these are only sparsely supplied with blood at rest. A maximal oxygen uptake of 4 l/min needs a diffusion capacity of 60 ml/min/mmHg, and an oxygen uptake of 6 l/min a capacity of 100 ml/min/ mmHg as a prerequisite (Shephard, 1969).

Diffusion starts to decrease after the age of 20 (Riley & Cournand, 1951). Apart from age and the body surface, the diffusion capacity is also influenced by the position of the body. It is about 15–20% greater when lying (compared to sitting), and almost 15% more when sitting (compared to standing). The reason for this is an orthostatically-induced reduction of lung perfusion, especially in the upper parts of the lung, when standing or sitting.

In healthy, endurance-trained males and females the greater the maximal oxygen uptake, the higher the diffusion capacity in that both physiological capacities are size related. Intense physical exercise leads both to a lower oxygen content in venous mixed blood and to an acceleration of the rate of blood flow. As a consequence of the latter, the contact time between the alveolar air and the lung capillaries is reduced. In the border area of performance capacity, the contact time is no longer sufficient for complete saturation of the erythrocytes with oxygen. A reduction of P_{O_2} and oxygen saturation in the arterial blood can actually be registered in people capable of high performance. Here, the high peripheral oxygen depletion in endurance-trained athletes may play a role.

Distribution in the lungs

By distribution, we understand the quality of air distribution in the lungs. The ventilation/perfusion relationship is so controlled that, for example, alveoli excluded from ventilation due to pathological reasons also experience a general close-down of blood supply. In this way, a decrease of oxygen saturation is prevented. If, however, the oxygen saturation at rest amounts to only 96–98%, this is primarily the consequence of arteriovenous short circuits of various types.

During exercise, the lung capillary blood is increased by the opening of resting capillaries, and the distribution quality is improved. Alveoli which are only slightly ventilated at rest become involved in an intensive gas exchange. In addition, the increase in pulmonary arterial pressure plays a part. As a consequence, in light and moderate physical exercise, the arterial P_{O_2} generally increases over the initial resting pressure in order to decrease during maximal aerobic exercise.

Respiratory control during physical exercise

During physical rest, respiration is controlled by both chemical and nerve mechanisms. Certain of these mechanisms, however, are not yet clearly understood; such as the interaction between the known chemo-sensitive reflex zones of the arterial beds, and the integration of afferent impulses with stimuli that work directly on the respiratory centre and thus ensure precise adjustment to the performance situation. Major factors affecting the respiratory centre are the P_{CO_2}, H^+ concentration, P_{O_2} and neurogenic forces. Elevation of the H^+ concentration and the P_{CO_2}, and a reduction of the P_{O_2} have the effect of increasing ventilation.

As a result of related experimental investigations, Hartung *et al.* (1966) proposed that the adjustment of $\dot{V}_E$ during exercise is largely determined by the intracellular H^+ concentration.

The only chemoreceptors with a certain control function for ventilation are situated in the arterial system and the brain stem. To what extent carbon dioxide-sensitive receptors exist in the pulmonary artery, bringing about increased ventilation as a result of increased carbon dioxide release in the blood as a sequel of the raised lactate content from heavier muscular activity, has to remain open (Wasserman, 1978).

Respiration as a factor limiting performance

The ventilatory capacity is not exhausted, even by intensive dynamic exercise using large muscle masses. The $\dot{V}_E$ reaches, at the most, 70–80% of the maximal voluntary ventilation under these conditions. The $\dot{V}_E$ can, additionally, be voluntarily raised.

These findings are clear evidence against a performance-limiting effect of ventilation as such. On the other hand, at altitude, especially above heights of 3000–4000 m, hyperventilation may contribute to limit performance capacity. To what extent the oxygen need of muscles used for respiration can have an effect on performance limitation has yet to be established.

If the arterial P_{O_2} in top athletes in endurance sport at the borders of performance capacity sinks by 15 mmHg or more, the shortening of the contact time of the erythrocytes in the lung capillaries may have a considerable part to play in limiting performance. This could be especially true under altitude conditions.

References

Hartung, M., Venrath, H., Hollmann, W., Isselhardt, W. & Jaenckner, D. (1966) *Über die Atmungsregulation unter die Arbeit*. Westdeutscher Verlag, Köln, Opladen.

Hollmann, W. (1961) Zur Frage der Dauerleistungsfähigkeit. *Fortschr. Med.* **17**, 439.

Hollmann, W. & Hettinger, Th. (1980) *Sportmedizin— Arbeits- und Trainingsgrundlagen*. Schattauer-Verlag, Stuttgart.

Riley, L. R. & Cournand, A. (1951) Analysis of factors effecting partial pressures of oxygen and carbon dioxide in gas and blood of lungs theory. *J. Appl. Physiol.* **4**, 77.

Shephard, R. J. (1969) *Endurance Fitness*. Toronto University Press, Toronto.

Wasserman, K. (1978) Breathing during exercise. *New Engl. J. Med.* **298**, 780.

Wasserman, K. & McIlroy, M. B. (1964) Detecting the threshold of anaerobic metabolism in cardiac patients. *Am. J. Cardiol.* **14**, 844.

Further reading

Comroe, J. H. (1966) The lung. *Science* **214(2)**, 56.

Dejours, B. (1966) *Respiration*. Oxford University Press, Oxford.

Hollmann, W. (1963) *Höchst- und Dauerleistungsfähigkeit des Sportlers*. Barth-Verlag, Munich.

Knipping, H. W. (1929) Die Untersuchung der Ökonomie von Muskelarbeit bei Gesunden und Kranken. *Z. Exp. Med.* **66**, 517.

Rossier, P.H., Bühlmann, A. & Wiesinger, K. (1958) *Physiologie und Pathophysiologie der Atmung*. Springer-Verlag, Berlin.

2.4 Metabolic capacity

W. HOLLMANN, H. LIESEN & A. MADER

Introduction

The ability of a muscle to perform long-duration exercise depends, among other things, on the supply of sufficient blood, oxygen and nutrients. The type of contraction of the muscle and the degree of loading play a significant role in the metabolic process. Dynamic exercise for periods longer than 2 min is characterized by dominant aerobic metabolic processes; static exercise, even of moderate intensity, and dynamic exercise in the maximal border area are characterized by intensive anaerobic metabolism. The aerobic metabolic processes take place in the mitochondria (intramitochondrial metabolism), and the anaerobic processes in the muscle cell plasma (extramitochondrial metabolism).

In muscular activity, chemical energy is changed to mechanical work. The efficiency is about 30–35%; by far the greatest part of the released energy is in the form of heat.

High-energy phosphate breakdown The breakdown of ATP (adenosine triphosphate) to ADP (adenosine diphosphate) and phosphate, with the simultaneous release of energy, is the basis for muscle contraction and relaxation. The muscle cell store of ATP is, however, very limited. In resting muscle it is about 5–6 mmol/kg, which is sufficient for one to three muscle contractions or 1–2 s duration of exercise under heavy muscular demand. The organism is thus engaged in the constant reconstitution of ATP. It takes place so quickly that even after exhausting exercise the ATP level is scarcely reduced. Creatine phosphate (CP) provides the depot, and is available in amounts three to four times greater than the ATP in the muscle cell. CP breakdown is controlled by the enzyme creatine phosphokinase (CPK), which adjusts its activity to the current ATP consumption. In dynamic exercise, CP breakdown takes place more or less linearly with the power production and, under static loading, linearly with the force developed. The energy-rich phosphate remainder of CP is altered to ADP, thus producing new ATP.

In all, the energy of this phosphate is sufficient for about 6–8 s of maximal muscle exercise. In maximal load intensities, the ADP is altered via the myokinase to both ATP and adenosine monophosphate:

$$2\,ADP \rightarrow ATP + AMP.$$

The latter is broken down to inosine monophosphate, and a small percentage to adenosine. A higher concentration of ADP and AMP under severe load activates phosphofructokinase, i.e. glycolysis. About 70–80% of the CP resting level of 16–25 mmol/kg musculature can be split to produce energy. Under especially intensive continuous muscle demand, an almost complete emptying of the CP stores can occur. The breakdown of ATP to ADP produces about 42 kJ/mol. Mechanical work of 16.4–21.6 J_{mech} (1.6–1.99 m kg; 3.9–5.3 cal) can be obtained from 1 mmol of CP. The time constant for reconstitution of the high-energy phosphates is about 24–28 s.

High-energy phosphate repletion

The stores of energy-rich phosphates can be restored or stabilized in two ways: (a) without the help of oxygen, via the anaerobic breakdown of carbohydrate to lactate (glycolysis); or (b) in the presence of oxygen, via the oxidation of nutrients. The first process produces the anaerobic lactic acid energy-supply system. It involves the rephosphorylation of creatine to CP and the reconstitution of ATP from ADP through the conversion of glycogen to lactate. The mechanical work that can be obtained from this is limited by lactate accumulation in the exercising

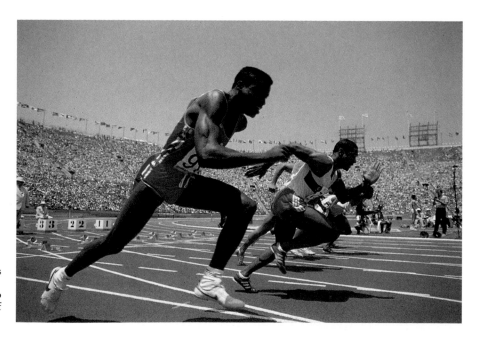

Fig. 2.4.1 The shorter the sprint event in track, the greater the dependence on high-energy phosphates as an energy depot. © The Los Angeles Times 1984 (National Photo Pool), photo by Joe Kennedy. Courtesy of the IOC archives.

musculature, and the associated acidosis in the whole organism. On average, 16–20 mmol/l lactate can be tolerated in the blood. A blood lactate level of 1 mmol/l can produce a mechanical workload of 1.6 m/kg bodyweight or cover an oxygen deficit of about 2.8–3.3 ml/kg.

Anaerobic metabolism

The maximum amount of work that can be mobilized by glycolysis with 18.5 mmol/l lactate, approximates 24 000 J (2500 m kg) for an 84 kg person and 27 500 J (2800 m kg) for a 95 kg person. In this estimate, 1 mmol/l lactate is taken to be equivalent to 3.3 ml oxygen/kg.

The anaerobic lactic acid energy-supply system is assisted by extra-mitochondrial NAD (nicotinamide adenine dinucleotide), which acts as a hydrogen acceptor. If there is not enough oxygen available, the pyruvate is reduced to lactate by taking a hydrogen atom from the NADH. The oxidized NAD can act as a hydrogen acceptor again, leading to further oxidation of glycogen and the delivery of energy for the reconstitution of the energy-rich phosphates. The blood lactate level reaches its maximum value with maximal dynamic exercise lasting 40–45 s. The importance of the aerobic mechanism increases with prolongation of the exercise bout.

Aerobic metabolism

The alternative way to supply energy is through the aerobic metabolic capacity (respiration), which is based on the oxidative rephosphorylation of ADP to ATP in the respiratory chain of the mitochondria by the oxidation of hydrogen. This mechanism is dependent on the combustion of carbohydrate or free fatty acids; only a small part is played by the utilization of protein. In a complicated breakdown process in the mitochondria (citric acid cycle), fractions of carbohydrate (pyruvate) and free fatty acids have their hydrogen withdrawn and the remaining carbon eliminated as carbon dioxide. The hydrogen proceeds along the respiratory chain in the form of the reduced co-enzymes $NADH_2$ and $FADH_2$, which consist of lipoproteins with various cytochromes and metals. The flow of two electrons through the chain produces the energy for ATP formation. At the end of the chain, each pair of electrons is bound to two protons and oxygen. The oxygen enters the muscle cells via pulmonary respiration and the blood.

Oxidative energy supply is not burdened with the accumulation of end products, because of the simple and complete absorption of carbon dioxide and oxygen through the vascular system and pulmonary respiration. Because of the high sensitivity of the mitochondrial respiratory chain to even minor ATP dephosphorylation, a practical adjustment of respiration in proportion to the existing energy requirement of the cell (operating at a level below maximal dynamic exercise) is theoretically guaranteed for as long as required.

Oxidative phosphorylation has priority over glycolysis (Pasteur effect). This is achieved by an increased dephosphorylation threshold for the activation of anaerobic glycolysis in comparison to that for respiration.

The lactate formed in the exercising musculature is largely transferred to the blood. Resting musculature which is not involved in the exercise can remove lactate from arterial blood and oxidize part of it. Further sites and pathways for lactate removal are: chemical alteration in the liver, heart muscle and the kidneys, as well as elimination in sweat and urine. The transfer of lactate from the active musculature to the blood increases almost linearly with the intramuscular lactate production.

Energy substrates   The type of nutritive substance burned depends on the quality and quantity of the exercise, on the nutrition, and on the state of training. In the first few minutes of exercise with increasing power production, carbohydrate metabolism predominates; however, the oxidation of fat gains in importance in prolonged submaximal demand. At first, the intracellular reserves are used. The fat reserves are practically inexhaustible, because fatty acids can be delivered by the vascular system in sufficient quantities for demand. This is not the case with glucose, although mobilization of the liver glycogen does meet some of the demand. In submaximal exercise with about 70% of the maximal oxygen uptake, the amount of energy obtained from carbohydrate breakdown is about 70% at the beginning of loading; after about 30 min of exercise, it is still about 50%. The better the state of endurance training, the greater the

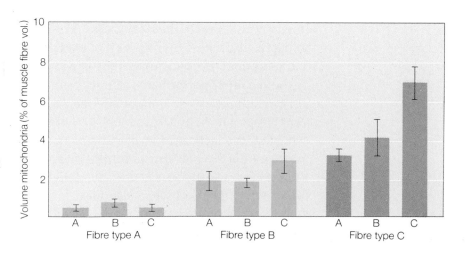

Fig. 2.4.2 Volume of mitochondria in the vastus lateralis muscle of untrained people (left bars, A), physically active people without any endurance training (middle bars, B), and endurance trained athletes (right bars, C).

percentage of free fatty acids which are burned, with a sparing effect on the glycogen deposits.

The proteins (amino acids) are more important in the process of continuous structural reorganization than in the supply of energy.

The metabolic capacity of trained skeletal muscle improves in the following ways:

1   Increase in the number and size of the mitochondria (Fig. 2.4.2).
2   Increased activity by some anaerobic, but mainly aerobic, enzymes.
3   Increased myoglobin content.
4   Increased combustion of free fatty acids, with a reduced demand on the enlarged glycogen stores.

Oxygen uptake

The transition of the cardiopulmonary system from rest to physical activity—elevated cardiac output, enlarged respiratory minute volume, redistribution of blood mainly to the exercising musculature, dilation of blood vessels and the capillary system in the exercising muscles—improves both the substrate supply of the muscle and the oxygen supply. In submaximal exercise, depending on the quality and quantity of the exercise, 2–6 min pass before the oxygen supply corresponds to the exercise intensity. If the latter remains constant, the steady state condition occurs. The time needed to reach the steady state of oxygen uptake is designated the initial phase. At the end of the exercise, the oxygen uptake reverts to the initial resting value after a few minutes, similar to an exponential–function curve.

The oxygen deficit is the amount of oxygen which was needed, but not taken up, during the initial transition period in relation to the exercise intensity and level of the steady state. The oxygen uptake excess over the initial resting value after the end of exercise is called the oxygen debt.

In untrained people, only a quasi-steady state occurs above about 50% of the maximal performance capacity. In this state there is a constant oxygen uptake, with a simultaneous slow increase of pulse rate and ventilation. When approximately 50% of the maximal oxygen uptake is achieved, the lactic acid level starts to rise with further increases in the exercise intensity. At this point the musculature needs more ATP than the aerobic restitution system can deliver. Consequently, an aerobic carbohydrate breakdown is also used to provide energy. In the border area of aerobic capacity, anaerobic glycolysis covers about 10% of the energy demand in the musculature.

With a submaximal to maximal intensity of aerobic exercise, the blood lactate level only reaches its highest value some minutes after cessation of exercise. The reason for this is the delayed diffusion of lactate out of the muscle cells.

Maximal oxygen uptake

The maximal oxygen uptake is the highest oxygen value per unit of time that the human body is capable of when breathing air. It is dependent on the cardiopulmonary–metabolic capacity, with its size primarily determined by cardiac output, peripheral utilization (AVDO$_2$) and by the aerobic capacity of the working skeletal muscles.

The behaviour of the maximal oxygen uptake from childhood to old age in males and females is shown in Fig. 2.4.3. Before puberty there is only a slight superiority in boys in comparison to girls. Females reach their maximal value between the ages of 14 and 16 years, and males at 19 years. Up to the age of 30, the values remain largely unchanged. Beyond 30 years, a reduction appears in untrained people, males losing their performance capacity quicker than females (Fig. 2.4.4). By carrying out regular endurance training, for example starting at the age of 40, it is possible to maintain relatively high maximal oxygen uptake values; at the age of 60 it is still possible to have average values equal to those of untrained people more than 20 years younger (see Fig. 2.4.3).

Through endurance training the maximal oxygen uptake can be

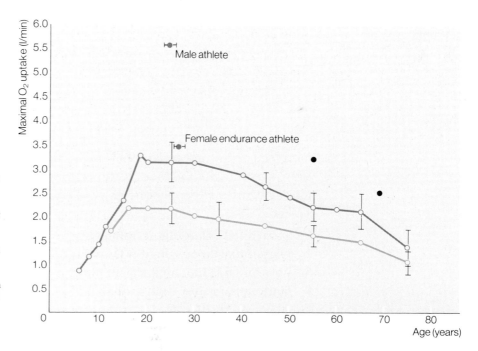

Fig. 2.4.3 Maximal oxygen uptake (l/min) in males (o———o) and females (o———o). For comparison the values of male and female world class athletes in endurance sports are drawn in (above 25 years of age). The black dots above the 55th and 66th years are mean values of endurance trained older people. All data were collected between 1955 and 1963.

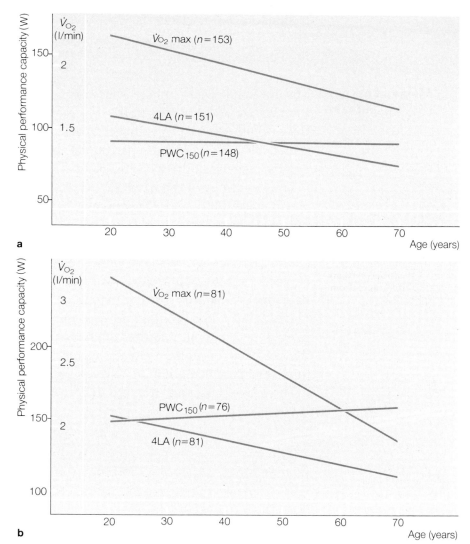

Fig. 2.4.4 Physical performance capacity (W) of untrained females (a) and males (b) between 20 and 70 years of age. The regression lines are related to maximal oxygen uptake ($\dot{V}_{O_{2max}}$), an arterial lactate level of 4 mmol/l (4 LA), and physical working capacity (PWC$_{150}$).

increased on average by 20–30%, and in certain exceptional cases by over 80%. According to the investigations done by Bouchard *et al.*, there are four categories of people carrying out endurance training (Bouchard & Thibault, 1986):

1 Low initial value, slight trainability.
2 High initial value, slight trainability.
3 Low initial value, high trainability.
4 High initial value, high trainability.

People in the last category are particularly able to attain maximal oxygen uptake values of about 100% over normal values. Approximately 80% of

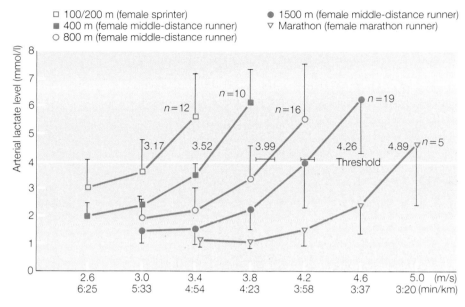

□ 100/200 m (female sprinter) ● 1500 m (female middle-distance runner)
■ 400 m (female middle-distance runner) ▽ Marathon (female marathon runner)
○ 800 m (female middle-distance runner)

Fig. 2.4.5 The anaerobic threshold of female sprinters, middle-distance runners (400, 800 and 1500 m) and marathon runners (from left to right).

the aerobic capacity is genetically fixed. According to calculations done by the authors, about one person in a thousand has the prerequisites to have a maximal oxygen uptake much greater than average (Hollmann & Hettinger, 1980).

While the average values for males are between 3000 and 3500 ml/min, world class athletes in endurance sports reach values of 6000–7000 ml/min. For the average female, the average value is 2000–2200 ml/min, but world class female athletes in endurance sports can reach values of more than 4000 ml/min.

The absolute maximal oxygen uptake should be differentiated from the relative maximal oxygen uptake (ml/kg bodyweight/min). The physiological norm of the relative maximal oxygen uptake for males from childhood to old age varies between 40 and 55 ml/kg/min. For females the corresponding values are between 32 and 38 ml/kg/min. If the maximal oxygen uptake is taken as being per kg lean body mass (LBM), hardly any significant difference can be shown between males and females. On average, these values are 46–49 ml/kg/min for men and 44–48 ml/kg/min for women. The bodyweight provides an index almost identical to that obtained from the nomogram method for establishing maximal oxygen uptake or LBM, especially fat-free body mass minus bone weight. People with noticeably higher amounts of fatty tissue also show an absolute increase in oxygen uptake if bodyweight is excluded as a factor.

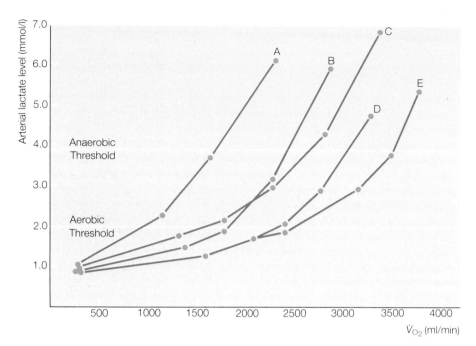

Fig. 2.4.6 The aerobic threshold (lower line) and the anaerobic threshold (upper line) of identical males ($n = 12$) during: (A) crank-turning exercise in a standing position, (B) pedalling exercise in a lying position, (C) bicycling, (D) stair climbing, and (E) treadmill running.

The highest maximal oxygen uptake values are reached in sports like bicycle road-racing, cross-country skiing and rowing. In track and field runs, sprinters have the lowest anaerobic threshold, while marathon runners have the highest (Fig. 2.4.5). The relative maximal oxygen uptake can reach values of 80–90 ml/min in cyclists and cross-country skiers. This is not the case for international class rowers, as their bodyweight is usually greatly above average. The absolute highest values for maximal oxygen uptake are reached in running uphill; measurements are highest if the slope is between 3 and 10%. The peak oxygen uptake measurements in this situation are 3–5% higher than those found when running on the flat; and values found in sitting cycle ergometer exercise are 5–10% lower. Lying pedalling exercise gives performance values 5–10% lower still, and standing arm-cranking exercise gives the lowest values (about 30–40% less than the exercise of horizontal running) (Fig. 2.4.6).

The specific conditions of a sport must be considered when examining the validity of statements on the absolute and relative maximal oxygen uptake values for the performance capacity of athletes in predominantly aerobic disciplines. Rowers, cyclists and swimmers do not have to carry their bodyweight during the exercise, as this function is assumed by the boat, bicycle or water. As a consequence they have to perform little or no work against gravity, and only have to overcome friction. The absolute maximal oxygen uptake value is therefore often of more significance in these events.

Anaerobic metabolic capacity

The basics of anaerobic capacity have already been presented. Elevated creatine phosphate levels have been demonstrated, amongst other findings, in weightlifters, sprinters and middle-distance runners, so the maximal athletic performance can be intensified or prolonged by several seconds and the competition results decisively improved. The creatine kinase level is raised either insignificantly or not at all during training, as the high activity of this enzyme obviously does not limit capacity in individual athletic performances.

The larger the energy-rich phosphate reserves, the longer a maximal running speed can be maintained. If anaerobic glycolysis takes over the supply of energy, the running speed has to be reduced due to the maximal possible energy flow rate. It is therefore advantageous if, for example, a 400 m runner starts mobilizing glycolysis energy as late as possible; this is possible with high phosphate reserves, recognizable by the lactate increase. In laboratory tests, the best 400 runners have the most delayed rises in lactate levels. The expected performance in competition can be extrapolated from the lactate level and the running time, provided that the blood lactate level increases by about 20 mmol/l in comparison to the pre-exercise level.

Performance improvements in sports like sprinting cannot be explained by adaptations in the anaerobic metabolism due to training. On the other hand, the forms of anaerobic training used in athletics lead to adaptations in the muscle fibres. Primarily, this is because of an increase in energy-rich phosphate and intramuscular glycogen, allied to an increased activity of some enzymes.

References

Bouchard, M. & Thibault, Chr. (1986) Übung und Training in Kindheit und Jugend. In W. Hollmann (ed) *Zentrale Themen der Sportmedizin.* Springer-Verlag, Berlin.

Hollmann, W. & Hettinger, Th. (1980) *Sportmedizin—Arbeits- und Trainingsgrundlagen.* Schattauer-Verlag, Stuttgart.

Further reading

Åstrand, P.O. & Rodahl, K. (1986) *Textbook of Work Physiology*. McGraw-Verlag, New York.

Berg, A. & Keul, J. (1981) Muscular enzyme activities in relation to maximum aerobic capacity in healthy male adults. *Aust. J. Sports Med.* **13**, 87.

Cerretelli, P., Bennie, D. W. & Pendergast, D. P. (1980) Kinetics of metabolic transience during exercise. *Int. J. Sports Med.* **1**, 171.

Danforth, W. H. (1965) Glycogen synthetase activity in skeletal muscle. *J. Biol. Chem.* **240**, 588.

Davies, R. E. (1965) On the mechanism of muscular contraction. *Biochem. J.* **1**, 29.

Di Prampero, P. E. (1981) Energetics of muscular exercise. *Rev. Physiol. Biochem. Pharmacol.* **89**, 143.

Gollnick, P. D., Armstrong, R. B., Saltin, B., Sauber, C. W., Sembrowich, W. L. & Shephard, R. (1973) Effect of training on enzyme activity and fiber composition of human skeletal muscle. *J. Appl. Physiol.* **34**, 107.

Hill, A. V. (1925) *Muscular Activity*. Williams & Wilkins, Baltimore.

Hollmann, W. (1961) Zur Frage der Dauerleistungsfähigkeit. *Fortschr. Med.* **79**, 439.

Howald, H. (1982) Training enduced morphological and functional changes in skeletal muscle. *Int. J. Sports Med.* **3**, 1.

Hultman, E. (1967) Muscle glycogen in man determined in needle biopsy specimens. Massed and normal values. *Scand. J. Clin. Lab. Invest.* **19**, 209.

Karlsson, J. & Saltin, B. (1970) Lactate, ATP, and CP in working muscles during exhaustive exercise in man. *J. Appl. Physiol.* **29(5)**, 598.

Keul, J., Doll, E. & Keppler, D. (1969) *Muskelstoffwechsel*. Barth-Verlag, Munich.

Kindermann, W. & Keul, J. (1977) *Anaerobe Energiebereitstellung im Hochleistungssport*. Hofmann-Verlag, Schorndorf.

Knuttgen, H. & Saltin, B. (1972) Muscle metabolites and oxygen uptake in short-term submaximal exercise in man. *J. Appl. Physiol.* **32**, 690.

Komi, P. V., Rusko, H. & Vihko, V. (1977) Anaerobic performance capacity in athletes. *Acta Physiol. Scand.* **100**, 107.

Liesen, H. & Hollmann, W. (1981) *Ausdauersport und Stoffwechsel*. Hofmann-Verlag, Schorndorf.

McGilvery, R. W. (1975) Substratutilisation bei muskulärer Tätigkeit. *Med. Sport* **15**, 65.

Mader, A., Heck, H. & Hollmann, W. (1976) Evaluation of lactic acid and anaerobic energy contribution by determination of post-exercise lactic acid concentration in ear-capillary blood in middle distance runners and swimmers. In *The International Congress of Physical Activity Sciences 1976, Quebec, Canada. Vol. 4. Exercise Physiology 1978*. Miami, Florida.

Mader, A., Liesen, H., Heck, H., Philippi, H., Rost, R., Schürch, P. & Hollmann, W. (1976) Zur Beurteilung der sportartspezifischen Ausdauerleistungsfähigkeit in Laber. *Sportarzt Sportmed.* **4–5**, 80, 108.

Margaria, R., Aghemo, P. & Rovelli, E. (1966) Measurement of muscular power (anaerobic) in man. *J. Appl. Physiol.* **21**, 1662.

Saltin, B. (1973) Metabolic fundamentals in exercise. *Med. Sci. Sports* **5**, 137.

2.5 The central nervous system

R. S. HUTTON

Introduction

In this brief review, the acute and chronic effects of exercise and/or repetitive activity on the central nervous system (CNS) will be discussed. Anatomically, the CNS includes the cerebrum, mid-brain, cerebellum, brain stem and the spinal cord; however, adaptations in the regulation of motor units (the 'final common pathway' as defined by Sherrington) by the indirect route, the γ-loop, should also be considered as part of the central nervous process in the control of movement.

Less is known about the adaptive processes in CNS structures in relation to acute exercise or long-term training than in other organ systems. This is in part due to the limited amount of experimental work in this area, and may also partly relate to the typical textbook rendition of the CNS as a steady-state system which is spared from the metabolic effects of exercise. Such changes in metabolic demands are typically viewed to be necessary to generate an adaptive response. It is only in recent years that exercise-induced alterations in neural substrate have been under consistent experimental investigation. The available literature on this subject is, therefore, limited and particularly patchy with respect to supraspinal neural structures.

Acute CNS adaptations to exercise

Spinal segmental responses to increased use are summarized in Fig. 2.5.1 which identifies the neural circuitry relevant to the following discussion (Hutton, 1984, 1985).

It has long been known that brief periods of high-frequency conditioning activation of α-motoneurons produce a heightened monosynaptic response to a test stimulus lasting several minutes. This is known as post-tetanic potentiation (PTP) of monosynaptic reflexes or of Hoffmann, tendon tap or stretch reflex responses (Fig. 2.5.1A). Its mechanism may involve temporarily enhanced neurotransmitter release at group Ia synaptic terminals and/or a brief decrease in 'branch point failure' (lack of

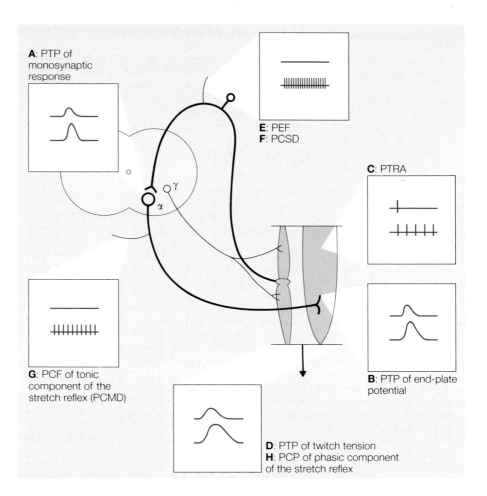

Fig. 2.5.1 Summary of acute adaptive responses of spinal segmental neural circuitry to brief periods of moderate to high levels of activation. α = α-motoneuron innervating a representative extrafusal skeletal muscle fibre. Together, the neural (α) and innervated muscle unit represent a motor unit. γ = γ-motoneuron innervating a representative muscle spindle intrafusal muscle fibre (muscle spindle capsule not shown). The γ-motoneuron and muscle spindle represent the γ-loop or indirect route for activating motor units through the Ia or group II afferent pathways. The arrow denotes muscle stretch. A–H: Neural or muscle electro-chemical or muscle force responses before (top traces) and after (bottom traces) a brief period of higher frequency levels of α–γ motoneuron activation. See text for explanation. Adapted from Hutton (1984) by Dr Shuji Suzuki and reproduced courtesy of Dr Suzuki from *Japn J. Phy. Fitness Sports Med.* (1983) **32**, 178, © The Japanese Society of Physical Fitness and Sports Medicine.

conduction down one or more branches of a terminal axon) of action potential propagation to terminal endings (Luschuer *et al.*, 1979). This phenomenon has been identified in humans (Hagbarth, 1962) but has not been conclusively demonstrated under conditions of natural drive of motor neuronal pools. PTP of the end-plate potential (Fig. 2.5.1B), caused by enhanced random release of neurotransmitter at the motor end-plate, and post-tetanic repetitive activity (PTRA) (Fig. 2.5.1C), a frequency-induced repetitive firing of muscle action potentials in response to a single neural stimulus, are other examples of enhanced input–output responses in spinal segmental circuitry in animals.

While these phenomena have not been conclusively isolated in humans, PTRA is certainly one possible mechanism to explain recent findings of enhanced irritability of EMG activity in the triceps surae of track athletes and sedentary controls following a maximum oxygen uptake treadmill test (Hutton & Doolittle, 1987).

A most dramatic effect of previous activation of motor units is seen in the PTP of twitch tension (Fig. 2.5.1D). As the name implies, brief periods of an interpolated higher activation frequency produce a greater force from motor units when stimulated at subsequent lower frequency levels of activation. Recent observations in both animals and humans (Burke *et al.*, 1976; Vandervoort *et al.*, 1983) suggest that PTP of sub-maximal muscle tension (maximum tension remains unchanged) might better be identified as 'post-activation potentiation'. This is because it has been shown to occur following a voluntary maximum contraction as well as a conditioning electrical stimulus, falling well within the physiological frequency range of activation of motor units. Intracellular properties in skeletal muscle fibres provide the potentiating mechanism (they are possibly involved in altering calcium concentration), and this may be interacting with PTRA which has been associated with adaptive responses at the terminal axon. The overall effect of this response is to optimize the tension-time integral of motor unit force production in response to lower levels of excitatory frequencies, that is more output in muscle force for less input of activation frequency (Burke *et al.*, 1976; Hutton, 1984).

Interestingly, the γ-loop or indirect route for activating motor units responds in kind to brief periods of higher frequencies of excitation. A higher level of γ-motoneuron activation is followed by an after-discharge to a test stimulus, thereby producing repetitive contractions of intrafusal muscle fibres and repetitive discharges of muscle spindle afferents. This response was originally called post-excitatory facilitation (PEF) (Fig. 2.5.1E). It results in a higher frequency of excitatory input to α-motoneurons over muscle spindle group Ia and/or II pathways. Collectively, the PEF multiunit afferent response has been termed the post-contraction sensory discharge (PCSD) (Fig. 2.5.1F). PCSD increases the excitatory drive to motoneurons, at static muscle lengths, through the tonic stretch reflex pathway (post-contraction facilitation, PCF of the tonic stretch reflex, as shown in Fig. 2.5.1G). The result of this after-effect of spindle discharge is a reflex-induced post-contraction moto-neuronal discharge (PCMD). The dynamic component of the stretch

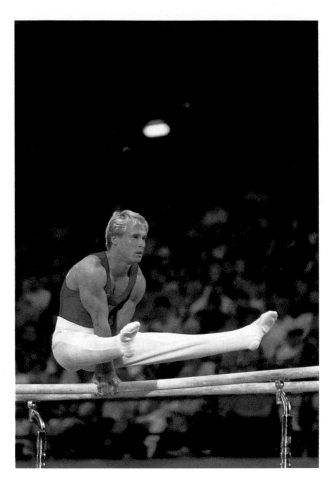

Fig. 2.5.2 The development of a successful performance of a highly complex gymnastic routine depends on central nervous system adaptation. © The Los Angeles Times 1984 (National Photo Pool), photo by Tony Barnard. Courtesy of the IOC archives.

reflex is enhanced when muscle stretch is applied after a previous higher intensity contraction. This increases muscle force during the initial change in muscle length.

Hence, all acute potentiated responses illustrated in Fig. 2.5.1 act in series on skeletal muscle fibres and serve to optimize input–output coupling at the spinal segmental level, leading to a greater submaximal force integral to lower driving frequencies to the α-motoneuronal pool. This might result in a perceived 'easing' of effort, a sensation that often accompanies the early stage of a submaximal continuous exercise regimen. One suspects that such adaptations are often confused with the presumed beneficial effects of warm-up, a thermal-dependent phenomenon.

The effect of the above observations is that a prior-maximum or near-maximum contraction of a muscle, which is about to be stretched, may predispose the muscle toward a higher level of activation and potential initial resistance to lengthening. This is a condition generally thought to result in the tearing of muscle tissue during stretch. In spite of this, many physical therapists and athlete trainers still argue, based on the proprioceptive neuromuscular facilitation (PNF) literature, that a maximum static contraction prior to stretch promotes relaxation in the same muscle. This has been shown not to be true (Moore & Hutton, 1980; Condon & Hutton, 1987). Instead, it would appear that levels of EMG activity prior to stretch correlate poorly with the actual increase in range of motion (ROM) achieved.

The design of experiments on stretching techniques must be carefully considered to avoid erroneous results. For instance, in many studies the magnitude of the stretching torque is not controlled across the stretching techniques being compared. Therefore the technique producing the greatest stretching torque, rather than the procedure promoting the lowest EMG activity, will yield the greatest ROM benefits. When the stretching torque is more closely controlled, acute adaptive changes in ROM produced by passive static stretch procedures are statistically comparable to the ROM achieved when compared to PNF procedures (Moore & Hutton, 1980; Condon & Hutton, 1987). Furthermore, when a stretching torque is aided by a voluntary contraction of the antagonist (a PNF procedure), co-contraction is consistently observed—as seen by increased EMG activity in the agonist. This occurs in spite of the observation of a decrease in the H-reflex, an electrically induced monosynaptic and oligosynaptic reflex, in the agonist. The latter is presumed to be due to α-γ co-activation in the antagonist with 'linked reciprocal inhibition' to the muscle about to be stretched (Etnyre & Abraham, 1986; Condon & Hutton, 1987). Presumed reciprocal inhibition, when unmasked by an electrical stimulus probe, is apparently obscured by other excitatory factors, e.g. a voluntary protective reaction by an athlete or patient in response to a large stretching torque induced by another person.

As is commonly known, muscle fatigue is induced through continuous exertion. An accurate definition of muscle fatigue is a decreased capacity to perform a maximum voluntary contraction regardless of the target force under investigation; for instance, fatigue effects caused by a repetitive 50% maximum voluntary contraction will not be seen until muscle tension declines below that level. In most of the research literature, declines in maximum muscle tension have been attributed to mechanisms intrinsic to the muscle cell. During fatigue, the well-known sigmoid increment in skeletal muscle tension to progressively higher frequencies of stimulation, producing a steep rise in tension within a relatively narrow-band-width of frequencies, is shifted to the left. Higher muscle tension is thereby produced by lower stimulation frequencies. This shift parallels mechanisms that progressively slow the contractile response of skeletal muscle to progressively higher stimulation frequencies. One might speculate, however, that some of the mechanisms discussed in Fig. 2.5.1 may assist in compensatory responses of the motor unit to fatigue. For example, it has recently been shown that the gain of the stretch reflex is enhanced both during, and following, a fatiguing muscle contraction (Nelson & Hutton, 1985; Windhorst *et al.*, 1986).

Less is known about supraspinal neural alterations during and after acute periods of exercise. Movement-related brain electroencephalographic (EEG) potentials (the readiness potential) have recently been shown to increase in size in parallel with an increase in force during rhythmical hand contractions (Freude & Ullsperger, 1987). With fatiguing contractions, readiness potentials were additionally increased in amplitude, suggesting a possible increase in CNS activation to spinal segmental levels. Clearly, short-term supraspinal CNS alterations to exercise remain a fertile area for future study.

Chronic CNS adaptations to exercise

Most of the research on neuromuscular adaptations to exercise has been focussed on skeletal muscle (see Chapter 2.1.1 and Part 5) with the underlying assumption that the functional properties of muscle fibres are largely determined by their neural innervation. This assumption is based on the following evidence (Hutton, 1983; Edstrom & Grimby, 1986):

1 The functional properties of muscle fibers are well matched to the physiological characteristics of their motor neuron, thus a motor unit is viewed to possess homogeneous neuromuscular properties.

2 Ensembles of motor units are determined ontogenetically and are divisible into faster and slower contracting populations with an attendant trimodal spectrum of tension-producing and fatigue-resistant capacities.

3 Muscle fibers belonging to a motor unit ensemble are mutable and convert when subjected to denervation and neural reinnervation by foreign motor neurons, e.g., as accomplished by cross-innervating a fast-contracting population of muscle fibers with motor neurons previously serving slow-contracting fibers, or vice versa.

4 Muscle fibers subjected to sufficient levels of use–disuse manifest significant changes in their structural, physiological, and histochemical properties, and such changes can be selective to subpopulations of

motor units. Thus it is possible for certain movement demands to rise above or fall below the activity thresholds for some motor unit ensembles but not for others.

(Hutton, 1983, p. 38)

In spite of these compelling indirect arguments, direct evidence of adaptive responses of motoneurons to chronic exercise is limited. While changes in axonal conduction velocity (Dirks & Hutton, 1984), some oxidative enzymes (Gerchman et al., 1975), cell size (Gilliam et al., 1977), and motor end-plate cholinesterase activity (Crockett et al., 1976) have been reported, the literature is fraught with controversy. For example, in a recent study of chronically stimulated motoneurons over 8 weeks (repetitive electrical 10, 20 and 40 Hz pulses, 50% of total time/day), no significant differences were found in cell size or histochemical staining of the oxidative enzyme succinic dehydrogenase, between the stimulated limb and the contralateral control limb in cats (Donselaar et al., 1986). However, the imposed activity was antidromic (opposite in direction to normal activation), and these findings may simply reflect the importance of increased synaptic activity in producing the chronic adaptations previously reported. The general trend in research has been for heavy resistance training to favour faster motoneuron conduction velocities (suggesting an increase in axonal cross-sectional diameter and cell size) and no change in oxidative enzymes or end-plate activity, while endurance training lowers conduction velocity, increases oxidative enzyme activity and enhances end-plate cholinesterase activity in fast twitch muscle fibres. These adaptations appear specific to motor unit types and cannot be generalized across motor unit populations.

A consistent finding in the literature on humans is the potentiating effect of strength training on electrically-induced EMG reflexes while subjects maintain a voluntary contraction (Milner-Brown et al., 1975; Sale et al., 1983). These reflex responses are labelled V_1 or M_1 (a short latency reflex of about 23–37 ms and comparable to the Hoffmann reflex under relaxed conditions), V_2 (an intermediate latency reflex of about 47–65 ms) and V_3 (a long latency reflex of 74–90 ms). Both the V_2 or M_2 and V_3 or M_3 reflex responses have latency periods long enough to be mediated through supraspinal structures, and capable of involving the motor cortex for the V_2 response (the transcortical reflex) and the cerebellum and motor cortex for the V_3 response. Although damage to these structures or the spinal cord above the spinal segment under investigation appears not to abolish these responses, supraspinal adaptations may nevertheless exist in parallel with spinal segmental contributions.

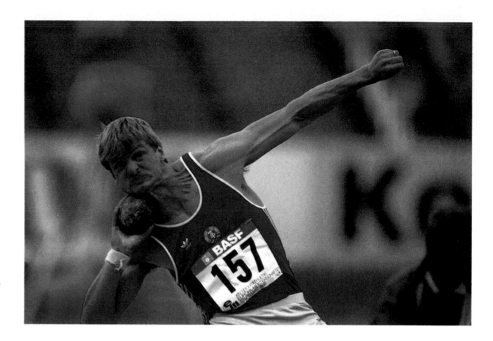

Fig. 2.5.3 In addition to muscle hypertrophy, strength training for such events as the shotput may potentiate EMG reflexes which will further increase the rate of force development. Photo by Leo Mason.

Strength training leads to a potentiated V_1 and V_2 reflex and possibly increases the V_3 response as well, although the observance of the latter reflex is more variable across untrained or trained subjects. Sale *et al.* (1983) have argued that strength training may increase a person's ability to voluntarily raise the excitability of motoneurons. Milner-Brown *et al.* (1975) suggest that, for V_2 or V_3 responses, supraspinal connections from motor cortex to spinal motoneurons may be enhanced to produce a significant increase in synchronization of motor unit recruitment (normal motoneuron recruitment is asynchronous). These explanations are not mutually exclusive but, in either case, these adaptive responses favour a faster mobilization of muscle force, as would be demanded by an activity such as weight training. It is interesting to note that these trained reflex responses are reversed with detraining and, in the case of the V_1 and V_2 reflexes, both show depressed amplitudes below control levels after 5 weeks of immobilization (Sale *et al.*, 1982). The above effects of exercise on proprioceptive mediated responses are summarized in Table 2.5.1.

The responsiveness of the monosynaptic component of the spinal stretch reflex to training has been well-demonstrated in limb muscles of monkeys (Wolpaw, 1985). Monkeys can be trained through operant conditioning to slowly change the amplitude of their spinal stretch reflex under conditions where the stimulus (stretch or electrical), initial muscle length, and motoneuronal tone are controlled. This change in the stretch reflex amplitude occurs over weeks and months and is relatively specific

Table 2.5.1 Effects of exercise on proprioceptive-mediated responses.

| | Acute | | | | Chronic | | | |
| | Isometric | | Isotonic | | Isometric | | Isotonic | |
Reflex	A	H	A	H	A	H	A	H
Hoffmann or V_1 (M_1) response	–	–	?(–)	?(–)	?(+)	?(+)	+	+
Tendon tap response	+	+	?(+)	?(+)	?(+)	?(+)	?	?
Stretch reflex response	+	?(+)	?(+)	?(+)	?(+)	?(+)	?	?
Long latency response								
V_2 (M_2)	?	?	?	?	?(+)	+	?(+)	+
V_3 (M_3)	?	?	?	?	?(+)	+	?(+)	+

A, animal observation; H, human observation; –, inhibition; +, excitation; ?, no evidence (speculated response).

to the agonist muscle trained. The direction of change in amplitude depends on the reward contingency, i.e. whether an increase or decrease in amplitude is rewarded. Furthermore, the adapted response persists for days following spinal transection above the trained cord segments, suggesting that adapted memory substrate exists in the spinal cord. These studies reflect the need for prolonged, repetitive training before certain alterations in neural circuitry may become manifested.

The tonic vibration reflex (TVR) is known to involve a significant polysynaptic component. A TVR is induced by a high-frequency vibration applied to the muscle tendon. Recently, endurance-trained athletes have been shown to have depressed TVR amplitudes and a lowered rate of change in amplitude following maximum aerobic capacity tests (Hutton & Doolittle, 1987). Similar results were not found in untrained subjects involved in normal levels of daily activity. This finding may reflect a conditioned interaction of supraspinal input on spinal segmental circuits.

Brain plasticity in response to exposure to increased environmental complexities has been the subject of considerable research. Typical dependent variables are brain weight or weight of brain subcomponents, dendritic branching and synaptic density. Enriching the environment in which animals are reared has been shown to quantitatively increase these variables, suggesting a cause and effect relationship in influencing neuronal development. Few investigators, however, have tried to dissociate the effects of an enriched environment on animal-brain morphology from effects that may be attributed to alterations in motor behaviour induced by the same environment. In this respect, mice subjected to physical activity (e.g. running, climbing, swimming) during late postnatal development show significantly higher brain weight than inactive controls (Pysh & Weiss, 1979). Histological examination of the cerebellum revealed significantly greater dendritic fields, branch length, synaptic density of dendritic spines, and total number of spines per unit length per cell. Others have concluded that acquisition of motor skills is a component of environmental complexity treatment, but that it is not the single cause for the observed changes in brain weight (Ferchmin & Eterovic, 1977).

A promising new approach to the study of central neural adaptations to exercise is to examine neurochemical alterations. For example, it has been reported that 12 weeks of endurance treadmill conditioning significantly increases D_2 dopamine receptor binding in the striatum of rats (Gilliam et al., 1984). Furthermore, endurance training may decelerate the effects of age on the deterioration in nigrostriatal dopamine neurons and striatal D_2 dopamine receptors.

As future studies on the CNS become available, the role of exercise in neural development and ageing will probably play a more central role in the study of exercise physiology. These findings should contribute greatly to our growing knowledge of the health benefits to be derived from an active life-style.

References

Burke, R. E., Rudomin, P. & Zajac III, F. E. (1976) The effect of activation history on tension production by individual muscle units. *Brain Res.* **109**, 515.

Condon, S. M. & Hutton, R. S. (1984) Soleus muscle electromyographic activity and ankle dorsiflexion range of motion during four stretching procedures. *Phys. Therapy* **67**, 24.

Crockett, J. L., Edgerton, V. R., Max, S. R. & Barnard, R. J. (1976) The neuromuscular junction response to endurance training. *Exp. Neurol.* **51**, 207.

Dirks, S. J. & Hutton, R. S. (1984) Endurance training and short latency reflexes in man. *Scand. J. Sports Sci.* **6**, 21.

Edstrom, L. & Grimby, L. (1986) Effect of exercise on the motor unit. *Muscle Nerve* **9**, 104.

Etnyre, B. R. & Abraham, L. D. (1986) H-reflex changes during static stretching and two variations of proprioceptive neuromuscular facilitation techniques. *Electroencephalogr. Clin. Neurophysiol.* **63**, 174.

Donselaar, Y., Kernell, D. & Eerbeek, O. (1986) Soma size and oxidative enzyme activity in normal and chronically stimulated motoneurones of the cat's spinal cord. *Brain Res.* **385**, 22.

Ferchmin, P. A. & Eterovic, V. A. (1977) Brain plasticity and environmental complexity: role of motor skills. *Physiol. Behav.* **18**, 455.

Freude, G. & Ullsperger, P. (1987) Changes in bereitschaftspotential during fatiguing and non-fatiguing hand movements. *Eur. J. Appl. Physiol.* **56**, 105.

Gerchman, L. B., Edgerton, V. R. & Carrow, R. E. (1975) Effects of physical training on the histochemistry and morphology of ventral motor neurones. *Exp. Neurol.* **49**, 790.

Gilliam, P. E., Spirduso, W. W., Martin, T. P., Walters, T. J., Wilcox, R. E. & Farrar, R. P. (1984) The effects of exercise training on 3H-spiperone binding in rat striatum. *Pharmacol. Biochem. Behav.* **20**, 863.

Gilliam, T. B., Roy, R. R., Taylor, J. F., Heusner,

W. W. & Van Huss, W. D. (1977) Ventral motor neuron alterations in rat spinal cord after chronic exercise. *Experientia* **15**, 665.

Hagbarth, K.-E. (1962) Post-tetanic potentiation of myotatic reflexes in man. *J. Neurol. Neurosurg. Psych.* **25**, 1.

Hutton, R. S. (1983) Central and peripheral neural adaptations with use–disuse. In B. B. Wolman (ed) *International Encyclopedia of Psychiatry, Psychology, Psychoanalysis and Neurology.* Aesculapius Publishers, New York.

Hutton, R. S. (1984) Acute plasticity in spinal segmental pathways with use: implications for training. In M. Kumamoto (ed) *Neural and Mechanical Control of Movement.* Yamaguchi Shoten, Kyoto, Japan.

Hutton, R. S. (1985) Neuromuscular physiology. In R. P. Welsh & R. J. Shephard (eds) *Current Therapy in Sports Medicine 1985–1986.* B. C. Decker, Philadelphia.

Hutton, R. S. & Doolittle, T. L. (1987) Resting electromyographic triceps surae activity and tonic vibration reflexes in subjects with high and average–low maximum oxygen uptake capacities. *Res. Quart. Exerc. Sport* **58**, 280.

Lüschur, H-R., Ruenzel, P. & Henneman, E. (1979) How the size of motoneurones determines their susceptibility to discharge. *Nature* **282**, 859.

Milner-Brown, H. S., Stein, R. B. & Lee, R. G. (1975) Synchronization of human motor units: possible roles of exercise and supraspinal reflexes. *Electroencephalogr. Clin. Neurophysiol.* **38**, 245.

Moore, M. A. & Hutton, R. S. (1980) Electromyographic investigation of muscle stretching techniques. *Med. Sci. Sports Exerc.* **12**, 322.

Nelson, D. L. & Hutton, R. S. (1985) Dynamic and static stretch responses in muscle spindle receptors in fatigued muscle. *Med. Sci. Sports Exerc.* **17**, 445.

Pysh, J. J. & Weiss, G. M. (1979) Exercise during development induces an increase in Purkinje cell dendritic tree size. *Science* **206**, 230.

Sale, D. G., McComas, A. J., MacDougall, J. D. & Upton, A. R. M. (1982) Neuromuscular adaptation in human thenar muscles following strength training and immobilization. *J. Appl. Physiol.* **53**, 419.

Sale, D. G., MacDougall, J. D., Upton, A. R. M. & McComas, A. J. (1983) Effect of strength training upon motoneuron excitability in man. *Med. Sci. Sports Exerc.* **15**, 57.

Vandervoort, A. A., Quinlan, J. & McComas, A. J. (1983) Twitch potentiation after voluntary contraction. *Exp. Neurol.* **81**, 141.

Windhorst, U., Christakos, C. N., Koehler, W., Hamm, T. M., Enoka, R. M. & Stuart, D. G. (1986) Amplitude reduction of motor unit twitches during repetitive activation is accompanied by relative increase of hyperpolarizing membrane potential trajectories in homonymous α-motoneurons. *Brain Res.* **398**, 181.

Wolpaw, J. R. (1985) Adaptive plasticity in the spinal stretch reflex: an accessible substrate of memory? *Cell. Mol. Neurobiol.* **5**, 147.

2.6 The endocrine system

H. WEICKER

Sympathoadrenergic regulation

The sympathoadrenergic system is involved in the regulation of many cardiocirculatory and metabolic functions during physical exercise, especially at the onset of exercise, but also during the adaptation to variant intensities and duration. The peripheral stimulation is executed by the catecholamines norepinephrine (NE), epinephrine (EPI) and, to a minor degree, by dopamine (DA), acting in close cooperation with their specific adrenoceptors. The great adaptability of the sympathetic system is a result of the catecholamines, which do not just act as hormones secreted from the adrenal medulla, but also as neurotransmitters released from sympathetic nerve endings or synapses close to their receptors. Dopamine, and to a lesser extent NE, are neurotransmitters eliciting the cerebral sympathetic regulation. The effect of the adrenoceptors on target cells originates both in the cardiocirculatory system where β-receptors are present on the heart muscle, and in the α- and β-receptors on the resistance and capitance vessels.

In the heart the increase of catecholamines improves the contractility; this is achieved through an increased Ca^{++} release from the sarcoplasmatic reticulum, and also by the adjustment of the heart rates, the coronary circulation, and the increase of the stroke volume according to the physiological need. The adrenoceptors of the arterial vessels regulate the blood distribution, the arterial resistance and the vessel tone of the veins. The catecholamines trigger metabolic functions by receptor stimulation and postreceptor reactions in which the adenylyl cyclase and cAMP system are strongly involved.

The significance of the sympathoadrenergic regulation is essential for glycogenolysis and gluconeogenesis in the liver, muscular glycolysis, and lipolysis in fat cells, as well as in the intramuscular triglyceride depots. It adjusts the airflow of the respiratory tract in the bronchioles by dilatation of the smooth muscles via β-receptors. Thus it improves gas exchange in the alveoles, important for optimal ventilation. Due to the conjugation of catecholamines by sulphate or methyl groups, the efficiency of liberated free catecholamines can be reduced, thus preventing adrenergic overstimulation since the conjugates have no receptor affinity. However, free catecholamines can also be liberated from the sulpho-conjugates, which increases the sympathoadrenergic potency without making new secretion necessary. Catecholamine metabolites, particularly vanillinic acid, are secreted through the kidney together with sulpho-conjugates which cannot be metabolized, in contrast to the methyl conjugates. Furthermore, catecholamines can be re-uptaken at the pre-synaptic membrane, sympathetic synapses and nerve endings, causing a feedback regulation of neurotransmitter secretion.

The secretion rate of neurotransmitters as well as that of hormones depends more on the intensity of exercise than on its duration. It can also be increased by emotional strain followed by an EPI increment in the plasma. Metabolic demands increase the secretion from the adreno-medulla, which shows a training-dependent increase in function, eliciting an elevation of the EPI blood level.

There exists a close interaction between NE and the angiotensin–renin system which is important for the regulation of the blood distribution and the resistance in arteries and capitance vessels. This is found, for instance, during the hormonal counter regulation of the orthostatic reaction. The elevated NE secretion reduces the glomerular filtration rate (GFR) and sodium excretion through the kidney. It therefore provides a volume-regulating support for the ADH and aldosterone functions.

Recent results indicate a close relationship between neurotransmitter and hormonal systems and a tremendous number of neuro- and gastro-intestinal peptides. The peptides are able to modulate the primary function of the hormones and neurotransmitters, both in their receptor inter-action and the postreceptor mechanisms.

Sex and pituitary hormones

The function of the sex hormones, the gonadotropins, and their releasing factors are also important for exercise efficiency and mental adjustment. Testosterone, oestradiol, and, to a minor extent, progesterone have an anabolic effect which provides the protein synthesis in skeletal muscles—increasing the muscle mass and force. They enhance the morphological training effects and inhibit catabolic destruction. Physical and mental overstrain can disturb the central gonadotropin regulation and its trigger function on the gonadal hormones.

Many studies have been carried out to elucidate 'sports amenorrhoea' which had primarily been regarded as a harmless physiological variation

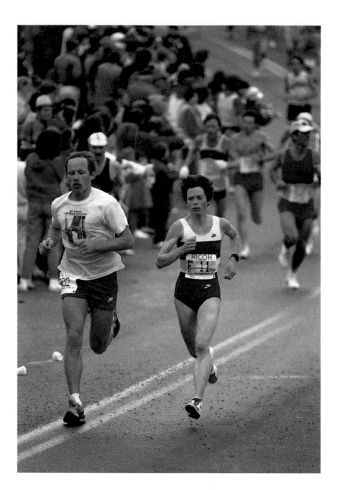

Fig. 2.6.1 Performance differences between male and female athletes are due in great part to sex hormone influences. Courtesy of *Runner's World Magazine*, photo by Christie C. Tito.

of the gonadal rhythm with a functional change in the menstrual cycle with no serious consequences. Investigations of pulsatile gonadotropin disturbance, however, have shown that strenuous exercise of long duration not only shortens the luteal phase but also the physiological secretion of oestradiol and, therefore, impairs the anabolic balance especially in the bones. This dysfunction could be a reason for spontaneous stress fractures in the extremities, and could also be a factor causing a deterioration of the course of an inovulation osteoporosis years after finishing sports participation. Whether emotional strain can facilitate the onset of anorexia nervosa and sports amenorrhoea is still a matter of unresolved discussion. High levels of training, strenuous competition, emotional strain and the beginning of a top athletic career before menarche are all able to disturb the gonadotropin rhythm and the pulsatile regulation.

Among the pituitary hormones, adrenocorticotropin (ACTH) plays a prominent role in the stimulation of supra-adrenal hormones. During exercise a load-dependent increase occurs and leads to the secretion of cortisol, enhancing the catabolic reaction of metabolism. In contrast to ACTH which peaks twice in double loads, cortisol shows a considerably lower response in the second load due to its longer half-life time. ACTH also partially stimulates the catecholamine release from the adreno-medulla and has, to a certain extent, lipolytic effects on the fat cells. Prolactine secretion also follows physical exertion. Vasopressin (ADH) liberation is not only triggered by volume and osmoreceptors, but also by a reduction in hypothalamic and hypophysial blood flow. Atrial natriuretic factor (ANF) secretion from myoendocrine cells of the right atrium inhibits the ADH liberation. On the other hand, ADH enhances the efficiency of corticotropin-releasing factor (CRF) followed by an ACTH increase. The growth hormone (STH) supports the anabolic reaction enhancing the amino acid uptake in the cell and, therefore, supports the protein synthesis in the muscle.

Glucoregulatory hormones

Intensive training also has an effect on carbohydrate metabolism and causes a decrease in insulin production; insulin is the most important glucoregulatory hormone and the strongest inhibitor of gluconeogenesis and lipolysis. Insulin secretion is reduced by adrenergic impulses on the β-cells of the pancreatic islet tissues by epinephrine. The insulin receptor numbers increase after long endurance training, which facilitates the stimulation of the glucose transporter on muscle and fat cell membranes.

The catecholamines and glucagon are the main insulin antagonists in the hepatogen glycogen formation. They stimulate glycogenolysis, triggering the cAMP system and phosphorylase-A which increase the glucose output from the liver. These hormones are important for the maintenance of the glucose homeostasis needed for neural and cerebral functions. The interaction of the glucoregulatory hormones with soma-tostatin has been explored in recent investigations which have shown its significance for carbohydrate metabolism.

Thyroid hormones, water and electrolyte balance

The thyroid hormones, T_3 and T_4, as well as their releasing factors, are not only important for the basic energy demand of the organism but also for the adaptation to work. They are especially important during aerobic energy production since T_4 increases the flux rate through the respiratory chain according to the ATP requirement. The water balance and electrolyte concentration are regulated by various hormones. The renin–angiotensin–aldosterone system is important for the regulation of the resistance in the vascular bed with respect to tone and volume. They trigger the renal flow rate supported by NE. Aldosterone is responsible for the sodium reabsorption, which is mainly stimulated by angiotensin and mineral concentration, especially of potassium. ADH secretion is stimulated by volume and osmoreceptors and is responsible for the water reabsorption in the distal tubulus.

Conclusion

Experimental results obtained in animal research and investigations in humans have augmented our knowledge in this field during the last decades. This knowledge can, therefore, be used with confidence for practical training advice as well as in advice on physical and mental adjustment to the strain of competition.

Further reading

Adlercreutz, H., Härkönen, M., Kuoppasalmi, K., Näveri, H., Huhtaniemi, I., Tikkanen, H., Remes, K., Dessypris, A. & Karvonen, J. (1986) Effect of training on plasma anabolic and catabolic steroid hormones and their response during physical exercise. *Int. J. Sports Med.* (Suppl. 1), **7**, 27.

Alén, M. & Suominen, J. (1984) Effect of androgenic and anabolic steroids on spermatogenesis in power athletes. *Int. J. Sports Med.* (Suppl.) **5**, 189.

Bieger, W. P., Weiss, M. & Weicker, H. (1981) Insulin affinity and hormone-dependent activity of human circulating monocytes after exercise. In J. Poortmans & G. Niset (eds) *Biochemistry of Exercise IV-A.* University Park Press, Baltimore.

Bonen, A. (1984) Effect of exercise and training on reproductive hormones. *Int. J. Sports Med.* (Suppl.) **5**, 198.

Bonen, A., Ling, W. Y., Belcastro, A. N., Simpson, A. A., MacIntyre, K. P., Neil, R. E. & MacGrail, J. C. (1981) Effects of acute and chronic exercise on the circulating concentrations of progesterone, estradiol, FSH and LH. In J. Poortmans & G. Niset (eds) *Biochemistry of Exercise IV-B.* University Park Press, Baltimore.

Cousineau, D., Péronnet, F., Picard, D., Jacks, B., Ledoux, M., Nadeau, R. & de Champlain, J. (1981) Plasma catecholamine response to prolonged exercise after muscle glycogen depletion and overloading. In J. Poortmans & G. Niset (eds) *Biochemistry of Exercise IV-B.* University Park Press, Baltimore.

Dale, E., Alexander, C. R., Gerlach, D. H. & Martin, D. E. (1981) Hormone profiles of women long-distance runners. In J. Poortmans & G. Niset (eds) *Biochemistry of Exercise IV-B.* University Park Press, Baltimore.

Galbo, H. (1981) Catecholamines and muscular exercise; assessment of sympathoadrenal activity. In J. Poortmans & G. Niset (eds) *Biochemistry of Exercise IV-B.* University Park Press, Baltimore.

Galbo, H. (1983) *Hormonal and Metabolic Adaptation to Exercise.* Georg Thieme Verlag, Stuttgart, New York.

Keizer, H. A. (1986) Exercise- and training-induced menstrual cycle irregularities (AMI). *Int. J. Sports Med.* (Suppl. 1), **7**, 38.

Keizer, H. A. & Bonen, A. (1984) Exercise-induced changes in gonadotropin secretion patterns. *Int. J. Sports Med.* (Suppl.) **5**, 206.

Keizer, H. A. & Kuipers, H. (1987) Hormonal responses in women as a function of physical exercise and training. *Int. J. Sports Med.* (Suppl.), (in press).

Keizer, H. A., Poortmans, J. & Bunnik, G. S. J. (1981) Influence of physical exercise on sex hormone metabolism. In J. Poortmans & G. Niset (eds) *Biochemistry of Exercise IV-B.* University Park Press, Baltimore.

Kuoppasalmi, K., Näveri, H., Kosunen, K., Härkönen, M. & Adlercreutz, H. (1981) Plasma steroid levels in muscular exercise. In J. Poortmans & G. Niset (eds) *Biochemistry of Exercise IV-B.* University Park Press, Baltimore.

Luyckx, A. S., Pirnay, F., Krzentowski, G. & Lefebvre, P. J. (1981) Insulin and glucagon during prolonged muscular exercise in normal man. In J. Poortmans & G. Niset (eds) *Biochemistry of Exercise IV-A.* University Park Press, Baltimore.

Reybrouck, T., Amery, A., Lijnen, P., Fagard, R., Billiet, L., Moerman, E. & De Schaepdryver, A. (1981) Daytime changes of plasma catecholamines, renin, lactate and hemodynamic variables at rest and during exercise and the effect of previous graded submaximal exercise. In J. Poortmans & G. Niset (eds) *Biochemistry of Exercise IV-B.* University Park Press, Baltimore.

Weicker, H. (1986) Sympathoadrenergic regulation. *Int. J. Sports Med.* (Suppl. 1), **7**, 16.

Weicker, H., Barwich, D., Bauer, D. & Zachmann, L. (1984) Changes in sexual hormones with female top athletes. *Int. J. Sports Med.* (Suppl.) **5**, 200.

Weicker, H., Rettenmeier, A., Ritthaler, F., Frank, H., Bieger, W. P. & Klett, G. (1981) Influence of anabolic and catabolic hormones on substrate concentrations during various running distances. In J. Poortmans & G. Niset (eds) *Biochemistry of Exercise IV-A.* University Park Press, Baltimore.

Winder, W. W. & Premachandra, B. N. (1981) Thyroid hormones and muscular exercise. In J. Poortmans & G. Niset (eds) *Biochemistry of Exercise IV-B.* University Park Press, Baltimore.

Wurster, K. G., Zwirner, M., Keller, E., Schindler, A. E., Schrode, M. & Heitkamp, H. (1984) Discipline specific differences in the responses of pituitary, gonadal, and adrenal to maximal physical exercise in female top athletes. *Int. J. Sports Med.* (Suppl.) **5**, 203.

PART 3

ASSESSMENT OF PHYSICAL AND FUNCTIONAL CAPACITY

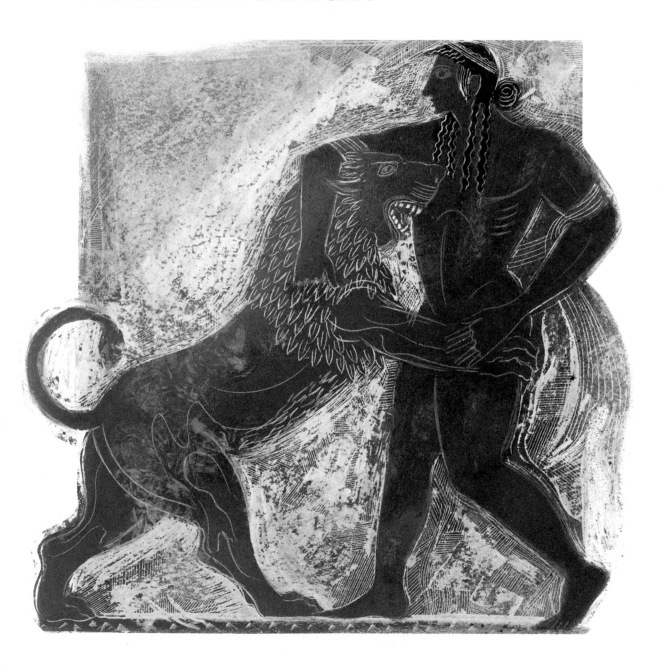

3.1 General physical capacity

I. DRĂGAN

Introduction

General physical capacity is the possibility of an active muscular system to deliver—by anaerobic glycolysis or oxidative phosphorylation—the necessary energy for the greatest possible mechanical work and to maintain it as long as possible. This capacity increases through sports training which improves the basic physical qualities: speed (acceleration), strength (force), resistance, endurance, skill, etc. Sports activities involve motor acts, muscular contractions which result from the transformation of chemical energy into mechanical energy, at the level of active muscles. The reserves of ATP (adenosine triphosphate) can convert the energy for 4–6 s, that is four to six muscular contractions. Energy resulting from the division of creatine phosphate (CP) at muscular level is used for the restoration of ATP; this can assure energy for about another 15 to 20 muscular contractions, or 15–20 s. If the exercise continues, the necessary energy is delivered by muscular glycogen (which helps the regeneration of high-energy phosphates) which can assure the continuation of exercise for about 45–60 s, despite a lack of oxygen. This results in an increase in lactic acid which induces a decrease in blood pH and therefore an inhibition of glycolysis. In the presence of oxygen the lactic acid is metabolized and used as an energy source at all levels of function. When there is sufficient oxygen, the recovery of the energetic substratum is closely correlated to the oxygen consumption, and the exercise can continue.

Depending on the oxygen needs and supply, physical exercises become predominantly aerobic or anaerobic. Aerobic efforts are of low, medium or submaximal intensity and occur under real or apparent equilibrium between oxygen need and supply. Aerobic exercise lasts from more than 3 min to many hours. Anaerobic efforts are of high intensity (maximal), of short duration (efforts up to 10–15 s duration without significant lactate accumulation and efforts up to 45–60 s involving large lactate build-up) and occur with an increasing lack of oxygen (the oxygen deficit is replenished after exercise). The mechanical efficiency of anaerobic exercise is much lower than that of aerobic exercise (16% compared to 23–25%).

Assessment of aerobic capacity

$\dot{V}_{O_2 \, max}$ is the most expressive parameter of aerobic capacity, and it can be estimated by two methods: (a) direct, using spiroergometric methods; and (b) indirect, using an Åstrand–Ryhming nomogram. The spiro-ergometric methods use gas analysers (open or closed circuit), and the exercise is performed on a cycle ergometer or on a treadmill. It is usual to start with a load of 75–100 W (1 W/kg) and to increase the power production every 3 min by 50 W until exhaustion; another methodology is to perform one submaximal exercise for 6 min in order to reach the steady state. The capillary lactate level is measured at the start, after each step of exercise and 10 min after the exercise has finished. For the indirect determination of $\dot{V}_{O_2 \, max}$, the basic principle used is the linear correlation between heart rate and $\dot{V}_{O_2 \, max}$ during a submaximal exercise lasting 6 min. This exercise is performed on a cycle ergometer or by a step test with the steps 40 or 50 cm high (see Fig. 3.1.2 and Table 3.1.1), the heart rate during the exercise is generally between 120–170 beats/min.

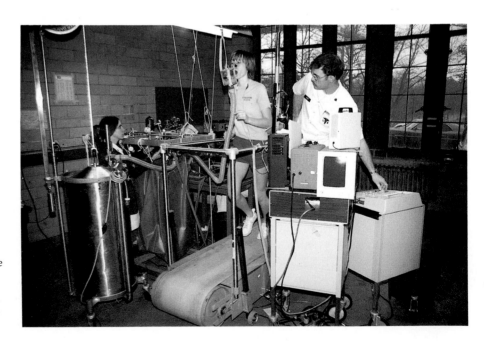

Fig. 3.1.1 Assessment of the maximal oxygen uptake of an athlete is frequently performed during grade running on a motor-driven treadmill. Courtesy of J. A. Vogel.

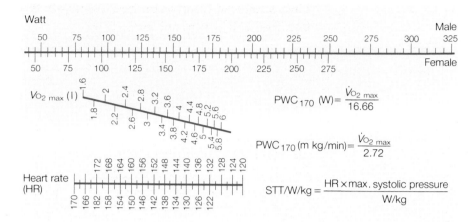

Fig. 3.1.2 Nomogram for the evaluation of $\dot{V}_{O_2}$ and PWC$_{170}$ by the indirect method (Åstrand–Ryhming).

The difference between direct and indirect determination seems to be $\pm 10\%$. For the interpretation of $\dot{V}_{O_2\ max}$ (direct method) we suggest the following scale:

Excellent (100%)—$110 - 0.4 \times$ bodyweight
Very good (95%)—$104.5 - 0.30 \times$ bodyweight
Good (84.2%)—$92.6 - 0.34 \times$ bodyweight
Medium (70%)—$77 - 0.20 \times$ bodyweight.

For the interpretation of $\dot{V}_{O_2\ max}$ (indirect method) see Table 3.1.1.

Table 3.1.1a Åstrand test: relationship between heart rate and $\dot{V}_{O_2\ max}$ (ml, STPD) in men and women.

	Heart rate	100 W	125 W	150 W	175 W	200 W	225 W	250 W
Men	120	3600	4050	4800	5500	6350	7100	—
	126	3200	3700	4400	5000	5800	6500	7200
	132	2900	3400	4000	4600	5300	6000	6600
	138	2700	3100	3700	4200	4900	5400	6100
	144	2500	2850	3400	3900	4500	5000	5700
	150	2300	2700	3100	3650	4200	4800	5300
	156	2200	2500	2900	3350	3800	4400	5000
	162	2000	2350	2800	3200	3600	4100	4600
	168	1900	2200	2600	3000	3400	3900	4400
Women	120	4100	4750	5450	—	—		
	126	3600	4200	4950	5600	—		
	132	3300	3800	4500	5100	5700		
	138	3000	3450	4100	4600	5100		
	144	2700	3200	3800	4200	4800		
	150	2500	2900	3500	3900	4400		
	156	2300	2700	3200	3600	4100		
	162	2200	2500	3000	3400	3800		
	168	2000	2350	2800	3200	3600		

Table 3.1.1b Standard values for the interpretation of $\dot{V}O_{2\ max}$ (ml/kg) in men (women = +20%).

Bodyweight (kg)	Low	Medium	Good	Very good	Excellent
50.1–55.0	<52	52–63	63–74	74–86	>86
55.1–60.0	<50	50–62	62–73	73–84	>84
60.1–65.0	<49	49–60	60–71	71–82	>82
65.1–70.0	<48	48–59	59–69	69–80	>80
70.1–75.0	<47	47–57	57–68	68–78	>78
75.1–80.0	<46	46–56	56–66	66–76	>76
80.1–85.0	<44	44–54	54–64	64–74	>74
85.1–90.0	<43	43–53	53–63	63–72	>72
90.1–95.0	<42	42–51	51–61	61–70	>70
95.1–100.0	<41	41–50	50–59	59–68	>68

The requirements for $\dot{V}O_{2\ max}$ in élite athletes are as follows:

Excellent—long-distance runners, rowing, cycling (road), 3 km and 1 km skating, long-distance skiing, kayak canoeing

Very good—runners (800 m to 1500 m and up to 5 km), swimmers (200 m to 1500 m), sports games, decathlon, skating (speed), cycling (velodrom), modern pentathlon, boxing, lawn tennis

Good—swimming (100 m), judo, wrestling, skating (500 m), fencing, bowling, table tennis

Medium—track and field (springs, sprint, throwings), Alpine skiing, riding, gymnastics, diving, weight lifting, shooting, bob-sleighing.

The cardiovascular reserves of performance can be appreciated by the heart volume/oxygen/heart rate max, the heart volume equivalent. The lower the equivalent the higher the cardiovascular reserves. The prediction of future cardiovascular reserves can be made by using the criteria in Table 3.1.2. Other tests, such as PWC_{130} (Ausdauergrenze–Hollmann) or PWC_{170} (Wahlund) can also be performed to assess aerobic capacity (Drăgan et al., 1982). Table 3.1.3 shows the PWC_{170} (m kg) extrapolated from the indirect method of determining $\dot{V}O_{2\ max}$ (Åstrand method).

Table 3.1.2 Criteria used to predict cardiovascular performance.

Heart volume (ml/kg)	Oxygen/HR_{max}	Heart volume equivalent	Prediction of aerobic capacity
Small (<11)	Small (14–20)	Medium (40–50)	Future potential
Medium (11–14)	Great (21–40)	Small (<40)	Very good
Large (14–17)	Great (21–40)	Great (50–60)	Very little
Very large (17)	Medium (15–27)	Great (60+)	Limited

Table 3.1.3 Indirect estimation of PWC_{170} from the $\dot{V}O_{2\,max}$.

Men		Women	
$\dot{V}O_{2\,max}$ (ml/min)	PWC_{170} (m kg)	$\dot{V}O_{2\,max}$ (ml/min)	PWC_{170} (m kg)
1600	520	1600	490
1700	575	1700	532
1800	612	1800	563
1900	643	1900	600
2000	673	2000	643
2100	722	2100	673
2200	765	2200	710
2300	814	2300	753
2400	857	2400	796
2500	900	2500	838
2600	936	2600	882
2700	967	2700	918
2800	998	2800	942
2900	1028	2900	978
3000	1071	3000	1016
3100	1108	3100	1065
3200	1144	3200	1095
3300	1181	3300	1132
3400	1224	3400	1181
3500	1255	3500	1224
3600	1285	3600	1261
3700	1322	3700	1297
3800	1359	3800	1328
3900	1408	3900	1365
4000	1438	4000	1389
4100	1482	4100	1438
4200	1530	4200	1499
4300	1548	4300	1530
4400	1573	4400	1561
4500	1616	4500	1610
4600	1652	4600	1652
4700	1687	4700	1683
4800	1714	4800	1714
4900	1744	4900	1744
5000	1775	5000	1775

Assessment of anaerobic capacity

The assessment of anaerobic capacity is still under discussion, compared to that of aerobic capacity, where the methods of assessment are now well established and validated by WHO. There are many methods available (neuromuscular, gas exchange, biochemical, ergometric, etc.), including those recommended by Dransfeld and Mellerowicz (1958), Margaria (1966), Georgescu (1969) and Hebbelinck (1969) (discussed in Drăgan *et al.*, 1982). However, the authors recommend the test discussed by Szögy in 1986 (Szögy & Böhmer, 1986). This is performed on

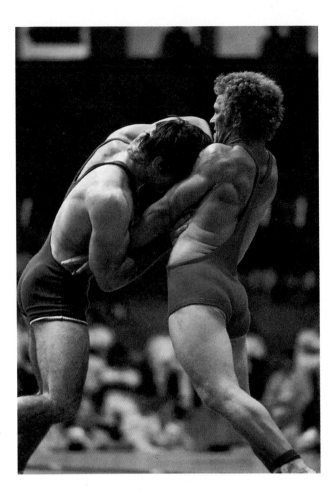

Fig. 3.1.3 The energy demands of championship wrestling require a high development of both aerobic and anaerobic capacities. Courtesy of the IOC archives.

a speed-dependent ergometer (Minjhard, Monark, Ergostat Fleisch, Siemens–Elema, etc.) and contains two separate tests as follows:

1 *First phase* (preponderant alactacid phase). This consists of the determination of the capillary lactate level on rest; and the recording of the maximal number of revolutions during 15 s on a cycle ergometer, at an exercise intensity of about 600 W for 100 r/min. The highest watt reached in 5 s is used as a parameter of anaerobic power. In the sixth minute after exercise the capillary lactate level is again determined in order to calculate the delta (Δ) lactate. The alactacid quotient (AQ) is calculated using the formula*

$$AQ = \frac{\text{TWP 15 s (kJ)}}{\Delta \text{ lactate (mmol/1) 15 s}}$$

where TWP is the total work performed in 15 s, and kJ is (work × time (s))/ 1000.

* The formulae given in this chapter for AQ, LQ and AI have been suggested by A. Rosetti, A. Lăzăvescu & I. Drăgan (Bucharest Sports Medicine Center, 1986) but are not published.

The higher the quotient the higher the alactacid energy reserves (ATP and CP). For the interpretation of $W_{max}/5$ s expressed in m kg, the following scale can be used:

Excellent (100%)—335 + 7.66 × bodyweight
Very good (95%)—319 + 7.27 × bodyweight
Good (84.2%)—283 + 6.44 × bodyweight
Medium (70%)—236 + 5.35 × bodyweight.

The demands for anaerobic power (5–10 s) are as follows:

Excellent—cycling (velodrom)
Very good—track and field (sprint, springs, throwings), rowing, kayak canoeing, weight lifting, sports games, skating (speed), lawn and table tennis
Good—runners (middle and long distance), biathlon, boxing, bob-sleighing, riding, gymnastics, decathlon, swimming (50 m), judo, wrestling, modern pentathlon, fencing, Alpine skiing, etc.
Medium—diving, shooting, etc.

2 *Second phase* (preponderant lactacid phase). This follows after a 1 h recovery period, and consists of the measurement of the capillary lactate level on rest; and, at the same exercise pattern as phase I, the subject must perform a maximal number of revolutions during 45 s using the same cycle ergometer. The total work performance during 45 s (TWP 45 s) is considered as the parameter of anaerobic endurance. The lactate level is again determined on the sixth minute after exercise. For the estimation of the lactacid quotient (LQ) the following formula is used

$$LQ = \frac{TWP\ 45\ s\ (kJ)}{\Delta\ lactate\ (mmol/l)\ 45\ s}.$$

The higher the quotient the higher the lactacid energy reserves, caused by a high alactacid or a high aerobic energy rate. We can also estimate TWP 45 s, expressed in m kg, multiplying the number of revolutions performed during 45 s by the kg load of each revolution. Again, there is a scale for interpreting the TWP 45 s:

Excellent (100%)—56.83 − 0.207 × bodyweight
Very good (95%)—53.99 − 0.196 × bodyweight
Good (84.2%)—47.85 − 0.174 × bodyweight
Medium (70%)—39.78 − 0.145 × bodyweight.

The demands for TWP 45 s are as follows:

Very good—biathlon, rowing, kayak canoeing, cycling, sports games, skating (short distances)

Table 3.1.4 Scale of performance reserves based on a number of parameters.

Type	Physical performance	Lactacid power	Aerobic power	Reserves
1	↑	↓	↑	↑ High
2	↓	↓	→	→ Potential
3	↑	↑	↘	↘ Exhausted?
4	↓	↑	↓	↓ Little

Good—track and field (except long-distance runners), bob-sleighing, boxing, weight lifting, judo, swimming (200 m to 1500 m), wrestling, modern pentathlon, skiing, tennis, etc.

Medium—long-distance runners, riding, gymnastics, fencing, bowling, diving, shooting.

The alactacid index (AI) is given by

$$AI = \frac{\% \text{ m kg 15 s}/\% \text{ m kg 45 s}}{\% \; \Delta \text{ lactate 15 s}/ \; \% \; \Delta \text{ lactate 45 s}} = 0.8.$$

The higher the index (>1) the greater the alactacid reserves.

The reserves of performance can be predicted by using a system which takes into account many parameters (physical performance, W or m/s, lactacid power, and aerobic power) (see Table 3.1.4).

References

Drăgan, I. *et al.* (1982) *Sports Medicine.* Sports-Tourism Ed., Bucharest.

Szögy, A. & Böhmer, D. (1986) *A two phase test for anaerobic capacity evaluation in laboratory and field.* XXIIIrd World Congress of FIMS, Brisbane.

Further reading

Åstrand, P. O. & Ryhming, I. (1954) A nomogram for calculation of aerobic capacity from pulse rate during submaximal work. *J. Appl. Physiol.* **7**, 32.

Conconi, F., Ferrari, M., Ziglio, P. G., Droghetti, P. & Codecă, L. (1982) Determination of anaerobic threshold by a non-invasive field test in runners. *J. Appl. Physiol. Respir. Environ. Exerc. Physiol.* **3**, 52.

3.2 Special performance capacity

G. NEUMANN

Basis of special performance

Endurance
Endurance is a decisive precondition for sports performances in many kinds of sports. Every endurance performance is based on complex mechanisms of regulation, significant ones being the energy processes and the control and regulation processes (information processes). Practically it seems to be useful to subdivide endurance into short term, medium term and long term. All cyclical endurance performances with a duration of between 35 s and 2 min belong to the short-term group; endurance performances from 2 to 10 min are grouped in the medium-term group; and all workloads lasting more than 10 min belong to the long-term endurance group. The latter has to be subdivided again into several time spans: long-term endurance group I comprises exercise performances with a duration between 10 and 35 min; group II between 35 and 90 min; group III between 90 and 360 min; and group IV more than 360 min (Table 3.2.1).

Table 3.2.1 The utilization of the functional systems of athletes during intensive endurance exercise of different duration (STE, short-term endurance; MTE, medium-term endurance; LTE I–IV, subdivisions of long-term endurance).

Functional system	Measured value	STE (35 s–2 min)	MTE (>2–10 min)	LTE I (>10–35 min)	LTE II (35–90 min)	LTE III (90–360 min)	LTE IV (>360 min)
Coronary circulation	Heart rate (beats/min)	185–200	190–210	180–190	175–190	150–180	120–170
Oxygen uptake	% $V_{O_2\,max}$	100	95–100	90–95	80–95	60–90	50–60
Energy exchange	% Portion: Aerobic	20	60	70	80	95	99
	Anaerobic	80	40	30	20	5	(1)
Energy consumption (1 kcal = 4.19 kJ)	kJ/min	250	190	120	105	80	75
	kJ total	380–460	460–1680	1680–3150	3150–9660	9660–27000	>27000
Breakdown of glycogen	% Glycogen in muscle	10	30	40	60	80	95
Lipolysis	Free fatty acid (mmol/l)	0.5	0.5	0.8	1.0	2.0	2.5
Glycolysis	Lactate (mmol/l)	18	20	14	8	4	2

In intensive short-term endurance exercises a high activation of the central nervous system can be observed (by electroencephalographic measurements). High portions of fast twitch fibres (FTF) are recruited into the motor programme. Energy is supplied anaerobically and comes from the local energy stores of the working muscles (ATP, CP, glycogen). The creatine phosphate level is important for the starting phase of exercise.

Medium-term endurance also requires a high activation of central nervous structures. Fast twitch and slow twitch fibres (STF) are recruited for the motor programme. Local energy stores are used, and in addition extramuscular stores, for instance the liver glycogen, must be provided for performance. In intensive workloads of 5–6 min duration high demands are put, simultaneously, on the anaerobic and the aerobic metabolisms. The cardiopulmonary system, especially the maximum oxygen uptake, is stressed to the highest possible level.

Long-term endurance is provided mainly by STF. The metabolism is regulated in a steady state. Since the energy stores in the muscles are not sufficient, liver glycogen and free fatty acids are also included in the energy supply. The longer the exercises last, the more important the aerobic capacity becomes. In exercise bouts lasting more than 1 h the aerobic glucose oxidation is increasingly substituted by free fatty acids. Endurance exercises lasting several hours are always a stress on the metabolism, and the increased cortisol secretion results in glycogenolysis,

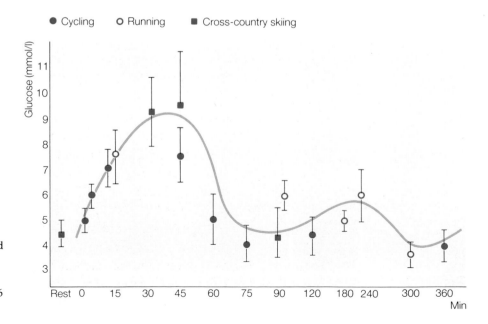

Fig. 3.2.1 Glucose concentration level in blood immediately after competitions in endurance sports (cycling, running, cross-country skiing) ($n = 6$ to 12).

Table 3.2.2 Adaptations to endurance training.

Formation of a stereotype motor programme in the STF

Increase in aerobic glucose utilization and increased participation of fats in energy metabolism

Extension of the energy stores (glycogen in muscle and liver, triglyceride in muscle)

Breaking down of about half the body fat deposits (e.g. in men from 15–20% down to 6–12% of the body mass)

Increased utilization of gluconeogenetic metabolic paths

Elevated activity of oxidative key enzymes in the STF

Increase in capillarization

Adaptation in oxygen uptake, transport and utilization systems (increase in $\dot{V}_{O_2\ max}$)

proteolysis and lipolysis. The elevated cortisol secretion promotes gluco-neogenetic metabolic processes. If carbohydrates are not available in sufficient quantities, the generation of ketone bodies is raised because the fatty acids cannot be broken down adequately by means of the β-oxidation. The adaptation to repeated endurance training sessions lasting several hours is characterized by an elevation of the substrate levels (glycogen in the liver and muscles, triglycerides in muscles, etc.). Adaptations to endurance training are summarized in Table 3.2.2.

Speed   Speed is a complex ability that is necessary to perform fast motor actions in the shortest possible time; it depends on central nervous motor programmes which are activated by intense will power. The organism can react quickly in different ways: in the speed of a single movement and motor response, or by achieving a high locomotor speed. A high locomotor speed is reached in exercises lasting 3–15 s. When starting to run from a resting position, the highest speed is reached between 35 and 80 m (6–10 s).

Fast movements are performed by recruiting the FTF, and because of their function and metabolic qualities these fibres constitute the most favourable preconditions for speed performances; for instance, successful sprinters have more than 60% FTF, as a result of their genetic aptitude. In speed training the FTF become hypertrophic, and the substrata reserves of ATP, AMP and CP are used. Glycolysis starts straight away, with the lactate concentration being 10–14 mmol/l after a 100 m sprint. Locomotor and reaction speeds can be improved through training. Reaction speed can be triggered by optic, acoustic or tactile impulses and is needed, to a greater or lesser extent, in almost all kinds of sports. The speed of a single movement is expressed by the frequency of the movement (frequency of walking, rowing, pedalling, etc.). The muscles must be prepared for speed performances by warming-up and stretching exercises.

Strength   Strength is another complex ability, which is required to execute muscle movements against external resistances or forces. Power, speed and endurance must be considered when discussing maximal force development. Power is the capability to give maximum acceleration to a body or competition implement or to counteract resistances with high speed. Strength endurance involves the execution of endurance performances against increased external resistances (e.g. ascents, gliding conditions, wind). The ability of maximum strength is needed to develop maximum voluntary forces in overcoming large external resistances.

The release of force in sports performances depends on the spectrum of muscle fibres recruited for the movement. The lowest levels of force development are reached by recruiting STF, and it can be maintained for long periods. Higher strength performances are possible by recruiting FTF in the motor programme; however, these fibres fatigue faster. The energy supply for strength performances is principally produced by high-energy phosphates (ATP, CP) and the anaerobic glycogen depletion in muscle. The supporting motor system (tendons, fibres, ligaments, cartilage, bones) also plays an important role in strength performances. The structure system adapts more slowly than muscle to strength training; and excessive loading can, therefore, frequently lead to problems in the structure system (e.g. chondropathia patellae, llumbalgia).

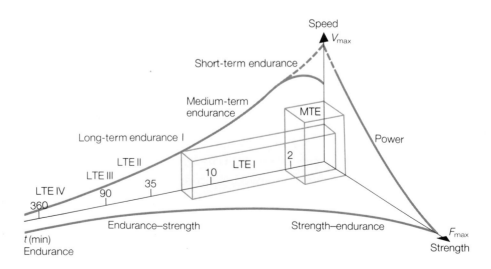

Fig. 3.2.2 Model of the relationships between endurance, strength and speed.

Coordination   Coordination is a basic precondition for sports activities. The coordinative abilities are individually developed control processes that make the motor performance possible in time and space. The term coordinative skills is also used, and it implies 'prefabricated', partly automated motor acts of high quality. The mental state of an athlete can clearly influence the execution of sports acts demanding high levels of coordination. In a state of high excitement (adrenergic stress), errors in the coordination of movements may occur. The sense organs of the athlete are important for coordination, both individually and through their interaction. The ability of differentiation of the optic, kinaesthetic, vestibular and acoustic sense organs influences the impulses (information) received and, therefore, influences the athletic performance. The motor programmes that are stored in the central nervous structures are known as the motor memory. The motor memory is trainable; it can be adapted and optimized for stable motor programmes that are specific to a particular sport. The

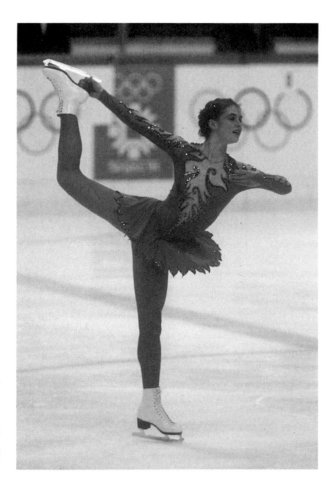

Fig. 3.2.3 While both aerobic and anaerobic energy release are necessary for figure skating performance, the dominant factor is the coordination of the activity of the muscles as controlled by the central nervous system. Courtesy of the IOC archives.

coordination abilities which are usually required in all types of sports include: balance, reaction ability, rhythm, orientation (in space) and differentiation (kinaesthetic).

Energetic conditions

The existing capacity of the athlete must be able to ensure sufficient energy for the demands of each sports performance. Changes in this energy supply capacity can be achieved through training and depends upon the demands of the sport. Changes in the aerobic and anaerobic capacity are particularly important in most types of sports. Adaptation develops through changes in the epigenetic regulation level, and this results in the use of previously unused capacity.

The adaptation to athletic training also raises the general, unspecific resistance of the athlete, and this promotes specific changes in the body's systems. The general adaptation comprises nervous, hormonal and immunological processes, which, biologically, combine to ensure muscle performance. If the homoeostasis of the systems are disturbed by effective exercise impulses, peripheral (autoregulative) and general central nervous regulation levels exert a modifying and coordinating influence. Repeated, heavy exercise makes it necessary to surpass the existing limits of the functional range of the systems; consequently the nervous central system control is rearranged, the muscle structure is changed and the organism adapts, on the whole, to the new exercise intensity. It takes about 4–6 weeks of endurance, strength or speed training to improve the efficiency of the muscle system; muscle hypertrophy becomes stable after approximately 6 weeks.

Aerobic capacity   The maximum oxygen uptake is a representative, measurable value used to evaluate the respiratory, cardiac, haemodynamic and muscle functional systems. The $\dot{V}_{O_2\ max}$ characterizes the functioning and capacity of the whole oxygen transport system, including oxygen uptake, transport and utilization. There is a fundamental relationship between the $\dot{V}_{O_2\ max}$ value and the athletic fitness level, especially when comparing trained and untrained people. If, however, there are only small performance differences in a group of athletes involved in the same kind of sports, no relationship between $\dot{V}_{O_2\ max}$ and sports performance can be found. The measurement of $\dot{V}_{O_2\ max}$ is of greatest practical importance in the endurance sports, although a high $\dot{V}_{O_2\ max}$ does not automatically mean a good level of athletic fitness. Alternatively, an athlete can be very fit, but

Table 3.2.3 Typical values for $\dot{V}_{O_2\ max}$ of élite athletes from different sports.

	Men ((ml/kg)/min)	Women ((ml/kg)/min)
Endurance sports		
Long distance running	75–80	65–70
Cross-country skiing	75–78	65–70
Biathlon	75–78	—
Road cycling	70–75	60–65
Middle-distance running	70–75	65–68
Skating	65–72	55–60
Orienteering	65–72	60–65
Swimming	60–70	55–60
Rowing	65–69	60–64
Track racing	65–70	55–60
Canoeing	60–68	50–55
Walking	60–65	55–60
Games		
Football (soccer)	50–57	—
Handball	55–60	48–52
Ice hockey	55–60	—
Volleyball	55–60	48–52
Basketball	50–55	40–45
Tennis	48–52	40–45
Table tennis	40–45	38–42
Combative sports		
Boxing	60–65	—
Wrestling	60–65	—
Judo	55–60	50–55
Fencing	45–50	40–45
Power sports		
Sprint (200 m track)	55–60	45–50
Sprint track and field (100 m, 200 m)	48–52	43–47
Long jump	50–55	45–50
Competition consisting of several events (decathlon, septathlon)	60–65	50–55
Nordic combination (15 km ski walking and ski jumping)	60–65	—
Weight lifting	40–50	—
Discus throwing, shot putting ·	40–45	35–40
Javelin throwing	45–50	42–47
Pole vaulting	45–50	—
Ski jumping	40–45	—
Technical-acrobatic sports		
Down-hill skiing (Alpine disciplines)	60–65	48–53
Figure skating	50–55	45–50
Gymnastics	45–50	40–45
Rhythmic gymnastics	—	40–45
Sailing	50–55	45–50
Shooting	40–45	35–40

have a low $\dot{V}_{O_2 \, max}$ as it is possible to complete heavy endurance performances by utilizing aerobic metabolism to a greater extent.

Typical $\dot{V}_{O_2 \, max}$ values for élite athletes are given in Table 3.2.3; these have changed very little during the last 30 years. For instance, in 1958 the successful cross-country skier, S. Jernberg, had a $\dot{V}_{O_2 \, max}$ of 70 ml/min/kg, while the long-distance runners and world record holders of the seventies (Bedford and Keino) had $\dot{V}_{O_2 \, max}$ values between 82 and 85 ml/min/kg. This, therefore, means that the improvement in endurance performances cannot be a result of an increase in $\dot{V}_{O_2 \, max}$. One of the most essential improvements, achieved under modern intensive training methods, can be explained by the fact that the oxygen available is utilized better by the muscles. As well as this, the muscles are trained in a highly specific way and obtain better contraction characteristics by adaptations in the contractile proteins (actin, myosin, troponin, tropomyosin) and through changes in the central nervous and neuromuscular control mechanisms. When the muscle contracts more efficiently, a bigger forward drive is obtained within a certain span of time, and consequently the athletes are faster.

Meanwhile, the methods used to evaluate aerobic capacity have been improved by measuring the oxygen uptake during submaximal workloads together with the metabolic lactate value. Practically, the problem is to ascertain the degree to which $\dot{V}_{O_2 \, max}$ is utilized in aerobic metabolism. The lactate concentration level of 3–4 mmol/l is generally chosen as a criterion of the oxygen uptake at the aerobic/anaerobic threshold. Untrained people start utilizing glycolytic metabolism in exercises surpassing 60% of the maximum oxygen uptake. Endurance-trained athletes can utilize $\dot{V}_{O_2 \, max}$ to a higher intensity level; they only need to utilize anaerobic metabolism when exercises exceed about 80% of the $\dot{V}_{O_2 \, max}$. Exercise training can push these limits further, for instance for marathon runners. This means that very well-trained runners can utilize up to 90–95% of their already high $\dot{V}_{O_2 \, max}$ in aerobic metabolism (Fig. 3.2.4). Thus, the steady and economical utilization of oxygen uptake can be used as a criterion for assessing aerobic capacity.

Anaerobic capacity   The anaerobic capacity comprises the ability of muscle to perform under alactic or lactic conditions. There are only a few kinds of sports which stress single paths of energy turnover, most using a combination of anaerobic capacity (alactic or lactic) and aerobic capacity. The graduated use of alactic, lactic and aerobic ATP resynthesis leads to the situation in short intensive exercise bouts, with a duration of about 6–10 s, where glycolysis starts from the first second of exercise.

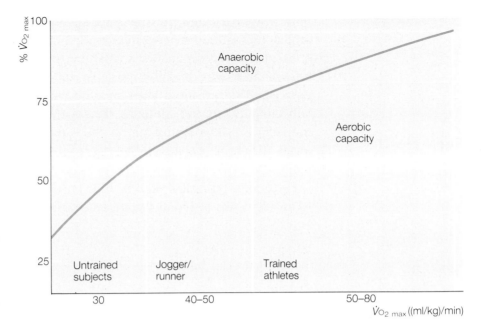

Fig. 3.2.4 Development of aerobic capacity depending on fitness level and related to percentage of $\dot{V}_{O_2\,max}$ utilization under aerobic conditions (lactate less than 3 mmol/l).

A precondition for the increase in anaerobic capacity is a change in the pattern of the neural system with more FTF being used in the motor programme. The oxidative and glycolytic metabolic performance of these fibres is also adapted according to the demands of the sport. The speed of anaerobic mobilization can be raised by changes in the calcium mechanism (T-system). Compared to an endurance athlete, a sprinter can make faster and more intense use of his or her anaerobic metabolic possibilities. The speed needed for a sport is decisive for the adaptation and ability to mobilize anaerobic metabolism.

Anaerobic capacity can be determined by measuring the lactate level and physical performance. An indirect evaluation is provided by the shift to the left of the lactate performance curve at the aerobic–anaerobic transition.

Functional metabolic transition In order to determine the regulatory conditions occurring on the aerobic–anaerobic threshold, Hollmann (1963) defined the 'oxygen prolonged performance limit' or the point of the 'optimal respiratory efficiency'. Following investigation into the partial values of respiration and gaseous interchange, Wasserman *et al.* (1973) introduced the term 'anaerobic threshold'. The aerobic–anaerobic transition is a significant one in the functioning of several systems and not just a category of diagnosis. It is a complicated transition because there are several changes occurring in both the aerobic and the anaerobic systems. Functional systems of the athlete that influence performance adjust themselves to a higher level of stress; they regulate in such a way that they enhance the rate of energy release and thus make it possible to endure higher intensities of exercise. The threshold level and functional transition period depend substantially on the athlete's fitness. Biological factors exerting an immediate influence on the aerobic–anaerobic transition include the level of aerobic capacity, the degree of recovery, and the training methods used.

Endurance training methods, which due to their higher intensity lead to an elevation of blood lactate levels up to 3–6 mmol/l, result in the

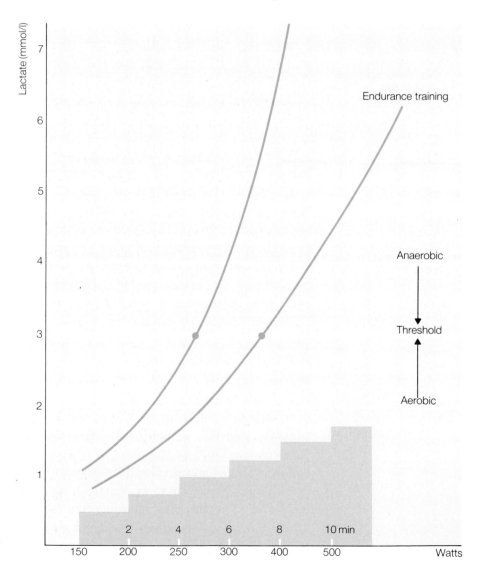

Fig. 3.2.5 Typical shift to the right of the aerobic–anaerobic threshold after an endurance training session.

clearest adaptation in the aerobic–anaerobic threshold (Fig. 3.2.5). The most significant connection between the level of the aerobic–anaerobic transition measured and an endurance performance can be seen in marathon running. The running time for 42 195 km becomes shorter as the aerobic threshold level rises (Neumann, 1983). With extensive aerobic training or glycogen deficiency, the mobilization of glycolysis is diminished. As a result of this type of training a lower lactate concentration level is measured in laboratory tests. The elevation of the lactate performance curve is flatter and the maximal lactate level is 2–4 mmol/l lower.

Tables 3.2.2 and 3.2.3 present the adaptations to endurance training and typical values for $\dot{V}_{O_2\,max}$ per unit body mass for athletes from different sports.

Reactivity of the immunological status

Intense sports competition and psychological stress have a depressive effect on the immune system. According to the stress concept of Selye, a very strong and differentiated reactivity is observed in the immune systems of athletes performing very intense or unaccustomed physical activity. Intensive athletic training affects the plasmaproteins and the cellular reactions; this co-response can be used to evaluate the athlete's stress tolerance. The biological resistance is stimulated through varying the workloads. Prolonged endurance exercises of high intensity (competition) exert an influence on the acute phase proteins and the immunoglobulins (Liesen et al., 1977; Neumann et al., 1982). Due to the elevation of intravascular haemolysis, particularly in running exercises, haptoglobins decrease by 40% on average. The concentration of leucocytes, lymphocytes and monocytes is raised without any detectable inflammation; the eosinophilic granulocytes, however, decrease (eosinopenia). These changes in the cellular blood constituents of the plasmaproteins and immunoglobulins can still be observed after 2 to 3 days. This is particularly true for marathon runners. The T-lymphocytes show an intense reaction to heavy athletic exercise, and release numerous cytotoxins. The decline in reactivity of T-lymphocytes with heavy, particularly if repeated, intensities of exercise can be shown by the lymphocyte transformation test. The lymphocyte transformation test shows a level in untrained people at rest of 60–90%, this falls in athletes to 55 ± 15%. After marathon running the test level diminishes to about 20%; in the same way the immunoglobulins IgA and IgG fall significantly for 1 to 2 days.

The depression of the immunological potential disturbs the immuno-logical protecting force of the organism following heavy athletic exercises for a short time. The diminished unspecific and specific immune protection can favour the development of infections. Investigations into the changes of the immune system following athletic exercise are only just beginning, nevertheless they have great practical importance.

References

Hollmann, W. (1963) *Höchst- und Dauerleistungsfähigkeit des Sportlers.* J. A. Barth, München.

Liesen, M., Dufaux, B. & Hollmann, W. (1977) Modification of serum glycoproteins in the days following a prolonged physical exercise and the influence of physical training. *Eur. J. Appl. Physiol.* **37**, 243.

Neumann, G. (1983) Metabole Regulation bei Lang-zeitausdauerleistungen. *Med. Sport* **23**, 169.

Neumann, G., Schubert, I., Wulf, E. & Zimmer, A. (1982) Zur Dynamik des Haptoglobins nach Lang-zeitausdauerbelastungen. *Med. Sport* **22**, 232.

Wasserman, K., Whipp, B. J., Koyal, S. N. & Beaver, W. L. (1973) The anaerobic threshold and respiratory gas exchange during exercise. *J. Appl. Physiol.* **35**, 236.

3.3 Physiological, medical, biomechanical and biochemical measurements

A. DAL MONTE & I. DRĂGAN

Physiological measurements

Neuromuscular measurements

1 Electroencephalography (EEG) expresses the electrical cortical activity of the nervous system, and is a very useful test for neurophysiological evaluation, especially in shooting, diving, fencing, aviation, motorcycling, chess, etc. The EEG test could also be used in boxing and other contact sports in order to assess possible preclinical damage of the nervous system. The test can be performed under standard conditions or using different stimuli, such as intermittent light, pharmacological, phonic, etc. stimulations; it can also be performed during exercise by teletransmission. The computerized evaluation of α- and β-rhythms is also of practical interest. There is a close correlation between EEG and sports type and fatigue or overtraining (early deterioration of EEG).

2 Electromyography (EMG) is a specific test which estimates: (a) neuromuscular excitability, important in neuromuscular sports; (b) the quality of muscular contraction by the estimation of evoked muscular potential —proximal and distal amplitude of contraction, A_p, A_d and distal latency, L_d; and (c) the velocity of nervus influxus inside motor or sensitive nerves. This list only covers the main tests used in sports medicine. The EMG test can also be performed during exercise by teletransmission, and correlates with fatigue and overtraining, and type of sport.

3 Reaction time (RT) measures the psychomotric reactivity, a quality which is more or less genetically determined. It can be measured on any limbs using acoustic or optic stimuli; the shorter the reaction time, the better the reactivity of the central nervous system. This test also correlates with type of sport and with fatigue and/or overtraining (deterioration). Good values are generally considered to be 14–16 hundredths of a second for acoustic stimuli (20–22 is satisfactory), and 16–18 hundredths of a second for optic stimuli (23–25 is satisfactory).

4 Neuromuscular coordination can be estimated by psychological tests or by a test performed on the Bettendorf pantograph, as described by Dal Monte (1983).

5 Muscular tonus (myotonometry) can be measured by some myotono-meters (based on the mechanical system). The state of the muscle in relaxation and contraction is examined; and the greater the difference between the two states the better the muscular tonus is.

Cardiovascular measurements

1 Heart rate (HR) is the most common and useful cardiovascular parameter used in sports medicine, both in the laboratory and in the field. It can be measured at rest, during exercise and afterwards (recovery), either directly or by teletransmission, and it is the simplest and most efficient test conducted in sports training.

2 Blood pressure (BP) is closely related to HR and is the second most practical parameter for the evaluation of cardiovascular function (measured in clinostatic and orthostatic positions, before, during and after exercise).

3 The electrocardiographic test (ECG) expresses the electric potential of cardiac muscle and is performed in sports medicine before, during and after exercise. Cardiovascular health and adaptation to exercise can be evaluated by examining some stress reactions, such as conductibility or excitability troubles, heart hypertrophy, repolarization troubles, etc. Sports doctors have thereby gained a better understanding of, and can give better scientific advice on, training.

4 Echocardiography is a morphologic and functional test which helps sports doctors achieve a more precise cardiovascular diagnosis, and at the same time is used for heart functional evaluation, especially concerning the left ventricle.

5 Heart volume (HV) evaluation, using two teleradiographies, represents another useful test for the estimation of heart reaction to exercise, especially in aerobic sports.

Respiratory measurements

1 Spirographic tests allow the estimation of vital capacity, VC (e.g. current volume, reserve inspiratory volume, reserve expiratory volume, maximal expiratory volume during 1 s (VEMS), Tiffeneau index, maximal inspiratory volume during 1 s, maximal voluntary ventilation).

2 Inspiratory and expiratory apnoea.

3 Maximal oxygen consumption on rest and during exercise.

4 Pulmonary ventilation.

5 The elimination of carbon dioxide and the respiratory quotient (RQ); for instance the increase of RQ from values under 1 to 1+ means that exercise has moved from a range where aerobic metabolism accounts for the energy demands to a range where anaerobic metabolism is dominant.

Liver, kidney and endocrine measurements These are performed through clinical examinations and biochemical tests, izotopical and/or echographic tests.

Psychological measurements They are necessary for a complete diagnosis of neuromuscular function. Sports physicians need information from the psychologist about psycho-reactivity (i.e. reaction time, using an Achillean reflexogramme, which is also an important test for evaluating thyroid function), attention (level of concentration), visual–motor coordination and equilibrium, intelligence, perseverance, general ability (skill), temperamental structure, resistance against psychological fatigue or stress, etc.

Medical measurements

Medical considerations of particular interest are previous medical treatment, and complete clinical and paraclinical examination (especially laboratory and radiology). Medical measurements must, of course, be conducted in particular conditions so that the whole functional system may be assessed.

Biomechanical measurements

Biomechanical measurements allow sports coaches to appreciate the bioenergetics and efficiency of sports movements; training can then aim to achieve a maximal energetic output with a minimal expenditure of energy, and avoiding at the same time possible fatigue and stress lesions in the locomotory system. Dal Monte (1983) described several techniques for biomechanical measurements: photographic (cronocyclophoto-graphic, stroboscopy, light traces (intermittent or continuous); cine-matographic (mono- or tridimensional, corrective, etc.); electrogonio-metric; dynamometric; electromyographic; and mixed (cinematographic–electrogoniometric, cinematographic–physiological, cinematographic–electromyographic–dynamometric–physiological, etc.).

Biomechanical measurements cover many areas: speed; velocity—reaction, displacement, repetition; neuromuscular coordination—technique, mobility, flexibility, amplitude of joint movements; muscular tenderness, elasticity and contraction; local resistance; force and strength; correction and efficiency of movements, etc.

Force, for practical reasons, is probably of the greatest interest in sports medicine, and it must be evaluated in a way of use to trainers. Tests, therefore, should be aimed at the analysis of various ways of expressing force, even if these do not correspond to the usual physiological definition.

In fact, the mechanical aspects of force are the essential ones to be considered, that is the speed of displacement (acceleration, a) of a mass (m) from which the intensity of the force to be applied can be derived ($F = ma$). Using this formula it is possible to identify: (a) shear force where the mass component prevails (resistance to be overcome, e.g. weight lifting); (b) fast force where the acceleration component prevails (high performance speed, e.g. jump); and (c) endurance force where neither component dominates (average intensity and speed, e.g. rowing). Shear force should be considered both as an absolute force, that is the maximum force which can be expressed by the athlete, and as a relative force, that is in relation to bodyweight.

Isometric dynamometry   This is used to measure shear force. The dynamometers used in the various laboratories can be classified in three basic types: mechanical, hydraulic, and electric and electronic. Regardless of type, however, all dynamometers should be totally dependable and insensitive to temperature changes, the length variations of the device should be minimal so

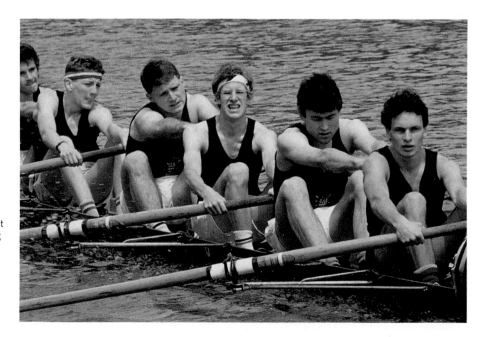

Fig. 3.3.1 Rowing is a sport requiring endurance during high-power output and, therefore, neither the force component nor the acceleration component of each muscle contraction dominates. Photo by Jim Chambers.

that measurements of muscular contractions can be taken in absolute isometric conditions, all friction must be reduced to a minimum, they should be easy to apply correctly to the muscular groups to be tested, and the support structure must be absolutely rigid. Since the force output of a single muscular group cannot be used as a general indication to evaluate the athletic capacities of a subject, some authors have suggested calculation of a dynamometric global index based on the sthenic degree of more than one muscular group. Morehouse (1972) used the following formula:

$$\text{ID} = \frac{LG + RG + LS + BS}{\text{Bodyweight}}$$

in which ID is the dynamometric index, LG is the left hand fingers flexors force, RG is the right hand fingers flexors force, LS is the force of the leg muscles and BS is the force of the trunk extensors. Drăgan *et al.* (1982) consider a similar index ($LG + RG$ + scapular force + lumbar force), but compare it to lean body mass determined by an indirect method (skin folds).

Isometric dynamography This uses an isometric dynamometer, electronic if possible, which can be connected to a computer. The parameter taken is the maximum isometric force (F_{max}) and, through a graphic illustration obtained either by mechanical means or by computer, it is possible to work out the correlation of the force signal with time. The Rome Sports Science Institute has measured the maximum force produced in 1 s ($F1_{max}$) in order to compare subjects with different muscular characteristics, in particular when dynamometric indexes have been derived. Amongst these indexes, the most important are: the relative force index ($F1_{max}$/bodyweight); the $t30$–$t50$–$t60$–$t90$ index (time taken to reach 30–50–60–90% of the $F1_{max}$, respectively); the reactivity coefficient or Verchoshansky's index ($F1_{max}/t_{max}$ × bodyweight); and the modified Verchoshansky's coefficient ($F50_{max}$ × $1/t50$). With the analysis of such derived indexes it is possible to obtain useful indications of the capacity of rapid muscular contraction, the 'explosive force'.

Concentric contraction dynamometry or eccentric–concentric dynamometry All the tests described above evaluate muscular sthenia of the isometric type. This parameter, although important, does not provide a full picture of muscular mechanics as it represents a type of contraction which is not usual in sports activities. In order to complete dynamometric evaluation it is therefore necessary to measure the force involved in muscular contractions of the concentric type.

In order to do this isokinetic dynamometers are used. The athlete subjected to an isokinetic dynamometric test must try to push a lever using maximum strength and speed. This lever is kept moving, at a previously set and constant speed, by a suitable motor. The dynamometer measures the force (the couple) applied by the subject to the lever. On the basis of the ratio between force and contraction speed, the greater the speed of the moving lever, the smaller the force applied (and vice versa). This test can be performed on various articulations (knee, shoulder, elbow, etc.). Isokinetic dynamometers are, however, expensive and complex devices.

Recently a system has been perfected by Bosco *et al.* (1983), the Ergo jump, for the evaluation of the explosive force of the lower limb extensors which, although it is limited to these muscular groups and is an indirect evaluation method, is easy to use and is reliable. This test analyses the heights reached by athletes in two different trials: (a) the squatting jump which is a vertical standing jump from a half-squatting position (knee articulation angle 90°) with the hands on the hips. This exercise is mainly performed using the contractile component of the extensor muscular groups of the lower limbs and it therefore gives an indirect measure of the explosive force; and (b) the countermovement jump, a vertical jump with a preceding spring, with bending of the knees to about 90° and hands on the hips. During this exercise, besides the contractile component, there is also, to a remarkable degree, the capacity of using the potential elastic energy stored during the stage of muscular stretching (eccentric–concentric dynamometry) and the coordination capacity of the athlete.

Force–velocity (F–V) curve

The most complete application of the methods described above is the construction of the *F–V* curve of a given muscular group. Generally, it is carried out with isokinetic dynamometers at various angular velocities. For the lower limb extensors it is possible, however, to use the jump test. This test consists in the performance of a series of jumps, with complete rest between one jump and the next one, from a half-squatting position. With the exception of the first jump, which is performed with no added loads, the following jumps are performed with increasing additional loads chosen according to the athlete's bodyweight. The load is applied to the athlete through a weight lifting bar or a loaded vest. For each jump the maximum vertical velocity is measured and then correlated with the relative overload, thus obtaining a typical curve of the contractile qualities of the athlete being tested. This procedure can be repeated for jumps performed with countermovement (see above), thus obtaining a second curve which, compared with the first, is moved to the right as the elastic component was also activated. According to various authors, the definition of the F–V curve is useful in order to identify the muscular typology of the subjects, as well as to allow a fuller analysis of training effects.

Conclusion   The following ergometers can now be used in sports medicine: step-test; cycle ergometers; treadmill; crank ergometers; simulating ergometers for kayak canoes (Dal Monte); ergometers for rowing (Gyessing–Nilsen and Dal Monte); ergometers for canoeing (Dal Monte); ergometers for Canadian canoes (Dal Monte); ergometers for cross-country skiing (Dal Monte); ergometers for swimming (Dal Monte, Stockholm Swimming Flume, etc.). It would therefore be impossible to present all the biomechanical measurements in this chapter. The authors feel that speed is best evaluated through neuromuscular measurements, resistance and endurance through cardiorespiratory and metabolic tests, and coordination through psychological and neuromuscular tests, and have therefore concentrated on these measurements of force.

Finally, Table 3.3.1 presents guidelines for classifying men and women in terms of power capacity.

Table 3.3.1 Guidelines for classifying men and women in terms of power capacity (measured in (m kg)/s).

	Age groups (years)				
	15–20	20–30	30–40	40–50	Over 50
Men					
Poor	Under 113	Under 106	Under 85	Under 65	Under 50
Fair	113–149	106–139	85–111	65–84	50–65
Average	150–187	140–175	112–140	85–105	66–82
Good	188–224	176–210	141–168	106–125	83–98
Excellent	Over 224	Over 210	Over 168	Over 125	Over 98
Women					
Poor	Under 92	Under 85	Under 65	Under 50	Under 38
Fair	92–120	85–111	65–84	50–65	38–48
Average	121–151	112–140	85–105	66–82	49–61
Good	152–182	141–168	106–125	83–98	62–75
Excellent	Over 182	Over 168	Over 125	Over 98	Over 75

From Mathews & Fox (1976); data from Kalamen (1968) and Margaria *et al.* (1968).

Biochemical measurements

The assessment of some biochemical parameters before, during and after sports efforts, is important in the methodology of investigation, due to the fact that severe changes of the homoeostasis can affect physical capacity and so become a limiting factor of performance. The evaluation of metabolic economy during exercise depends particularly on biochemical measurements, e.g. acid–alkaline and hydroelectrolyte balances, and basal conditions during and after exercise. The micro Astrup method is used in the study of adaptative biochemical changes during different kind of exercises as it allows the estimation of pH, P_{CO_2}, $^-HCO_3$, base excess, standard bicarbonate reserve, carbon dioxide, P_{O_2} and sulphur dioxide (blood).

pH Normal values of blood pH are in the range 7.35 to 7.45 (7.38–7.42); the higher the intensity of exercise the lower the pH values (e.g. up to 6.9–6.8 after a 400 m or 800 m run on track or field). In long-distance events the decrease of blood pH is more moderate (7.15–7.25). The severe decrease of blood pH (under 7) might explain the limitation of performance in aerobic sports. The variations in blood pH correlate significantly with the changes in blood lactate and base excess, both during exercise and in the recovery period. The faster the restoration of blood pH after exercise, the better the recovery of the body and the lower the residual fatigue.

Base or alkaline excess (BE) This represents the excess or deficit of acids or bases (alkaline radicals) and is the main metabolic parameter of acid–alkaline balance. The high correlation with blood lactate ($r = 0.98$) during or after exercise, confirms the value of this parameter in the biochemical measurement of physical capacity by the micro Astrup method. Keul *et al.* (1969) have established a conversion formula between blood lactate and BE (0.54 − BE/1.25). BE can also be used as an indicator of metabolic economy during exercise. The lower the BE/W/kg, the better the metabolic economy during exercise (effort performed on a cycle ergometer or treadmill; a value of 2 is excellent and 4–5 is bad). BE represents the deficit of alkaline radicals in the body as a result of the accumulation of organic acids (lactic, pyruvic), free fatty acids and cetoacids, formed during intense exercise; therefore, it reflects the whole mechanism of adaptation to exercise. Normal values of BE are between −2.3 and +2.3. After 400 m or 800 m events (track and field) the values of BE can decrease up to 30 mmol/l, while after 5 km or 10 km the values are between 6 and 12 mmol/l.

Standard bicarbonate or alkaline reserve (SB)

This represents another metabolic parameter used for the estimation of metabolic acidosis induced by maximal exercise. Normal values are between 22 and 26 mmol/l. The decrease of SB during exercise results mainly (95%) from the increase in lactic and pyruvic acids and 5% from the increase in free fatty acids. The lowest values (5–10 mmol/l) have been registered in middle- and long-distance runners.

Blood lactate

Blood lactate is the final product of muscular glycolysis and is used for biochemical measurement of physical capacity, both anaerobic and aerobic. The blood concentration of lactic acid depends directly on the intensity of exercise and expresses the metabolic adaptation to effort. A high level of blood lactate represents a limiting factor of performance. Normal values vary between 0.7 and 1.8 mmol/l. After 400 m or 800 m events (track and field) the capillary lactate can increase up to 30–34 mmol/l, while after 10 km or marathon races the values are lower (6–12 mmol/l). In élite athletes, the higher the aerobic capacity, the lower the capillary lactate, especially compared to untrained athletes (higher values). The dynamic follow-up of blood lactate and acid–alkaline balance parameters during sports efforts and competitions, allows us to measure the metabolic economy before, during and after exercise. These parameters also allow us to appreciate the anaerobic capacity, the alactacid and lactacid quotients, the resistance against hypoxia and the efficiency of medication used in athletes (ergotropic, trophotropic).

Creatine phosphokinase (CPK)

This enzyme intervenes in the muscular metabolism and is important in strength and speed efforts, such as springs, shot put, throwing, weight lifting, wrestling, boxing, etc. In these sports the high level of catecholamine secretion induces an increase in CPK activity; for instance 8 h after wrestling, judo or boxing competitions, the figures of serum CPK can be three to four times higher than basal values (normal values on rest are between 0.1 and 0.7 IU, as measured by the Bergmayer enzymatic method). After short and intense exercise the values can increase up to eight times, this increase is evident 8 h after exercise and lasts 24–48 h.

Serum urea

Serum urea is an indicator of protein metabolism, and it often increases after long-duration exercise or hard training (especially strength). The determination of serum urea the day after training or a competition is an important criterion for the estimation of residual metabolic fatigue and, of course, of metabolic recovery. Periodic measurement of serum urea can help in the planning of future training, especially with regard to volume.

Serum creatinin This represents another important factor in the measurement of exercise, and levels increase slightly after hard efforts. Normal values are between 0.7 and 1.5 mg% for men and 0.5 and 1.3 mg% for women as measured by the Jaffé method. The urinary excretion of creatinin is still high 12–24 h after long-duration exercise, in proportion to the effects induced by the exercise on muscular tissue. This excretion correlates with body-weight (especially with muscular mass), and must therefore be taken into account when considering the urinary creatinin during the 24 h period.

Plasma proteins Plasma proteins represent an important metabolic factor which correlates with strength and endurance efforts. Normal values are 7.2 ± 0.9 g% for men and 6.9 ± 0.8 g% for women as measured by the Weichselbaum method.

Free fatty acids (FFA) FFA are significant in long-distance events, when the decrease after training or competition might signify the utilization of fat as an energy source. (1-Carnitine can induce a better utilization of FFA during long-term exercises by facilitating the entrance of FFA across the mitochondrial membrane into mitochondria, at the place of β-oxidation of fat.) Normal values of FFA are from 0.40 to 0.75 mmol/l as measured by the Dohl method. High values of FFA on rest are considered by some authors as a sign of a better metabolic state (higher reserves of energy).

Electrolytes **1** Calcium intervenes in the neuromuscular excitability (normal values in serum between 4.5 and 5.6 mmol/l; Ca^{++} levels between 2.1 and 2.7 mmol/l; using the flame photometer). The decrease of total or ionized calcium below normal values is found in the tetanic syndrome. Long-term efforts in high temperatures induce a higher excretion of calcium by perspiration and/or urine excretion, a fact which justifies the periodic follow-up of calcium in elite athletes, especially in long-distance efforts.
2 Magnesium, a co-factor in numerous enzymatic systems implicated in vital cell functions (ATPasis, cholinesterasis, phosphatasis), intervenes in the proteic biosynthesis and in contraction and neuromuscular excitability. Normal values are between 1.7 and 2.5 mg%, using the Métais–Schirardin method. An increase of magnesium excretion in urine and sweat is registered during long-distance races. It is therefore of interest to periodically follow-up the variations in serum magnesium, especially in endurance athletes.
3 Sodium (normal values 101 ± 3 mmol/l in serum and 100–220 mmol/ 24 h in urine, using the flame photometer) and potassium (normal

values 3.9–5.1 mmol/l in serum and 40–100 mmol/24 h in urine, using the flame photometer) should also be measured from time to time in élite athletes. This is especially so in endurance athletes or in long-distance runners and cyclists during the summer.

Haemoglobin (Hb) Because of the role of Hb in cellular oxidation, it represents a significant factor in aerobic sports. The close correlation between Hb and $\dot{V}_{O_2\,max}$ makes Hb an important parameter in the assessment of physical capacity and sports form. Normal values of Hb are between 14 and 16 g%, using the Drabkin method; values of 17 or 18 g% are usual in athletes performing aerobic sports.

Urine tests Measurements of pH, density, proteinurine, haematurine, cylindrurine and urobilinogenurine can all give an indication of a person's adaptation to exercise. The Donaggio test (2 ml urine + 1 ml thionin 1‰ soln + 2 ml ammonium molybdate 4%) is a qualitative test which shows the increase of urine mucoproteins, which signify a stress reaction induced at the corticorenal gland level as a result of metabolic fatigue. The intensity of colour (violet) indicates the degree of positive reaction (+, ++, +++), while negative reaction is indicated when the coloured substance falls to the bottom of the bottle leaving the urine clear. The quantitative determination of urine mucoproteins can be performed by using the Biserte–Montreuil method (normal values are 50–250 mg/24 h) and the interpretation of results are the same as in the Donaggio test. Lower values after exercise indicate a better metabolic economy.

The following are other urine tests of interest in sports medicine:

1   17-Cetosteroids represent the final metabolites of androgenic hormones (normal values are 8–20 mg/24 h for men and 7–14 mg/24 h for women using the Dreckter method). The higher the urinary excretion after exercise, the higher the reaction of the corticorenal gland as a result of greater stress.

2   Vanillylmandelic acid levels can be used to estimate the main urinary metabolites of catecholamines (normal values are 1.6–8 mg/24 h) which correlate physical and especially psychological stress. The higher the values after exercise, the higher the stress of the adrenal gland (Pisano–Cannellian method).

3   Urine catecholamines (normal values of noradrenaline are 10–50 μg/24 h and of adrenaline, 4–9 μg/24 h) can also be used for biochemical measurement of exercise.

Other tests such as serum aldolasis (normal values are 1.8–4.8 IU, using the Richterich method), serum sialic acid (normal values are 50–70 mg%, using the Dische–Winzler method) or serum glycoproteins (normal values are 80–130 mg%, using the Winzler method) can also be of practical interest in some circumstances. Low increases after exercise indicate better levels of fitness.

Conclusion   This section has summarized the most important biochemical measurements available which can help sports doctors to assess physical capacity and functional adaptation to exercise. This should lead to better sports training and, therefore, sports form.

References

Bosco, C., Luhtaner, P. & Komi, P. V. (1983) A simple method for measurement of mechanical power in jumping. *Eur. J. Appl. Physiol.* **50**, 2, 73, 282.

Dal Monte, A. (1983) *La Valutazione Funzionale dell'Atleta.* G. C. Samsoni Editore Nuova, Firenze.

Drăgan, I. *et al.* (1982) *Sports Medicine.* Sports-Tourism Ed., Bucharest.

Kalamen, J. (1968) *Measurement of maximum muscular power in man.* Ph.D. Thesis, Ohio State University.

Keul, J., Doll, E. & Keppler, D. (1969) *Muskelstoffwechsel.* J. A. Barth, München.

Margaria, R., Anghemo, P. & Rovelli, E. (1966) Measurement of muscular (anaerobic) power in man. *J. Appl. Physiol.* **21**, 1662.

Mathews, D. K. & Fox, E. L. (1976) *The Physiological Basis of Physical Education and Athletics*, 2nd edn. W. B. Saunders, Philadelphia.

Morehouse, L. E. (1972) *Laboratory Manual for Physiology of Exercise.* C.V. Mosby, Ontario.

Further reading

Manta, I., Cucuianu, M., Benga, G. & Hogărdău, A. (1976) *Biochemical Methods in Clinical Laboratory.* Ed. Dacia, Cluj-Napoca, Romania.

3.4 Exercise testing and ergometers

A. DAL MONTE

Ergometers

Step test   A very common test of physical performance is the step test; it consists of one or more steps which the subject has to climb at a set speed and in various ways according to the different tests used. The action of climbing represents the actual physical challenge. The available types of step tests are extremely ill-suited to the specific functional evaluation of most sports disciplines. In particular, the muscle and circulation work done by the lower limbs in these tests are totally unnatural to all types of athletes.

These types of tests have the following drawbacks:

1 It produces localized fatigue in the muscular groups utilized to make the whole body perform the action of climbing steps between 30 and 50 cm high (depending on the type of step test).
2 It does not allow the involvement of the cardiorespiratory system with the muscle and peripheral circulatory systems in conditions similar to those of competition.
3 The test is often disliked by athletes, who alter the significance of the test by performing it irregularly and incompletely without raising their centre of gravity the necessary 50 cm to define the work done. This can result in an incorrect evaluation of the test results.
4 In spite of the use of the available types of optical and acoustical timers, not all subjects, even in the case of excellent athletes, are able to keep up with the necessary climbing and descent rates.

The step test, therefore, even if dependable in cardiology as it involves a below maximal and easy exercise intensity, is not suitable for a specific functional evaluation of athletes. On the other hand, however, it is very simple and allows mass screenings of population samples performing unspecified sports activities and, in particular, it can be used to carry out aptitude tests on young people.

Cycle ergometer   Cycle ergometers are of use in sports medicine, but are also subject to certain limitations. They are a non-specific evaluation test and can therefore be applied in various sports (see Wingate test and aerobic metabolism tests below).

The cycle ergometer is obviously of particular use in cycling sports. It must be adjusted so that cyclists can simulate their athletic motions as closely as possible. For a correct evaluation of cyclists the following adjustments should be made on the cycle ergometer:

1 The handle bar should be adjustable in height and of a racing design.
2 The saddle should also be of the racing type, and it should be adjustable both vertically and horizontally, so that the distance between the handle bar and the saddle as well as the distance between the handle bar and the pedals can be varied.
3 The pedal cranks should be racing-style with foot stops, and be adjustable in length.

Cycle ergometers with a set pedalling rate are not suitable. Set torque models (such as the Fleish or Monark) are available, with the power proportional to pedalling rate; these are useful when it is necessary to measure the highest mechanical power of the subject. Other devices have a set power independent of the number of pedalling movements, and are suitable for those cases when the power demand is to be set by the operator and metabolic parameters are to be measured.

It is therefore advisable to use multiple braking system devices, choosing the adjustable torque and constant power system (Fig. 3.4.1) (so that the athlete may, up to a certain point, suit the pedalling action to

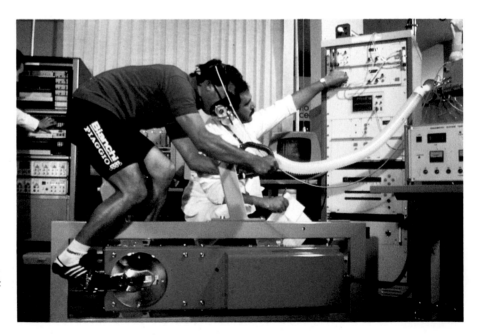

Fig. 3.4.1 Cycle ergometer used in the Institute of Sport Science (Department of Physiology and Biomechanics).

his or her own anthropometric, muscular and technical features) in the case of metabolic measurements ($\dot{V}_{O_2\ max}$), and the set torque system for mechanical measurements (Wingate).

Treadmill This is an ergonometric device which is widely used as it involves natural movements such as marching and running. In the evaluation of the athlete, however, the treadmill has to be used in such a way as to simulate the specific discipline practiced, so as to achieve a performance with peripheral muscular and vascular work as close as possible to training and competition situations.

If this is to be achieved, in the author's opinion, the treadmill should be used level, even if this means doing without a simple and sufficiently exact calculation system, from a physical point of view, for the evaluation of the quantity of work performed in a unit of time (i.e. the power produced by the athlete in the test). The work performed by a particular subject on the treadmill can be evaluated as follows:

$$\text{m kg/min} = \frac{\text{weight in kg} \times \text{m/h} \times \%\,\text{gradient}}{60\ \text{min}}.$$

According to this formula, an athlete running at 4 km/h and on a 25% gradient performs at an exercise intensity equivalent to a subject going at a speed of 20 km/h on a 5% gradient. These two situations can not be equated in the athlete, as with the first load (high gradient and low speed) he/she would soon stop with symptoms of local muscular stress; in the second case, the performance would last longer and would involve a higher oxygen uptake value, and local stress phenomena would appear only at a late stage.

The muscular and peripheral vascular system involvement in the level treadmill race can be compared, biomechanically and physiologically, to a race on track. In fact, it has been shown (Dal Monte) that at high speeds (over 20 km/h) the energy costs of treadmill (with no gradient) and track work do not show significant differences from a statistical point of view.

The treadmill should be only used on gradients in the case of specific evaluation requirements.

Crank ergometers There are two types of basically different handle ergometers: one directly resulting from the replacement of pedals with a common double manual crank cycle ergometer, and another actioned by the subject through a single large crank with both hands and in a standing position. In the latter case the crank radius and consequently the circle drawn during the performance of the ergonometric tests are much greater than in the former.

The single crank ergometer does not simulate actions regularly performed by athletes in their training, and is therefore not suitable for a specific functional evaluation of athletes. The double crank ergometer can now be considered a specific ergometer for sailing boat crew members of the 12 m International Rating (American Cup). In this discipline some crew members use the 'grinders', real cranks which, through a system of gear change, are used to stretch the sheets of the prow sails.

Simulating ergometer of the kayak canoe (Dal Monte)

This consists of a modification of the double crank ergometer, which uses a common cycle ergometer as the basic device (Fig. 3.4.2). It can be used for the specific functional evaluation of canoers on condition that the normal cranks are replaced by a system capable of reproducing, as closely as possible, the typical movement of the kayak canoe. This is possible if the two cranks are long and placed obliquely, so as to show a gradient simulating the continuity of the paddle oar loom. This is achieved with a system of two blades joined through a central bar, called a loom, of variable length depending on the athlete's height. The ergometer is also provided with a stand on which a seat and a canoe pedalling set are fixed, so that the athlete can be placed in the same position as he or she would take in a boat.

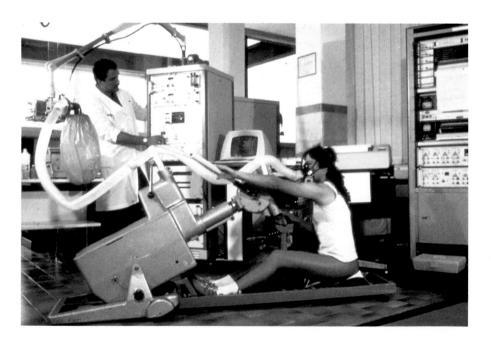

Fig. 3.4.2 Ergometer for the kayak canoe.

Oar ergometer for canoeing (Gjessing– Nilsen)

In this ergometer (Fig. 3.4.3) the rests of the athlete (foot rests and carriage) and their kinematics reproduce exactly those of the boat. The handgrip, set at the end of a sliding bar along an oscillating support, however, can only move on a sagittal plane, whilst the real oars can move around a rotation centre at rowlock level.

The resistance of the oar in the water is simulated by a belt brake winding around a pulley. This pulley uses a 'free' drive system and always turns in the same direction, even during the pickup stage. The propelling force is not directly applied to this pulley but to another one with a spiral-shaped cable where the metal tension rod connected with the handgrip rests. The two pulleys are connected through a drive chain.

The braking force can be adjusted by moving a weight along the traction lever of the belt. This device allows more independence than the set braking torque from friction coefficients and movement speed.

Although the resistance torque is practically constant, the active force

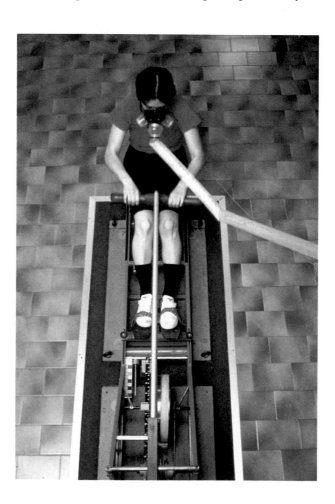

Fig. 3.4.3 Rowing ergometer (Gjessing– Nielsen) for the specific functional evaluation of a rower in a laboratory.

varies according to the position of the handgrip, as an approximate simulation of the variation of the resistance of the oar through the water. In reality this resistance also depends on the kinematics of the athletic movement, so that it is under constant control of the athlete.

Oar ergometer for rowing (Dal Monte)

This is an oar ergometer which allows a reproduction of the specific movement of the rower and, above all, of the oar going through the water. Unlike the oar ergometer of Gjessing, the system reproducing the blade going through the water consists of an actual oar fitted to a rowlock similar to that of a boat. With this, the rower can perform all types of possible movements on the fulcrum of the rowlock itself, just as it works in reality. There is a hydraulic braking system which reproduces the resistance of the oar through the water.

For the evaluation of an athlete it is possible to use either one or two oars, thereby reproducing the two most typical types of rowing—pair oars and double scull.

The force applied on the oar and the inertia movements on the pedals are recorded through strain gauges, whilst the angular variation is recorded on the rowlock with a goniometer. The calculation of the work performed is based on an integration of each individual oar stroke. With this method it is possible to evaluate the force application trend, both regarding quantity and the way it is applied at each moment of time, and not just with an average calculation per minute. Consequently, the performance of the athlete's rowing technique can be assessed in detail, as it would actually take place at a competition.

Ergometer for Canadian canoes (Dal Monte)

This type of ergometer is based on a device in which the athlete takes the same kneeling position as in the boat (Figs 3.4.4 and 3.4.5). The knee of the athlete rests on an anatomic support.

The mechanical reproduction of the specific movement is possible by using a belt braking system winding around a flywheel which will offer resistance when the blade is moved towards the back of the ergometer, but which allows free sliding in the starting phase. The device consists of two 2.5 m tracks, one on each side so that the subject can row on either side of the boat, on each of which, through the articulation, runs a blade. The blade is connected to a cable rotating on two pulleys (one at each end of the track), the first of which is integral with a flywheel. To complete the biomechanical study of the movement, a strain gauge is applied to each blade and this allows an analysis of the force applied at each active phase. A peculiarity of this ergometer is the possibility it affords to evaluate two athletes at the same time, one at each bearing.

Pattern of paddle stoke in strength – time diagram in athletes A and B

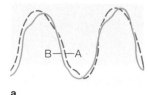

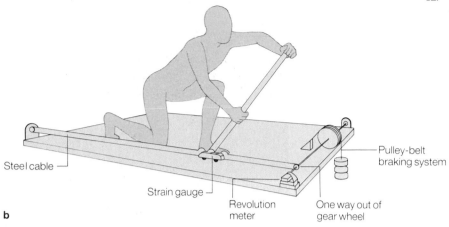

Steel cable

Strain gauge

Revolution meter

One way out of gear wheel

Pulley-belt braking system

a

b

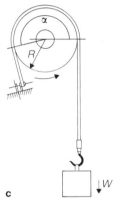

c

Braking torque on the pulley shaft;

$$M = W \cdot R \left(1 - \frac{1}{e^{f\alpha}}\right) \text{ e per } \alpha \gg 0: M = W \cdot R$$

where R = radius; W = weight

Eternal work performed by the athlete =

$$2\pi \cdot W \cdot R \cdot n + 2 \cdot r \cdot n + l \cdot s \cdot m$$

where n = number of turns of pulley;
m = number of strokes; l = length of strokes;
r and s = additional friction coefficients

$\alpha \approx 60'$

d

Reducing all the internal work to the swinging of trunk and head of the work is:

$$0.07\, P \cdot S \cdot (l - \cos \alpha) \cdot m + 6.7 \cdot 10^{-6} \cdot P \cdot S^2 \cdot \alpha_{rad}^2 \cdot m$$

where P = weight of the athlete; S = stature of the athlete; m = number of strokes per minute

Fig. 3.4.4 Diagrams illustrating the functioning of the ergometer for canoeing.

Ergometer for cross-country skiing (Dal Monte)

This device is placed on a treadmill and, to calculate the work performed by the upper limbs, it utilizes the same measurement system as described for the Canadian canoe. The only difference is the force sensor which consists of a linear transducer balanced by a calibrated spring and located near the stick handgrip (Figs 3.4.6 and 3.4.7). For the lower limbs, the device has two ski rollers at the front, two 2.5 m rails preventing lateral deviations during tests and, on the foot supports, two linear transducers to measure the forces acting on the feet.

The test is carried out with the subject skiing on the treadmill at various gradients and at different speeds; the work intensity of the test is achieved through the increase of the gradient and the braking effect of the flywheel. In this way, it is possible to calculate the work of the lower limbs using the formula described in Fig. 3.3.6 in connection with the

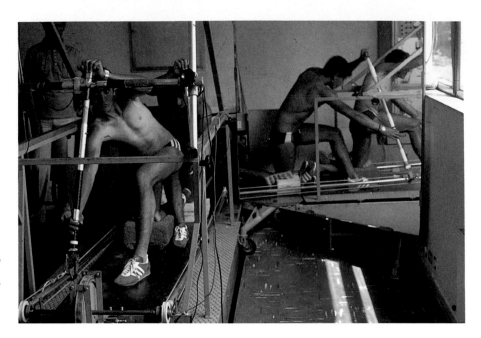

Fig. 3.4.5 Ergometer for canoeing. This instrument can be used simultaneously by two athletes, usually of the same crew. Each athlete works a paddle connected to a strength indicator. This way it is possible to calculate the crew's total work and compare the work of each individual crew member.

treadmill. The work performed by the upper limbs is calculated using the method described for the Canadian canoe ergometer, utilizing the same type of brake. Finally, the total work can be found by combining the mechanical energy produced by both upper and lower limbs.

Ergometers for swimming

The functional evaluation of swimming involves particular technical difficulties, which has led to the development of especially adapted ergometers. Amongst these is a very simple and cheap one—the Dal Monte type—with which it is possible to carry out work tests in the water of a normal swimming pool. At the same time the swimmer is kept in the closest possible conditions to those of real swimming.

In this system the athlete performs work tests covering the typical aspects of swimming. It consists of a counterweight which the swimmer has to keep in balance with the thrust of the different swimming styles (crawl, back-stroke, breast-stroke, dolphin-stroke). The brake, or counterweight, hangs from a rope wound around a large diameter pulley. The resistance is calculated according to the body surface, using the same technique as that for the calculation of the resistance in a submerged hull by the length/volume ratio.

The ergometric pools are more sophisticated and flexible. An example of these ergometers is the circular pool where the subject swims in a ring of water with a stable stand in the middle bearing the recording devices for the metabolic parameters. The best known swimming ergometer is

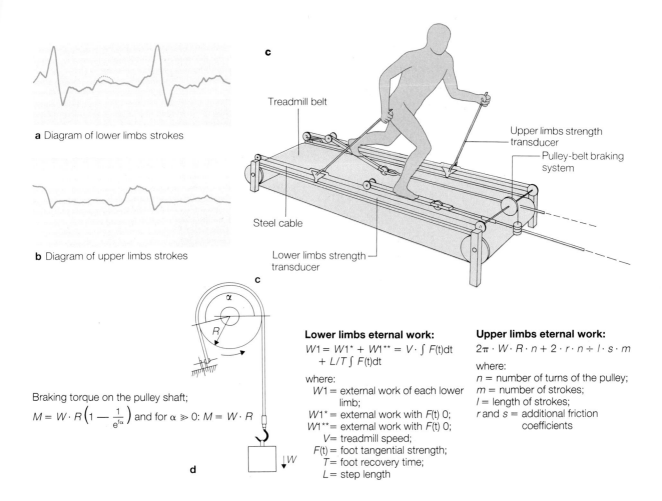

a Diagram of lower limbs strokes

b Diagram of upper limbs strokes

Treadmill belt

Upper limbs strength transducer

Pulley-belt braking system

Steel cable

Lower limbs strength transducer

Braking torque on the pulley shaft;

$$M = W \cdot R \left(1 - \frac{1}{e^{f\alpha}}\right) \text{ and for } \alpha \gg 0: M = W \cdot R$$

Lower limbs eternal work:

$$W1 = W1^* + W1^{**} = V \cdot \int F(t)dt + L/T \int F(t)dt$$

where:

$W1$ = external work of each lower limb;
$W1^*$ = external work with $F(t)$ 0;
$W1^{**}$ = external work with $F(t)$ 0;
V = treadmill speed;
$F(t)$ = foot tangential strength;
T = foot recovery time;
L = step length

Upper limbs eternal work:

$$2\pi \cdot W \cdot R \cdot n + 2 \cdot r \cdot n \div l \cdot s \cdot m$$

where:

n = number of turns of the pulley;
m = number of strokes;
l = length of strokes;
r and s = additional friction coefficients

Fig. 3.4.6 Diagram illustrating the functioning of the ergometer for cross-country skiing.

the Stockholm Swimming Flume which can be defined as a water treadmill. In this ergometer, in fact, it is the water that moves under the thrust of propellers in a longitudinal direction and the swimmer, swimming against the current, is in reality always in the same position relative to the outside and, therefore, also to the laboratory instruments.

At the Physiology and Biomechanics Department of the Sport Science Institute of Rome, there is a model of an ergonometric pool designed by Dal Monte; this is the final model of a design presented for the first time in 1964 (Fig. 3.4.8). This device consists of an open-water pipe section (measuring 6.70 × 3 m) with fluid put in motion by four fans connected to a 240 hp (180 kW) BMW boat engine. In this case, too, the swimmer moves in the opposite direction to the water so that in relation to the sides of the ergonometric pool he or she remains still. On a side section of the pool there is a special crystal window (measuring 2 × 1 m) from

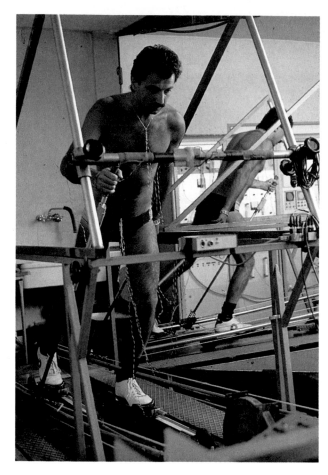

Fig. 3.4.7 Ergometer for cross-country skiing. This instrument allows the measurement of work by each limg (superior or inferior) using a linear vertical displacement transducer applied on the 'ski roller' and on the sticks. It is possible to evaluate the modulation and type of force applied.

which it is possible to observe and, if required, to film the movement of the athlete under the floating surface. It is also possible to connect the subject, through a telescopic arm and an inhalation mask, with an ergospirographic device to evaluate the metabolic and cardiovascular parameters in stress conditions. This pool is also used for other types of sports, such as flipper swimming, canoeing and windsurfing (Fig. 3.4.9).

Parameters recorded during functional testing

During exercise tests, many parameters can be recorded:

1 Continuous heart rate, recorded either by analogic graph or by digital counter. The heart rate (Fc) during muscular exercise is an extremely useful datum to indicate cardiovascular behaviour during: (a) nonspecific

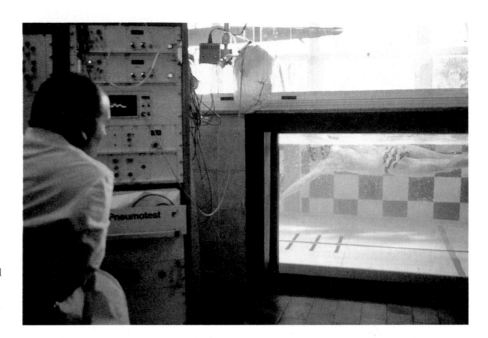

Fig. 3.4.8 Ergometric pool functioning in the Institute of Sport Science (Department of Physiology and Biomechanics).

ergonometric tests (step tests and similar); (b) specific tests based on a simulation of the disciplines practiced; or (c) field training.

2 Electrocardiogram, through which it is possible to keep under constant control the electric activity of the heart. Parameters include morphology and rate, as well as rhythm and re-polarization troubles.

3 Lung ventilation, with an analogue recorder of the ventilation flow. Lung ventilation does not, however, seem to represent a limit for agonistic performances of any duration and intensity, although it should still be considered carefully. In fact, if the litres of air ventilated through the lungs per unit of time is even, the energy cost of lung ventilation can vary remarkably in relation to the amplitude of the respiration act and to their rate. This therefore affects performance. The incidence of fatigue of respiration muscles is also presently being evaluated as a performance-limiting factor.

4 Oxygen uptake ($\dot{V}_{O_2}$), through an analyser capable of continuous and linear functioning, or possibly without long gaps or with known and set gaps, so that correct calculations can be made in connection with ventilation and heart rate. This expresses the oxidation processes taking place in the muscles. The oxygen uptake can vary in relation to the duration and intensity of the test. In fact, it is a well known fact that the highest oxygen uptake is achieved through rapidly exhaustive tests which also imply a very rapid accumulation of lactic acid and, obviously, a rapid exhaustion of the working capacity of the athlete. In some cases,

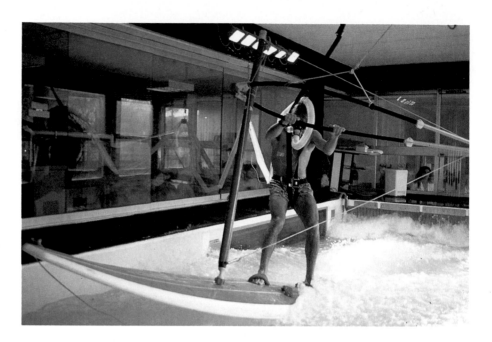

Fig. 3.4.9 Functional evaluation test of windsurfing in an ergometric pool.

especially for long-distance athletes who rarely utilize all their aerobic power, it is better to keep under control the systolic blood pressure (SBP) and the performance of the specific gesture, that is the energy cost of distance covered (in metres) by kg of bodyweight.

5   Production of carbon dioxide ($\dot{V}CO_2$), through an analyzer, again linear and continuous, presenting the same functional characteristics required for the oxygen analyser. The quantity of carbon dioxide produced can, within certain limits, give indications of the amount of lactic acid accumulated to be expelled. In fact, according to some researchers, the passage of the respiratory quotient (CO_2/O_2) from values inferior or equal to one to higher values, indicates that work is made not only through energy sources of the oxidating type, the aerobic sources, but also through a massive intervention of the anaerobic lactic acid sources.

6   Respiration flow, for the purposes of evaluating the economics and rationality of the ventilation of the lungs, through a pneumotachograph, again with linear and analogous action, recording continuously.

7   Blood lactate before, during and after the effort. The quantity of blood lactate is the only functional test involving a surgical act; this is presently used in most functional laboratories where athlete evaluations are being carried out. Obviously, it is fundamental in the SBP evaluation and in the evaluation of the functional possibilities of glycolytic metabolism.

8   The work done. For tests based on constant resistance ergometers

(oar ergometers, cycle ergometers, etc.) or for tests in which it is difficult or impossible to measure a metabolic parameter (ATP/CP) directly; it is the quantity of work done by the subject which has to be measured. Therefore the mechanical power is measured, which is considered to be the indirect expression of an athlete's metabolic and contractile muscular qualities. In constant resistance ergometers the work done is the ratio between such resistance, in general the torque necessary to overcome the sliding friction of a band on the surface of a flywheel, and the number of the turns made by the flywheel. In other cases, as in jumping and uphill races, the work is the product of bodyweight and displacement, against gravity, of the centre of gravity.

From these basic parameters it is possible to obtain the derived indexes, that is $\dot{V}_{O_2}/Fc$, $\dot{V}_{O_2}/kg$, R (respiratory exchange ratio), the respiration equivalent and the ratio between pneumotachogram and V, the mechanical power.

It should be noted that the parameter, $\dot{V}_{O_2}/kg$, is much more important than the absolute $\dot{V}_{O_2}$ when subjects are evaluated for sports involving elevation of their centre of gravity during the movement. In fact, in this case, the bodyweight becomes a limiting factor and must be considered when evaluating aerobic power.

The conventional recording method of associated ventilation and metabolic parameters, based on the collection of exhaled air in Douglas bags and its subsequent analysis through Haldane, Van Slyke or Shollander devices, is ill-suited to investigations following individual trends of athletes subjected to maximal ergonometric tests, which are often necessary to test top athletes.

Even if, from the point of view of the evaluation of athletes, the precision of data obtained with the Haldane device is technically and conceptually perfect, many researchers tend to prefer open circuit devices which are less precise, but present many advantages such as:

1   The possibility of utilizing extremely light breathing masks which are less bothersome and have a lower respiration resistance when the ventilation flow is very high.
2   The absence of two or four big, heavy and cumbersome corrugated pipes.
3   Continuous detection and recording in real time of the gas exchanges and of the metabolic costs.
4   The continuous and linear detection of lung ventilation.
5   The possibility of using, at the same time, the pneumotachogram graph.

Laboratory tests

Alactacid anaerobic metabolism

In spite of the many sports conditioned by aerobic metabolism, less attention has, in general, been paid to the extent of anaerobic power and capacity than to aerobic metabolism. Alactacid anaerobic capacity and power is the energy source most difficult to examine.

For an evaluation of the quantity of high-energy phosphates and of the enzymes causing their breakdown, the only direct methods presently available are muscular biopsy and, in part, nuclear magnetic resonance (NMR). The first method involves a surgical act and is not easy to carry out due to technical complexities and, sometimes, due to legal obstacles. The second method is too costly at present. For these reasons the tests used are those that indirectly evaluate the alactacid anaerobic power through the detection of the greatest quantity of work done in very short periods of time (up to 5 s). Some of these tests are: the Margaria step test; the cycle ergometer test of Cumming which lasts 30 s; the explosive power test with only one pedal stroke on 150° of angular movement (Ayalon); the Ergo jump 15 s test suggested by Bosco, or a modification of it suggested by the Institute of Sports Science; and the thrust test on the treadmill suggested by Dal Monte.

Margaria step test

This test bases the evaluation of the maximum alactacid power on the duration of time used to climb, two steps at a time, a 14-step stair as fast as possible, taking the time (t) used to climb from the third to the ninth step. The known data are the weight of the subject (F) and the height of the stair (S); it is then possible to obtain the mechanical power ($F \times S \times t-1$).

Ayalon test

The test suggested by Ayalon consists of an evaluation of the time used to perform half a pedal turn (more exactly 150°) with the left leg on the pedal of a set couple cycle ergometer braked by a load which can be set (2.9 kg) or proportional to the bodyweight of each athlete. The known parameters in this test are the resistance (F) applied to the flywheel and the space covered (S) equal to half the circumference of the flywheel.

Cumming test

The test suggested by Cumming consists of pedalling from a standing position on a set couple cycle ergometer, either with set resistance or, as in a later version, proportional to the bodyweight of the athlete, for 30 s at top speed. The highest alactacid anaerobic power is evaluated through the number of pushes on the pedals made in the fastest 5 s. In this case, the known data are force (F) and time, whilst the space (S) covered is to be found (number of pedal pushes × flywheel circumference).

Ergo jump 15 s   The test suggested by Bosco (Ergo jump 15 s) evaluates the mechanical power of the leg extensor muscles. The test consists of the evaluation of the off-the-ground time with a digital watch, Ergo jump (+/−0.000 s), during a series of vertical jumps executed one after the other for 15 s. The jumps are made on a plate connected to the timer and which automatically open and close the circuit.

To calculate the average power, the following formula can be used:

$$\text{Power } (W) = \frac{g^2 \times Tv \times 15\,s}{4 \times NS \times (15\,s - Tv)}$$

where $g = 9.81$, being the gravitational constant; Tv = total off-the-ground time automatically recorded by the timer; 15 s = total working time; NS = number of jumps performed; $15\,s - Tv$ = total time on the ground. During the short moments of contact with the plate, at each jump, the subject must bend his or her legs to make, with the knee, an angle of around 90°.

The modified Ergo jump 15 s consists of two trials in which the subject must perform jumps and their countermovements, without interruption, for 15 s. The two trials differ in the type of loading, which is short for one, with a thrust time equal to approximately 120 ms, and ample in the other, with a thrust time of approximately 270 ms. The two series of jumps are necessary to allow comparisons to be made, normalizing values at 120 ms and 270 ms through a linear regression, of the data, including subjects who performed the jumps with different thrust times.

It is possible to calculate a series of parameters relative to the performance, and the most significant ones are: the average height reached in the jumps, the average work performed, and the average power generated.

Dal Monte test   The Dal Monte test is based on the evaluation of the heaviest thrust applied by a subject, whilst running on an uphill (10%) treadmill ergometer, on a dynamometric bar placed before him/her. The duration of the test has been set at 5 s, and the position of the dynamometric bar has been experimentally set at the level of the centre of gravity of the body. The test is performed three times at the treadmill sliding speeds, which are different each time (2, 3 and 4 m/s).

The work done during the test is calculated by analyzing the dynamometric diagrams recorded and considering the lift of the bodyweight and the mechanical performance of the uphill racer. The choice of three different racing speeds offers all subjects the possibility of generating muscular power according to the best neuromotor pattern of each.

Lactacid anaerobic metabolism

What has been said concerning the evaluation of the alactacid anaerobic metabolism is also valid for lactacid anaerobic metabolism. In fact the methods commonly used are few: the evaluation of the quantity of oxygen debt (slow component), the evaluation of lactate concentration in the blood and in the muscles and, in the same way as above, the evaluation of the quantity of work done during tests of average duration (30–60 s).

The indirect evaluation of the lactic acid accumulated by the athlete during a functional test can be obtained collecting the air exhaled over a rather long period of time and starting from the moment the effort stopped. In this way it is possible to calculate, with checks carried out at short intervals, the decreasing curve of the lactic acid through the oxygen uptake in excess of the oxygen uptake of the athlete at rest.

The oxygen uptake of the athlete per unit of time before the work test, represents, with good approximation, his/her metabolism at rest. The difference of the two quantities of oxygen uptake gives, therefore, an acceptable evaluation of the oxygen debt incurred. In order to extract from the total debt the percentage of the lactacid debt, it is necessary to subtract the alactacid component which is much smaller quantitatively than the lactacid one.

In fact this evaluation is a rather gross approximation as it does not consider certain important aspects such as the quantity of lactate which becomes oxidized during rest, the result of the resynthesis of glycogen, the alterations of basic metabolism after the effort, the reforming of oxygen supplies in the tissues and blood, and the energy cost of ventilation and cardiac activity, which also remain high at rest.

In conclusion, it can be considered that the oxygen debt, or the oxygen uptake at rest, does not only reflect the action of the metabolism of the test, but also all those re-adaptation processes which occur during the period of rest.

The following tests are used in the indirect evaluation of lactacid accumulation. A number of other tests have been proposed in order to evaluate anaerobic metabolism; most of these take into consideration the time of exhaustion in a constant lead test (Curetou, 1951; Cummingham & Faulkner, 1969; Thomson & Garvie, 1981; Schuabel & Kindermann, 1983).

Wingate test

This test is a new version of the 30 s one suggested by Cumming in which the resistance load of the cycle ergometer was independent from the bodyweight. In the Wingate test performed on a set couple cycle ergometer, the load is equal to 40 g/kg bodyweight in the Fleish ergometer

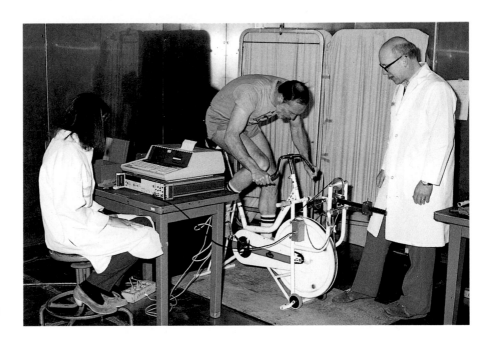

Fig. 3.4.10 The Wingate anaerobic test involves cycling against a predetermind resistance force as rapidly as possible for a period of 30 s.

and 75 g/kg bodyweight in the Monark ergometer. The subject must pedal for 30 s at top speed and the number of pedal pushes is recorded every 5 s (Fig. 3.4.10). Since the average braking couple and the number of pedal pushes are known, it is possible to calculate the average power of each fraction of 5 s and the total power. According to some researchers the test should be performed starting from a condition of rest, whilst others maintain that the subject must be pedalling (up to 100 revolutions/min) before the load is applied and the test starts.

Modified Wingate test The test is performed with the athlete pedalling for 30 s with a set load, which can vary according to the bodyweight of the subject, on a cycle ergometer (Dal Monte) built in such a way that the couple applied to the pedals and the pedalling rate can be directly measured. With these two parameters it is possible to calculate the power of the subject moment by moment. Computer processing gives the power applied to overcome the electromagnetic resistance and the power necessary to overcome the braking force represented by the flywheel inertia. The values obtained with this test are normally higher than those obtained with the conventional Wingate test as the latter does not consider either the additional friction or the inertia of the flywheel, which is only partly eliminated by allowing the athlete to start the flywheel before the beginning of the test.

Capillary blood samples are taken before and after the test to find the quantity of lactic acid produced.

With the data recorded during the test it is possible to evaluate:

1 The maximum power, presumably due to the alactacid anaerobic mechanism (see the alactacid anaerobic power test).
2 The average power, heavily conditioned by the lactacid anaerobic mechanism.
3 The decrease in total power which is a function of the special lactacid resistance of the subject.

Ergo jump 60 s This test is identical to the Ergo jump 15 s test but its duration (60 s) is such that it mainly refers to the lactacid anaerobic metabolism. Recently, research is being conducted into the convenience of reducing the duration of the test to 45 s to obtain values more closely related to the 'power' of lactacid metabolism. It has been found that most subjects in the 60 s test show a rapid and considerable reduction in performance after 45 s. This is probably due to the difficulty of withstanding lactate levels which are already high after the first 45 s of the test.

Moritani test The Moritani test, described in the paragraph concerning the laboratory measurement of the anaerobic threshold (below), makes it possible to obtain, according to its author, the value of the total anaerobic capacity of the athlete.

Aerobic metabolism Tests conducted under stress for the evaluation of aerobic metabolism can be performed subjecting the athlete to maximal or below maximal work. It is better to use maximal work tests if the objective is to examine the adapting capacity of the various organs and systems involved in muscular work when under maximum stress. If, however, the objective of the test is to show the progressive adaptation to submaximal loads (as in long-distance running) or to those typical of the sport practiced, it is preferable to use submaximal tests or tests simulating the competition. It is also advisable to use submaximal tests in the case of unhealthy subjects when it would be dangerous to use high workloads.

In particular, especially for maximal tests, it is important to consider the following aspects.

Performance technique Certain customary rules must be abided by: the athlete must be subjected to the test only if in perfect physical condition, well rested, if no alcohol or drugs have been taken recently and if he or she has not smoked. It is also necessary to perform some practice tests on the ergometer chosen, so that the subject becomes familiar with the device, the environment and the personnel. A warm-up period of 5–10 min is needed before the test starts.

The laboratory climatic conditions must be kept comfortable and constant; it is advisable that temperature does not exceed 20°C, that humidity is such as to allow good evaporation (40–50%) and that the air is not still, in order to avoid interference in the test caused by an excessive rise in the body core temperature. For longer tests, the American College of Sports Medicine recommends that the WBGT temperature (0.7 WB temp. + 0.2 black globe temp. + 0.1 DB temp.) should not exceed 28°C.

Specificity As indicated in the first part of the chapter (ergometers) the author is convinced that, to obtain a true evaluation of the athletic qualities of a subject with an ergospirographic test, the subject must perform the test simulating as closely as possible the typical movements that are performed during competition. The results of the evaluation tests carried out on swimmers (treadmill and pool) and canoers (crank ergometer and kayak) are also significant.

There is no doubt that sports activities indicate specific adaptations in the human body, and therefore these adaptations must also be studied just as specifically.

Test procedure Since functional evaluation is a very new discipline, the procedures applied to the tests suggested so far are as numerous as the researchers who have tried them.

In general, in maximal tests, both in tests interrupted when the maximum $\dot{V}_{O_2}$ is reached and when carried on to exhaustion, the triangular method is used. With this method the load is increased by a previously set step every 2 or 3 min. There are, however, differences concerning the quantity and the methods of increasing the load; for example, many researchers prefer to increase the treadmill load raising the treadmill rather than increasing the speed. In the same way there is a considerable difference in the quantity of watts increased at each step in tests carried out with cycle ergometers.

In the author's opinion, when higher functional levels of the athlete have to be reached, it is advisable to use methods with short-lasting steps (2 min) with big load increases. To define the moment when the test should be interrupted, it is important to establish if exhaustion of the subject has to be reached, thereby evaluating the maximum quantity of work which the athlete can perform and his or her capacity to accumulate lactate. In other cases it is better to interrupt the test according to a previously set trend of a certain parameter, for example, reaching a V_{O_2} plateau combined with continuous increases of power output.

In both cases, there are certain aspects which may invalidate the results obtained and which must be considered. For example, not all authors agree on the fact that during a test based on the increase of power output it is possible to reach a $\dot{V}_{O_2}$ plateau which can be considered as the maximum $\dot{V}_{O_2}$. On the other hand, there is no doubt that the capacity of a subject to bear fatigue depends largely on his/her psychic qualities and on the desire to 'participate' fully in the test.

In laboratory submaximal tests these problems do not arise because the exercise intensity is not exhausting in the short run, and because the object of the test is essentially that of evaluating the adaptation of the oxygen transportation and diffusion system as well as the performance of the technical movement without, therefore, investigating the maximum performance capacity of the athlete. The evaluation of maximum $\dot{V}_{O_2}$ is very useful when a research project is aimed at the analysis of the qualities necessary for a specific sports discipline, or when young athletes are tested for selection. On the other hand, however, the maximum $\dot{V}_{O_2}$ is not useful as a parameter when top athlete training programmes have to be set out.

To perform this evaluation, according to different objectives, the following tests can be utilized:

1   Triangular tests: tests with stepwise increases in intensity and duration to the point at which maximum acceptable intensity or the maximum $\dot{V}_{O_2}$ ($\dot{V}_{O_2}$ plateau?) is reached.
2   Rectangular tests: the athlete is subjected to one exercise intensity only, to be maintained as long as possible.
3   Trapeziform tests: the athlete is subjected to increasing exercise intensities, as in the triangular test and then, once the desired heart rate is reached or when the required exercise intensity is kept for a previously set time, he/she is subjected to a stable intensity.
4   Periodic load tests: the athlete must perform successive phases of rectangular tests with rest periods between tests.
5   Increasing intensity tests: with rest periods between one intensity and the next.
6   Time tests: the athlete must produce 'maximum power' in a period defined previously which usually corresponds to the average duration of a competition.

Particularly interesting is the possibility of subjecting the athlete, at least for some disciplines (e.g. rowing), to two tests: a non-specific one, of the increasing load type, to verify aerobic power; and the other, of the time type, which, performed on an oar ergometer, simulates the competition making it possible to verify the real involvement, in the discipline practised, of the metabolic systems of the athlete.

In the Physiology and Biomechanics Department of the Sport Science Institute, besides the conventional and non-specific triangular and trapeziform tests, it is possible to use a series of specific sports tests which attempt to simulate the competition, with aspecific ergometer and competition times.

The indications supplied so far concern laboratory tests carried out with $\dot{V}_{O_2}$ direct control methods. In the laboratory, indirect, submaximal tests can also be conducted to obtain the $\dot{V}_{O_2}$. They will be described in the section on field tests below.

The anaerobic threshold The only method to establish the anaerobic threshold is to get the subject to exercise for a number of rather long periods of time (at least 30 min), each time at constant intensity and taking the lactic acid blood level periodically during each test. Obviously, when intensities higher than the anaerobic threshold are reached, the athlete will finish the test with progressively accumulating lactate, or, if the chosen intensity is very high the athlete may stop before the test has ended. If the intensity is lower or just reaches threshold intensity, the athlete will be able to terminate the test without having accumulated lactic acid.

Such methods of evaluation are, however, impractical because they require a series of attempts before defining accurately the correct threshold value. It is not therefore possible to use it for athletes. The suggested techniques are based, in general, on increasing intensity tests.

Wasserman was the first to suggest the variations observed in the ventilation trend. Ventilation, during an increasing power production test, increases at a linear ratio, as compared with exercise intensity, up to a point beyond which the ventilation increase becomes clearly greater and out of proportion with the oxygen requirements of the body. According to Wasserman this depends on the fact that the increased production of carbon dioxide and the decrease of pH (index of increased blood acidity), consequent to the accumulation of lactic acid, which occur beyond the threshold, stimulate the control mechanisms of ventilation.

Other suggestions have been made and they are all based on Wasserman's original idea—that is on ventilation variations—as this is a parameter strictly related to internal metabolic balances.

The study of the lactic acid blood level curve using the increasing intensity test is now considered to be logical as the test is directly related to the phenomenon being measured. In the past, however, it was not accepted by many researchers because of the technical difficulties connected with blood sample taking, and because of the impossibility of identifying a standard value to use as a reference point.

In 1976 Mader suggested, on the basis of empirical observations, that the value of 4 mmol/l should be considered as the point on the lactic acid blood level curve corresponding to the crossing of the anaerobic threshold.

Still utilizing the lactic acid blood level curve caused by work, Stegman and Bunc perfected two methods for the definition of individual anaerobic thresholds. Both these researchers used the criterion of curve tangents. For further clarification on the methods used see the original texts.

In 1982, Karlsson, in a critical review concerning the anaerobic threshold problem, presented with great precision the OBLA (onset blood lactate accumulation) concept. He stated that the threshold should be taken—always during an increasing exercise intensity test—at the OBLA point, maintaining that this point can be understood as:

1   A sudden increase of the lactic acid blood level as compared to the trend of submaximal load values.
2   An increase in the lactic acid blood level as compared to a standard value (e.g. 2 mmol/l) considered as an indication of basal conditions.
3   A standard value fixed in advance (4 mmol/l).

A further method for the definition of the anaerobic threshold is suggested by Moritani. This method consists of three different tests on the cycle ergometer, each with a constant power production differing from the other two. The duration of the test is recorded, that is the longest period during which the athlete is able to maintain a certain pedalling rate (fixed in advance). Since the power and the duration of the test is known, it is possible to calculate the work done by the subject.

If the three points (corresponding to the time and the work of each test) are placed on a system of cartesian axes with time on the x axis and the work done on the y axis, it is possible to identify a line represented by the equation:

(Work limit = $a + b \times$ time limit).

The line thus drawn intercepts the y axis at a point higher than zero (value a in the equation).

According to Moritani, this value gives an indication of the anaerobic capacity, that is of the quantity of work that the subject can produce using only the anaerobic mechanisms. It is also evident that a character-istic of this line is the inclination on the x axis. This characteristic, represented by the *b* coefficient of the equation points, indicates the power corresponding to the anaerobic threshold, that is to the intensity of exercise that can be accepted without any accumulation of lactic acid.

One particular laboratory application, with immediate implications in the field, is currently being tested in the Institute of Sport Science using the ergometric pool. The swimmer is asked to swim to exhaustion at three speeds fixed in advance. Once the time taken has been recorded, it is possible to relate it to the distance covered.

Force   In the field of sports medicine, the evaluation of force must conform, essentially, with trainers' requirements. It is advisable, therefore, that tests should be aimed at the analysis of these various ways of expressing force even if the usual definitions of force used by sports technicians do not correspond to physiological definitions.

Force should essentially be seen in its mechanical aspects, considering the speed of displacement (acceleration $= a$) of a mass (m) from which the intensity of the force (F) to be applied can be derived; that is $F = ma$. On the basis of this formula, it is possible to identify:

1 Shear force: the m component prevails (resistance to be overcome, e.g. weight lifting).
2 Fast force: the a component prevails (high performance speed, e.g. jumps).
3 Endurance force: neither component prevails (average intensity and speed, e.g. rowing).

Shear force should be considered both as an absolute force, that is the maximum force which can be expressed by the athlete, and as a relative force, that is in relation to bodyweight.

Isometric dynamometry   The dynamometer is used to measure shear force and is described in detail on pp. 112–113. The force output of a single muscular group, however, cannot be used to evaluate the overall capacity of an athlete and a dynamometric global index based on the sthenics of a number of muscular groups has therefore been suggested. According to Dal Monte, the dynamometric global index is given by the sum of the dynamometric values of: the finger flexors, the muscles that lower the shoulder (according to Bethe), the lower limb extensors, and the back extensors.

If, instead of a global evaluation, the objective is the evaluation of a particular muscular group specifically subjected to a training process, the dynamometric test should be applied to that particular muscular group and, whenever possible, it should be carried out with the subject in a competition position.

Isometric dynamography

Using an isometric dynamometer it is possible to measure several parameters, which can be used in the analysis of the capacity of rapid muscular contraction (see p. 113).

Concentric contraction dynamography

Isokinetic dynamometers are used to measure concentric muscular contractions, which complements the above isometric measurements and provides a more complete picture of muscular mechanisms (see pp. 113–114).

Force–velocity curve

The *F–V* curve of a given muscular group can be constructed using the above measurements, and is useful in identifying muscular typology of athletes and in analysing effects of training. For fuller details see pp. 114–115.

Field tests

Besides the functional evaluation performed in the laboratory, another type of evaluation is being used more and more frequently, and this is performed on the athletes directly on the training field. Field tests can be performed without the complex devices and the specialized personnel which are a basic requirement for laboratory tests, and can be carried out more frequently. As a rule, they only require simple devices or measuring systems (tape measures, timers); sometimes instruments have to be more complex but they are always cheap and easy to use. Since the tests are easy to repeat, they can be used for long-term surveys looking at the trends of investigated parameters over time. This can be especially useful in verifying the effects of a certain type of training.

However, when a functional evaluation of top athletes is undertaken, some field tests requiring extremely complex investigations will need to be performed. In order to improve performance, specific physiological and biomechanical adaptations have to be investigated and analyzed, and the necessary measurements can be obtained only by direct evaluations made on the competition field. For these purposes, it is therefore necessary that tests are essentially competition tests or, in any event, such as to allow a study of physiological (heart rate, lactate, $\dot{V}O_2$, etc.) or biomechanical (force, velocity, acceleration, displacements, etc.) parameters at the moment when the athletes perform their exercises.

In the Physiology and Biomechanics Department of the Institute of Sport Science, in order to carry out this research, a mobile laboratory has

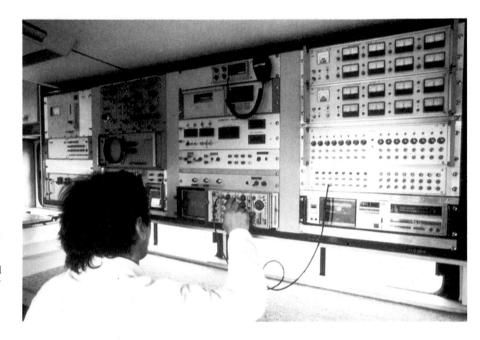

Fig. 3.4.11 View of the inside of the second mobile unit from the Institute of Sport Science, showing some of the apparatus used for respiratory tests and for the survey, printing and monitoring of radio-transmitted data.

been set up. This laboratory receives information supplied by sensors placed on the body or equipment of the athletes through the radio and records it on tape (Fig. 3.4.11). This system can obviously be used only for a few top athletes, whilst conventional field tests have wider applications.

Alactacid anaerobic metabolism

This area has attracted no particular interest on the part of physiologists. The Margaria step test and Bosco Ergo jump 15 s (see above) can be considered field tests in terms of their simplicity and cheapness. Another test to be considered for the evaluation of this energy system is short-distance sprinting (30–50 cm). This is a complex athletic exercise for which both motor coordination and rapidity of movement are extremely important, but with which it is possible, through a simple time-measuring operation, to obtain an evaluation parameter which is easy to check and showing with acceptable precision the amount of quickly available energy of the subject.

Lactacid anaerobic metabolism

In the field evaluation of this energy system for which, as for alactacid tests, no sufficient investigations have been carried out so far, it is possible to use some of the tests already described, like the Ergo jump 60 s and the Moritani test. The latter, which was created as a laboratory test, is presently being subjected to a series of checks for its use on the field.

A specific evaluation test can be the performance of racing trials on set distances lasting between about 30 and 60 s (200–1000 m according to the speciality), with blood samples taken for an analysis of the lactate produced. This type of method can supply data on the efficiency of the lactacid system and, with suitable follow-ups, on the possible modifications occurring due to training activities. It is obvious that this type of test requires the use of systems for the analysis of the lactic acid accumulated. These systems, however, can be carried out with portable devices easy to find on the market.

Aerobic metabolism

Maximal tests

1   *Cooper test.* A conventional field test for the evaluation of physical fitness is the 12 min Cooper test. This test must be mentioned because it is extremely popular, but it is not free from drawbacks because it belongs to the maximal test category and requires a total and exhaustive participation on the part of the athlete tested. The parameter taken is the longest distance which can be covered by an athlete in 12 min, a parameter which is considered to be the expression of the aerobic power of the athlete. Although, according to the author, the test should be a self-evaluation on the part of the subject under examination, it should be noted that only individuals well trained for racing can find their own rhythm and are psychologically prepared for a really maximal performance. Also, the duration of the test and the effort required necessarily imply an involvement of the lactacid metabolism, so that this test cannot be considered as an exclusively aerobic one. In conclusion, then, this test is not advisable, as originally intended, for subjects of any age. And, as a maximal test it subjects the cardiocirculatory system of untrained subjects to efforts which cannot be considered 'physiological'.

2   *Shuttle or Léger test.* This is a test of the 'increasing loads' type (1 min steps) performed over a distance of 20 m, achieved by running backwards and forwards. The test comes to an end when the subject has reached exhaustion point; the evaluation of $\dot{V}_{O_2 \text{ max}}$ is made on the basis of the highest velocity reached. This test is based, in the same way as the Cooper test, on the observation (Cavagna–Margaria) that the energy cost of the race for each kg of bodyweight does not depend on velocity and, therefore, that a higher speed corresponds to a higher aerobic power. The same limitations apply as do in the Cooper test.

Submaximal tests   Some authors have created some nomographs for an indirect calculation of $\dot{V}_{O_2}$ based on the supposedly linear ratio between $\dot{V}_{O_2}$ and Fc. With this method it is possible to define Fc in one or two submaximal tests (with simple ergometers—step tests or cycle ergometers) lasting sufficiently long to reach a steady state (3–5 min). The mechanical power produced by the subject and its metabolic equivalent being known, the $\dot{V}_{O2\ max}$ can be extrapolated on the basis of the Fc_{max} of that subject (evaluated according to age).

The nomographs are rather approximate as they are conditioned by two assumptions which are not always constant for all subjects:

1   The linear ratio between heart rate and $\dot{V}_{O2}$ at maximal rates.
2   The energy cost of the exercise chosen.

Indirect methods for the definition of $\dot{V}_{O2\ max}$ are particularly suited for quick selections carried out on large populations or to obtain differential measurements of $\dot{V}_{O2\ max}$ on the same subjects in different experimental or environmental conditions.

Amongst the best known nomograms are the Åstrand and Margaria nomograms. The former is based on the detection of heart rate in only one exercise test. The standard error in this predicting method for the maximum oxygen uptake in submaximal exercises is approximately 10% for individuals of the same age and sufficiently well trained. It increases to 15% for individuals with little training and belonging to different age groups, even if the age-correcting factor is used in the calculation of $\dot{V}_{O2\ max}$. Untrained subjects are often underestimated, whilst athletes in their best form tend to be overestimated.

In the Margaria nomogram, heart rate is detected during two or more moderate or submaximal exercises.

Defining the anaerobic threshold   1   The Conconi test is based on the definition of the ratio between locomotion velocity and heart rate in athletes subjected to increasing loads in track or road tests. The anaerobic threshold is represented by the point (defined as deflection velocity, vd, or starting heart rate, Fci) where this ratio changes from linear to curvilinear.

Up to now this test, which is carried out in the same typical training and competition conditions of the various sports disciplines, has been used for racing, marching, cross-country skiing, cycling, roller skating, ice skating, canoeing and rowing.

It has been proved (Conconi) that vd is correlated with the average velocity of middle-distance and long-distance competitions. vd, and even more Fci, is conveniently used to personalize training work.

Conconi's test, which shows ample correlations with SBP, measured with several constant load tests for 30 min ($R^2 = 0.80$), in an experiment conducted at the Institute, does not always give objective results as it requires the subjective action of an operator to define the deflection point. It is also required that athletes subjected to this test have gained familiarity with it.

2 The Moritani (modified) test is aimed at defining the anaerobic threshold or the critical power, with reference to the maximum power which can be produced by muscles with the energy created by aerobic processes only. As previously indicated this is a laboratory test which some authors (Mognoni) have tried to use on the field. Modified in this way it consists of the performance of at least three separate tests at the highest possible speed, each a different distance, but such that the racing time varies between 40 and 300 s.

Placing the data on a system of cartesian axes, with time as the x coordinate and the distance covered on the y coordinate, it is possible to obtain a line crossing the y coordinate at a point over zero (value a in the equation, see above). In field tests, as in laboratory ones, value a should indicate the anaerobic power, that is the quantity of work which the subject can produce using only anaerobic mechanisms. It is equally clear that this line is characterized also by its inclination on the x coordinate. This characteristic, represented by coefficient b in the equation, indicates the power corresponding to the anaerobic threshold, that is the intensity of work which can be borne without an accumulation of lactic acid.

Further checks on this test are presently being carried out to verify its reliability and validity on the field.

Alternate aerobic–anaerobic metabolism

Those sports, defined as alternate or mixed, in which more metabolic mechanisms are present in varying intensity and duration, are difficult to evaluate in their entirety because of the impossibility of distinguishing the action of the various metabolisms. Two field tests have been devised at the Institute of Sport Science for the purpose of evaluating the basic qualities of athletes in these sports:

1 Capacity of producing high levels of muscular power.
2 Capacity of quick recovery after performance.
3 Capacity of repeating the same performance after a short interval of time.

Dal Monte five sprints test

This test is made up of five sprints, from standing starts, over distances of 50 m for men and 40 m for women and goal-keepers (for certain team games), to be covered at the highest possible speed at intervals of 1 min one after the other.

The parameters taken are the following:

1 Time (power) used to perform the five sprints from a standing start (maximum time for each sprint 7 s).

2 Heart rate (recovery capacity) taken before the test, between the 40th and the 55th second after each sprint, between the 60th and the 90th second after the fifth sprint, and, lastly, at the end of the third minute after the end of the test.

If the same times are taken between the first and fifth sprints, it means that the subject is endowed with particular endurance (capacity to repeat power performances many times one after the other).

Alternate test This is a modification of the above described five sprints test and of the Bosco Ergo jump 15 s. It consists of 12 series of jumps, performed with countermovement, with 20 s rest between one series and the other, with the exception of the intervals between the third and fourth, the sixth and seventh, and the ninth and tenth series, where the rest time is 30 s. This is the time necessary to take a sample of 20 μl of blood from the ear lobe for the detection of lacticaemia. The calculated parameters are those relating to the height of the jump, to the work and to the power, with the addition of those relating to the decrease of performance and to the quantity of lactate produced.

In carrying out the test, whenever possible, the measurement of lacticaemia can obviously be left out. In this case the evaluation is performed on mechanical parameters only.

Alternate and shuttle test In the case of sports for which high racing speeds are very important, a shuttle test can be utilized. It is featured by nine series of sprints, each made up by four repetitions over a distance of 9 m (covered therefore four times backwards and forwards). The interval between one series and the next is 20 s. The time used can be considered, with sufficient approximation, to be the expression of the subject's anaerobic power, whilst the achievement of steady results over the nine series can be considered as (special) endurance power.

Force

Maximal force The increasing load method is performed by lifting ten times the heaviest possible load corresponding to approximately 80% of the maximum force. Subsequently, after an adequate muscular rest, the load is gradually increased until a load is reached which the athlete can lift in one go. The weight that the athlete is able to lift six times in succession represents 85% of the maximal load, whilst the load which can be lifted four times represents 90% of the maximal load.

Explosive force   **1**   Long jump without run: a judo mat or something similar and a tape measure are required. The athlete, barefooted, bends his/her knees, moves the arms backwards, and with a strong thrust, jumps as far as possible. The result of the test is the length of the jump.

2   The Abalakov test: for this test an automatic stop tape measure is required. This should be fixed to the floor by one end and to the athlete's waist by the other. The athlete must then perform, from a half-squatting position, the highest possible jump he/she is capable of, using, in the thrust, the upper limbs. With the tape measure it is possible to find the height reached by the subject.

Force–velocity curve   For a description of this test see the earlier section on laboratory tests and the paragraph dealing with force evaluation.

Endurance   The lifting test needs a horizontal bar at approximately 190 cm from the floor and a timer. The athlete under study must catch the bar with both hands with palms forward, and then raise the body to bring the chin over the bar. The aim of this test is to find the maximum time that the subject can hold this position.

References

Cummingham, D. A. & Faulkner, J. A. (1969) The effect of training on aerobic and anaerobic metabolism during a short exhaustive run. *Med. Sci. Sports* **1**, 65.

Curetou, T. K. (1951) *Physical Fitness of Champion Athletes*. University of Illinois Press, Urbane.

Schuabel, A. & Kindermann, W. (1983) Assessment of anaerobic capacity in runners. *Eur. J. Appl. Physiol.* **52**, 42.

Thomson, J. M. & Garvie, K. J. (1981) A laboratory method for determination of anaerobic energy expenditure during sprinting. *Can. J. Appl. Sport Sci.* **6**, 21.

Further reading

Cooper, K. H. (1968) *Aerobics*. M. Evans & Co., New York.

Dorgo, I.(1986) *A new test for estimating recovery in elite athletes* (Free communication). XXIIIrd World Congress of FIMS, Brisbane.

Reindell, H., König, K. & Roskamm, H. (1982) The equivalent of heart volume. In I. Drăgan *et al.* (eds) *Sports Medicine*. Sports-Tourism Ed., Bucharest.

PART 4

ENVIRONMENTAL CONDITIONS

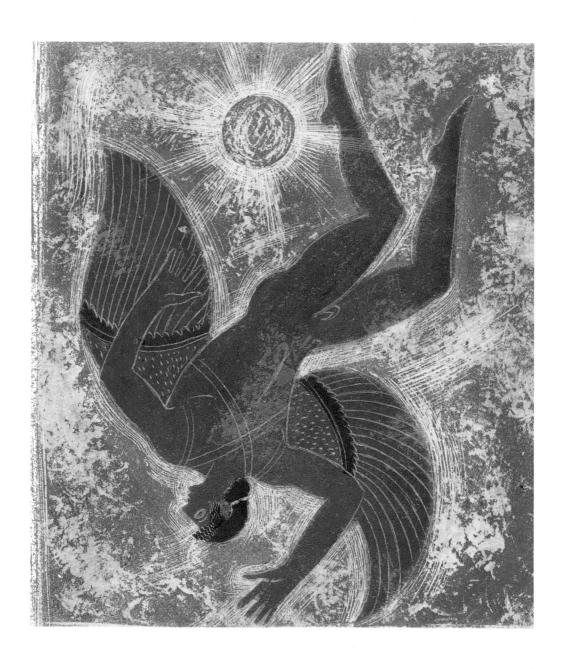

4.1 Heat

R. J. SHEPHARD

The main environmental factors which influence sport performance in a warm climate (Shephard, 1976, 1982) are dry bulb (DB) temperature, solar radiation, wet bulb (WB) temperature and air or wind movement over the body surface. The DB temperature and air movement influence heat loss or gain by convection; radiant heat exchange occurs with the atmosphere or the walls of a building; and heat loss resulting from evaporation of sweat depends on the WB temperature, air movement over the skin surface and the permeability of any clothing that is worn. Direct conduction of heat is usually a minor consideration unless a competitor collapses onto a hot track.

Maintenance of body temperature

As a homeotherm, the athlete tries to maintain a constant body temperature in the face of wide variation in environmental conditions and body heat production. In cold or temperate conditions, the DB temperature is lower than that of the skin; the heat gain from internal metabolism (and possibly some radiation on a sunny day) must match losses by convection, evaporation of moisture from the lungs, insensible perspiration, and possibly radiation to a cold atmosphere or building. When environmental temperatures exceed those of the skin (commonly 32°C), heat is also gained by convection from the environment, and the only method for dissipating heat becomes the evaporation of sweat.

The metabolic heat production varies with the strenuousness of the activity, rising from some 300 kJ/h at rest (4.186 kJ = 1 kcal) to as much as 4.5 MJ over the first hour of strenuous effort. Depending on the type of exercise, 10–25% of this metabolism is utilized for the performance of external work, and the remainder heats the body or is dissipated to the environment. The main avenue of dissipation during vigorous sport is the evaporation of sweat, even in a cool climate. Some heat is also stored through a rise of mean body temperature; equilibrium rectal temperatures of 37.5, 37.7 and 37.9°C have been reported for energy outputs of 419, 670 and 975 kJ/m²/h respectively (Lind, 1963). Such increases in body temperature are well tolerated and indeed help in both heat dissipation and a speeding up of metabolic processes. A modest 'warm-up' of this order also reduces further the chances of musculoskeletal injury and of cardiac dysrhythmias (Barnard *et al.*, 1973). Well-trained athletes tolerate much higher rectal temperatures than non-athletes, but nevertheless in warm or hot environments the rise of body temperature can exceed the desired upper limit of 40°C, resulting in illnesses such as heat hyperpyrexia, heat stroke or heat exhaustion.

Upper limits must thus be prescribed for the environmental conditions under which strenuous activities can be permitted (Shephard, 1976; Noble & Bachman, 1979), and officials should have the knowledge and the authority to stop contestants who show signs of impending heat stroke.

Humidity and performance

Given the importance of sweat evaporation to the dissipation of heat, it is not surprising that performance in a warm climate is strongly influenced by relative humidity and air or wind speed. In some sports such as North American football, impermeable protective clothing has added a fatal additional component to an already dangerous heat load (Buskirk, 1968).

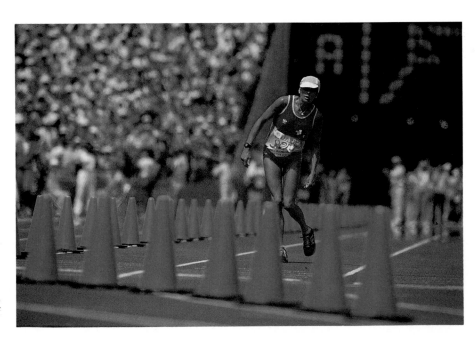

Fig. 4.1.1 Competition in long-lasting events (such as a marathon) under conditions of high environmetal temperature, humidity and radiant load can cause dehydration, high body core temperature, loss of coordination and disorientation. © The Los Angeles Times 1984 (National Photo Pool), photo by Jay Dickman. Courtesy of the IOC archives.

About 1 MJ of heat can be stored as the body temperature rises to 41°C, while each litre of sweat that is evaporated dissipates 2.43 MJ. In sustained efforts such as football, hockey, running and long-distance rowing, 1.0–1.2 litres of sweat must be evaporated every hour to assure thermal equilibrium (Shephard, 1982). Unfortunately, even under favourable conditions of low relative humidity 50% or more of the total sweat secretion rolls to the ground unevaporated, so that body fluid losses may reach 2 l/h.

There is an increase of heart rate in all forms of submaximal effort, with a deterioration of maximum oxygen intake and endurance performance. Dehydration reduces cardiac stroke volume and, as the maximum minute volume of cardiac output falls, the blood flow to exercising muscles diminishes and an increasing proportion of energy needs are met anaerobically. Lactic acid accumulates in both blood and muscles, and the onset of fatigue is hastened. Initially, an increased proportion of the total blood flow may be diverted to the cutaneous circulation, but as dehydration develops, the cutaneous circulation is also curtailed, further hampering the processs of heat elimination. As activity is continued, sweat output also decreases due to a maceration of the skin and a blockage of the exits from the sweat glands (Shephard, 1982). The combined effect of all these reactions is to reduce the performance of athletes in the heat, particularly in endurance events.

Convection and radiation

Experiments on the laboratory treadmill give a misleading impression of thermal loads on the track, since running or cycling forces a stream of air over the body even in the absence of wind; this can be helpful both to convection and to the evaporation of sweat.

Radiant heating depends on the position of the sun relative to the body. In bright sunshine, loads may reach 360 kJ/h when the sun is directly overhead, rising to 900 kJ/h in the late afternoon when the sun is lower (Shephard, 1982). If the track is hot, there may also be low temperature radiation from the ground.

Acclimatization

Body responses to a hot environment are considerably modified by acclimatization. While the well-trained athlete already has some heat tolerance by virtue of physical condition, further acclimatization develops with 7–10 days of residence in a hot climate and subjective comfort increases. There is also an increase of venous tone and of central blood volume. However, the main change is in the sweating response; sweat is produced earlier and in greater quantities after acclimatization, while its salt content is reduced (Shephard, 1982). In consequence, there is a smaller rise in rectal temperature and heart rate for a given set of environmental conditions, heat loss is increased, less strain is placed on the heart and circulation, and athletic performance is improved.

If the athlete normally lives in a cool environment, some acclimatization is possible by wearing impermeable clothing and/or exercising in a climatic chamber for 3–4 h/day. However, the acclimatization takes about twice as long to achieve and is less effective than exposure to the natural environment. Most of the adaptation to heat is lost within 2 months of return to temperate conditions, although reacclimatization seems to occur more rapidly than the adjustment to an initial exposure.

Prevention of injury

As with most medical problems, prevention is better than cure (Shephard, 1976; Noble & Bachman, 1979). The cornerstone of prevention is the setting of precise limits for competition. Other important factors are the provision of appropriate clothing, maintenance of fluid balance and the provision of sufficient minerals. Vulnerable individuals include the obese, the unfit, the dehydrated, those who are unacclimatized, the very young and very old, those who have an initial fever, and those with a history of heat stroke.

Limits to competition　　Although interests such as television may clamour for competition in the afternoon sun, it is better to organize events in the early morning or the cool of evening, and avoiding the summer months in the warmer parts of the world. The worst situation arises on a hot day with a high relative humidity, high solar radiation and little wind, especially if it is early in the summer before competitors have become heat acclimatized.

The stress of a given environment is commonly calculated as the wet bulb/globe thermometer index (WBGT):

Outdoors WBGT = 0.7 (WB) + 0.2 (GT) + 0.1 (DB)
Indoors WBGT　= 0.7 (WB) + 0.3 (DB)

where GT is the globe temperature, a measure of radiant heating recorded from a thermometer enclosed in a black or grey metal sphere. The index as calculated, however, makes no allowance for air movement. A relative air speed of 5 m/s can lower the effective temperature by 5–7°C (less in warm environments).

When organizing distance races such as marathon competitions, it is recommended that the event be cancelled if the WBGT exceeds 28°C. There is a high risk of heat illnesses in vulnerable individuals if the WBGT lies in the range 23–28°C, a moderate risk if the WBGT is 18–23°C, and a low risk at lower temperatures (Noble & Bachman, 1979). Wyndham and Strydom (1972) have suggested that no unacclimatized athlete should run for more than 30 min if the WBGT has reached 25°C.

Clothing Loose fitting and lightweight white clothing can protect the body against solar radiation, and it can also conserve sweat that would otherwise roll to the ground. Football fatalities in the USA have often been associated with the wearing of nylon uniforms. While these are easy to wash, they have the serious disadvantage of not allowing the passage of sweat. Natural fibres are much more effective than synthetic materials in this regard.

Fluids Sweating may amount to at least 2 litre over the first hour of strenuous activity, dropping to about 1 l/h over more prolonged effort. The first 1.5–2.0 litre can be derived from water associated with the glycogen molecule and water formed by metabolism (Kavanagh & Shephard,

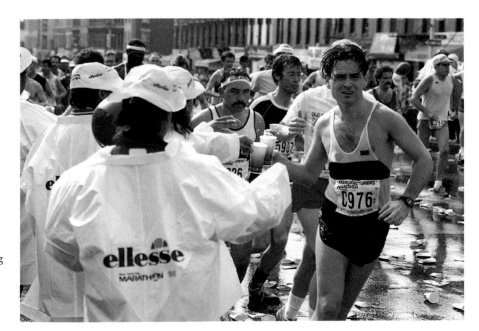

Fig. 4.1.2 Frequent hydration is essential during a long-lasting event, especially under conditions of thermal stress. Courtesy of *Runner's World Magazine*, photo by Robert Gerheart.

1978). However, if the loss amounts to more than 2.5–3.0% of body mass, working capacity is adversely affected, with a greater rise of body temperature and a larger increase of exercise heart rate. It is then imperative that the fluid is replaced if performance is not to deteriorate and the risk of heat illnesses is not to increase. Rules that prohibit an adequate fluid intake should not be tolerated.

Many of the commercially available replacement fluids contain minerals and carbohydrate, but because they are then hyperosmotic the rate of gastric emptying is slowed and the volume of fluid which can be ingested and absorbed is limited. In terms of the volume absorbed, the most effective fluid is tap water (Kavanagh & Shephard, 1978), although it is important to check this for potability as an attack of gastroenteritis can have disastrous effects upon performance. About 500 ml can be drunk shortly before an event, and thereafter 150–250 ml at 15 min intervals. Larger volumes merely remain in the stomach and cause gastric discomfort. Small amounts of glucose or glucose polymer (up to the equivalent of 5% glucose) and small amounts of salt can be added to improve flavour without seriously reducing the rate of fluid absorption.

Heat can also be dissipated (and thus sweat conserved) by evaporating water applied to the skin and clothing. Athletes should thus take advantage of opportunities to run under showers or hoses during a distance race.

Mineral ion losses   Sweat contains quite large amounts of sodium chloride (Verde *et al.*, 1983). The normal salt loss is about 12 g/day, but a competitor who sweats hard can lose up to 8 g/h from a total pool of some 175 g. Problems of a cumulative deficit can thus arise through several weeks of competing in a very hot climate. A deficit can be readily detected (Wyndham & Strydom, 1972) through a decrease in the salt content of the urine (Fantus test) and a progressive reduction in body mass (due to an associated decrease of body water). A sodium ion loss of 0.5 g/kg causes the athlete to become tired and irritable, with complaints of giddiness, fainting and cramps. Because of the reduced plasma volume, there is a decrease in maximum cardiac output and maximum oxygen intake. If the deficit is allowed to reach 0.75 g/kg, there is apathy, stupor and a marked fall of blood pressure (Wyndham & Strydom, 1972).

With acclimatization, the loss of salt in both sweat and urine is reduced through an increased output of the hormone aldosterone. The needs of an acclimatized athlete can be satisfied (Malhotra *et al.*, 1959) by a small increase in the normal dietary intake of salt (to about 16 g/day). However, the unacclimatized athlete may need deliberate sodium supplements.

These are best provided as salt drinks; salt tablets either pass through the intestines unabsorbed, or produce a bolus of highly salinized blood with an increased renal excretion of sodium ions. During competition, the blood concentration of sodium and other mineral ions rises, and at this stage water is more important to the body than mineral replacement. During the subsequent recovery period, however, minerals lost in sweat must be replaced (Kavanagh & Shephard, 1978). A concentration of 0.1% sodium chloride can be added to water without an appreciable change in its taste. Higher concentrations are not well accepted, and may merely discourage the drinking of an adequate volume of fluid. After the first 10 days in the tropical milieu, specific supplements are no longer necessary.

In addition to sodium ions, sweat contains such minerals as potassium, calcium, magnesium and iron (Verde *et al.*, 1983). The potassium concentration is 1.5–2.0 times that found in the plasma. Moreover, the increased output of aldosterone with acclimatization, while conserving sodium ions, merely increases the loss of potassium. Fortunately, body potassium reserves are substantial, and most commercial preparations of table salt contain potassium. A cumulative deficit is thus unlikely unless athletes have been training and/or competing in the hot environment for many days. During vigorous exercise, serum potassium levels rise because of leakage of potassium from the working muscles. As with sodium ions, the appropriate time for replacement of losses is thus in the recovery period rather than during the exercise bout (Kavanagh & Shephard, 1978).

Heat pathologies

Heat collapse   Heat collapse is the commonest thermal problem encountered on a hot day; it is found in both athletes who omit a warm-down and spectators who have stood for a long period. There is essentially a loss of consciousness due to an inadequate cerebral blood flow, and the condition is easily treated by adopting a supine position, with elevation of the legs, tepid sponging and administration of oral fluids. It is nevertheless important to check that the loss of consciousness is not an expression of cumulative salt deficiency or heat stroke. One important warning criterion is the rectal temperature; any reading over 41°C must be treated as heat stroke until the diagnosis is disproved (Wyndham & Strydom, 1972). The oral temperature is not a safe guide, as hyperventilation may have led to a local cooling of the tongue.

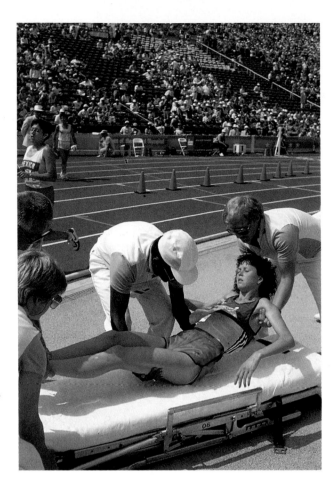

Fig. 4.1.3 Rapid treatment of heat collapse is essential, including placement of the athlete in the supine position and elevation of the legs to regain cerebral blood flow. © The Los Angeles Times 1984 (National Photo Pool), photo by Pat Downs. Courtesy of the IOC archives.

Heat stroke   Heat stroke is a dangerous and potentially fatal failure of the heat-regulating mechanisms and requires hospital admission. There may be a clouding rather than a loss of consciousness, sometimes with hallucinations, muscle twitching, convulsions and loss of control of the body sphincters. If untreated, the rising core temperature can lead to irreversible damage in the brain, kidneys, liver and adrenal glands. Competitors should be warned to watch for early symptoms, including excessive sweating, headache, nausea, dizziness and disturbance of consciousness. A partner should also monitor their condition. Emergency treatment is directed to rapid cooling by tepid sponging and fanning of the body.

During recovery, intravenous bicarbonates are needed to counter metabolic acidosis, hydrocortisone and intravenous fluids are given to counter a falling blood pressure, and dialysis may be needed if there is renal failure. However, if recovery is rapid, and there is no sign of organ damage, the patient can be allowed to run again within 1 week.

References

Barnard, R. J., MacAlpin, R. N., Kattus, A. A. & Buckberg, G. D. (1973) Ischemic response to sudden strenuous exercise in healthy men. *Circulation* **48**, 936.

Buskirk, E. R. (1968) Problems related to the conduct of athletes in hot environments. In *Physiological Aspects of Sport and Physical Fitness.* Athletic Institute, Chicago.

Kavanagh, T. & Shephard, R. J. (1978) Fluid and mineral needs of post-coronary distance runners. In F. Landry & W. A. R. Orban (eds) *Sports Medicine.* Symposia Specialists, Miami.

Lind, A. R. (1963) A physiological criterion for setting environmental limits for everyday work. *J. Appl. Physiol.* **18(1)**, 51.

Malhotra, M. S., Sharma, B. K. & Sivarama, R. (1959) Requirements of sodium chloride during summer in the tropics. *J. Appl. Physiol.* **14**, 823.

Noble, H. B. & Bachman, D. (1979) Medical aspects of distance race planning. *Physician Sportsmed.* **7(6)**, 78.

Shephard, R. J. (1976) Environment. In J. G. P. Williams & P. Sperryn (eds) *Sports Medicine*, 2nd edn. Arnold, London.

Shephard, R. J. (1982) *Physiology and Biochemistry of Exercise.* Praeger, New York.

Verde, T., Shephard, R. J., Corey, R. & Moore, R. (1983) Sweat composition in exercise and heat. In N. Bachl, L. Prokop & R. Suckert (eds) *Current Topics in Sports Medicine.* Urban & Schwarzenburg, Vienna.

Wyndham, C. H. & Strydom, N. B. (1972) Korperliche Arbeit bei hoher Temperatur. In W. Hollmann (ed) *Zentrale Themen der Sportmedizin.* Springer, Berlin.

Further reading

Leithead, C. S. & Lind, A. R. (1964) *Heat Stress and Heat Disorders.* Cassell, London.

4.2 Cold

R. J. SHEPHARD

Sudden immersion in cold water can cause involuntary gasping, inhalation of water and laryngospasm. It may also provoke cardiac arrhythmias. Generalized hypothermia (Pugh, 1972; Shephard, 1985) is a problem when swimming in cold water, in boating accidents and in hill walking. A substantial drop of body temperature has also been observed in the later stages of some marathon races conducted at near-freezing temperatures. Local cooling leads to loss of proprioceptive skills (with an increased risk of injury) and to frostbite of the extremities; it is particularly common in downhill skiing, where a high speed of descent displaces the still film of warm air around the body surface.

Heat exchange

The general principles are the same as for a warm environment, although the importance of heat losses by convection plus the warming and humidification of respired air are much increased (Shephard, 1982). Heat stores can be depleted by a cooling of the body, but physical efficiency is impaired if the core temperature drops by 1°C, and consciousness is impaired at the lower safe limit of 35°C. There is a selective loss of heat from the peripheral tissues through a process of peripheral vasoconstriction, and for this reason some 2 MJ of heat can be lost before the critical temperature of 35°C is reached. Possible tactics for avoiding a dangerous drop in core temperature include an increase of clothing, an increase of voluntary physical activity, involuntary movements (shivering) and non-shivering thermogenesis.

Clothing It might seem a simple matter to wear additional clothing until a comfortable body temperature is restored. However, arctic clothing is heavy and restricts mobility, so that it is not popular for active sports. Furthermore, the need for insulation varies widely with the intensity of the activity that is being undertaken. For instance, if clothing is effective

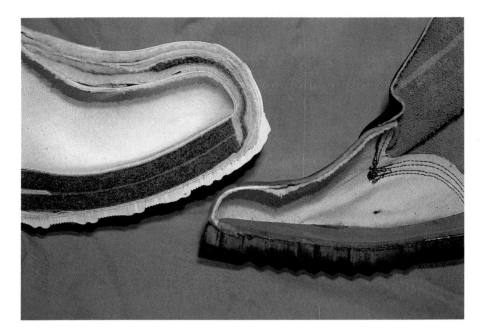

Fig. 4.2.1 Selection of all apparel for cold-weather sport is a question of compromise between insulaton, as exemplified in the boot on the left, and mobility, as in the boot on the right (Longitudinal sections). Courtesy of M. Hamlet.

when resting under cold conditions, it may lead to sweating once activity is begun. As the clothing becomes saturated with sweat its insulating properties are destroyed. It is therefore very important to choose clothes where the amount of insulation can be varied according to the needs of the moment. In severe hypothermia, involuntary urination can also reduce the insulation of clothing.

Body movement pumps cold air beneath clothing unless the neck, wrist and ankle openings are firmly closed. In a number of hill-walking disasters, insulation has been further reduced because clothes have become soaked with rain or mist. If temperatures are above freezing it is important for the outermost layer to be waterproof, while at lower temperatures it is important that it be windproof (Pugh, 1972).

Voluntary activity   Since at least 75% of metabolic energy consumption appears as heat, it might seem simple to increase the amount of physical activity until thermal comfort is attained. This may be difficult in practice, because the effects of body movement (including pumping of air through the clothing and disturbance of the still film around the body surface) increase body heat needs, sometimes by as much as six to seven times (Burton & Edholm, 1969). Voluntary heat production may also be limited by injury, lack of food, poor initial fitness, or exhaustion due to high winds and more vigorous colleagues.

Shivering Shivering involves the involuntary contraction of one group of muscles against their antagonists. In moderate work, it can boost oxygen consumption by as much as 1 l/min, with a 20 kJ/min rise in heat production (Pugh, 1972; Nadel *et al.*, 1974). However, the capacity to shiver wanes as local glycogen reserves become depleted, and anyway the uncontrolled shaking movements preclude skilled activity. Indeed, shivering can be an important factor in the occurrence of accidents to both climbers and divers. The acclimatized subject shivers less in any given environment, apparently allowing the temperature of the peripheral tissues to drift lower with a view to decreasing heat losses from the core (Shephard, 1985).

Non-shivering thermogenesis In the absence of formal shivering, body heat production can still be boosted by various forms of non-shivering thermogenesis, particularly the breakdown and resynthesis of neutral fat. One tissue which is adapted to this role in animals is brown fat; however, it is less certain that adult humans have significant quantities of this type of fat (Shephard, 1985).

Cold and performance

Performance of short-term events is adversely affected by what is in essence the absence of a warm-up. Muscle tone and viscosity are increased and the speed of contraction is slowed, leading to delayed relaxation of the antagonist muscles. Speed and power events are thus performed poorly, and there is an increased risk of injuries due to failure of relaxation, impaired proprioceptive function and hypothermic or hypoglycaemic confusion. There may be a small increase of maximum oxygen intake due to peripheral vascular constriction, and an increased physical solution of oxygen in the blood, but any benefit from these changes is offset by the added costs of increased muscle viscosity, shivering, heavy clothing and the need to move over snow or wet terrain. With more prolonged exposure, blood volume is depressed by a cold diuresis and inadequate fluid intake.

Acclimatization

With repeated local or general exposure, cold environments become progressively less unpleasant (Shephard, 1985). However, acclimatization seems less obvious than in the heat. Prolonged exposure may lead to an increased output of thyroxine and development of a thermogenic reaction to the secretion of noradrenaline, but the main response of the acclimatized person is a peripheral vasoconstriction in the cold. This increases the effective insulation obtained from muscle and subcutaneous fat.

Cold pathologies

Cold exhaustion   Cold exhaustion and collapse occur as a response to falling blood sugars and decreasing core temperatures. Cerebral function begins to fail at 35°C, with a slowing of pace, unsteadiness, muscle weakness, cramps and stumbling (Shephard, 1982). If shelter and food are found at this stage recovery is rapid, but if ignored a failure of shivering and a loss of vasoconstrictor tone lead to an accelerating loss of control over body temperature. At the same time, hypoventilation with disturbances of acid–base balance and leakage of potassium ions from hypoxic tissues increase the risk of ventricular fibrillation or cardiac arrest. Anxiety, irritability, apathy or loss of purpose rapidly lead to loss of consciousness. Confusion may cause loss of direction, injury, or removal of clothing through a paradoxical feeling of warmth. A significant mortality occurs if the rectal temperature drops below 32°C; if temperatures cannot be measured, severity should be gauged from mental changes and loss of coordination.

Evacuation by stretcher can be dangerously slow, and if the person can walk, the best emergency treatment is probably to remove water from drenched clothing by rolling in dry snow, a brief rest in a temporary wind shelter, administration of hot and sweet fluids, provision of extra clothing and escort to a place of safety. If injured, or the distance is too great, the most effective approach is probably to share a well-insulated sleeping bag with a rescuer. Intravenous 4% dextrose can be given if available. Struggling must be avoided in the severely hypothermic, as this merely pumps very cold and hyperkalaemic blood into the central circulation.

If hypothermia is severe, there remains an appreciable risk of later circulatory, respiratory and renal failure, and evacuation to hospital must be attempted as soon as the journey can be withstood.

Frostbite   Frostbite is a local destruction of superficial tissues, caused by freezing of extracellular water and dehydration damage to the exposed parts. This usually occurs at a skin temperature of about −1 to −2°C. Contributory

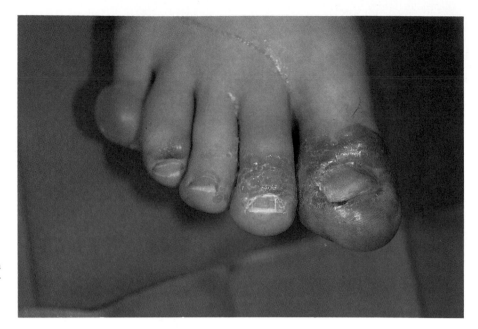

Fig. 4.2.2 Deep second-degree of early third-degree frostbite of the toes common to tight-fitting boots of cross-country skiers and mountaineers. Courtesy of M. Hamlet.

factors include contact with cold metal, overtight garments, an intense local vasoconstriction (more likely in an unacclimatized person who is a cigarette smoker), a very low air temperature (-20 to $-30°C$) and excessive air movement over the affected part (skiing, or exposure to a high wind).

The immediate treatment should be a rewarming of the affected area by warm ($42°C$) water, body heat or expired air, unless there is a danger of refreezing. The part should then be kept cool to minimize both metabolic demand on the damaged tissues and secondary vascular occlusion by oedema. Smoking must be avoided. If the skin is destroyed measures are needed to avoid secondary infection, while α-receptor blocking agents such as phenoxybenzamine hydrochloride (10 mg/day) can be given to improve the circulation. Late gangrenous changes reflect vascular occlusion and hypoxia.

Effects of cold water   A fall into near-freezing water can be fatal in as little as 15 min, since both conduction and convection of heat occur more rapidly in water than in air (Hayward *et al.*, 1975). Unless close to shore, the optimum tactic is to minimize the exposed body surface by huddling in the foetal position. Attempts at swimming reduce tissue insulation (by increasing blood flow to the limbs) and also increase the movement of cold water over the skin surface. If rewarming is too rapid, there may be adverse effects as cold blood suddenly surges from the peripheral to the central circulation.

References

Burton, A. C. & Edholm, O. G. (1969) *Man in a Cold Environment*. Hafner, New York.

Hayward, J. S., Eckerson, J. D. & Collis, M. D. (1975) Effect of behavioral variables on cooling rate of man in cold water. *J. Appl. Physiol.* **38**, 1073.

Nadel, E. R., Holmér, I., Bergh, U., Åstrand, P. O. & Stolwijk, J. A. J. (1974) Energy exchanges of swimming man. *J. Appl. Physiol.* **36**, 465.

Pugh, L. G. C. E. (1972) Accidental hypothermia among hillwalkers. In G. R. Cumming, D. Snidal & A. Taylor (eds) (1972) *Environmental Effects on Work Performance*. Canadian Association of Sport Sciences, Ottawa.

Shephard, R. J. (1982) *Physiology and Biochemistry of Exercise*. Praeger, New York.

Shephard, R. J. (1985) Adaptation to exercise in the cold. *Sports Med.* **2**, 59.

4.3 Altitude

R. J. SHEPHARD

Despite the paucity of medical problems which have been encountered during competitions in Mexico City and other cities at high elevations, the potential dangers of altitude competition are a continuing concern of sports physicians (Jokl & Jokl, 1968; Shephard, 1974). At the XXth World Congress of Sports Medicine (Melbourne, 1974), the FIMS thus approved a resolution urging extreme caution at altitudes of more than 2290 m (8700 feet), with an absolute prohibition of contests above 3050 m (10 000 feet).

An athlete who is to compete at altitude will want advice on likely acute changes in performance (Goddard, 1967; Margaria, 1967; Jokl & Jokl, 1968), with prescription of an optimum acclimatization schedule (Goddard, 1967) and counsel regarding possible residual benefits of altitude training (Richardson, 1974). The physician must also be prepared to treat specific altitude pathologies such as mountain sickness and pulmonary oedema, while watching for possible aggravation of general medical conditions (Jokl & Jokl, 1968; Shephard, 1974).

Performance at altitude

Gravity The acceleration due to gravity diminishes by some 0.3 cm/s^2 for every 1000 m of altitude. A high competition site thus confers an advantage on many classes of athlete, including jumpers, pole vaulters, hurdlers and throwers. However, even at 4000 m, the benefit (0.13%) is smaller than that obtained from a change of latitude, gravitational forces increasing by 0.53% from the equator to the poles.

Wind resistance The wind resistance encountered by athletes is largely due to turbulent air movement over the body surface, and it is thus proportional to $\frac{1}{2} pv^2$, where p is the density of the atmosphere, and v is the relative velocity of air movement. Density decreases by 19.9% at 1830 m, 25.7% at 2440 m and 31.2% at 3050 m. At sea level, wind resistance accounts for some 11% of the energy expended in running 5000 m; thus the decrease of atmospheric density boosts the potential 5000 m performance by about 3.4% at an altitude of 3000 m. Since work against turbulent resistance is proportional to the third power of relative air speed, the advantage of high-altitude competition is much larger in the faster events, about 14.3% in a 100 m run, and even greater in cycling, skiing and speed-skating contests.

Temperature The ambient temperature decreases by about 2°C for every additional 300 m of altitude. Wind velocities also tend to be greater at high and exposed sites. A day that seems comfortable at sea level can thus produce conditions where performance deteriorates and hypothermia develops at an altitude of 3000 m.

Oxygen partial pressure The partial pressure of respired oxygen decreases in parallel with the diminution in atmospheric density. Thus, there is some 31% less oxygen per unit volume of air available to the athlete at 3000 m than at sea level. Such hypoxia has little direct impact on the performance of the sprinter, provided that a somewhat longer recovery interval is allowed between heats. However, the endurance competitor is appreciably handicapped. Advantages due to a lesser wind resistance and reduced gravitational forces are outweighed by hypoxia if an event lasts for more than 1 min, and a substantial loss of performance is seen in 5 km and 10 km races. In Mexico City (2240 m), times for the last two events are commonly about 8% poorer than at sea level. The corresponding diminution in the partial pressure of atmospheric oxygen is about 24%, indicating that various physiological mechanisms provide even a temporary altitude resident with some compensation against hypoxia.

Acclimatization

If an athlete remains at high altitude, the body makes further adjustments that restore performance towards its sea-level value; this diminishes the likelihood that medical problems will develop during competition. Specific adaptations include a reduction in the bicarbonate content of the blood and tissues, an increase of haemoglobin levels, a restoration of blood volume and an increase in the activity of the various tissue enzymes. It is necessary to examine the time course of these changes in order to advise the athlete on an appropriate acclimatization schedule.

The bicarbonate content of the cerebrospinal fluid is reduced within a few hours of moving to altitude, and parallel adjustments of blood and tissue buffers occur over the next week. These changes allow the competitor to slightly hyperventilate without developing intermittent ventilation and other symptoms of carbon dioxide lack. The oxygen content of the arterial blood is partially restored, and perhaps a fifth of the lost endurance is regained. A slight adverse effect on sprint (anaerobic) performance might be anticipated from the loss of buffers, but this is hard to demonstrate in practice.

An increase in the haemoglobin content of the blood improves oxygen transport in the face of the low inspired partial pressure of oxygen. Increases in red cell count and haemoglobin concentration have been described within a few days of reaching altitude, but these seem due mainly to haemoconcentration. A true increase of red cell mass develops much more slowly, over the course of several months. The team physician should check both the haemoglobin and the serum iron levels of competitors while they are at sea level, since fads of diet, iron losses in the sweat, depressed formation and an increased breakdown of red cells can all predispose the endurance athlete to the additional handicap of an overt anaemia or a latent iron deficit.

Other tissue adaptations to altitude include an increase in the myoglobin content of the muscles, and an augmentation in the activity of various enzyme systems. These responses occur over 1 or 2 weeks, helping to compensate the sprinter for loss of tissue-buffering capacity, and speeding recovery from exhausting exercise.

Plasma volumes often diminish during the first few weeks at altitude. The stroke volume of the heart is reduced, while the maximum cardiac output is depressed yet more by some diminution of maximum heart rate and possible effects from a high blood viscosity. There are associated deteriorations of maximum oxygen intake and endurance performance.

In prescribing an optimum acclimatization schedule, a balance must be struck between useful respiratory adaptations and the disadvantages of a possible cumulative fluid loss. At altitudes below 2250 m, respiratory gains seem to outweigh the circulatory losses, and most authorities recommend a 3–4-week period of acclimatization. During this time, the athlete must be guarded against unfamiliar microorganisms, the psychological problems of living away from home, and the practical risks of interruption to a well-established training plan. At 3000 m, the cumulative loss of plasma fluid cannot be ignored, and it may be wise to compete within 72 hours of reaching altitude. Opportunity is thus allowed for recuperation from the journey, adjustments of cerebrospinal bicarbonate levels, and recovery from any mountain sickness, but competition is completed before there has been time for a serious decrease of maximum cardiac output. The main disadvantage of a short stay at altitude is that the athlete has little chance to learn the peculiarities of the course or an appropriate competitive pace. An early pre-contest site visit is thus desirable.

The native of high altitude has a clear advantage when endurance competitions are conducted at great heights, and this constitutional endowment may also be of some help under sea-level conditions. Specific characteristics include a high haemoglobin level, and a limited response of carotid body chemoreceptors to oxygen lack; the latter feature reduces the likelihood of hyperventilation, excessive carbon dioxide washout and intermittent breathing during vigorous effort.

High-altitude training camps Since sea-level residents ultimately adapt well to competition at moderate altitudes, and there is some evidence that high-altitude natives have a persistent advantage in endurance competitions at sea level, some teams have elected to prepare themselves for major international events through varying periods of altitude training. The physiological objective has been to time the return to sea level so that the altitude polycythaemia is preserved, but body buffers are restored to their initial values. While there is a theoretical possibility of gaining some advantage of oxygen transport 4 to 20 days following altitude exposure, this must be set against such practical disadvantages as the curtailment of training and the learning of an incorrect pace while at altitude. If athletes are in peak condition prior to a mountain sojourn, the net result of an altitude camp thus seems either no change or even a small deterioration in maximum oxygen intake and times for endurance competition. Most teams now seem disillusioned about altitude training, except where competition is planned at altitude and a long period of residence is possible at an agreeable training site.

A few authors have experimented with hypoxic training at sea level, for instance by having soccer players rebreathe through long tubes. Any physiological benefits from this approach have been slight, with difficulty in distinguishing an increased tolerance of hypoxia from a habituation to hypercarbia. The impact upon performance has further been offset by a disruption of normal training.

Altitude pathologies

Mountain sickness Mountain sickness can be quite difficult to diagnose, as the symptoms are non-specific, including headache, insomnia, irritability and a variety of gastrointestinal disturbances. There is an increase of extracellular fluid, with a tendency to cerebral oedema and an alteration in the volume and composition of the intestinal secretions. These changes are secondary to hyperventilation and the associated acid–base disturbances.

During moderate recreational activity, the threshold for the development of mountain sickness seems to be an altitude of 2500–3000 m. Moreover, some authors have argued that the heavy training schedule of an international athlete may increase the risk, so that typical symptoms can develop at a mere 1800 m. At the altitudes of interest to sports physicians, the disorder only lasts 2–3 days, and most patients respond well to conservative treatment. Training schedules should be lightened temporarily, and symptomatic therapy given for headache and sleeplessness. Carbonic anhydrase-inhibiting diuretics such as acetazolamide (250 mg qds) are best avoided. While the immediate symptoms are reduced by administration of this drug, the course of acclimatization is slowed, and the induced loss of fluid further aggravates the deterioration of performance due to a shrinking plasma volume.

Chronic mountain sickness is unlikely at the altitudes where competitions are held. If symptoms persist, this may reflect a compounding of the initial episode with an intercurrent gastrointestinal infection, irrational fears of altitude, discouragement from poor track times, or loss of condition due to the interruption of training schedules.

Pulmonary oedema An intense pulmonary oedema occasionally develops within 9–36 h of reaching altitude. Among recreational athletes, the threshold altitude

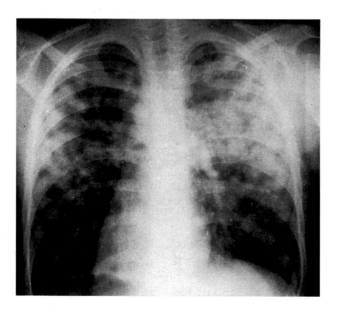

Fig. 4.3.1 Pulmonary oedema is one of the most serious adverse responses to travel to altitude and the accompanying hypoxic conditions. Courtesy of Altitude Research Division, USARIEM.

seems about 2500 m, but since unusually vigorous exercise is a precipitating factor, competitors could possibly encounter this disorder at lower elevations. Circumstances predisposing to high-altitude oedema include recent respiratory infection, pulmonary venous constriction (secondary to oxygen lack), peripheral vasoconstriction (secondary to hyperventilation), an increase of total blood volume and pulmonary hypertension (secondary to previous residence at altitude) and an increase of left ventricular diastolic pressure (secondary to myocardial oxygen lack). The syndrome is thus most commonly encountered in people with past experience of altitude who have returned to engage in vigorous physical activity without allowing adequate time for readjustment to the low partial pressure of oxygen.

The patient presents with an acute dyspnoea, a blood-stained, watery phlegm, chest discomfort, cough, nausea and vomiting. There are the usual physical signs of alveolar exudate (including poor air entry, dullness to percussion and basal râles), ECG evidence of right ventricular strain, and intense pulmonary vascular congestion with diffuse pulmonary opacities.

If neglected, such cases can prove fatal. However, there is usually a good response to bed rest, oxygen and antibiotics for the prevention of secondary infection.

General medical conditions

At moderate altitudes, problems of oxygen transport can be accommodated by the simple expedient of moving a little more slowly. However, the athlete who attempts to sustain the same pace as at sea level inevitably increases the risk of developing general medical conditions, including myocardial infarction and cardiac arrest. Even slight reductions of arterial oxygen saturation increase the likelihood that exercise will induce cardiac arrhythmias and manifestations of cerebral hypoxia such as central scotomata, impairment of colour vision and disturbances of coordination. The hazards remain small for a young and healthy, medically-screened athlete, but nevertheless, the danger is appreciably greater than at sea level, particularly for the masters' competitor. Black athletes should be checked for sickle-cell disease, since several deaths from splenic rupture have occurred at altitudes of around 2500 m.

If patients with diseases affecting the oxygen transport system (anaemia, angina, heart failure or chronic respiratory disease) visit a mountain resort, their exercise prescription should be reduced. Patients with a history of epilepsy may require additional sedation while at altitude.

Ultraviolet radiation is greater at altitude than at sea level; and, in particular, when such radiation is reflected by snow it can cause problems of sunburn and temporary blindness. Barrier creams and dark glasses should be used as necessary.

Conclusion

Both the practical experience of high-altitude competitions and the theoretical considerations presented above support the FIMS position that problems attributable to altitude are unlikely below 2300 m. Between 2300 and 3000 m, there is an increasing chance that the more vulnerable members of a team could develop mountain sickness, pulmonary oedema, and other medical problems such as cardiac arrhythmias and cerebral hypoxia. On present knowledge, the likelihood of occasional incidents above 3000 m seems sufficient to justify the categoric prohibition of major competitions in such an environment.

References

Goddard, R. F. (ed) (1967) *The Effects of Altitude on Physical Performance.* Athletic Institute, Chicago.

Jokl, E. & Jokl, P. (1968) *Exercise and Altitude.* Karger, Basel.

Margaria, R. (ed) (1967) *Exercise at Altitude.* Excerpta Medica Foundation, Amsterdam.

Richardson, R. G. (ed) (1974) Altitude training. *Br. J. Sports Med.* **8**, 1.

Shephard, R. J. (1974) Altitude training camps. *Br. J. Sports Med.* **8**, 38.

4.4 Air pollution

R. J. SHEPHARD

The athlete is exposed to above average quantities of air pollutants, since endurance exercise increases the respiratory minute volume up to 20-fold. Furthermore, in order to accommodate the large tidal volume of all-out performance, the mouth is opened widely, bypassing the normal mechanism for the filtration of particulates and soluble vapours in the nose. Finally, the maximum utilization of the respiratory and cardio-vascular systems may uncover functional changes which are not detected in a lightly-stressed, sedentary peer.

The supposed response to air pollutants must be distinguished from the effects of drying of the airways and respiratory muscle fatigue. The inhalation of large volumes of cold and dry air can provoke an exercise-induced bronchospasm, particularly in subjects with sensitive airways. Partly for this reason, and partly because of respiratory muscle fatigue, there may be a small (10%) decrease of maximum voluntary ventilation over the course of a marathon race (Shephard, 1987).

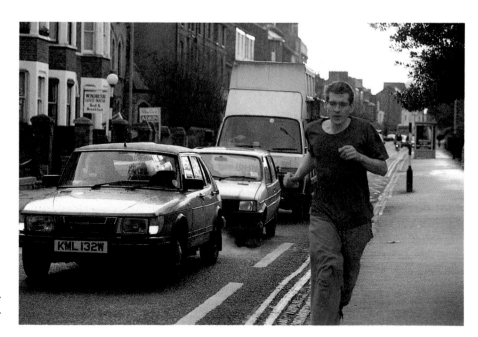

Fig. 4.4.1 Sports, such as running or jogging, conducted in urban environments can expose the athlete to a number of pollutants caused mainly by motor vehicles and industry. Photo by Jim Chambers.

Air pollutants fall into two main categories—reducing and oxidant forms of smog (McCafferty, 1981; Shephard, 1984). The reducing smog is produced by burning carbon fuels, such as soft coal. Depending on the height and sophistication of local smoke stacks, it consists of smoke particles, sulphur dioxide and the much more toxic sulphur trioxide. The acute response to high concentrations of this mixture is a bronchospasm; this could increase the work of breathing, and thus impair performance. Several world disasters have demonstrated the long-term lethal potential of reducing smog when it is discharged from low-level smoke stacks into a cold and humid environment. The victims are usually the very young and the very elderly. Factors contributing to death include a paralysis of the tracheal ciliae, an increased bronchial production of mucus and airway collapse, followed by an upper respiratory tract infection. The athlete who is exposed to reducing smoke might thus be at increased risk of developing a respiratory infection, with consequent interruption of training and the potential hazard of a viral myocarditis.

Oxidant smog is a very complex chemical mixture, formed from vehicle exhaust under the influence of sunlight. Constituents include carbon monoxide, hydrocarbons, ozone and various oxides of nitrogen. Carbon monoxide (Shephard, 1983) can increase the risk of cardio-vascular death in the elderly, and the combination of carbon monoxide exposure, the performance of maximal exercise and the excitement of intense competition could conceivably cause a similar catastrophe in a young athlete. If carbon monoxide is administered, oxygen transport is impaired by the formation of carboxyhaemoglobin and there is a left-ward shift of the oxygen dissociation curve. Goldsmith (1970) reported slower times in swimming competitions when urban carbon monoxide concentrations exceeded 30 ppm, although it is difficult to be certain whether these changes in performance were due to the carbon monoxide, to other constituents of the smog, or to associated changes in the weather. Ozone at the concentrations found in large North American cities (0.1–0.3 ppm) also inhibits respiratory effort and reduces maximum oxygen intake. Wayne *et al.* (1967) have noted that athletes fail to demonstrate the expected training response when oxidant levels are high. Exposure to nitrogen oxides causes some reduction in pulmonary-diffusing capacity at a concentration of 0.6 ppm, a level occasionally reached in Los Angeles. Finally, oxidant smog is intensely irritant to the eyes, and can thus disturb performance in events where fine vision is required.

The best tactic for the team physician is to minimize exposure to all types of smog (Shephard, 1984). Reducing smog accumulates in the low-lying areas of an older city; it is thus an advantage to choose a hotel which is situated on a hill. The sulphur-laden smoke particles take a long time to penetrate a building, particularly if the windows are kept closed; indoor concentrations are often only a third of those outside. It is therefore best to remain indoors if the night appears smoggy.

At least 80% of carbon monoxide is generated by vehicle exhaust and levels drop rapidly on moving a few metres away from busy roads. Car journeys should be made at times of day when the roads are not congested, and where possible air should not be drawn from the road into the vehicle. Care should be adopted in selecting travel routes. Tunnels should be avoided, and it should be remembered that the concentration of pollutants is often less on wide open motorways than in narrower city streets, where the traffic is moving more slowly and air movement is restricted by adjacent tall buildings. The body eliminates half of an accumulated burden of carbon monoxide in 3–4 h, this process being speeded by the prolonged breathing of oxygen and by exercise.

If radio reports indicate that high levels of ambient ozone are likely, training should be conducted in the early morning and late evening, when the levels of this pollutant are much lower. There have been suggestions that some protection against ozone might be obtained by requiring the ingestion of anti-oxidant chemicals such as vitamin C and vitamin E, but to date benefit has not been confirmed.

Some adaptation to carbon monoxide is possible through an increase of haemoglobin levels (this response is seen in the chronic smoker). There have also been reports that the response to ozone is reduced after 2–5 days exposure to concentrations of at least 0.3 ppm. Chronic exposure to reducing smog lessens sensitivity to this type of pollutant, although the mechanism seems to be an increase of mucus production, hardly a desirable attribute for a competitive athlete.

References

Goldsmith, J. R. (1970) Contribution of motor vehicle exhaust, industry and cigarette smoking to community carbon monoxide exposures. *Ann. NY Acad. Sci.* **174**, 122.

McCafferty, W. B. (1981) *Air Pollution and Athletic Performance.* C. C. Thomas, Springfield.

Shephard, R. J. (1983) *Carbon Monoxide: The Silent Killer.* C. C. Thomas, Springfield.

Shephard, R. J. (1984) Athletic performance and urban air pollution. *Can. Med. Assoc. J.* **131**, 105.

Shephard, R. J. (1987) The respiratory system as a limiting factor. In I. Jacobs (ed) Limiting factors in endurance effort. *Can. J. Appl. Sport Sci.* (Suppl.) **12**, 455.

Wayne, W. S., Wehrle, P. F. & Carroll, R. E. (1967) Oxidant air pollution and athletic performance. *JAMA* **199**, 901.

PART 5

THE PROCESS AND IMPLEMENTATION OF PHYSICAL TRAINING

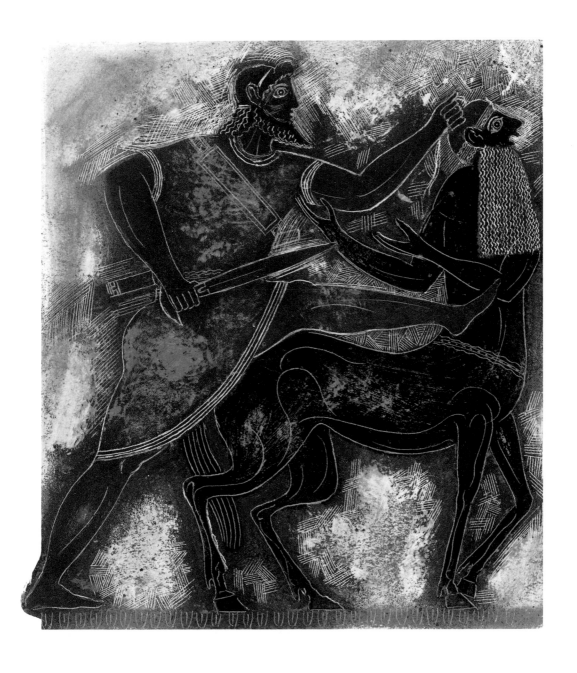

5.1 Strength and power

P. V. KOMI & K. HÄKKINEN

Introduction

Muscle strength and muscle power may be defined quite differently and their meaning can therefore also be different. Physiologically and also biomechanically their separation is somewhat difficult, because strength itself depends on the neural activation level and its value is time dependent. Power is also closely associated with activation and time. For these reasons, rather than trying to define the terms according to strict principles of physics, muscle strength and power can be understood in the way they have evolved in the practical training terminology. Strength expresses the muscle's ability to exert high forces, and power refers to the explosive nature of force production. Explosive strength may be synonomous with power.

There is no question that strength and power are essential elements in physical performance. For example every sport contains elements which require strength and power from our muscles. Depending on the specific type of activity, the requirement for strength and power are also specific. This has led scientists and coaches to experiment and think of the training methods which would suit most optimally the specific needs for strength and power development. This chapter focuses on some of the basic principles of strength and power training with the major emphasis on an attempt to explain the possible interactive processes which are — if not responsible — at least associated with the phenomenon of increase in strength or power.

Overload principle

In normal subjects muscle strength can be easily increased by almost any method, provided that the training loads used exceed those of normal daily activities. In fact, the greater the training load, the greater the strength increase will be. This so-called overload principle has been referred to in the literature as early as the late 1800s (Roux, 1895), and defined more clearly later (Hellebrandt & Houtz, 1956). Figure 5.1.1

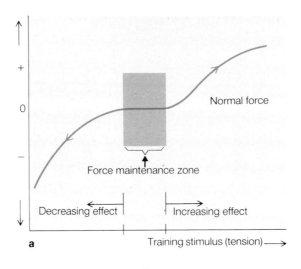

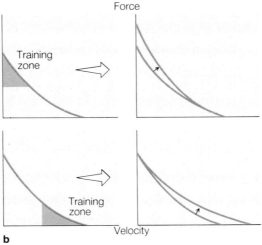

Fig. 5.1.1 Two important principles in strength and power training. (a) Overload principle, which emphasizes that increase in force is a function of the tension level, which must be higher than that in regular daily activities. From Komi (1975). (b) Force–velocity principle, which puts emphasis on the specific portion of the curve for selection of training loads.

presents schematically a more current view of this principle. The force maintenance zone refers to the situation where daily tension levels of specific muscles are sufficient to maintain the muscle's force capacity at the same level. If the exercise training loads increase there will be a training effect and strength increases correspondingly. On the other hand, if the regular muscular activity (tension) levels are lower than normal, the force capacity decreases (underload principle). The tension level is therefore crucial in the principle and it would be attractive to speculate that eccentric muscle contractions could be useful for strength training, because in this type of muscle action the force production capacity is the highest (see Chapter 2.1). Eccentric muscle training can indeed be very beneficial (Komi & Buskirk, 1972) provided that training is progressive and excessive muscle soreness is avoided.

Training tensions above the maintenance zone belong, therefore, to the strength training zone. The training zone can be defined more practically as loads ranging, for example, between 60 and 100% of the maximal voluntary strength performance. In strength athletes the corresponding zone could be limited to 80–100%. In this connection maximal refers to the maximal amount of weight that can be lifted for a single repetition (1RM). 2RM would be a slightly lighter load which could be lifted twice. On average, a load that can be lifted ten times (10RM) corresponds approximately to the load of 75% of 1RM.

Force–velocity principle

Training modes can be designed more strictly from the exact measurements of the conventional force-velocity (F–V) curve. Figure 5.1.1b presents a hypothetical model for such a principle. If the training loads are selected from the force end of the curve so that the loads are higher but the movement velocity lower (because of the high load) then the training effect is primarily in that particular part of the force–velocity curve. On the other hand, if the training zone is close to the velocity end of the curve, then the training effect is also primarily in the velocity characteristics. Depending on the training status of the individual, the response may not necessarily always follow this principle. For example, a subject weak in initial force and speed capacity can easily improve both components regardless of the area he or she chooses as the training zone from the F–V curve.

The preceding discussion on the principles of strength training did not include such aspects as frequency of training sessions per week, number of repetitions, rest pauses between exercise bouts, etc. All these aspects are important to consider when planning the strength-training programme. It is, however, beyond the purpose of this chapter to go into the details of these aspects, which are all of different importance in the programme depending on the specific practical purpose. For example, body building actually requires a different training programme to weight lifting. A sprint runner must apply different strength training principles to the hammer thrower, etc. For these reasons, it is more useful to look at the various structures in the neuromuscular system, in which adaptations may occur, in such a way that they might help in understanding the complex questions of, for example, specificity of strength and power training.

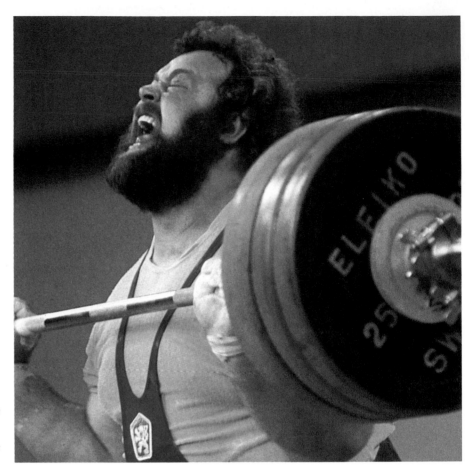

Fig. 5.1.2 A daily training programme for the development of strength must consider the forces to be developed in a bout and the number of repetitions for each bout, the rest pause between bouts and the frequency of bouts. Courtesy of the IOC archives.

Component analysis of strength and power training

Strength increase is not synonymous with hypertrophy. In fact it is possible that, especially in initially untrained subjects, a major part of the strength increase can often be attributed to an increase in neuromotoric activation of the muscle, because the measured integrated electromyographic activity (IEMG) may change parallel to the increase in muscle strength (Fig. 5.1.3a). Although EMG has not been used in many strength-training studies there are a number of reports which have shown force increases without appreciable increase in muscle circumference or individual muscle fibre size. For a review on the subject, the

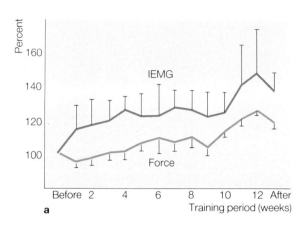

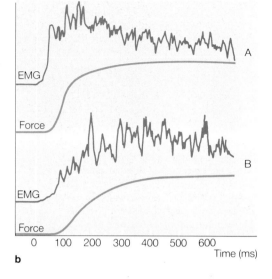

Fig. 5.1.3 (a) Increase in strength can often take place with a parallel increase in neuromotoric activation of the muscle. Young subjects (age range 13–15 years) trained four times a week with maximal isometric contractions of the knee extensor muscles. From Komi *et al.* (1978). (b) 'Parallelism' of rates of EMG and force developments during maximum isometric elbow extensors. The subject in A had a high rate of EMG increase, which was associated with rapid force increase. The subject in B had in both curves much slower rates of increase. From Komi (1986).

reader is referred to an article by Sale (1986). There seems to be an appreciable activation reserve, which can be mobilized with appropriate training (see Fig. 5.1.3b). There are several ways in which the training can change activation: (a) more activation to the prime movers; (b) an improved co-contraction of synergists; and (c) increased inhibition of antagonist muscles. Increased synchronized activation of motor units is reportedly a phenomenon which is characteristic of strength athletes (Milner-Brown *et al.*, 1975).

The current view of the mechanism of strength and power training also pays attention to the changes in the muscle tissue itself. Hypertrophy is a phenomenon which is characteristic of strength athletes, especially body builders. Increase in muscle mass comes primarily from the increase in the size of individual fibres, but probably not from an increase in the number of individual fibres (MacDougall, 1986). The latter idea is supported by the finding that body builders do not possess a greater number of muscle fibres in a specific muscle than their normal male counterparts (Sale *et al.*, 1987). Although the detailed mechanism is not known for the increase in fibre size, the necessary requirement for hypertrophy is that training loads are maximal or near maximal and that the total stimulus duration is sufficiently long.

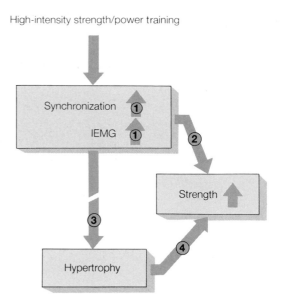

High-intensity strength/power training

Fig. 5.1.4 Schematic presentation of the sequence of events leading to an increase in muscle strength (or power) during the course of high-intensity training. Increases in synchronized firing of active motor units and increase in overall motor unit activity are assumed to take place simultaneously. Hypertrophy is a delayed process, but is an important contribution to the strength development. The numbers in circles refer to the order (time sequence) in which the specific changes and influences occur. From Komi (1986).

Muscle fibre hypertrophy is very probably a delayed process. The degree of hypertrophy is not only dependent on the type of training used, but its occurrence may follow the effects of the motor input; the preceding motor unit activation is a necessary condition for the hypertrophic myofibrillar changes. Figure 5.1.4 summarizes schematically the time course of the interaction between neural and hypertrophic factors. The early changes in strength training may be accounted for largely by

Fig. 5.1.5 Houk's component analysis of hypothetical stretch reflex (Houk, 1974). Stretch from L_0 to L_1 causes force to increase from F_0 to F_1. This change can be attributed to three functional components. (a) The muscular component, expressing the basic length–tension characteristics of the muscle. (b) The length–feedback component originating from the facilitatory spindle discharge. (c) The force–feedback component, which arises from inhibitory Golgi tendon organ discharge. The stiffness is defined by the slope of the force increase, and the length–feedback components either increase or decrease stiffness, respectively.

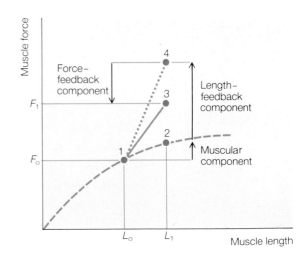

the neural factors with a gradually increasing contribution of the hypertrophic factors.

The component analysis can also be related to the stiffness regulation and stretch-shortening cycle (SSC); the basic concepts have been introduced in Chapter 2.1. One of the purposes of strength and power training is an improvement in muscle stiffness, especially in the explosive type of force production (power). Figure 5.1.5 presents a further, and more detailed, analysis of the various components which contribute to force production and muscle stiffness. The length–feedback component, which originates from muscle spindles, increases stiffness whereas the force–feedback component (from the Golgi tendon organs) decreases it. The final result is the line 1 to 4, the slope of which defines the stiffness. Figure 5.1.6 presents the possibilities which the training has on these two components plus the effects of neuronal adaptation and hypertrophy on the muscular component. The presented analysis is very relevant to the entire concept of strength and power training, including stiffness regulation. It could also be used as a basis for understanding the complexities of specificity of strength and power training.

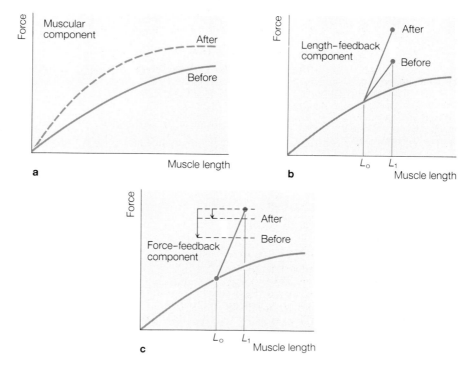

Fig. 5.1.6 Three objectives of strength/power training on the force–length relationship of human skeletal muscle. (a) The muscular component can be trained by increased motor unit activation (neuronal adaptation) and hypertrophy. The resulting influence is the shift to the left in the force–length curve. (b) The influence of the length–feedback component increases if training causes increases in muscle spindle discharge for the same stretch load. (c) The inhibitory effect (decrease in stiffness) from the Golgi tendon organ can be decreased by proper strength/power training. From Komi (1986).

Specificity of heavy-resistance strength and power training

A very important aspect from the scientific and practical point of view is the specificity of heavy-resistance strength and power (explosive) type of training on muscular performance during all types of muscle actions. This specificity can be demonstrated clearly by the specific training-induced shifts in the concentric force–velocity and isometric force–time curves, as well as by the specific shifts in the mechanics of various SSC exercises.

To support the hypothesis presented in Fig. 5.1.1b, typical heavy-resistance strength training which utilizes high training loads with slow contraction velocities, tends to improve primarily maximal muscular strength, i.e. in the high force portions of the *F–V* curve (e.g. Ikai, 1970; Coyle *et al.*, 1981; Häkkinen & Komi, 1985a). This can be seen from Fig. 5.1.7, which also demonstrates that the influence of heavy-resistance strength training becomes gradually smaller in the high velocity end of the *F–V* curve. The specificity in this regard is very consistent, as shown in Fig. 5.1.7b. When this kind of training is discontinued the decreases during detraining are greater in the high force end of the *F–V* curve. Experimental evidence is available to confirm that the specificity applies

Fig. 5.1.7 (a) Average force–velocity (load–vertical squat jumping height) curves of the leg extensor muscles during various concentric contractions before and after 24-week heavy-resistance (between 70 and 100% of the maximum) strength training. (b) Relative changes (± s.e.) in the heights of the vertical squat jumps (SJ) with loads of 0, 40 and 100 kg and in the maximal squat lift during the corresponding 24-week training period and the following 12-week detraining period in subjects (*n* = 11) accustomed to strength training. * = *P* < 0.05, ** = *P* < 0.01, *** = *P* < 0.001. Adapted from Häkkinen & Komi (1985a).

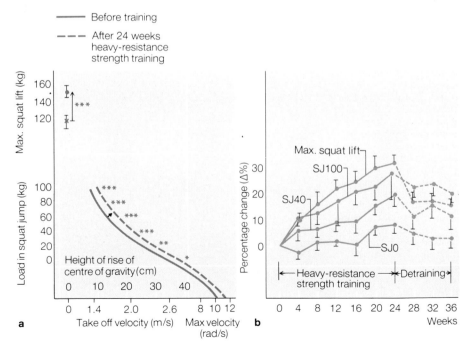

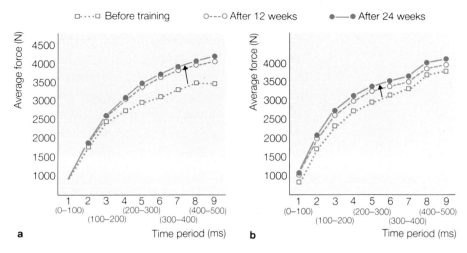

Fig. 5.1.8 (a) Average isometric force–(absolute) time curves in the explosive maximal bilateral leg extension before and after 24-week heavy-resistance (between 70 and 100% of the maximum) strength training. (b) Before and after 24-week explosive (power)-type strength training in subjects ($n = 11$ and $n = 10$) accustomed to strength training. From Häkkinen *et al.* (1985a, 1985b).

also to the velocity end of the *F–V* curve (Ikai, 1970; Coyle *et al.*, 1981; Häkkinen & Komi, 1985b) as well as to situations where higher loads are produced very explosively and with an exceptionally short duration (e.g. Schmidtbleicher, 1985).

In the isometric force–time curve the changes during heavy-resistance strength training are correspondingly in the high force portions of the curve, while the changes are gradually smaller in the very early parts of the force–time curve (Fig. 5.1.8a). The results in Fig. 5.1.8a also demonstrate that when 'pure' heavy-resistance strength training was intensively continued for several months no improvements or even some periodical shifts backwards in the very early parts of the curve were observed. In power training (Fig. 5.1.8b) the changes in the high force portions of the curve are smaller than those found in heavy-resistance strength training. Power training primarily influences the very early parts of the force–time curve (e.g. Viitasalo *et al.*, 1981; Komi *et al.*, 1982; Häkkinen *et al.*, 1985b).

Fig. 5.1.9 (a) Mean (± s.e.) heights of rise (of the centre of gravity) in drop jumps performed from different heights before and after 24-week heavy-resistance (between 70 and 100% of the maximum) strength training. (b) Before and after 24-week explosive (power)-type strength training in subjects ($n = 11$ and $n = 10$) accustomed to strength training. From Häkkinen & Komi (1985a, 1985b).

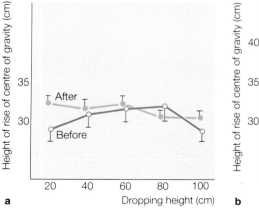

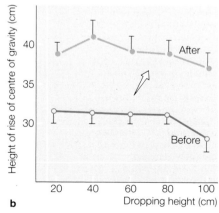

The specific effects of heavy-resistance strength and power training are very pronounced during SSC exercises, in which high contraction velocities are utilized. In contrast to heavy-resistance training, power training with various jumping exercises usually results in great increases in tolerance to, and utilization of, stretch loads (Fig. 5.1.9). These observations should be given special attention because of their relevance for practical purposes. The effective time taken by muscles to contract in normal movements and especially in athletic activities is very short.

Specificity of neural and hypertrophic adaptations

Strength and power training do not only increase neural activation in individuals with low initial force levels. This phenomenon can also be observed amongst strength athletes (Fig. 5.1.10). Prescription of training intensity is, however, more sensitive and difficult in this kind of subject group. When these strength athletes trained with submaximal loads of 70–80% of the maximum, the maximum IEMG decreased but it increased when the training loads were between 80–90% of the maximum or more. In strength athletes the training loading should be periodically varied and/or kept at progressively increasing levels to maintain training-induced increases in the maximal neural activation of the muscles (Häkkinen, 1985; Komi 1986).

In power training, in which the muscles are also highly activated in various training exercises but the time of this activation is short, the

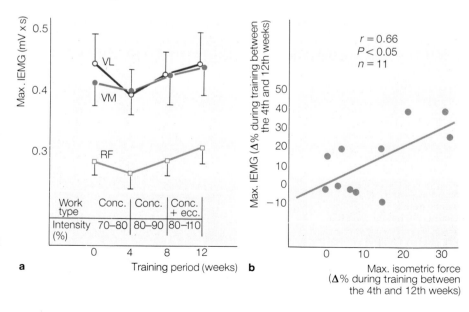

Fig. 5.1.10 (a) Mean (± s.e.) maximal IEMGs of the vastus lateralis (VL), vastus medialis (VM) and rectus femoris (RF) muscles in the bilateral maximal isometric leg extension in subjects (n = 11) accustomed to strength training during 12-week heavy-resistance strength training. (b) Relationship between the relative changes in the average maximum IEMG and the relative changes in maximal force between the fourth and 12th week during the corresponding training. Adapted from Häkkinen *et al.* (1985a).

increase in the maximal neural activation of the trained muscles is very specific. As presented in Fig. 5.1.11a, great increases may occur in the amount of neural input to the power-trained muscles during a short period of time—as indicated by the shift in the earlier portions of the IEMG–time curve. The positive correlation found between the individual changes in the 'early' IEMG and the changes in force production (power) during the early part of the isometric force–time curve (Fig. 5.1.11b) indicates strongly the importance of the neural component for this specific purpose (see also Schmidtbleicher, 1985). Explosive strength training improves muscle activation during the high-velocity concentric contractions and during the SSC exercises, in which high velocities are used. These increases occur parallel to increases in muscular power produced during the respective performances. These observations also deserve practical attention for the planning of training programmes, especially for various power-type athletic activities.

When a muscle of an initially untrained subject, in particular, is subjected to heavy-resistance strength training it will always respond by increasing its cross-sectional area during later training weeks/months. Training-induced hypertrophy in skeletal muscle takes place in both fibre types, although it may be greater in fast twitch muscle fibres (e.g. MacDougall *et al.*, 1977; Häkkinen *et al.*, 1981, 1985a; Komi *et al.*, 1982; Houston *et al.*, 1983). In strength athletes with a considerable training background, the response to heavy-resistance strength training is characterized by smaller muscular hypertrophy but also by its different time course in comparison to adaptations taking place among initially less

Fig. 5.1.11 (a) Average IEMG–time curves calculated from averaged IEMGs of the VL, VM and RF muscles produced during the first 500 ms in explosive maximal isometric bilateral leg extension in subjects ($n = 10$) accustomed to strength training before and after 12- and 24-week explosive (power)-type strength training. (b) Relationship between the relative changes in average 'early' IEMG and the relative changes in average 'early' force (power) (see Fig. 5.1.8b) after the corresponding 24-week training. From Häkkinen *et al.* (1985b).

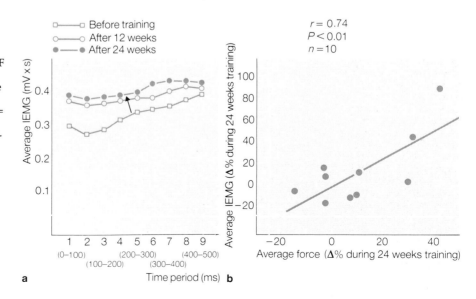

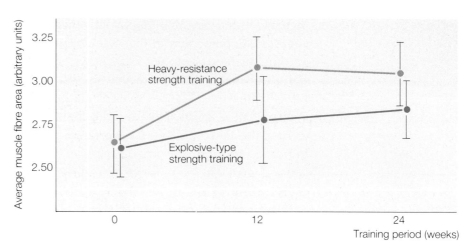

Fig. 5.1.12 Average (arbitrary units ± s.e.) total fibre area of the fast and slow twitch fibre types of VL muscle during 24-week heavy-resistance (between 70 and 100% of the maximum) strength training and during 24-week explosive (power)-type strength training in subjects ($n = 11$ and $n = 10$) accustomed to strength training. Adapted from Häkkinen (1986).

and/or untrained subjects (e.g. Häkkinen, 1985). As has been already speculated, the type of strength-training regimen may also be of some importance with regard to the degree of hypertrophy, because élite weight lifters are well known to differ with respect to their smaller muscle mass from those of élite body builders (e.g. Häkkinen *et al.*, 1986). The importance of the training regimen in inducing muscular hypertrophy is maybe even more drastic, when the effects of power training are compared to those of typical heavy-resistance strength training (Komi *et al.*, 1982; Häkkinen, 1986) (Fig. 5.1.12). Especially in previously well-trained subjects and/or athletes, power-type training does not necessarily result in muscular hypertrophy despite prolonged training periods. These findings further specify the suggested concept of specificity of heavy-resistance strength and power training. Since muscle hypertrophy is known to contribute to the increase in maximal strength, it is natural that the increase in maximal strength during heavy-resistance strength training is much greater than that induced by power training. The reason for the slight hypertrophy during power training may be due to the short total time the muscles are active. On the other hand, this observation can be considered as advantageous in several athletic activities, because muscle power can be increased without a corresponding increase in muscle mass and bodyweight. These advantages cannot, however, be seen unless the strength/power-training programmes have been well spaced and matched with the specific needs of the sports event.

References

Coyle, E., Feiring, C., Rotkis, T., Cote, R., Roby, F., Lee, W. & Wilmore, J. (1981) Specificity of power improvements through slow and fast isokinetic training. *J. Appl. Physiol.* **51(6)**, 1437.

Häkkinen, K. (1985) Factors influencing trainability of muscular strength during short term and prolonged training. *Nat. Strength Cond. Assoc. J.* **2**, 32.

Häkkinen, K. (1986) Training and detraining adaptations in electromyographic, muscle fibre and force production characteristics of human leg extensor muscles with special reference to prolonged heavy resistance and explosive type strength training. *Studies in Sport, Physical Education and Health.* University of Jyväskylä, Jyväskylä.

Häkkinen, K., Alén, M., Kauhanen, H. & Komi, P. V. (1986) Comparison of neuromuscular performance capacities between weight lifters, power lifters and body builders. *Int. Olympic Lifter* **5**, 24.

Häkkinen, K., Alén, M. & Komi, P. V. (1985a) Changes in isometric force- and relaxation-time, electromyographic and muscle fibre characteristics of human skeletal muscle strength training and detraining. *Acta Physiol. Scand.* **125**, 573.

Häkkinen, K. & Komi, P. V. (1985a) Changes in electrical and mechanical behaviour of leg extensor muscles during heavy resistance strength training. *Scand. J. Sports Sci.* **7**, 55.

Häkkinen, K. & Komi, P. V. (1985b) Effect of explosive type strength training on electromyographic and force production characteristics of leg extensor muscles during concentric and various stretch-shortening cycle exercise. *Scand. J. Sports Sci.* **7**, 65.

Häkkinen, K., Komi, P. V. & Alén, M. (1985b) Effect of explosive type strength training on isometric force- and relaxation-time, electromyographic and muscle fibre characteristics of leg extensor muscles. *Acta Physiol. Scand.* **125**, 587.

Häkkinen, K., Komi, P. V. & Tesch, P. A. (1981) Effect of combined concentric and eccentric strength training and detraining on force–time, muscle fiber and metabolic characteristics of leg extensor muscles. *Scand. J. Sports Sci.* **3(2)**, 50.

Hellebrandt, F. A. & Houtz, S. J. (1956) Mechanisms of muscle training in man. *Phys. Ther. Rev.* **36**, 371.

Houk, J. C. (1974) Feedback control of muscle: a synthesis of the peripheral mechanisms. In W. B. Mountcastle (ed) *Medical Physiology*, 13th edn, pp. 668–677. Mosby, St Louis.

Houston, M., Froese, E., Valeriote, St., Green, H. & Ranney, D. (1983) Muscle performance, morphology and metabolic capacity during strength training and detraining: a one leg model. *Eur. J. Appl. Physiol.* **51**, 25.

Ikai, M. (1970) *Training of muscle strength and power in athletes.* Presented at the FIMS Congress, Oxford, 1970.

Komi, P. V. (1975) Faktoren der Muskelkraft und Prinzipien des Krafttrainings. *Leistungssport* **1**, 3.

Komi, P. V. (1986) Training of muscle strength and power: interaction of neuromotoric, hypertrophic, and mechanical factors. *Int. J. Sports Med.* (Suppl.) **7**, 10.

Komi, P. V. & Buskirk, E. R. (1972) Effect of eccentric and concentric muscle conditioning on tension and electrical activity of human muscle. *Ergonomics* **15(4)**, 417.

Komi, P. V., Karlsson, J., Tesch, P., Suominen, H. & Heikkinen, E. (1982) Effects of heavy resistance and explosive type strength training methods on mechanical, functional and metabolic aspects of performance. In P.V. Komi (ed) *Exercise and Sport Biology*, pp. 90–102. Human Kinetics, Champaign.

Komi, P. V., Viitasalo, J., Rauramaa, R. & Vihko, V. (1978) Effect of isometric strength training methods on mechanical, electrical and metabolic aspects of muscle function. *Eur. J. Appl. Physiol.* **40**, 45.

MacDougall, J. D. (1986) Morphological changes in human skeletal muscle following strength training and immobilization. In N. L. Jones, N. McCartney & A. McComas (eds) *Human Muscle Power*, pp. 269–288. Human Kinetics, Champaign.

MacDougall, J., Elder, G., Sale, D., Moroz, J. & Sutton, J. (1977) Skeletal muscle hypertrophy and atrophy with respect to fibre type in humans (Abstract). *Can. J. Appl. Sport Sci.* **2(4)**, 229.

Milner-Brown, H. S., Stein, R. B. & Lee, R. G. (1975) Synchronization of human motor units: possible roles of exercise and supramaximal reflexes. *Electroencephalogr. Clin. Neurophysiol.* **38**, 245.

Roux, W. (1985) *Gesammelte Abhandlungen über Entricklungs—Mechanik der Organismen*, Vol. 1. Funktionelle Anpassung, Leipiz.

Sale, D. (1986) Neural adaptation in strength and power training. In N. L. Jones, N. McCartney & A. McComas (eds) *Human Muscle Power*, pp. 289–307. Human Kinetics, Champaign.

Sale, D. G., MacDougall, J. D., Alwoy, S. E. & Sutton, J. R. (1987) Voluntary strength and muscle characteristics in untrained men and women and male body builders. *J. Appl. Physiol.* **62(5)**, 1786.

Schmidtbleicher, D. (1985) Klassifizierung der Trainingsmethoden im Krafttraining. *Lehre der Leichtathletik* **24(1/2)**, 25.

Viitasalo, J. T., Aura, O., Häkkinen, K., Komi, P. V. & Nikula, J. (1981) Untersuchung von Trainingswirkungen auf die Krafterzeugung und Sprunghöhe. *Leistungssport* **11(4)**, 278.

5.2 Coordination and balance

K. TITTEL

Introduction

Coordination, as the cooperative interaction of the nervous system and the skeletal muscles, plays a decisive role in successful sports performance along with strength, power, speed and endurance. The early development of motor coordination has many implications for the competitor: (a) the determination of the eventual limits on the dynamics, efficiency and quality of performance; (b) the degree to which the metabolic energy-release mechanisms can be utilized; (c) the facilitation of appropriate and rapid responses in the control of body equilibrium to changing situations and conditions; (d) the assurance of the performance of certain activities with grace and beauty of movement; and (e) the protection of the competitor against injuries attributable to awkward movement and chronic overloading of bone, cartilage and other connective tissue. The optimal development of coordinative capability serves as the basis for successful motor learning in every sport and the eventual performance of movements and sports skills at the highest levels of mastery (Fig. 5.2.1). This is particularly important for such technical acrobatic sports as gymnastics, rhythmic gymnastics, diving and figure skating, as well as for technical events in track and field and other sports activities like swimming, wrestling, fencing, boxing and ball games.

Athletic activities require a well-tuned cooperation of all the factors contributing to performance, including coordinative, conditional and intellectual capabilities, as well as technical or tactical/technical skills and character/moral capacities. Investigational results should always consider this larger context. It is also, therefore, rather difficult to train coordinative capabilities systematically or through general principles as used in undifferentiated agility training. For instance, in basketball one needs to specifically train reactive, combinatory, changing, differentiating and orientational capabilities in a sport-specific way. Training methods should be selected in a way whereby those coordinative capabilities which are primarily trained are those needed for a given sports event, and should improve technical/tactical skills and their practical application.

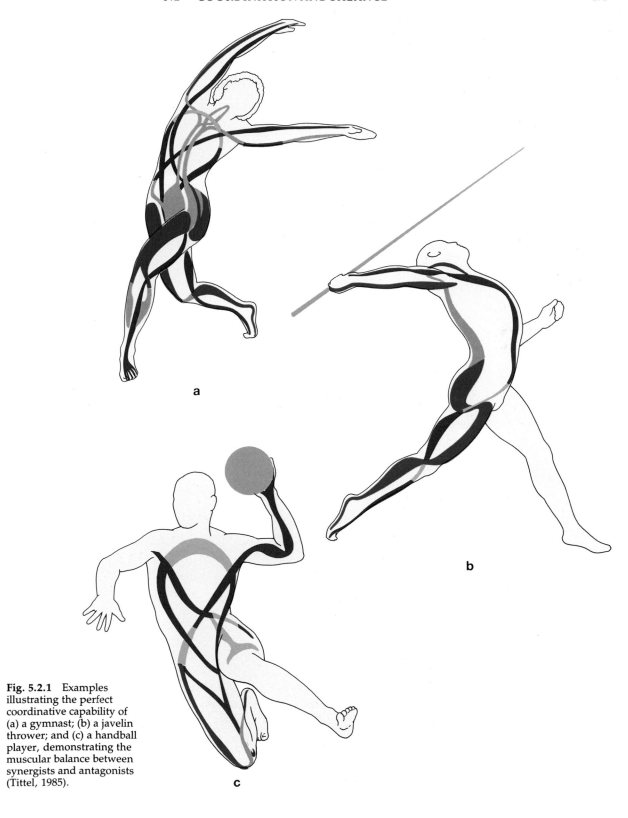

Fig. 5.2.1 Examples illustrating the perfect coordinative capability of (a) a gymnast; (b) a javelin thrower; and (c) a handball player, demonstrating the muscular balance between synergists and antagonists (Tittel, 1985).

Motor coordination

In sports sciences, five fundamental coordinative capabilities can normally be distinguished which demonstrate, according to Hirtz (1981), a hierarchical order:

1 To spatially orientate oneself.
2 To kinesthetically differentiate.
3 To react.
4 To keep rhythms.
5 To maintain balance.

The two capabilities mentioned first present relatively consolidated and generalized process qualities of motor control of movements. The latter three relate to qualities using sensory and complicated programming and performance operations. Speed and endurance coordinative capabilities are border areas of the energetical-conditional capability complex, while motor learning, controlling, and adaptational capacities should be seen as being the principal aims of coordinative capabilities.

Seen from the sports medicine point of view, the coordination of a movement is mainly the internal organization of the optimal control of the motor system and its parts. At stake is the acquirement of motor skills, which can be found in an optimization of the cooperation of motor units in one muscle (intramuscular coordination) or in several muscles

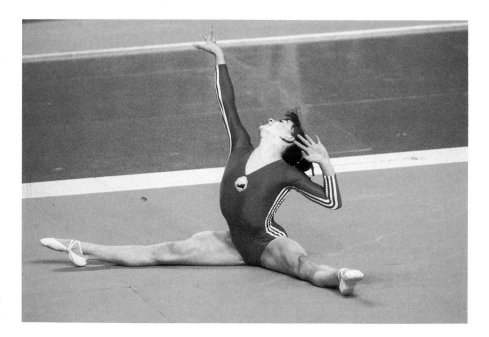

Fig. 5.2.2 Spatial orientation and kinesthetic differentiation are strongly in evidence during the performance of a champion gymnast. Courtesy of the IOC archives.

(intermuscular coordination) including internal or external feedback mechanisms. The basis of coordinative capabilities lies in the highest levels of the CNS and sensory motor subsystems. The cerebral cortex develops a motor programme which is called upon via pyramidal pathways and deeper brain structures, and leads to the corresponding skeletal muscles after switching motor nervous pathways in the spinal cord (Fig. 5.2.3). The muscles can thus perform purposeful activities supported by nervous irritational and inhibitional processes. Studies on the sensomotor transfer behaviour point to the fact that different regulating and controlling mechanisms come into effect at differing motor frequencies:

1   Slow motor frequencies are performed according to the 'follow-up regulation' from one point to the other.
2   'Programmed control' is utilized at increasing motor speeds. The limit lies between 0.5 and 0.8 Hz.

In both functional systems the following subfunctions and performances can be registered during the process of motor coordination:

1   Intellectual cognitive activities with information intake via the optical, acoustical or tactile-kinesthetic sensors, central nervous information

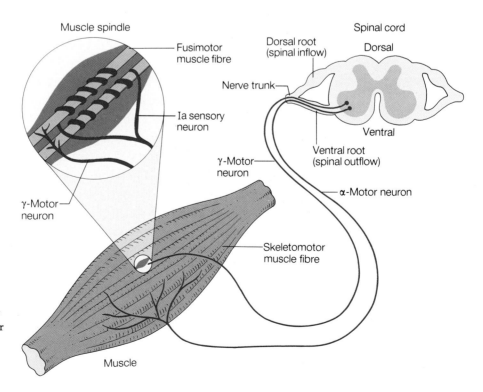

Fig. 5.2.3 Cross-section of the spinal cord in the lumbar region, with an enlarged detail of a muscle spindle (Edgerton, 1979).

processing (calling upon the motor memory), motor conception, complex motor anticipation and concentration.

2 Control and regulatory mechanisms to perform various motor coordinative activities—programming the motor answer and altering the contraction or relaxation of skeletal muscles, and regulating the components in a motor system by means of a 'debit–credit comparison'.

These mechanisms form part of the neurophysiological fundamentals of coordinative capabilities and their control (Farfel, 1977; Freund, 1983; Paerisch, 1984; Pickenhain *et al.*, 1985; Rühl & Wittekopf, 1985; Wittekopf & Beyer, 1986; Bernstein, 1987).

Neurophysiological fundamentals of coordinative capabilities

The working capacity of the sensors (acting as specific receptors or 'measuring devices') of the afferent nerval pathways and sensory centres and of the primary projectional fields in the cortex cerebri are essential presuppositions for the quality of information intake and processing (see Fig. 5.2.3). All those muscle groups which are responsible for motor reaction in the body are represented in the gyrus precentralis of the lobus frontalis. An electrical stimulation of it facilitates movements that are, however, rather disordered. This is because the corresponding 'control values' in the nervous cell complexes of the motor cortical areas and the subcortical regions (particularly in the formatio reticularis of the brain stem) and the cerebellum caused by the incoming information have not yet been triggered. This skeletal–motor target function is important for the regulation that follows to adapt cardiac, vascular and respiratory activities to muscular efforts. The transfer of that target function is supraspinally made in the vegetative core areas of the hypothalamus and medulla oblongata. It runs via two parts linked with each other—nervous and humoral—although in practice one pathway tends to be dominant.

The final aim of perfecting coordinative capabilities for a given motor process is the ingraining or 'tracking' of an optimal pattern which is generally termed the motor stereotype. This can be defined as the temporally–spatially identical performance of a given movement repetition conditioning the application of identical motor units at a constant impulse frequency. According to Pavlov (1953), who introduced that term in 1927, motor stereotypes characterize actional sequences which are mainly based upon trained conditioned reflexes, which may, however, not be transferred to human automatized movements. A decisive role is, for example, played by the requirement not only to ingrain an optimal motor stereotype in combat sports or ball games but also to adapt the trained motor pattern in newly occurring situations. Put the other way round, in human beings there are possibilities for modifications in the relatively stereotypical motor chains of automated movements, thus providing for a certain flexibility according to the anticipated action target and the unforeseen situation. It is now known that intermuscular coordination is due to clear variance even if the motor stereotype is highly established. It seems, therefore, to be more correct to use the term motor-dynamical stereotype.

Four stages may be defined in the development and training of optimal intermuscular coordination:

1   The beginner forms a picture of the motor process in the cortex cerebri by theoretical explanations and practical demonstrations using film loops, video tapes or sequence photos—mental training.
2   Collecting individual experiences of motor processes with corresponding irritation of stimulating processes.
3   Avoiding irrelevant co-actions of inadequate muscles.
4   Automation and stabilization of coordination (forming a motor-dynamic stereotype) with optimal intra- and intermuscular coordination.

Effect of age on training of coordinative capabilities

The consolidation of coordinative capabilities is highly affected by biological age. Longitudinal as well as cross-sectional studies by Hirtz (1979, 1981) with 2200 7- to 16-year-old pupils and 19- to 25-year-old students allowed the definition of certain categories of coordinative capabilities during ageing. It was found that stagnation , or even regression, can occur in developing coordinative capabilities during pubescence. This was characterized in particular by large differences in biological developmental levels or stage of somatotypical criteria. This statement can be confirmed by our studies on complex reactive, kinesthetic differentiation, spatial orientation and balancing capabilities with 13-year-old handball players. In addition to remarkable differences between biological and calendar ages (up to 6.1 years), body height (up to 44.1 cm), bodyweight (up to 48 kg) and muscular mass (up to 25.5 kg), a non-linear relationship could be seen between biological age and coordinative capabilities. Individuals who were biologically younger (biologically aged about 11 years) showed better coordination test results than children biologically aged 13 or 14 years. This result means that co-ordinative maturity occurs before sexual maturity. There was also a non-linear relationship between somatotypical characteristics and coordina-tive capabilities, shown by the better test performances achieved by the biologically younger players.

The following conclusions can be made:

1 It is necessary to consider biological age whenever coordinative capabilities are to be assessed, trained or perfected with adolescents.
2 During pubescence the perfection of coordinative capabilities is hampered because morphological and functional changes in the body result in a need for a 'tuning-up' of control and regulatory mechanisms. The timing of this is more reliably characterized by the biological age and the real development of somatotypical features than by calendar age.
3 A better potential for developing and training coordinative capabilities can be found prior to pubescence; the focus of learning must, therefore, lie at an earlier age with biologically advanced children than with retarded ones.

These variations in maturity and development of coordinative capa-bilities must be given special consideration when they are assessed and measured. Sometime around the eighth or ninth year the spatial com-ponent of the motor analyzer develops, as well as maximal motor frequency and speed coordination. During the 11th and 12th years reactive capability using acoustic and optical signals and rhythmic capacity are fully developed. The reason why the lower developmental dynamics are temporarily phasic lies in the generally restricted motor activity during the tenth and 11th years.

The training of coordinative capabilities (Israel, 1976; Willimczik, 1979; Winter, 1981), the effects of which result from the dominance of practis-ing the corresponding motor pattern, can be supported during child-hood and adolescence by changed external conditions, which include:

1 Adjusting boats, lengths and widths of sculls, oars or paddles in accordance with the somato-typical conditions of rowers and canoeists.
2 Altering dimensions or adjusting equipment in gymnastics (e.g. of bar thickness).
3 Reducing the weight of athletic equipment (e.g. shots, javelins, discs, hammers).
4 Adjusting ball sizes (handball), ball weights (football), net heights (volleyball), basket heights (basketball) and playing field sizes.

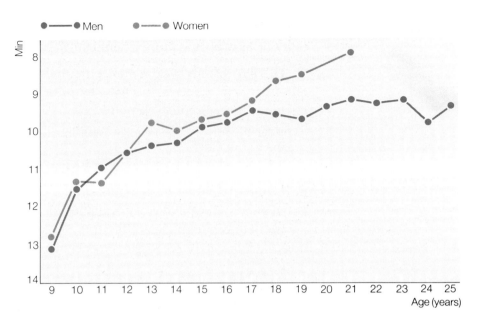

Fig. 5.2.4 Hand skill dependent on age and sex (Rutenfranz & Hettinger, 1959).

Varying the external conditions can enhance training but the alteration in weight or resistance should not be so large as to basically change the characteristics of rhythm or speed (and thus of the coordinatory structure).

Sex-specific differences These occur only during the 12th or 13th year of age (Fig. 5.2.4), as compared to conditional-energetical areas related particularly to spatial orientation, reaction and balance capabilities and maximum speed. According to Rutenfranz and Hettinger (1959), women show 10% better coordinative capabilities than men after 18 years of age and capabilities 6–7% better after 30 years of age (Müller & Vetter, 1954; Hettinger et al., 1976).

Measurement and evaluation of coordinative capabilities

Sports sciences (Ratov, 1972; Meinel & Schnabel, 1977; Blume; 1978; Hirtz, 1981) have concentrated on: teh egistration of cinematic values and trends, visual observations (supported by video or film recordings), and the construction of evaluational criteria. The following separate investigational opportunities are offered by sports medicine and those natural sciences cooperating with it to register and evaluate coordinative capabilities, despite their close functional interrelationship with total motorics (Wilke & Fuchs, 1969; Sologub, 1976; Hollmann & Hettinger, 1980; Bredow & Beyer, 1982; Beyer et al., 1983; Tittel, 1984, 1985; Pöthig et al., 1985).

Electromyography (EMG)

Electromyography provides an assessment of intramuscular coordination during a planned movement by offering an insight into:

1 The size of electrical action potentials, produced by the irritated muscular cell, whereas the EMG amplitude measures the mechanical response to an electrical stimulus.

2 The impulse frequency and number of motor units contributing by means of the EMG.

Simultaneous telemetric EMG recordings from several skeletal muscles during sport-specific movements provide information on the innervational efforts and the level of activities or their duration. The developmental of intermuscular coordination can be assessed from this information (Fidelus *et al.*, 1966; Kipke, 1966; Henrikson & Bonde-Petersen, 1974;

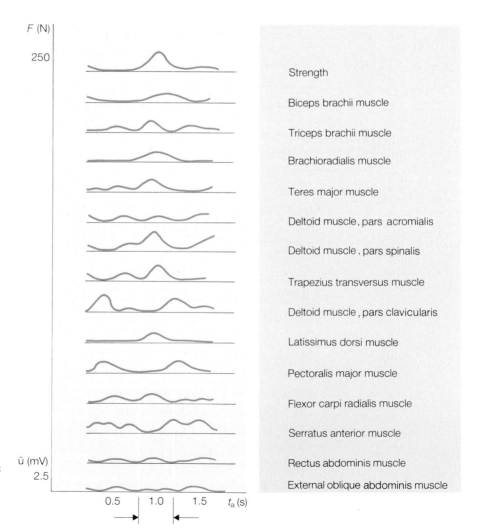

Fig. 5.2.5 Average EMG pattern of 14 single muscles in the arm, shoulder and trunk areas, and the corresponding pulling force and activity time using an arm force pull–press ergometer. F = pulling force; $\bar{u}$ = EMG amplitude; t_a = activity time. (Wittekopf & Rühl, 1984.)

Wittekopf & Rühl, 1984). Improvement in intermuscular coordination is shown by:

1 A decrease in electrical activities for a given load.
2 A reduction of overlapping between muscles participating in a movement.
3 Shorter and more precise functions of each muscle activated.

In publications available on 'topographic innervational pictures' during various sport-specific movements, very often the position used as a starting point is that a reliable relationship exists between the external dynamics of a movement and its muscular innervational pattern, which is, however, not true (Leipold-Büttner, 1979; Rühl & Wittekopf, 1985). Analysing, for example, the relationship between physical requirements of speed movements and the resistance to be overcome, remarkable differences can be found which can be registered very early by means of the Janda muscular functional test (Janda, 1986).

Figure 5.2.5 shows an average EMG pattern of 14 muscles in the arm, shoulder and trunk areas, and the corresponding pulling force and time under load (using an arm force pull–press apparatus). The inclusion of muscular efforts into motor phases allows assertions on synergistic or

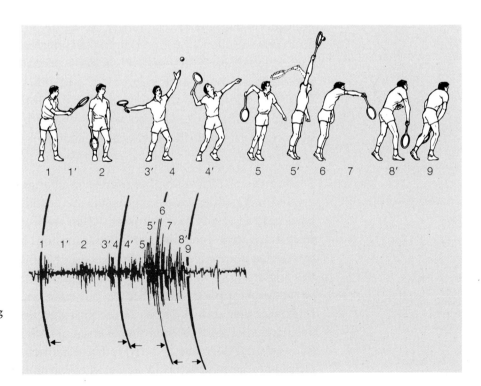

Fig. 5.2.6 Service of a tennis player demonstrating the different actions of specific main muscles and unspecific auxiliary and stabilatory muscles (Beillot & Rochcongar, 1982).

antagonistic active muscles, respectively, thus demonstrating once more that 'anatomical' antagonists might become functional synergists in certain conditions (Tittel, 1985). Furthermore, typical innervational patterns can be shown which—in accordance with their temporal sequence of action—provide for a differentiation of activated muscles into: (a) predominantly activated motor-specific main muscles; and (b) motorically unspecifically activated auxiliary and stabilatory muscles (Fig. 5.2.6).

The registration of pre-innervational phases (e.g. pars spinalis of deltoid muscle in Fig. 5.2.5) is also interesting because of their importance for powerful, explosive movements. Thus, a generally reliable assessment of the changed innervational level is possible, i.e. the substitution of the main muscles by auxiliary and stabilatory ones during changes in the temporal coordination of muscular efforts. In doing so, disturbances of the motor–dynamic stereotype can be diagnosed at a time when no changes in the external motor pattern can be observed.

Polymyography   Polymyography (according to Wyssochin, 1979) consists of a synchrone graphical registration of bio-electrical activity, strength (by means of dynamography) and muscle tonus (by means of tonography) of various muscle groups during arbitrary tensing and relaxing under isometric conditions (Fig. 5.2.7). The functional status of neuromuscular systems, and their variations through training at differing duration and intensities, can be objectively assessed by means of polymyography which has shown its reliability under laboratory and field conditions. In addition to that it is possible to diagnose troubles of intermuscular coordination caused by fatigue or overload, and to evaluate the efficiency of various training means and therapeutical measures or methods for recovery.

Electro-encephalography   During the last 15 years the interest in changes of biopotentials of the brain during athletic movements has increased—particularly stimulated by Anokhin (1960) and Bernstein (1987)—since they represent a complicated system–reaction that is programmed, regulated, and controlled by cortical neuronic systems. When certain methodical preconditions for the registration were kept to and automatic mathematical evaluative procedures applied, EEG studies provided statements on the level of intermuscular coordination. Thus, for example, it could be proved that an increasing perfection of motor-dynamic stereotypes is accompanied by a gradual decrease of activated cortical neurons and that regulating effects are more specifically directed towards the pyramidal cells in the

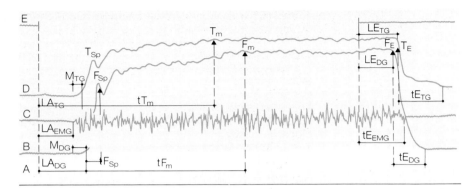

Fig. 5.2.7 Polymyography (Wyssochin, 1979) consisting of the synchrone graphical registration of the dynamogram (B), EMG (C) and tonogram (D); E is the signal for starting and concluding the load. Explanation of parameters: LA_{EMG} = latency time of exertion upon EMG; LA_{DG} = the same upon DG; LA_{TG} = the same upon TG; M_{DG} = latency time of muscle contraction (from first oscillations of EMG to ascent of DG curve); M_{TG} = the same (calculated upon EMG and TG); F_{Sp} = ascent amplitude of DG curve; tF_{Sp} = ascent time of strength from zero to F_{Sp}; T_{Sp} = size of first ascent of muscle tonus by reason of TG; F_m = maximum strength (calculated by the greatest amplitude of DG curve); tF_m = time up to F_m; T_m = maximum value of muscle tonus; tT_m = time up to T_m; LE_{DG} = latency time of relaxation upon DG; LE_{TG} = the same upon TG; F_E = size of muscle strength at the beginning of relaxation; T_E = size of muscle tonus at the beginning of relaxation; tE_{DG} = duration of relaxation (from F_E to zero); tE_{TG} = duration of relaxation (from T_E to zero); tE_{EMG} = total duration of relaxation upon EMG.

depths of the cerebral cortex, which is reflected in disappearing marked rhythms of surface EEG.

Muscular function test (according to Janda, 1986)

High levels of coordinative capabilities can only be achieved if an optimal relationship between muscular contractional and extensional capacities of synergists and antagonists exists. Investigational findings (Moore & Hutton, 1980; Berthold *et al.*, 1981; Tittel, 1984, 1986; Janda, 1986; Schmidt, 1986; Tauchel & Müller, 1986) point, however, to the fact that as early as from the eighth year of age muscular dysbalances can be found at unproportionally high levels, along with negative effects upon intermuscular coordination and the connective and supportive tissues (e.g. achillodynia, chondropathia retropatellaris or muscle traction fractures). Muscular dysbalances principally result from imbalanced training programmes. Strength exercises, for instance in a unilateral manner with extensor muscles (e.g. in rowing, throwing or shot putting), often neglect necessary stretching capacities in these muscles and their antagonists.

It should be remembered that a 'tonic' muscle, with its dominant supporting function, most frequently reacts to an overload during training by an obvious reduction of its length, whereas a 'phasic' muscle with its dominant motor function, reacts by a reduction of its force. Table 5.2.1 demonstrates those muscles which are particularly endangered with

Table 5.2.1 'Tonic' and 'phasic' muscles most liable to reduce in length or strength during training overloading.

Tonic muscles	Phasic muscles
Rectus femoris muscle	Rectus abdominis muscle
Calf muscles	Gluteus maximus muscle
Epaxial musculature	Gluteus medius muscle
Hamstring muscles	Trapezius muscle
Iliopsoas muscle	Rhomboid muscles
Tensor fasciae latae muscle	Serratus anterior muscle
Pectoralis major muscle	Prevertebral musculature

regard to reduction of length or strength. This is of importance in coordination training as a shortened tonic muscle inhibits its phasic antagonist thus preventing it from being optimally activated. Exercises to strengthen abdominal muscles are often erroneously performed, lifting the trunk with fixed feet; the already shortened iliopsoas muscle is thereby additionally reduced. This leads to a weakening of its phasic antagonists, the abdominal and buttocks muscles, thus reversing the original aim. Iliopsoas and rectus femoris muscles should therefore be excluded if a successful strength training with abdominal muscles is to be performed.

Janda (1986) has presented five basic stages for the assessment of muscular performances by the muscular function test. In sports medicine this can be restricted to the final three stages:

Stage 5 Optimal stretchability of the muscle or muscle group.
Stage 4 Slight shortening of the muscle; the range of movement necessary can be achieved by passive support.
Stage 3 Strong shortening of the muscle; because of a lack in stretchability the muscle can neither actively nor passively achieve the required range of movement.

The muscular function test is a semi-objective test procedure which provides (if performed three to four times per year at regular intervals) a sufficient evaluation of the strength and stretching capacities of muscle groups that cooperate functionally, thus assessing the developmental level and training state of intermuscular coordination. The advantage of the test lies in its small technological requirements (test plank-bed, goniometer, measuring scale in cm); its disadvantage is a degree of subjectivity, which might, however, be reduced by standardizing the test procedure and by repeating tests using one assessor. It is advisable to perform an EMG study at the same time as the Janda test.

Muscular dysbalances therefore result in a need for changes in training sessions: relaxing and stretching exercises should be included initially, particularly as the strength development of a muscle depends on its stretching status prior to contraction. It is possible to reduce the shortening of a muscle through a specific stretching programme over several years, e.g. in the iliopsoas muscle from 78% at the beginning to 30%, and the rectus femoris muscle from 81% to 39%. The amount of weakening muscular strength can be reduced by an individually adjusted strength programme, e.g. in the rectus abdominis muscle from 75% to 11% and in the gluteus maximus muscle from 63% to 0% (Dordel, 1975; Moore & Hutton, 1980; Rohde, 1984; Spring, 1985).

Spiroergometry and anthropometry

The assessment of oxygen consumption allows an indirect statement to be made on the quality of motor coordination for given movements per unit time (Bigland-Ritchie & Woods, 1974; Hollmann & Hettinger, 1980). Daily running loads from 15 to 30 min duration cause an obvious reduction of oxygen consumption after 2–3 weeks at a given rate with unchanged bodyweight. That oxygen saving can be as high as 15%. The reason why lies in the intermuscular coordination that has been improved by training, since cardiopulmonary findings which have been collected at the same time show no changes. Oxygen consumption is also closely related to anthropometric and biomechanical values, e.g. individual optimal stride length. This finding was put in dispute by Nurmi (Finland) who had an average stride length of 225 cm running the 1500 m race, as a stride length of between 190 and 200 cm would have been much more economic for his speed. Therefore, he could have saved oxygen and utilized it as an additional performance reserve. Even athletes with comparable physical capabilities like the former women sprinters Stecher (GDR) and Szewinska (Poland) differed quite remarkably in their bodyweights, body heights and coordinative style. Szewinska ran with an accentuated stride length whilst Stecher ran with an accentuated step frequency, as seen in those sprinters who dominate the scene today.

Posturography

Hierarchically structured and functionally intertwined proprioceptive and visual systems contribute to the adjustment of body balance. These systems become more differentiated during programmed training and can be assessed by means of posturography. Deviations from an erect posture are continuously registered as the athletes try to keep balance. The test is repeated once with open, and once with closed, eyes with movement in vertical, frontal and transversal directions by means

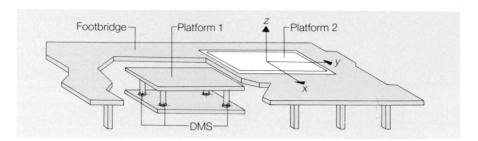

Fig. 5.2.8 Measuring platform with expansion stripe (Baumann, 1968) for the registration of deviations around transversal (x), frontal (y) and vertical (z) axes. DMS = densiometric stripe.

of a computerized system and a measuring platform (Fig. 5.2.8). This platform is placed upon piezo-electrical quartz crystals and is movable around three axes. From the curves gained, the quality of the capability to maintain balance can be evaluated.

According to studies made so far (Rossberg & Talsky, 1970; Dichgans & Brandt, 1980; Gundlach, 1985) practice sessions that apply stronger vestibulary stimulation have positive effects upon the vestibulospinal motorics, particularly important for gymnasts, ballet dancers and divers, who have to deal with multidimensional vestibulary sensations. After 12 days of rotational stimulation vestibulary reactions dwindled away, resulting in greater reliability of gymnastic exercises performed on the beam or horse.

Nystagmography This method can also be utilized for measuring the capability to maintain balance and to assess possible trainability (Wilke & Fuchs, 1969; Tokita & Fukuda, 1971; Krüger *et al.*, 1983). This procedure can, for example, be performed as thermic habituation by daily rinsing of the ear tube with 10–20 ml water at different temperatures (e.g. 17°C and 47°C) and then measuring the latency time and duration of the nystagmus. Research demonstrates a clear reduction of experimental nystagmic reaction after 2 weeks (Fig. 5.2.9).

In addition to these measuring procedures, applied mainly to register individual coordinative capabilities, some investigational methods shall be cited finally which have been reliable particularly in exercise medicine, neurophysiology and in psychology to test sensomotor performances. These are:

1 The O'Connor test (or ball test) to assess the coordinative capability of skillfulness.
2 Tapping (registering the maximum possible tapping frequency of an individual for 2 min) to assess basic psychomotor speed.

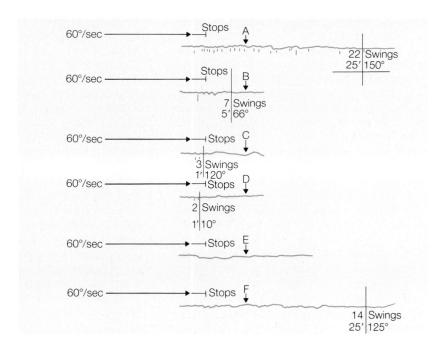

Fig. 5.2.9 Nystagmogram before, during and after vestibulary stimulations. After 12 days reactions dwindled away (Rossberg & Talsky, 1970). A = test before vestibulary stimulation (vst); B = after 5 days vst; C = after 7 days vst; D = after 12 days vst; E = termination of vst; F = 3 weeks after termination of vst.

3 Flicker-fusion frequency to register the optical analyser's capacity to discriminate as an expression of the actual activity condition of the central nervous system.

4 The impedance audiometry (significantly related to the latter flicker-fusion frequency) where the investigational results are clearly dependent on the loads applied.

5 Tachistoscopic studies to register short-period optical signals (e.g. by colour slides) to assess individual speeds of perception and processing.

All these technological possibilities to register and evaluate fundamental coordinative capabilities stress that high coordinative qualities, which are always specific, can be usefully trained as early as possible. This calls for the continuous cooperation of the sports physician with the coach or trainer and in particular with the athletes.

References

Baumann, W. (1976) Ortsfeste Kraftmeßplatte mit Dehnungsmßstreifenprinzip (DMS). In W. Hollmann & Th. Hettinger (eds) *Sportmedizin—Arbeits- und Trainingsgrundlagen*, p. 143. Schattauer-Verlag, Stuttgart.

Beillot, J. & Rochcongar, P. (1982) Électromyographie globale et applications en Médecine du Sport. In F. Commandré & Y. Bence (eds) *Explorations Fonctionnelles Neuro-musculaires en Médecine du Sport*, pp. 47–71. Masson, Paris.

Bernstein, N. A. (1987) *Bewegungsphysiologie*, 2nd edn. Barth-Verlag, Leipzig.

Berthold, F., Jelinek, W. & Albrecht, R. (1981) Die Bedeutung des Muskelfunktionstests nach Janda für die sportärztliche Praxis. *Med. Sport* **21**, 171.

Beyer, L., Wittekopf, G. & Schumann, H. (1983) Möglichkeiten und Grenzen in der medizinischen Bestimmung der Koordinationsfähigkeit. *Bericht Tag. Ges. Sportmed. DDR* **25**.

Bigland-Ritchie, B. & Woods, J. (1974) Integrated EMG and oxygen uptake during dynamic contractions of human muscles. *J. Appl. Physiol.* **36**, 465.

Blume, D. D. (1978) Zu einigen wesentlichen theoretischen Grundpositionen für die Untersuchung koordinativer Fähigkeiten. *Theor. Prax. Körperkult.* **27**, 29.

Bredow, E. & Beyer, L. (1982) *Koordinative Leistungsvoraussetzungen aus Sportmedizinischer Sicht.* Konf. Sektion Sportwiss., Greifswald.

Dichgans, J. & Brandt, T. (1980) Visual-vestibular interaction. In J. Held, H. W. Leibowitz & H. L. Teuber (eds) *Handbook of Sensory Physiology.* Springer, New York.

Dordel, H. J. (1975) Die Muskeldehnung als Maßnahme der motorischen Leistungsverbesserung. *Sportunterricht* **24**, 40.

Edgerton, V. R. (1979) The nervous system. In R. H. Strauss (ed) *Sports Medicine and Physiology*, pp. 49–62. W. B. Saunders, Philadelphia.

Farfel, V. S. (1977) *Bewegungssteuerung im Sport.* Sport-Verlag, Berlin.

Fidelus, K., Stache, H. J. & Schille, D. (1966) Elektromyographische Untersuchungen der Beuge- und Streckmuskulatur des Kniegelenks beim Muskelkrafttraining. *Med. Sport* **6**, 111.

Freund, H. J. (1983) Motor unit and muscle activity in voluntary motor control. *Physiol. Rev.* **63**, 387.

Gundlach, H. J. (1985) Posturographische Untersuchungen zur Differenzierung des quasi-statischen Gleichgewichtsverhaltens von Sportlern verschiedener Disziplinen. *Med. Sport* **25**, 69.

Henrikson, J. & Bonde-Petersen, F. (1974) Integrated electromyography of quadriceps femoris muscle at different exercise intensities. *J. Appl. Physiol.* **36**, 218.

Hettinger, Th., Eissfeld, G., Olbrich, K. H. & Seibert, U. W. (1976) Geschicklichkeit und deren Übbarkeit. In W. Hollmann & Th. Hettinger (eds) *Sportmedizin— Arbeits- und Trainingsgrundlagen*, pp. 146–152. Schattauer, Stuttgart.

Hirtz, P. (1979) Stand und Entwicklung der koordinativ-motorischen Leistungsfähigkeit von Kindern und Jugendlichen. *Theor. Prax. Körperkult.* **28**, 103.

Hirtz, P. (1981) Koordinative Fähigkeiten— Kennzeichnung, Alternsgang und Beeinflussungsmöglichkeiten. *Med. Sport* **21**, 348.

Hollmann, W. & Hettinger, Th. (1980) *Sportmedizin— Arbeits- und Trainingsgrundlagen.* Schattauer, Stuttgart.

Israel, S. (1976) Die Bewegungskoordination frühzeitig ausbilden. *Körpererz.* **26**, 11.

Janda, V. (1986) *Muskelfunktionsdiagnostik*, 2nd edn. Volk und Gesundheit-Verlag, Berlin.

Kipke, L. (1966) Das elektromyographische Bild des am Trainingsgerät imitierten Armzuges der Freistilschwimmer. *Med. Sport* **6**, 116.

Krüger, S., Gundlach H. J. & Dahl, D. (1983) Untersuchungen zur Frage der vestibulären Habituation— eine Studie an Wasserspringern. *Med. Sport* **23**, 309.

Leipold-Büttner, W., Haberland, M. & Wittekopf, G. (1979) Untersuchungen über den Zusammenhang von bioelektrischer und mechanischer Muskelaktivität bei dynamischer Muskelarbeit der oberen Extremität. *Wiss. Z. Dtsch. Hochsch. Körperkult.* **20**, 141.

Meinel, K. & Schnabel, G. (1977) *Bewegungslehre.* Volk und Wissen, Berlin.

Moore, M. A. & Hutton, R. S. (1980) Electromyographic investigation of muscle stretching technique. *Med. Sci. Sports Exerc.* **12**, 322.

Müller, E. A. & Vetter, K. (1984) Die Abhängigkeit der Handgeschicklichkeit von anatomischen und physiologischen Faktoren. *Arbeitsphysiol.* **15**, 255.

Paerisch, M. (1984) Neue Aspekte zur kontraktilen Dynamik von Muskeln. *Med. Sport* **24**, 225.

Pavlov, I. P. (1953) *Ausgewählte Werke.* Akademie Verlag, Berlin.

Pickenhain, L., Beyer, L. & Meischner, U. (1985) Neue Erkenntnisse zur Steuerung der Bewegungskoordination beim Menschen. *Med. Sport* **25**, 225.

Pöthig, D., Ries, W., Roth, N., Pögelt, B., Kucher, A., Pankau H. & Winiecki, P. (1985) Experimentelle Untersuchungen zum psychomotorischen Grundtempo im Alternsgang. *Med. Sport* **25**, 73.

Ratov, I. P. (1972) *Untersuchungen der Sportlichen Bewegungen und der Möglichkeiten zur Steuerung der Veränderungen ihrer Charakteristik mit Einsatz von Technischen Mitteln* (Russian). Diss, Moscow.

Rohde, J. (1984) Die Selbstbehandlung von Muskeldysbalancen. *Z. Physiother.* **36**, 305.

Rossberg, G. & Talsky, D. (1970) Untersuchungen zur Trainierbarkeit des Gleichgewichtssystems. *Sportarzt Sportmed.* **6**, 136.

Rühl, H. & Wittekopf, G. (1985) Die motorische Koordination bei automatisierten Bewegungsabläufen. *Med. Sport* **25**, 138.

Rutenfranz, J. & Hettinger, Th. (1959) Untersuchungen über die Abhängigkeit der körperlichen Leistungsfähigkeit von Lebensalter, Geschlecht und körperlicher Entwicklung. *Z. Kinderheilkd.* **83**, 65.

Schmidt, H. (1986) Muskuläre Dysbalancen und deren Beeinflussung durch Sport. *Med. Sport* **26**, 145.

Sologub, J. B. (1976) *Elektroencephalographie im Sport.* Barth-Verlag, Leipzig.

Spring, H. (1985) Was bringt das Stretching? *Schweiz. Z. Sportmed.* **33**, 21.

Tauchel, U. & Müller, B. (1986) Untersuchungen zu Muskelfunktionsstörungen im Kindesalter und die Bedeutung des arthromuskulären Gleichgewichts für die sportliche Belastung. *Med. Sport* **26**, 120.

Tittel, K. (1984) Morphologische Grundlagen für die Funktionsdiagnostik des Bewegungsapparates. *Z. Physiother.* **36**, 11.

Tittel, K. (1985) *Beschreibende und Funktionelle Anatomie des Menschen*, 10th edn. Fischer-Verlag, Jena-Stuttgart.

Tittel, K. (1986) Funktionell-anatomische und biomechanische Grundlagen für die Sicherung des arthro-muskulären Gleichgewichts im Sport. *Med. Sport* **26**, 2.

Tokita, T. & Fukuda, T. (1971) Telemetrische Übertragung der Augen- und Kopfbewegungen bei Körperdrehungen von Ballettänzern. *Med. Sport* **11**, 367.

Wilke, J. & Fuchs, H. (1969) Untersuchungen über Veränderungen der vestibulären Erregbarkeit durch sportliche Übungen und über die Habituation als Methode zum vestibulären Training bei Turnern. In F. W. Oeken & J. Wilke (eds) *Hör- und Gleichgewichtsorgan*, pp. 1–40. Barth-Verlag, Leipzig.

Willimczik, K. (1979) *Die Motorische Entwicklung im Kindes- und Jugendalter.* Hofmann-Verlag, Schorndorf.

Winter, R. (1981) Grundlegende Orientierungen zur entwicklungsmäßigen Vervollkommnung der Bewegungskoordination. *Med. Sport* **21**, 194, 254, 282.

Wittekopf, G. & Beyer, L. (1986) Physiologische Aspekte des motorischen Lernprozesses. *Med. Sport* **26**, 144.

Wittekopf, G. & Rühl, H. (1984) Beispiele oberflächenelektromyographischer Untersuchungen zur Beurteilung der muskulären Koordination sportlicher Bewegungsabläufe. *Med. Sport* **24**, 229.

Wyssochin, W. W. (1979) Die Polymyographie—eine Methode zur Untersuchung des Funktionszustands des neuromuskulären Systems bei Sportlern. *Med. Sport* **19**, 361.

5.3 Flexibility

M. HEBBELINCK

In simply moving a part or segment of the body the two most important factors involved are the power or amount of force present and the amplitude or range of motion. The former is indicative of the amount of function of the muscles crossing over the joint, and the latter of the amount of motion between the joint surfaces. Harris (1969) suggested five hypothesized factor structures (Fig. 5.3.1) based on single and combined segments moving in the different planes according to the degrees of freedom of the different joints. According to Holland (1968), flexibility is an erroneous term and suggests the use of the terms mobility or range of movement, whereas Fleischman (1964) distinguishes extent (or static) and dynamic flexibility. Extent flexibility refers to the amplitude of movement, while dynamic flexibility signifies the ability to move

Fig. 5.3.1 Hypothesized factor structures. From Harris, 1969.

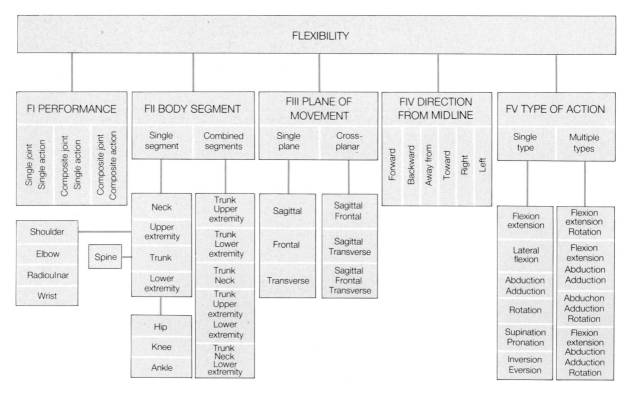

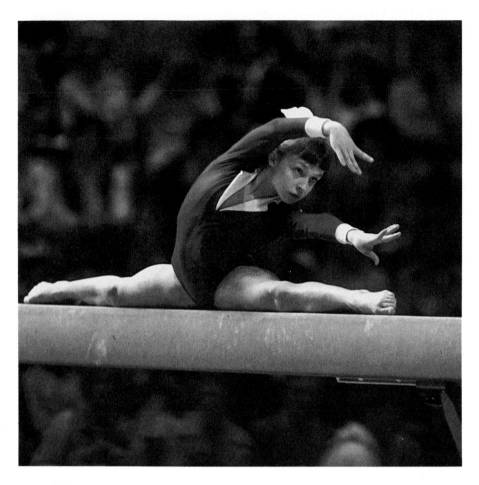

Fig. 5.3.2 Flexibility is specific to the sports activity but the ranges of most movements in women's gymnastics must be great for the élite performer. Courtesy of the IOC archives.

part or parts of the body quickly or make rapid and repeated movements involving muscle suppleness. From a factor-analytical study of Harris (1969) it appears, however, that these speeded movements are not measuring flexibility.

In most habitual daily activities, as well as in elite sports and recreational sports, flexibility (or absence of stiffness) is an important factor for physical performance. Flexibility or range of movement has also been considered an important factor for the prevention of injuries of athletes. One can distinguish two types of flexibility: (a) single joint motion, consisting of the direct measurement of the excursion of a limb or a segment of the body when only one joint is involved (e.g. flexion or extension of the wrist); and (b) composite, consisting of range of movement when using more than one joint or more than one type of action within a single joint (e.g. arm and shoulder extension in throwing).

Flexibility is not a general factor, but refers rather to a number of specific abilities, varying from one segment of the body to another or from one specific movement to another. The hurdler and gymnast, the pole vaulter and swimmer, all need flexibility, but the quality and intensity of the range of movement in each of the types of sport will be different and highly specific. While these examples may illustrate the specific requirements for different sports, it may be equally important to emphasize the importance of an optimum mobility of the various body segments to be present in order to meet the daily requirements of physical fitness and well-being.

Under normal conditions, the range of movement is restricted by the bone structure of the joint, cartilage tissue, length of the ligaments, and muscles, tendons and other connective tissues which cross the joints. The range of movement may, however, also be limited by the contact of muscle, fat, and remaining tissues compressed between the articulating segments of the bones. Age, body type, professional activities, gender, and factors such as temperature, humidity, warming-up, circadian variation, psychological stress or relaxation, and active or passive execution of the movement may influence the range of movement (Reilly, 1981). Extreme hypermobility and joint laxity may be due to intensive flexibility training prior to the calcification of the growth plate. Excellent reviews have been made on the anatomical and physiological factors determining range of motion (Holland, 1968) and on the effects of training and disease on connective tissue (Booth & Gould, 1975).

Stretching exercises

Over the past three decades researchers have devoted considerable attention to the application of flexibility exercises, particularly stretching. In order to achieve a greater range of movement, exercises are devised to stretch any major muscle group of the human body. All that is needed is time and sound anatomical and sports technical knowledge to explore the various locked joint positions related to the specific movements. Various methods can be used, for example, prolonged static or held stretch in which the participant voluntarily contracts the opposite group of muscles from those he/she is stretching, or a second method, called ballistic or rebounding stretch, in which a body movement forces a muscle or a group of muscles into a series of elongations one after another. In addition to ballistic and static stretching a third method is used in which active stretching is brought about by rhythmic movements. Passive stretching exercises are also used, in which the muscle elongation movements are done with the subject's own bodyweight or with the assistance of a partner, trainer or physiotherapist. Considerable comparative studies have been made on the advantages and disadvantages of the various stretching techniques, but no clear-cut conclusion has been reached (Borms, 1984).

De Vries (1974), who pioneered much of the scientific work in the area of flexibility and athletics, came to the conclusion that controlled static stretching exercises might be preferred since: (a) there appears to be less risk of injury (muscle soreness and connective tissue trauma); (b) the antagonistic muscles are fully relaxed; and (c) it requires less energy expenditure than the ballistic method. Often static as well as ballistic exercises are used in a warm-up, where all major joint complexes can be systematically mobilized. Particular sports call for their own specific emphasis and a considerable variety of stretching exercises can be achieved by changing the initial posture. A number of the stretching exercises used are of the Hatha Yoga type and more recently, with the revival of the fitness idea, not only coaches and athletes but also a larger public has become interested in stretching. The book by Beaulieu (1981), *Stretching For All Sports*, displays an impressive number of useful exercises and gives more than 600 references as well as a solid theoretical introduction to the subject.

Muscle tone and the capacity of muscle to relax are important features of motor performance. Amplitude of movement and an optimum prestretching may enhance the contraction force. This can be observed, for instance, in javelin and discus throwing. Physiologically, myotatic or stretch reflexes play an important role in the development of greater muscular power. The muscle spindle is activated when a muscle is passively stretched and evokes reflex contraction in the muscle concerned. It facilitates the contraction of the muscle stretched and at the same time it ensures a protective function in securing appropriate postural adjustments or evasion from extreme positions. Within the last few years a technique based on the principle of proprioceptive neuromuscular facilitation evolved as an alternative to the two traditional methods (static and ballistic stretching) for increasing flexibility. In principle this method, called the contract–relax technique (Wallin *et al.*, 1985) includes three phases. First, the muscle is stretched not quite fully to the end of its physiological range. At this time a maximal isometric muscle contraction is carried out and held for 7–8 s. After this comes 2–5 s of relaxation; then the muscle is passively fully stretched to the limit of its physiological range and held there for 7–8 s.

Flexibility exercises have to be incorporated in the preparatory part of a training session and have to be preceded by a general warm-up (callis-thenics and light jogging) of at least 10 min. Throughout the flexibility routine the amplitude of an exercise has to be increased progressively.

As mentioned before, strength has to be considered in a positive relationship to flexibility. This also holds true for neuromuscular co-ordination and flexibility. However, many coaches and athletes believe that strength gains may limit flexibility or hinder suppleness, or vice versa that substantial gains in flexibility may have a deleterious effect on strength. Such beliefs are mostly based on the observation that increment in muscle bulk may limit the range of movement. This may be true in extreme cases, but generally the capacity of a muscle to stretch cannot affect its ability to perform; swimmers or gymnasts who are both strong and flexible are proof of this concept. It should, however, also be realized that too much flexibility, either inherited or acquired, may hinder skillful performance, and that limiting the mobility of other joints may positively influence such performance. A correct ratio between strength and flexibility exercises must be respected according to the specificity of the athletic activity. It should also be noted that the emotional and psycho-logical status of the athlete plays an important role in maintaining and developing flexibility. The individual under stress may display an attitude of tenseness that could be manifested in a certain degree of joint rigidity. This state of anxiety is often reflected in an involuntary increase of muscular tone. Techniques that aid the individual in willed relaxation must be considered along with flexibility or stretching exercises.

Measuring flexibility

Since flexibility is not a general factor of athletic performance, but rather specific to each joint or group of joints, it is clear that simple tests such as the sit-and-reach test provide very limited information about parts of the body other than the subject's flexibility of the trunk and hips and forward bending. Several tests of this nature have been developed for assessing the flexibility of different parts of the body in different postures.

More accurate estimates of flexibility can be made using:

1 Goniometry; a goniometer consists of a 180° protractor, which may have two extended arms, one fixed at the zero line and one mobile, or just one mobile arm which can be locked in any position. The centre point of the goniometer is aligned with the centre of the joint and readings are taken in extreme positions.

2 Flexometry; the 'Leighton' flexometer (Leighton, 1966) contains a rotating circular dial marked off in degrees and a pointer counterbalanced to ensure it always points vertically. It is strapped on the appropriate body segment and the range of motion is determined in respect to this perpendicular.

3 Electrogoniometry; the electrogoniometer or 'Elgon' consists of two extended arms rotating around the knob and housing of a potentiometer. The two arms are secured to the moving body segments. Displacement and velocity are continuously recorded during motion so that changes in joint angles throughout a movement are monitored.

Besides these three commonly used goniometers, many other devices and apparatus have been developed, especially for use in physical therapy and physical medicine. The standardization of the clinical goniometry has been elaborated under the auspices of the American Academy of Orthopaedic Surgeons (1965).

References

American Academy of Orthopaedic Surgeons (1965) *Measuring and Recording Joint Motion*. American Academy of Orthopaedic Surgeons, Chicago.

Beaulieu, J. E. (1981) *Stretching For All Sports*. Athletic Press, Pasadena.

Booth, F. W. & Gould, E. W. (1975) Effects of training and disease on connective tissue. In J. H. Wilmore (ed) *Exercise and Sports Science Review*, Vol. 3. Academic Press, New York.

Borms, J. (1984) Importance of flexibility in overall physical fitness. *Int. J. Phys. Educ.* **21**, 15.

De Vries, H. A. (1974) *Physiology of Exercise*, 2nd edn. C. Brown, Dubuque.

Fleischman, E. A. (1964) *The Structure and Measurement of Physical Fitness*. Prentice-Hall, Englewood Cliffs.

Harris, M. L. (1969) A factor analytic study of flexibility. *Res. Q. AAHPER* **90**, 62.

Holland, G. L. (1968) The physiology of flexibility: a review of the literature. *Kinesiol. Rev.* **1**, 49.

Leighton, J. R. (1966) The Leighton flexometer and flexibility test. *J. Assoc. Phys. Ment. Rehab.* **20**, 86.

Reilly, T. (1981) The concept, measurement and development of flexibility. In T. Reilly (ed) *Sports Fitness and Sports Injuries*, pp. 61–69. Faber & Faber, London.

Wallin, D., Ekblom, B., Grahn, R. & Nordenborg, T. (1985) Improvement of muscle flexibility. A comparison between two techniques. *Am. J. Sports Med.* **13**, 263.

5.4 Speed and acceleration

A. THORSTENSSON

Speed and acceleration are important ingredients in many sports. Speed in a sports context can have several different meanings, one being instantaneous speed, for example the speed at take-off in a jump, or at release in a throw, another being average speed over a 100 m dash or, for that matter, over a marathon race. It is obvious that quite different factors are limiting in these situations and that the training has to differ accordingly. Here speed will mean maximal speed and thus apply to sports events where the highest possible speed is strived for in a single short-lasting effort or in repeated maximal efforts together lasting less than about 10 s. Acceleration means change in velocity over time and in this context the aim is to achieve the highest possible rate of velocity increase.

Many factors will influence the ability to reach high speed and acceleration. These include biomechanical factors as well as properties of the muscles and the nervous system (Table 5.4.1). The purpose of this

Table 5.4.1 An overview of factors influencing maximal velocity and acceleration during short-term physical efforts. The factors are listed roughly in the same order as they are discussed in the text (except the general factors, most of which are not discussed).

Biomechanical		Muscular	Neural	General
$v_f = v_0 + a \cdot t$	(1)	Mechanics	Neuronal properties	Dimensions
$F = m \cdot a$	(2)	force–velocity	excitability	
$F \cdot t = m \cdot v_f$	(3)	type of contraction	conduction velocity	Age
$M = F \cdot l$	(4)	stretch-shortening	transmission	Sex
$M = I \cdot \alpha$	(5)	force–time		Training
$I = \Sigma m \cdot r^2$	(6)	force–length	Coordination	
$M \cdot t = I \cdot \omega_f$	(7)	Morphology	recruitment	Drugs
$v = \omega \cdot r$	(8)	fibre orientation	synchronization	Fatigue
		fibre-type composition	agonist–antagonist	Motivation
		elastic component		
		Metabolism		
		energy stores		
		enzyme activities		

The abbreviations used in the biomechanical formulae are: v_f = final velocity; v_0 = initial velocity, a = linear acceleration; t = time; F = force; m = mass (inertia); M = moment of force (torque); l = lever arm length; I = moment of inertia; α = angular acceleration; r = radius (distance from centre of gravity to axis of rotation); ω_f = final angular velocity; v = instantaneous linear velocity; ω = instantaneous angular velocity. Each formula has a number which is referred to in the text.

chapter is to review some of these factors, and their implications for performance and training in events demanding high speed and acceleration. Based on this information some ideas about present and future training methods will be presented. Naturally several of the principles for training of speed and acceleration will be similar to those for strength, power, flexibility and coordination.

Biomechanical considerations

The magnitude and direction of the final speed reached after a period of acceleration will directly determine, for example, the height and length in a jump or in a running step. In turn, the magnitude of the final speed will depend on two factors, namely the size of the acceleration and the time during which the acceleration lasts (formula 1, Table 5.4.1). Often, but not always, the possibility to increase the time is limited and would rather lead to a decrease in performance. Thus, the ability to accelerate becomes critical. To accelerate a body takes an unbalanced force and the acceleration is directly proportional to the magnitude of the force and inversely proportional to the mass (inertia) of the body to be accelerated (formula 2). Consequently, the mass of the body and its segments has to be taken into account. This becomes even more evident when considering that the muscles, which are the prime generators of force, act over joints by producing torques or moments of force (formula 4). These moments are in turn resisted by moments of inertia (formulae 5 and 6). Thus, the length of lever arms and the distance from the centre of gravity to the axis of rotation also become critical.

Individual differences in dimensions can probably explain some of the variation in performance. The dimensions are essentially determined by heritage and could be one basis for selection. However, it is not clear which criteria should be used for such a selection. In sprinting, for example, the advantage of being short (low moments of inertia) in the frequency domain is counterbalanced by the disadvantage as far as the step length is concerned. In events where the whole body or part of it is to be accelerated, as in a jump, it is an advantage, everything else being equal, to be light in relation to the force-producing capacity. Thus, it is desirable that the training should result in an increased force but with as little muscle hypertrophy as possible (cf. below).

Another consequence of the above-mentioned biomechanical principles is that the angular velocity of a segment can be modified by voluntarily changing the moment of inertia. By keeping body parts close to the centre of rotation (low moment of inertia) the velocity of rotation can be increased without changing the applied torque (formulae 5 and 7). On the other hand, the linear speed is proportional to the radius at any point in a rotational movement (formula 8). Consequently, to attain a high linear velocity for any rotational speed the radius should be made as long as possible. Clear examples of these two principles are present in the wind-up and release in a discus throw or in a tennis serve. When the acceleration of several segments contribute to the final speed, such as when producing a reaction force from the ground in a jump, the proper timing of these segmental accelerations becomes important (cf. coordination below and Chapter 5.3).

It is clear from the above that a good technique, that is a proper utilization of biomechanical principles and passive forces, is critical for maximizing the output, the final speed, of a certain force application. Thus, training of technique has a central role in the programme for improving maximal speed and acceleration. Relatively small details in technique can be decisive between otherwise equal performers. Recent advances in biomechanical methodology, such as computerized movement recording systems and force plates will lead to improvements in technique analysis and training.

Fig. 5.4.1 The application of biomechanical principles to the refinement of a sports technique, as in speed skating, can increase speed and decrease energy cost. Courtesy of the IOC archives.

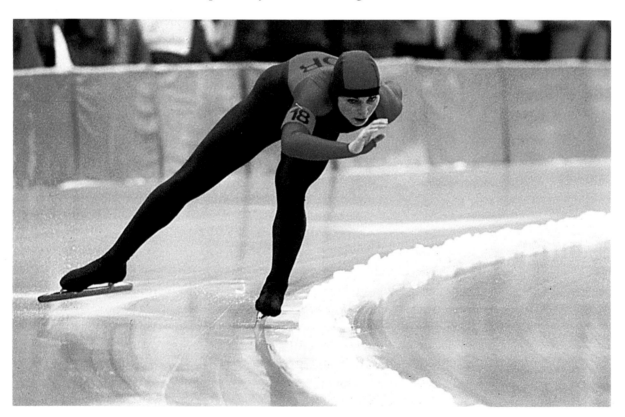

Muscle properties

The muscles are the prime generators of the force necesssary for athletic achievements. It is therefore worthwhile to discuss some factors related to the ability of the muscle to produce force under different circumstances.

Muscle mechanics

Force–velocity

The speed of muscle contraction has a marked effect on the force-generating capacity of a muscle (Fig. 5.4.2). The type of contraction also plays a major role. During concentric contractions, that is when a muscle is allowed to shorten while contracting, the maximal force declines gradually with increasing speed, whereas the opposite is true during eccentric contractions, when the active muscle undergoes lengthening (Fig. 5.4.2). Even though the speed dependency is less under eccentric conditions it is clear that the maximal eccentric force is higher than the concentric at all comparable speeds. Since the amount of muscle activation is reported to be similar in both situations, passive elements must come into play in the eccentric case. Although these elements are as yet not well identified, it is likely that training with eccentric contractions will lead to an increased quality and/or quantity of these passive (elastic) structures which might be important for fast production (cf. below). Some caution is warranted in the execution of this type of training since the extremely high forces can lead to tissue damage. It is well known that excessive eccentric exercise leads to muscle soreness (Fridén, 1983).

It should be remembered that force–velocity (or rather torque–velocity) curves like the ones in Fig. 5.4.2 have most often been obtained under isokinetic conditions, which means that maximal voluntary strength (torque) is measured at different constant angular velocities. Some limitations of this technique might affect the applicability of the results. Most natural movements are not isokinetic, but consist of accelerations and decelerations. However, it seems as if the actual speed is decisive for the force output and not the manner in which it is reached. This has been demonstrated in recent experiments on a new dynamometer, providing controlled accelerations and decelerations (Thorstensson, unpublished preliminary observations).

Another circumstance is that the force–velocity curve is dependent on the level of activation of the contracting muscles. During a certain athletic movement the activation is not always maximal, which means that the force–velocity curve for a muscle can have different shapes depending on the actual movement, such as in a step during running (Chapter 2.1). Also, the range of speeds provided by the available isokinetic devices are limited as compared to the highest speeds attained

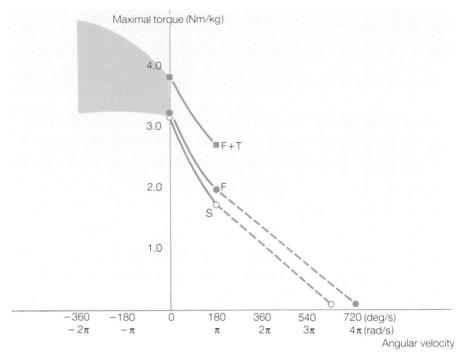

Fig. 5.4.2 Torque–velocity relations are shown schematically for intact human muscle. The curves are based on measurements during maximal voluntary knee extensions (modified from Thorstensson, 1976 and unpublished data). Torque is expressed per kg of bodyweight. Since angle-specific torque is analysed (at 60° of knee flexion, i.e. close to the angle for peak torque) and since angular velocity should roughly mirror contraction velocity of the active muscles, the torque–velocity curves are taken to represent force–velocity relationships. To the right of the y axis are concentric contractions performed by different subject categories. S = a group of normal, habitually active males with a predominance of slow twitch fibres (relative area of FTF is 40%); F = a corresponding group with a high proportion of fast twitch fibres (relative area 60% FTF); F + T = a group of Swedish national team sprinters and jumpers who had a high relative area of fast twitch fibres (70% FTF) and also several years experience of systematic training. The curves for the S and F groups are extrapolated with straight lines to the speed values reached with only the inertia of the shank resisting the movement. Corresponding data for the F + T group are not available. The pale green area to the left of the y axis denotes eccentric (lengthening) contractions where corresponding information is scarce at present.

in fast movements (cf. Fig. 5.4.2). However, one should remember that most natural movements are accelerated or decelerated starting or stopping at near zero velocity and that the highest force is produced closer to the lowest than to the highest speed. Therefore, isokinetic devices, recently also including possibilities to measure eccentric strength, are useful tools to evaluate force–velocity relationships and training programmes. Speed-specific training effects have been demonstrated after low load–high speed type of training (Chapter 5.1).

Stretch-shortening cycle   One way of changing the force–velocity curve during concentric conditions is to let the concentric contraction be preceded by an eccentric one. Such a stretch-shortening cycle (SSC) has repeatedly been shown to shift the

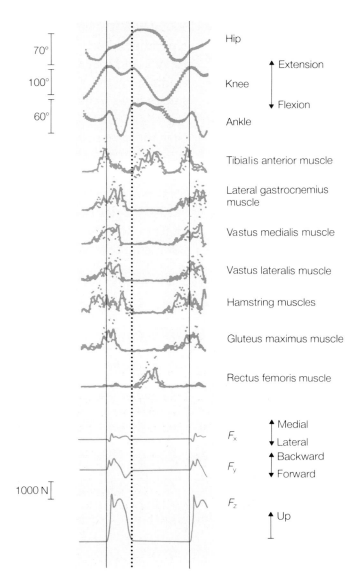

Fig. 5.4.3 An example of leg movements, muscle activity patterns (EMG) and reaction forces from the ground for a sprinter (bodyweight 75 kg) running at a constant speed of 8 m/s (modified from Nilsson *et al.*, 1985 and unpublished data). The stride cycle is normalized between consecutive foot strikes of the ipsilateral foot (continuous vertical lines). Ipsilateral toe off is indicated by a dotted vertical line. The contralateral support phase is represented by a horizontal bar at the bottom. The actual cycle duration was 500 ms and the support time was 145 ms. Calibration bars for displacements and forces are given to the left and arrows to show the direction of angular displacements and reaction forces are presented to the right. The EMG signals have been filtered, rectified and individually normalized, which means that no quantitative comparisons between muscles can be made. The curves for angular displacements and EMG are means for six consecutive strides. Points around the curves indicate ± 1 s.d.

concentric force–velocity curve to the right (e.g. Bosco, 1982; cf. Fig. 5.4.2), thereby improving performance. This phenomenon occurs spontaneously in many natural movements, such as jumping, running and throwing, and is a way of increasing the efficiency of movement (Cavagna, 1977). Compare, for example, the activity of the knee-extensor muscle vastus lateralis and the concomitant flexion movement during the early stance in running in Fig. 5.4.3. The SSC has certainly been included in training programmes before but during recent years it has been systematized into a special type of training, plyometrics, which has been shown to result in improvements of, for example, jumping performance (e.g.

Bosco, 1982). There appears to be room for much improvement and experimentation before this type of training is optimized. Factors such as the rate and magnitude of loading in the eccentric phase as well as the duration of the coupling time between the eccentric and concentric phases need to be investigated further.

Force–time   Time for force production is often limited in sports events. In sprinting, the support phase may last for only about 100 ms and the actual push-off phase only for half of that time (Figs 5.4.3 and 5.4.4). It is therefore important to be able to produce force fast. The rate of force production in a muscle is dependent on several factors. Some of them are more easily understood when viewing the muscle as a simple model consisting of a contractile component and an elastic component in series. During the

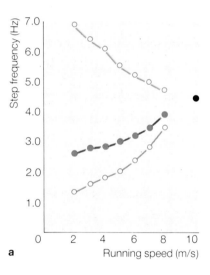

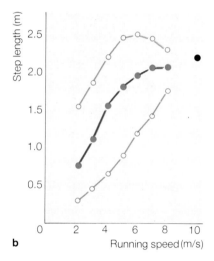

Fig. 5.4.4 Step frequency (a), step length (b) and support time (c) for a group of normal, habitually active young males during running at different constant velocities on a motor-driven treadmill. A step is defined as the interval between a foot strike and the next strike of the contralateral foot. The continuous lines show the average values for normal running. The area between the green lines represents the range between the means for the extreme values which the subjects were able to attain when asked to run with the highest and lowest step frequencies possible at each speed. Modified from Nilsson & Thorstensson, 1987). Values at supramaximal running speed (10 m/s) from Mero (1987) are also included for comparison (solid black circles); these data were obtained in towing experiments.

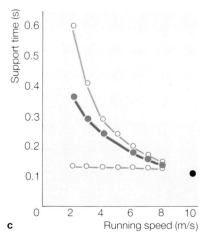

time it takes to reach a maximal or a certain submaximal force level during isometric or concentric contractions the series elastic components are stretched by a shortening contractile component. Notice that the contractile components also shorten during an isometric contraction. The stiffer the elastic component, the faster the rate of force production. Passive elastic components are involved in eccentric contractions and in the SSC (cf. above). In the latter a stiffer elastic component is obtained by an active contraction of the muscle prior to a load that causes stretch. In running, for example, the knee and ankle extensors are activated prior to ground contact (Fig. 5.4.3). Training with eccentric contractions or SSCs might improve the force–time characteristics of a muscle. However, rate of force production, particularly in the contractile component, could also be improved by performing isometric or very heavy load training provided that it is carried out explosively. It appears that the rate of force development is crucial, and not so much the actual amplitude of the force.

Force–length Muscle length affects force production. The force–length relationship varies for different muscles, but usually the longer the distance between origin and insertion for a certain muscle the higher the active force that can be attained. Forces arising in the parallel elastic components of antagonistic muscles resisting passive stretch might limit the range of motion and result in a lesser ability to utilize optimal lengths for force production in the synergistic muscles. Proper flexibility training should lead to a restoration of a maximal physiological range of motion. Hypermobility, on the other hand, could possibly lead to a decrease in stiffness of the elastic components and thus be negative for the performance (cf. above).

Muscle morphology and metabolism

Fibre orientation The ability of a muscle to produce a high maximal contraction speed is, among other things, related to its architecture both with respect to the internal arrangements of sarcomeres and myofibrils and the orientation of muscle fibres. A muscle with a high number of sarcomeres arranged in series can attain higher maximal speeds than a muscle with a low number, everything else being equal; whereas the number of myofibrils and thereby sarcomeres in parallel are decisive for the force output. A muscle with its fibres arranged in parallel can produce a higher maximal speed, but less force per unit cross-sectional area than a muscle with an oblique fibre orientation (Sacks & Roy, 1982). The geometry differs between muscles and probably to some extent between individuals. It is mainly genetically determined but it has been argued, although not conclusively demonstrated, that the muscle hypertrophy associated with heavy strength training might change the orientation of muscle fibres and thereby impair the maximal speed of contraction.

Type of fibre   The relative number of different types of muscle fibres also seems to affect force–velocity–time relationships of a muscle (Fig. 5.4.2). Thus, although the case is not as clear as in animal muscle preparations, a high percentage of fast twitch fibres (FTF or type II fibres) appears to be essential for performance of high speed and acceleration. Even though there is a relatively large variation among athletes in explosive events, individuals with a dominance of slow twitch fibres are never found. Both the ability to maintain high force at high speed and to produce force at a high rate during isometric contractions have been shown to correlate positively with percentage of FTF (Thorstensson, 1976; Viitasalo, 1980; cf. Fig. 5.4.2). No corresponding correlation is present for maximal isometric strength. The observed statistical correlations are, however, relatively low and considerable variation is present.

The metabolic and microstructural basis for muscle fibre classification (different forms of the myosin ATPase enzyme) appears to be mainly genetically determined and hard to influence by training (cf. Thorstensson, 1976). Since these properties seem to be more related to speed and force production than to endurance, the genetic influence is likely to be more pronounced in explosive than in endurance events. Thus, selection would play a major role in this context. Although it seems hard to change slow into fast fibres, strength and speed training could change the relative fibre distribution by selectively increasing the cross-sectional area of fast fibres (Thorstensson, 1976). The problem then becomes to find optimal training programmes to engage mainly, if not only, the FTF type. An interesting issue, not yet looked into, is to what extent muscle properties, e.g. fibre-type composition, affect the trainability of a muscle.

Biochemical   The biochemical characteristics of muscle fibres are thus to a certain, but *characteristics*   varying, degree influenced by training. Depending on the intensity and duration of the training regimen, different metabolic pathways are utilized. In events demanding maximal efforts of short duration the total energy cost might be small, but since energy has to be delivered fast, only some pathways are possible. Since the energy sources for these pathways are very limited, local depletion in certain fibres might occur after only a few seconds. However, no study has so far shown any major increases in quickly available energy sources such as the phosphagens, ATP and creatine phosphate, or in enzymes involved in their metabolism, such as actomyosin ATPase, creatine kinase or myokinase (adenylate kinase). In a study of sprint training on a treadmill increases in the order of 20–30% were observed for these enzymes (Thorstensson *et al.*, 1975). This is in contrast to the much larger local adaptations seen in muscle metabolic properties after endurance training (Saltin & Gollnick, 1983). However, relatively few studies have been reported on adaptations to speed training, and not all critical metabolic steps have been investigated.

Neurophysiological aspects

As indicated several times above, properties of the nervous system have to be considered when discussing the ability to produce speed and acceleration. High excitability of motoneurons, fast conduction velocity and efficient transmission of nerve impulses between neurons as well as at the motor endplate are important factors (cf. Chapter 2.5). These properties influence the possibility of utilizing stretch reflex potentiation of force during an SSC (Chapter 2.1 and above) as well as critical performance variables such as reaction time. To what extent these variables are trainable is still essentially unknown.

Coordination The term coordination is often discussed in relation to speed and acceleration (cf. Chapter 5.3). A proper coordination is essential both on the micro and macro level, that is both the activation of different motor units and of different muscles have to be timed accurately to achieve optimal performance. An activation of as many motor units as possible, preferably fast ones, in a synchronous fashion would be advantageous for rapid force production. Moreover, proper timing of the activation of different synergistic muscles and avoidance of unnecessary activation of antagonistic muscles producing counteracting torques are essential for maximal speed and acceleration. Such modifications of the activation pattern appear to occur gradually with training (cf. Chapter 5.3). However, very few studies have specifically investigated technique training from this point of view. It should be remembered that all antagonistic muscle activity, as for example observed with EMG recordings, is not counterproductive, but is rather needed to stabilize joints or to decelerate a limb to provide for transfer of energy from one segment to another, such as during the swing phase of a step in sprinting (cf. Fig. 5.4.3). It is felt that much progress can be expected in the area of coordination training not least by the development of high-speed movement recording systems with the possibility of immediate feedback to the athlete and coach.

Stride characteristics

It has been discussed whether the limitations for sprinting performance lie in the ability to move the limbs in an alternating fashion at a high frequency or in the ability to take very long steps. From the results shown in Fig. 5.4.4 it is evident that neither the highest possible frequency nor the longest possible steps are utilized at maximal speed. Using the peak values in Fig. 5.4.4a and b would give totally unrealistic values for maximal speed. The actual combination of frequency and amplitude at maximal speed is a compromise. Both factors ultimately depend on the ability of the muscles involved to produce a high force in a short time (Fig. 5.4.4c; cf. Fy in Fig. 5.4.3). The ability to maintain a high frequency and a consistent movement pattern throughout a sprint race might also be a limiting factor. Training regimens aiming at overcoming normal limits have included downhill running, towing after a vehicle, running shielded from wind resistance or with tail wind, running on a motor-driven treadmill at supramaximal speeds, etc. In all cases the objective evaluation of the results have, however, been poor.

Sprinting represents a rather stereotyped movement pattern. In other sports, such as team handball, soccer, etc., the ability to switch from one motor pattern to another becomes important. The player has to make quick changes in direction of progression from side to side and from forward to backward, depending on the situation. Training and testing methods for this type of agility are still essentially unexplored.

Conclusion

In summary, the ability to produce high maximal speed and acceleration depends on an optimal combination of biomechanical, muscular and neural factors. Some of these factors have a strong genetic component. Knowledge of the different factors is a prerequisite for estimating their relative importance and for constructing selective tests for their evaluation. The next challenge is to formulate better criteria for optimization of training regimens. The aim is to make the training more specifically directed towards the factors most critical for a certain performance and towards improvement of specific weaknesses in a certain individual. This forms a continuing challenge for researchers in several fields as well as for coaches and athletes.

References

Bosco, C. (1982) Stretch-shortening cycle in skeletal muscle function. *Studies in Sport, Physical Education and Health* **15**. University of Jyväskylä, Finland.

Cavagna, G. A. (1977) Storage and utilization of elastic energy in skeletal muscle. *Exerc. Sport Sci. Rev.* **5**, 89.

Fridén, J. (1983) Exercise-induced muscle soreness. *Umeå University Medical Dissertations* **105**. University of Umeå, Sweden.

Mero, A. (1987) Electromyographic activity, force and anaerobic energy production in sprint running. *Studies in Sport, Physical Education and Health* **24**. University of Jyväskylä, Finland.

Nilsson, J. & Thorstensson, A. (1987) Adaptability in frequency and amplitude of leg movements during human locomotion at different speeds. *Acta Physiol. Scand.* **129**, 107.

Nilsson, J., Thorstensson, A. & Halbertsma, J. (1985) Changes in leg movements and muscle activity with speed of locomotion and mode of progression in humans. *Acta Physiol. Scand.* **123**, 457.

Sacks, R. D. & Roy, R. R. (1982) Architecture of the hindlimb muscles of cats: functional significance. *J. Morphol.* **173**, 185.

Saltin, B. & Gollnick, P. D. (1983) Skeletal muscle adaptability: significance for metabolism and performance. In L. D. Peachey (section ed.) *Handbook of Physiology, Section 10*, pp. 555–631. American Physiological Society, Bethesda, Maryland.

Thorstensson, A. (1976) Muscle strength, fibre types and enzyme activities in man. *Acta Physiol. Scand.* (Suppl.) **443**, 1.

Thorstensson, A., Sjödin, B. & Karlsson, J. (1975) Enzyme activities and muscle strength after sprint training in man. *Acta Physiol. Scand.* **94**, 313.

Viitasalo, J. (1980) Neuromuscular performance in voluntary and reflex contraction. *Studies in Sport, Physical Education and Health* **12**. University of Jyväskylä, Finland. ●

PART 6

ANTHROPOMETRY

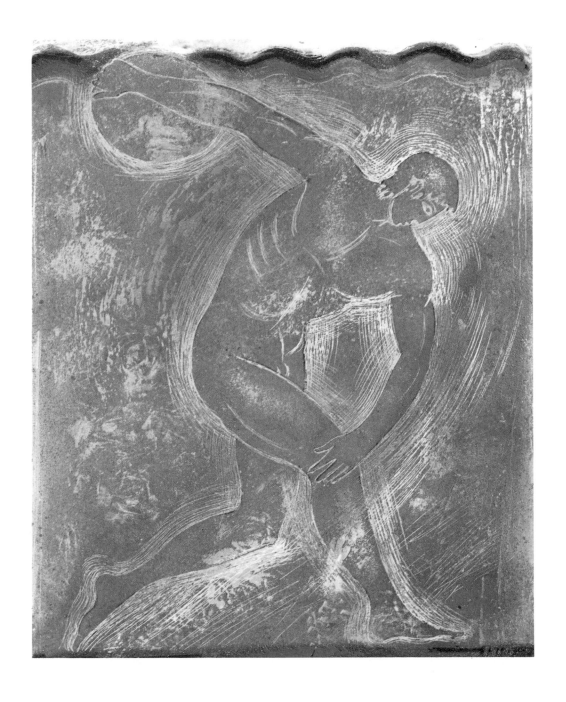

6.1 Anthropometry applied to sports medicine

W. D. ROSS, E. H. DE ROSE & R. WARD

The study of human structure extends to antiquity. Hippocrates 400 BC defined one of the first biological classification systems and identified pathological correlates. He also tried to define body composition, using elements like blood, yellow bile, black bile and mucus. His concept in terms of health and harmonious development of structure is a theme which persists to the present day.

In recent years the quantitative interface between human structure and function has received increasing attention and an impressive body of research literature has appeared. Many investigators have adopted the term kinanthropometry for this area of research. For Tittel (1978), the term serves to identify the biomechanical factors involved in expressing centripetal force from the limbs to the body or centrifugal force from the body to external objects. It also provides the proscenium for the drama of growth, development and ageing. In sports medicine, such research has particular relevance in assessing physique status and monitoring change. Regardless of age of the individual or level of commitment to any recreational or professional sports activity, there are structural constraints which may affect performance or relate to health and well-being.

With the infinite variety of human physique, some activities and sports are more suited to some individuals than to others. The study of the interface between structure and function constitutes a basic tool for the identification of athletic potential; it also transcends élite sport. Regardless of the level of participation or mode of the challenge, the sports physician may be called upon to assess growth and development, particularly in assessment of physique and monitoring body composition.

Such study involves the multivariable identification of the highly complex individual. The advance of the field is absolutely dependent upon the evolution of theoretical and methodological approaches to data management. This in turn presupposes: (a) technical competence in measurement; (b) comprehensive measurement protocols; (c) efficient, cost-effective data assembly, resolution and report systems; and (d) conceptual and theoretical appreciation of the use and limitations of various analytic stratagems.

Effective application of such research requires a cooperative relationship between scientists and coaches and an appreciation of the specific requirements of each sport. For example, the sport of lightweight rowing evokes a whole new set of circumstances where the assessment of physique is a crucial aspect of training.

Instruments

Anthropometric instruments for obtaining weight, stature (height), lengths, breadths, girths and skinfold thicknesses can range in price and sophistication. Most of the instruments can be purchased or constructed in non-specialized machine shops. An inexpensive basic kit is shown in Fig. 6.1.1.

Weight scale Bodyweight, representing body mass, is a critical measure. Rather simple instruments may suffice. Ideally, these should be accurate to 0.1 kg. A simple procedure for calibration is to weigh very accurately a set of plates used in weight lifting and adjust the scales accordingly through the range of subjects measured.

Stadiometer Stature and sitting height may be obtained by using elaborate wall-mounted or portable stadiometers. In the simplest form, this is a triangle device providing a right-angled plane to obtain a mark on a paper

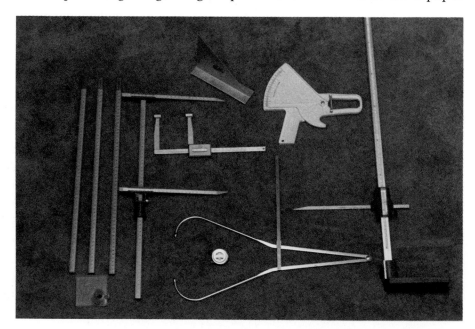

Fig. 6.1.1 Basic anthropometric kit consisting of weight scale, triangular headboard, anthropometric tape, skinfold calipers, bone calipers and anthropometer.

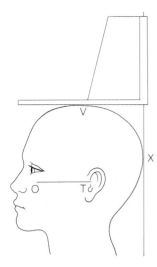

Fig. 6.1.2 Position of the head in the Frankfort plane. Orbitale (inferior margin of the eye socket) and tragion (notch above the tragus of the ear at the anterior margin of the zygomatic bone at that point) on a line horizontal to the long axis of the body.

attached to a wall. Measurement to the mark is made with a metallic tape and read to the nearest 0.1 cm.

The measurement of stature requires rigorous technique. Technically, stature is the vertical distance from the floor to the vertex of the head when oriented in the Frankfort plane. The vertex is the highest point on the skull when the head is positioned so the line joining the orbitale and tragion is horizontal or at a right angle to the long axis of the body as illustrated in Fig. 6.1.2. The barefooted subject stands erect with heels together and arms hanging naturally by the sides. The heels, buttocks, upper part of the back and usually, but not necessarily, the back of the head are in contact with the vertical wall.

When two measurers are available, one positions the subject and gives instruction to take a breath and stretch up while cupping the subject's head and applying gentle traction to the mastoid processes. The other measurer assures the subject's heels are not elevated, brings down the headboard, crushing the air firmly and contacting the vertex, and marking the level or reading the scale.

With some care, a single measurer can achieve sufficiently objective measurements of stretch stature by positioning the subject's head in the Frankfort plane and applying traction (a practice trial), and then making the measurement unaided with the subject taking a deep breath and stretching up. The head must remain properly orientated. Occasionally, the cue 'stretch up, lower your shoulders, head up' will help achieve the correct positioning.

Anthropometer Projected lengths (from the floor to a landmark), direct lengths and various breadths can be obtained by anthropometers which may be purchased or made in non-specialized machine shops. The constructed instrument is scaled by affixing an anthropometric tape to permit reading to the nearest 0.1 cm from a simple parallax-correcting slider (Ross, 1985b).

Bone caliper Bone widths require a sturdy caliper which permits firm pressure on broad pressure plates. Easily obtainable vernier scale or electronic engineers' calipers can be adapted for obtaining bone widths (Carter, 1980). Essentially, this is accomplished by fitting larger branches, 10 cm long with circular pressure plates 15 mm in diameter.

Skinfold caliper Skinfold thicknesses, consisting of a compressed double thickness of skin and entrapped adipose tissue, may be obtained with various instruments. A pressure of 10 g/mm^2 exerted by a Harpenden skinfold caliper or the inexpensive Slim Guide caliper is deemed appropriate for most applications. Recent studies have shown negligible systematic differences; however, varying manufacturing standards may introduce error. The actual compression can be measured by hanging known weights to the jaw surface (surface area × tension = 10 g/mm^2). The Harpenden caliper can be interpolated to the nearest 0.1 mm through a 5 cm range and the Slim Guide can be interpolated to the nearest 0.5 mm through an 8 cm range. They have similar dynamic action and both are adequate. Variance at the same site is primarily a function of the technique not the instrument.

Anthropometric tape   Girths are obtained by an anthropometric tape. The objective is to obtain a perimeter measure without compressing the skin. This requires the anthropometrist to develop a light touch which will vary with the characteristics of the subject. The ideal tape is flexible, about 7 mm wide, 2 m long, made of steel or non-extensible material, with a high-contrast white or yellow background and clear millimetre increments with un-equivocal figures. The tape should have about a 7 cm stub end from the zero mark. The best tape is automatically retractable into its housing. The tape, with the housing always held in the right hand, is extended by the left, with readings at the zero line to the nearest 0.1 cm. The anthropometrist holds and snubs the tape by a pinch grip of the thumbs and index fingers, while the pinning and levelling is done with the third digits.

Measurements and interpretation

Precision and accuracy of measurement   Precision is the degree of consistency or reliability of a measurement. This is largely achieved through practice. Some measurement protocols call for three sequences of all the measurements with the median (any identical pair or mid-score) used in the assessment. This practice permits test–retest comparisons. If desired, the technical error of measurement is found by comparing differences of repeated measures expressed as the square root of the sum of the squares of the differences of the measures divided by twice the number of subjects ($[\text{sum } d^2/2n]^{0.5}$). Unlike physiological tests, anthropometric test–retest reliability correlation coefficients (r) are close to 1.0 and are not discriminatory enough for this purpose.

Accuracy of measurement is a matter of how closely the measurement approximates the true value. Having properly calibrated the instruments, accuracy of measurement is usually assessed by comparison with a 'criterion anthropometrist' who is well-experienced in the specific techniques and whose technique does not vary from written specifications for each laboratory based on some standard reference (Stewart, 1952; Martin & Saller, 1966; Tittel & Wutscherk. 1973; Weiner & Lourie, 1981; Carter *et al.*, 1982; Ross & Marfell-Jones, 1982; Cameron, 1986; Lohman *et al.*, 1987; Ross *et al.*, 1987).

Landmarks and conventions

The landmarks shown in Fig. 6.1.3 are largely the classical procedures of Martin (1928) as further defined and specified for use in the 1968 Mexico and 1976 Montreal Olympic Games Anthropological Project (MOGAP) described by Martin & Saller (1966), Ross *et al.* (1978) and Carter *et al.* (1982) with augmented descriptions by Ross and Marfell-Jones (1982), Ross *et al.* (1983) and Ross *et al.* (1987).

Conventionally, measurement techniques are described in terms of

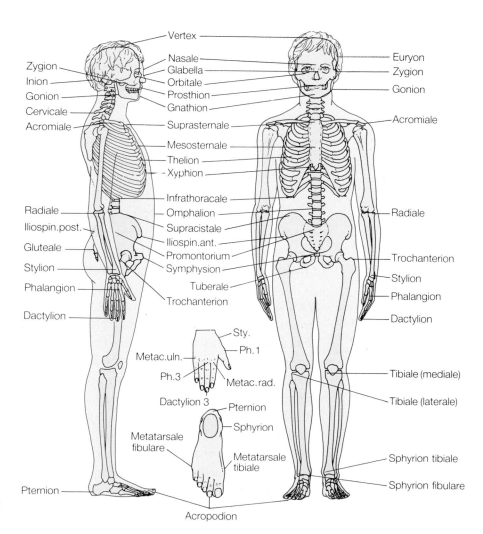

Fig. 6.1.3 Anthropometric landmarks.

the landmarks with orientation from the anatomical position of the subject (standing, palms facing forward).

The measurement proforma

Modern data assembly is facilitated by use of standard proforma, a data assembly plan compatible with computer operations, particularly those evolving for microcomputer spreadsheets. The proforma shown in Fig. 6.1.4, provides for single or multistation data assemblies as in the Montreal Olympic Games (Borms *et al.*, 1979; Carter *et al.*, 1982). Each item is numbered and arrayed to facilitate computer entry.

In general, the measurement protocol is designed to keep changing of instruments to a minimum. Sequencing with respect to the anthropometrist, is from superior to inferior, left to right, with turning and positioning of the subject accordingly. Haste, failure to take frequent rest breaks, extraneous talk, noise and poor lighting, heating and ventilation contribute to error.

Although the number of items in the sample proforma provides for a comprehensive physique assessment, it is not optimal for all purposes. One could make a reasonable case for inclusion of both right- and left-side measures since bilateral asymmetry is often encountered, and direct, rather than indirect, measures of segmental lengths since these are preferred to projected measures as discussed by Day (1984, 1986). Mid-thigh girth, wrist breadth, symphysion–gluteale diameter, and various measurements of head, face, hands and feet could well be included in adaptations of the sample proforma.

It is axiomatic that every measurement proforma or clinical record should include date of birth of the subject and the date the measurements were taken. The convention of converting the entries to decimal fractions of years should be a standard operation.

Cross-sectional norms and prototypes: assessment of status

Data obtained at any given time may be compared to cross-sectional norms or prototypical samples. This provides an individual assessment of physique status for age, sex, ethnic origin or activity stratum of the population sampled. In some instances, where large cross-sectional surveys are not available or have a restrictive measurement protocol, a small, intently studied sample may serve as a reference group—sometimes referred to as a prototypical sample (Eiben, 1972; DeGaray *et al.*, 1974; Ross *et al.*, 1980b; Carter *et al.*, 1982; Ross & Marfell-Jones, 1982). One of the uses of data assembled on Olympic athletes is that it may be used as a general reference, as done in studies of Venezuelan athletes by Perez (1981).

Fig. 6.1.4 (*opposite*) Measurement proforma including provision for replicated measurements, and designated spaces for numerical data entry and decimal fractions of year recording procedure. Proforma designed by Kinanthropometric Research Associates, Simon Fraser University.

Basic anthropometric proforma

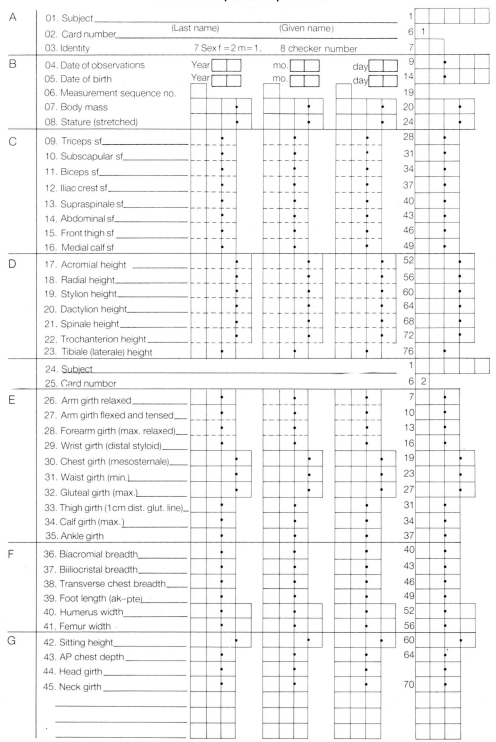

Fig. 6.1.4

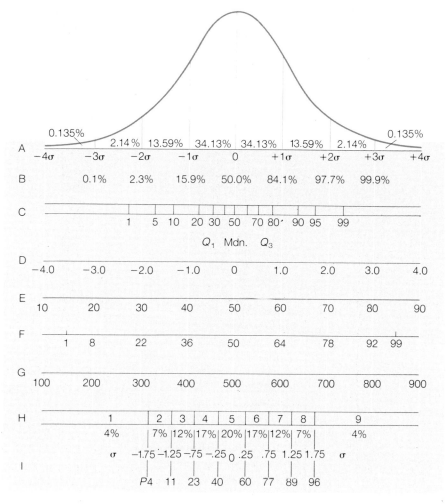

Fig. 6.1.5 Standard scores and scaling options for construction of cross-sectional norms. A = standard deviations; B = cumulative percents; C = percentile scale showing Q_1 (P25), median (P50) and Q3 (P75); D = sigma scale; E = T-scores; F = hull scores; G = T-score × 100; H = stanine scores based on standard deviation distances; I = stanine scores based on percentile transformations at P4, 11, 23, 40, 60, 77, 89, 94. From Ross & Ward (1986).

Norm tables   Norms categorized for age, sex, ethnicity and other identifying characteristics, permit the identification of individual physique status. When the distribution for a given item is relatively normal, various standard scores (as shown in Fig. 6.1.5) may be used for scaling. Because of the essential skewness in skinfold caliper thicknesses and some performance test items, percentile scaling is often preferred—as in the use percentile transformed standard nine (stanine) scores (Ross & Ward, 1986).

Somatotype   The standard somatotype photograph illustrated in Fig. 6.1.6 is primary source data. Identified with age, height and weight, the somatotype provides the best single description for the classification of human shape. The somatotype compresses a great deal of information into a three-component rating (endomorphy–mesomorphy–ectomorphy) which may be displayed on a two-dimensional grid as a somatoplot, or conceived of as a somatoplot in three-dimensional space.

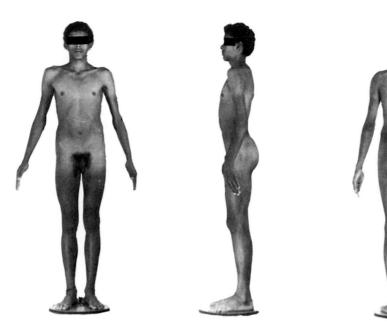

Fig. 6.1.6 Somatotype photoscopic rating of a Pan-American and Olympic winner of the 800 m running race, studied at age 17.09. The result using the procedure described by Sheldon *et al*. (1954) was 2, 3, 5. Courtesy of LAPEX-UFRGS.

The anthropometric procedures for calculation of a Heath–Carter somatotype from data on the proforma and plotting it on a somatochart are summarized below:

1 Endomorphic component (relative adiposity). This is obtained by finding the sum of triceps, subscapular and supraspinale skinfold in millimetres. A correction for stature of the subject (h) option may be used, i.e. $X = $ sum $(170.18/h)$.

Endomorphy $= 0.1451\, X - 0.00068\, X^2 + 0.0000014\, X^3 - 0.7182$.

2 Mesomorphic component (relative musculoskeletal robustness) from the following equation:

Mesomorphy $= 0.858\,(H) + 0.601\,(F) + 0.188\,(A) + 0.161\,(C) + 4.5$

where H is humerus breadth (cm); F is femur breadth (cm); A is corrected arm girth: A cm $-$ (triceps mm/10); and C is corrected calf girth: C cm $-$ (medial calf mm/10).

3 Ectomorphic component (relative linearity or stretched outness), obtained from the reciprocal of the ponderal index:

$\text{PI} = h/(w^{0.333})$.

If PI is greater than 40.75, ectomorphy $= 0.732\, \text{PI} - 28.58$. If PI is equal to or less than 40.75, ectomorphy $= 0.463\, \text{PI} - 17.63$.

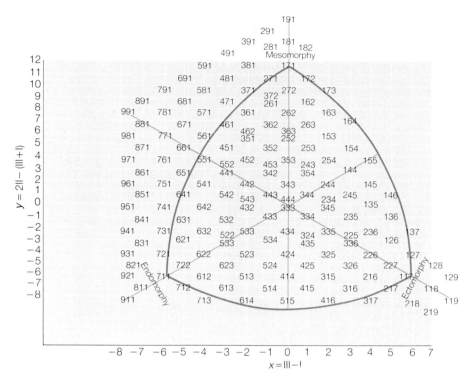

Fig. 6.1.7 Somatochart with x and y axes in ratio 1 : $3^{0.5}$ used for plotting $x =$ ecto − endo, and $y = 2 \times$ meso − (ecto + endo) co-ordinates for the somatoplot.

After defining each of the components, it is possible to plot them as a single point on a somatochart, a Reauleaux triangle used by Sheldon, as shown as Fig. 6.1.7. The triangle is partitioned by three axes intercepted in the centre, forming angles of 120°. The axes define three areas of dominance: endomorphy to the west, mesomorphy to the north and ectomorphy to the east. Plotting coordinates on an x–y somatochart grid where the ratio of x to y axis is ($3^{0.5}$: 1) is as follows:

$x =$ ecto − endo

$y = 2 \times$ meso − (ecto + endo).

Somatotype means, somatoplots on a two-dimensional somatochart, dispersion distances as well as somatopoints and attitudinal distances in three-dimensional space and various analytical methods are discussed by Carter *et al.* (1983).

As shown in the somatochart in Fig. 6.1.8, male athletes distribute in the upper part of the chart ranging from distance runners in the east to weight throwers displaced to the extreme northwest. In the biomechanical schema of Tittel (1978), this would be from sports most dependent on centripetal forces to those most dependent on centrifugal forces. Female athletes are lower on the chart with vectors to the male counterpart in the same sport generally pointing to the northeast in an ectomesomorphic direction.

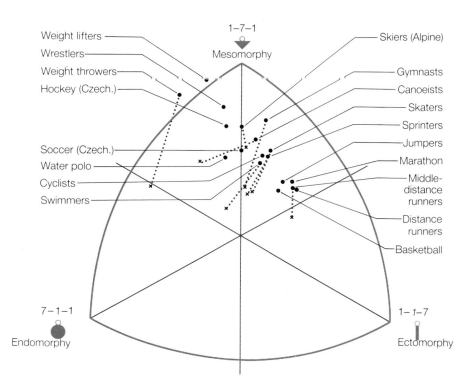

Fig. 6.1.8 Somatochart distribution of male (●) and female (×) athletes showing ● to × vectors for similar sports. Data from Chovana & Zrubak (1972); De Garay *et al.* (1974); Chovanova (1975); Ross *et al.* (1977b); and Carter (1984).

Proportionality

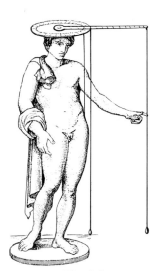

Fig. 6.1.9 The definer, a device used to measure human proportionality of the type designed by Leone Battista Alberti.

The use of artists' work to assess human proportionality is part of our artistic legacy. As early as the fifth century BC, Polyclitus, the Greek sculptor, using aesthetic criteria from selected models eclectically crafted his much copied *Doryphorus* or spear bearer. These copies have served as the artistic canon for ideal male proportions ever since.

The intellectual and artistic giants of the Renaissance, Leonardo da Vinci (1452–1519), Albrecht Durer (1471–1547) and Andreas Vesalius (1514–64) were also students of human form and proportionality. Kinanthropometrists feel a special kinship to a slightly earlier artist, Leone Battista Alberti (1404–71). As shown in Fig. 6.1.9 drawn from copies, he used a device called a definer to quantify proportionality characteristics. The definer was essentially a cap with a circular protractor. Alberti dropped plumb lines at given radii and measured to projected landmarks from the plumb line at measured heights. His model was a cylinder; its size was immaterial.

In much the same way, an arbitrary unisex reference human or phantom, proposed by Ross and Wilson (1974) is used as a metaphorical model. *z*-Values obtained, as shown in Fig. 6.1.10, are departures from the model, much as were the projections in Alberti's cylinder. The phantom is a calculation device, not a norm. How two individual's

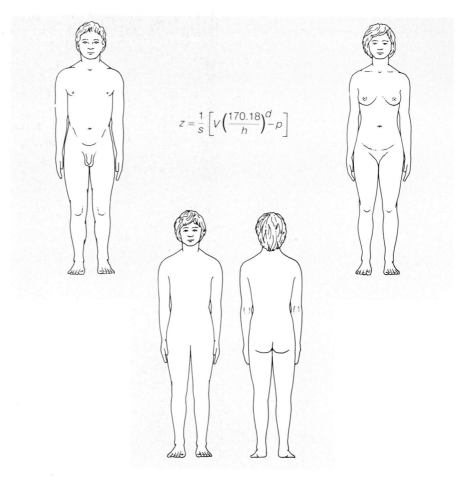

$$z = \frac{1}{s}\left[V\left(\frac{170.18}{h}\right)^d - p\right]$$

Fig. 6.1.10 The phantom, a unisex reference human used as a sample independent model with ascribed measures (*p*) and standard deviations (*s*). Usually, all items are adjusted geometrically to the phantom stature (170.18) using the subject's obtained height (*h*) with dimensional exponents *d* = 1 for all linear measures (lengths, breadths, girths, thicknesses), *d* = 2 for all areas (surface area, cross-sectional areas) and *d* = 3 for all volumes and masses (of whole body and its parts, bodyweight).

biacromial breadth compares to the phantom tells us something about the proportional difference in shoulder breadth and this is quite independent of the model. Any variable can be selected as a standard and one of several similarity systems may be used to ascribe dimensional exponents. Routinely, stature as the standard is scaled geometrically in the general formula for the phantom *p* and *s* specifications (Ross *et al.*, 1980a, 1983; Ross & Ward, 1982a, 1982b, 1984; Ross, 1985a).

Phantom *z*-values As inferred from the formula, the phantom scales every subject to the same stature and adjusts all measures geometrically. This is similar to projecting an image on a screen where the changing focal length does not alter the proportionality of the parts. A *z*-value is the deviation from the phantom *z*-value 0.00 in terms of the standard deviations for the particular item. A *z*-value of 1.0 means that item is one standard deviation above the phantom value. A *z*-value of −1.0 indicates the item is one standard

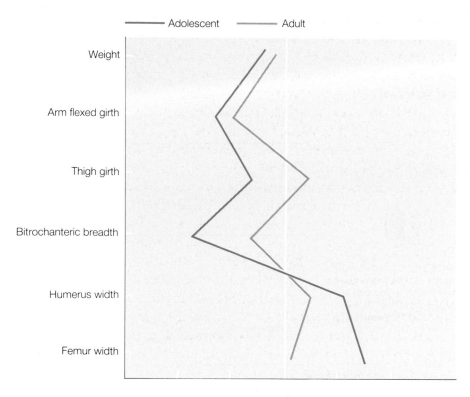

Fig. 6.1.11 Proportionality profiles showing phantom z-values for one adolescent (age 15.08) and one adult (age 28.35) male soccer players. The boy's proportionally larger bone diameters and smaller girths over muscular parts are characterisic of the normal growth pattern (De Rose *et al.*, 1984).

deviation below the phantom value. Because the phantom is a unisex reference, scores above and below 3.0 are often encountered, particularly in variables which are skewed. For example, a neonate's head girth is proportionally very large, over 40 phantom z-values (Faulhaber, 1978).

Comparison of individuals

As shown in Fig. 6.1.11, an outstanding 15-year-old male soccer player was compared to a mature international class player on a proportionality grid with a 0.0 centring line. The 15-year-old was proportionally lighter, smaller in arm and mid-thigh girth and bitrocanteric width (hips), but was proportionally larger in the humerus and femus widths. Despite both being outstanding players, the difference was typical of a 15-year-old and a mature athlete. The boy's proportionally larger bone diameters and smaller girths over muscular parts is characteristic of the normal growth pattern. One can infer the boy is less muscular than his older peer and this would be a matter for further monitoring.

Comparison of an individual and prototype

To illustrate a comprehensive analysis, data obtained by Copley (1979) on Stan Smith, the 1972 Wimbledon Champion, was compared to a prototypical sample of non-athletically selected university male students as shown in Fig. 6.1.12. Stan Smith's profile for trunk and right-side limbs were shown as a broken-line graph displayed on sample means

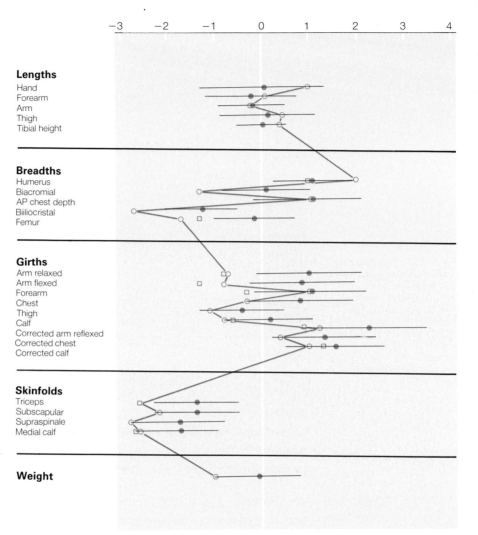

Fig. 6.1.12 Proportionality profile of USA tennis player, Stan Smith, compared to prototypical reference of male Canadian university students. Means and standard deviations of prototypical z-values are displayed as horizontal graphs. Stan Smith's profile for trunk and right-side limbs are shown as a broken-line graph displayed on sample means (●) and unbroken line horizontal standard deviation bars. The unbroken line profile of Stan Smith shows linearity of build typical of tall subjects. Left-side z-values are shown as □ (Copley, 1984).

and unbroken-line horizontal standard deviation bars. Thus, in a single display one can note Stan Smith's hand, forearm, thigh lengths and tibial height were proportionally large with respect to the prototype, but not the arm length. His proportional right humerus breadth and chest breadth were comparatively large, whereas his biacromial, biiliocristal and femur breadths were proportionally small as one notes in comparing tall individuals with their smaller peers (Ross *et al.*, 1987). His dominant right upper limb humerus breadth was much larger than the left, whereas, in the lower limb, the left femur breadth was the largest. His skinfolds and bodyweight were proportionally small with respect to the prototype. Proportionality profiles of this type focus on salient aspects of physique and reflect the individual adaptation reflecting the type of sport and style of the athlete.

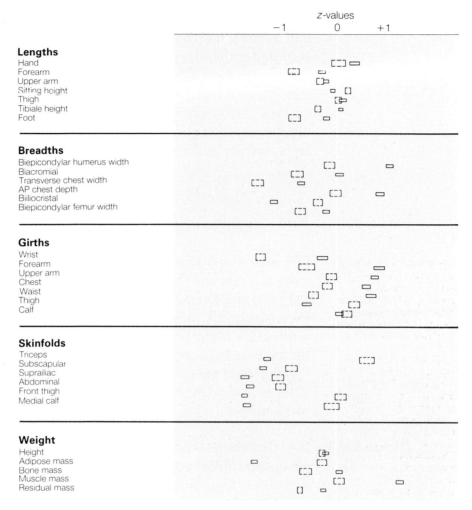

Fig. 6.1.13 Phantom mean and standard error of z-values illustrates sexual dimorphic proportionality pattern in prototypical male and female samples of Canadian university students. By convention, non-overlapping of adjacent standard error bars is regarded as a significant difference. Broken line boxes are plus and minus one standard error of z-values from mean for females, unbroken solid boxes show similar distances from male mean.

Group comparisons In making group comparisons, differences between mean values are conventionally recognized as being significant when adjacent standard errors of z-bars (standard deviation/$n^{0.5}$), do not overlap, for example:

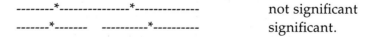

This is only an approximate test of significance at about the 5% probability level. It does not take into account the degrees of freedom for multiple comparisons or obviate the need for strict statistical tests when the difference is a crucial issue.

As shown in Fig. 6.1.13, females differ in a characteristic way from males—as indicated for the items where adjacent standard error bars do not overlap. Females have smaller hands and feet, shorter forearms and legs, and longer torsos. They have smaller breadths, except for hips, as indicated by the larger biiliocristal breadth. They are smaller in uncorrected girths, except for the thigh girth where they are larger and calf girth where there is no apparent difference. They have larger skinfolds than men and typically greater proportional limb skinfold values than in the torso measurements. Unlike a male pattern, the dysplagic pattern in females regardless of selectivity and training is: (a) lower body muscularity; and (b) limb adiposity.

Body composition

Weight for height The individual interpretation of weight for height or use of the Quetelet index (w/h^2) or body mass index (BMI) as an indicator of obesity is neither as simple or informative as it ostensibly appears (Garn, 1986; Garn et al., 1986; Martin et al., 1986; Ross et al., 1984, 1987). Variance in bodyweight is not a simple function of adiposity but reflects the basic morphology of the individual. The practice of sports medicine would be greatly enriched if bodyweight were studied longitudinally and viewed as a measure of size which must be explained by changes in the various structures and tissue masses.

Densitometry It is commonly observed at swimming pools and the beach that fat people tend to float in water and lean people sink. The relative floatability of a person is therefore used to estimate his or her percent body fat. The principle of buoyancy phenomena has been appreciated from the time of Archimedes (287–212 BC). If one knows the mass and density of an object, and the densities of its constituent parts, one can calculate the mass of each.

Since pioneering studies of Behnke (1942), the density characteristics of humans have been explored mainly as an indirect method for assessing percent fat. The implicit assumption is that the human body is composed of two compartments, a fat compartment with a density of 0.90 g/ml and a lean body mass (LBM), everything else, with a density of 1.10 gm/ml. Ostensibly simple, but technically demanding, human density can be determined by underwater weighing or water displacement with appropriate corrections for entrapped air using gas analytic procedures.

At issue, however, is the necessary assumption of constant densities of fat and LBM. While one could contend that the density of human fat, ether-soluble lipids, is not constant the variance is relatively small compared to that of the LBM. Thus, the major scientific issue is delineated by the assumption of a constant density of the LBM for individual assessment. For this to be true, one should expect two conditions to be generally true as well: (a) the constituent tissues of the LBM are in fixed proportions; and (b) each of these has constant densities.

The anatomical evidence is not supportive of the first condition. In six male and seven female unembalmed cadavers, the dissected muscle mass ranged from 41.9 to 59.4%, bone from 16.3 to 25.7% and the remainder from 24.0 to 32.4% (Clarys *et al.*, 1984; Martin 1984; Martin *et al.*, 1986). The proportional differences in constituent tissues is hardly surprising to human biologists and clinicians who are always confronted by human variability. The second condition, the assumption of constant densities of the constituent tissues of the LBM, is also refuted by the cadaver evidence. In 25 embalmed and unembalmed male and female cadavers the density of bone ranged from 1.164 (s.d. 0.037) gm/ml for the pelvis to 1.570 (s.d. 0.100) gm/ml for the mandible. The overall coefficient of variance in bone density was about 4% in the cadaver study. Dual-photon absorptiometric studies of young adults have shown larger variances of bone mineralization (Mazess *et al.*, 1984). The evidence of proportional contribution of the constituent tissues and the appreciation of density variance led Martin (1984) to estimate a coefficient of variation of the density of the LBM of at least 2%.

The error of assuming a constant density of the LBM is clearly signalled when negative values, zero, or values as low as 2 and 3% fat are predicted for athletes (Pollock *et al.*, 1977; Adams *et al.*, 1982). Over-estimates of a similar magnitude would not be so easily detected as being in error. As for bodyweight, density is best used in monitoring change rather than hazarding predictions of percent fat.

Skinfold caliper prediction of percent fat

The use of skinfold calipers to predict percent fat in formulae validated by density criteria is doubly indirect. In addition to assuming constant densities in a two-compartment model, five other assumptions are required: (a) constant compressibility of the skinfold; (b) skin thickness negligible or a constant fraction of the skinfold; (c) fixed adipose tissue patterning; (d) constant fat fraction of the adipose tissue; and (e) fixed proportion of internal to external fat. Martin *et al.* (1984) refute each of these assumptions.

The constants used with the sum of skinfold thicknesses does not necessarily alter the information. A skinfold is the thickness of a compressed double fold of skin and entrapped adipose tissue. The obtained measure can be used directly to assess adiposity without adorning illusions about percent fat, as illustrated by Carter (1982). We are entirely in agreement with the following conclusion by Johnston (1982):

> At present it seems human biologists are better off to continue to use anthropometry itself, rather than attempt to make estimates of whole body composition from available equations. Even if equations could prove useful estimates of mean parameters for samples, it seems clear they are not reliable for individual prediction.

Fractionation models   Since the work of Jindrich Matiegka (1921), a number of fractionation models have been developed. Drinkwater and Ross (1980) and De Rose *et al.* (1984) proposed working systems for physique appraisal. Drinkwater (1984) also has proposed an experimental model partitioning the body into four regions and fractionating skin, adipose tissue, muscle, bone and residual tissues. These models are predicated on assumptions for changing volumes to masses, and while not as vulnerable to gross error as the densitometric system, there are inherent limitations.

The O-scale system   A geometrical adjustment to a standard stature and simple scaling of the sum of skinfolds and bodyweight provides for a physique assessment system (Ross & Ward, 1984). Adiposity (*A*) and proportional weight (*w*) ratings are expressed as stanine scores for 34 male and female categories, every year from age 6 to 17, 18 and 19 years, and in 5-year increments until age 70, as shown in Tables 6.1.1 and 6.1.2.

Recognizing the essential skewness in skinfold data, the originators of the system used percentile transformed standard score equivalents with standard nine, or stanine, divisions at P4, 11, 23, 40, 60, 77, 89 and 96 which encompasses percent expectancies of 4, 7, 12, 17, 20, 17, 12, 7 and 4 for each rating interval.

The norms were based on comprehensive data assembly on 1236 children and young adults from one laboratory (Ross *et al.*, 1980b) and over 19 000 adults from the nationwide Canadian YMCA LIFE (life-style inventory and fitness evaluation) project conducted by Bailey and Mirwald (Bailey *et al.*, 1982). The intent was to base norms on a sample of 'best off' subjects as perhaps being the most appropriate for assessing and monitoring health status as suggested by Tanner (1976).

Unlike phantom which is a sample-independent scaling device, the O-scale ratings and profile is always related to a size-adjusted norm for the given subject's age and sex. To illustrate, O-scale adiposity (*A*) ratings from Table 6.1.3 entry of ((sum of triceps, subscapular, supraspinale, abdominal, front thigh and medial calf skinfolds) × (170.18/obtained

Table 6.1.1 O-scale proportional weight ratings for females and males.

Age	1	2	3	4	5	6	7	8	9
Females									
6	53.1	54.4	57.4	60.2	63.8	66.7	71.3	72.9	
7	51.3	53.8	56.2	57.6	60.8	64.1	68.9	72.8	
8	51.7	54.3	55.8	57.3	59.8	62.7	66.6	71.6	
9	49.9	52.0	54.4	56.5	59.7	63.2	67.7	72.2	
10	47.6	51.2	53.2	55.8	60.0	63.7	71.1	75.8	
11	46.6	49.3	52.0	53.8	58.2	65.0	70.7	74.7	
12	46.2	49.2	51.8	54.8	59.6	63.9	72.8	80.2	
13	46.0	49.8	52.2	56.3	59.9	65.3	71.8	77.0	
14	46.3	50.2	53.3	56.7	60.3	64.8	71.8	78.0	
15	47.2	50.3	54.2	57.2	60.5	64.3	71.0	76.3	
16	47.3	52.2	55.3	57.7	60.8	63.8	70.8	75.0	
17	49.0	52.8	55.8	58.4	61.6	64.4	70.0	75.3	
18–19	51.8	54.8	57.5	60.4	63.5	66.8	71.0	77.8	
20–24	52.2	55.2	57.6	60.8	64.2	68.3	72.9	80.0	
25–29	52.5	55.2	57.7	61.0	64.8	68.9	74.8	83.0	
30–34	52.3	55.3	58.5	61.5	64.8	69.1	74.8	84.5	
35–39	53.1	56.2	58.8	62.4	66.3	70.7	76.7	88.0	
40–44	54.4	57.6	60.8	63.8	68.1	73.2	80.2	89.2	
45–49	55.2	58.7	62.0	65.2	69.8	74.6	82.3	91.8	
50–54	54.2	57.8	62.2	65.3	69.6	74.3	82.7	93.0	
55–59	55.5	59.1	62.5	66.8	72.8	78.1	84.4	95.5	
60–64	56.3	59.0	63.8	67.4	71.9	77.5	85.4	93.5	
65–69	53.3	58.7	65.3	69.2	74.8	78.8	84.3	91.7	
Males									
6	55.2	56.8	59.9	62.6	64.8	66.7	69.6	73.9	
7	49.5	55.1	56.7	59.8	63.2	65.2	67.5	69.3	
8	49.8	54.2	55.8	57.9	60.5	63.4	66.7	67.8	
9	49.4	53.3	55.1	57.4	59.7	62.5	66.1	69.1	
10	50.1	53.1	54.3	57.2	59.5	61.8	66.8	71.9	
11	48.1	50.4	53.5	55.8	59.6	63.3	70.2	75.7	
12	46.3	50.6	52.8	54.9	58.3	62.2	67.3	74.4	
13	46.2	48.8	51.4	54.2	57.2	61.6	67.0	73.2	
14	46.6	48.8	51.3	54.2	57.3	60.8	64.5	71.3	
15	46.8	49.2	51.4	54.3	57.5	61.2	66.8	71.7	
16	47.1	49.8	52.7	55.3	58.3	61.4	66.8	71.7	
17	47.9	50.8	53.5	56.3	59.3	62.4	67.5	71.8	
18–19	49.5	52.8	56.4	59.0	62.5	64.5	67.8	70.8	
20–24	51.3	54.8	57.8	61.8	65.6	69.4	74.6	80.1	
25–29	53.1	56.2	59.8	63.2	67.5	71.4	76.4	84.3	
30–34	53.8	57.7	61.2	64.6	68.7	73.2	78.3	85.2	
35–39	55.2	58.6	61.8	65.4	69.7	73.8	79.0	86.2	
40–44	55.6	59.1	62.7	66.4	69.7	73.8	78.9	86.0	
45–49	55.6	59.6	63.5	66.8	70.8	75.0	79.7	86.8	
50–54	55.9	59.9	63.4	66.6	70.7	74.8	79.6	86.3	
55–59	56.6	60.4	63.5	66.7	71.3	76.1	80.7	87.8	
60–64	55.9	60.3	63.3	66.3	70.5	74.8	79.8	87.3	
65–69	53.0	57.5	62.1	66.5	69.5	73.9	77.8	81.3	

Table 6.1.2 Fourth, 50th and 96th percentiles for advanced O-scale measurements and z-values for the 20–25-year-age group.

	Measurements			z-Values		
	4th	50th	96th	4th	50th	96th
MALES						
Weight	59.0	75.0	97.5	−1.4	−0.1	2.0
Height	166.9	179.7	191.5	—	—	—
Skinfolds						
Triceps	4.6	8.9	18.9	−2.4	−1.5	0.6
Subscapular	6.9	11.4	25.6	−2.1	−1.2	1.5
Biceps	2.8	4.4	10.4	−2.6	−1.9	1.0
Iliac crest	6.6	13.7	34.4	−2.3	−1.3	1.6
Supraspinale	4.1	9.0	25.6	−2.5	−1.5	2.1
Abdominal	3.8	15.2	42.5	−2.7	−1.3	1.9
Front thigh	5.7	12.5	25.8	−2.6	−1.8	−0.2
Medial calf	4.0	8.2	18.5	−2.6	−1.7	0.4
Girths						
Arm relaxed	25.9	31.3	36.5	−0.9	1.2	3.3
Arm flexed	28.2	33.1	38.2	−1.0	0.9	3.1
Forearm	25.4	28.0	31.3	−0.6	1.0	3.1
Wrist	15.3	16.6	19.6	−2.3	−0.6	2.4
Chest	88.6	97.6	114.2	−0.4	1.1	3.5
Waist	70.5	80.9	100.5	−0.8	1.1	5.2
Gluteal	88.5	97.6	110.3	−1.8	−0.3	1.7
Thigh	51.0	58.4	66.3	−1.6	−0.2	1.6
Calf	33.0	37.0	42.5	−1.8	0.1	2.1
Ankle	18.2	22.1	26.6	−3.2	−0.5	2.5
Bone widths						
Humerus	6.2	7.1	8.0	−1.3	0.7	2.8
Femur	8.6	9.7	10.9	−2.6	−0.5	1.6
Skinfold-corrected girths						
Arm relaxed	24.5	28.6	32.0	0.7	2.5	4.4
Chest	85.0	94.7	107.2	0.1	1.5	3.5
Thigh	46.4	54.3	60.7	−0.6	1.1	2.6
Calf	29.9	34.4	39.2	−0.8	1.2	3.4
FEMALES						
Weight	47.5	58.2	74.3	−1.3	−0.1	2.0
Height	154.2	165.5	176.4	—	—	—
Skinfolds						
Triceps	8.4	15.3	27.0	−1.5	0.1	2.9
Subscapular	7.2	12.2	25.4	−1.9	−0.9	1.9
Biceps	3.8	7.3	15.2	−2.0	−0.2	3.9
Iliac crest	6.8	11.4	26.0	−2.2	−1.4	0.6
Supraspinale	5.5	11.0	24.2	−2.1	−0.8	2.3
Abdominal	6.8	15.5	32.7	−2.3	−1.1	1.2
Front thigh	11.0	22.4	39.2	−1.8	−0.4	1.7
Medial calf	7.6	15.2	28.0	−1.7	0.0	2.7
Girths						
Arm relaxed	22.2	26.7	31.5	−1.8	0.3	2.6
Arm flexed	23.5	27.1	32.0	−2.3	−0.6	1.6
Forearm	21.3	23.3	26.5	−2.3	−0.8	1.4
Wrist	13.6	14.5	16.3	−3.3	−1.9	0.8
Chest	78.4	83.8	96.0	−1.5	−0.1	2.5

Table 6.1.2 *continued*

	Measurements			z-Values		
	4th	50th	96th	4th	50th	96th
Waist	61.0	67.9	81.7	−2.0	−0.4	2.9
Gluteal	84.8	93.7	106.2	−1.1	0.3	2.6
Thigh	47.8	55.9	63.8	−1.4	0.3	2.4
Calf	30.6	34.8	39.7	−1.5	0.3	2.6
Ankle	18.5	20.8	23.9	−2.1	−0.2	2.4
Bone widths						
Humerus	5.3	6.0	6.8	−2.8	−0.7	1.5
Femur	7.9	8.9	10.0	−2.8	−0.7	1.9
Skinfold-corrected girths						
Arm relaxed	18.3	22.0	25.4	−1.6	0.2	2.1
Chest	75.4	80.6	88.7	−1.1	0.2	1.9
Thigh	40.6	48.6	55.1	−1.2	0.7	2.5
Calf	25.7	29.9	34.5	−1.8	0.3	2.7

height)) and proportional weight (w) ratings from Table 6.1.2 entry of (obtained weight × (170.18/obtained height)^3) were shown as before and after assessments for a programme of exercise management and dietary constraint for a young woman. As shown in Fig. 6.1.14, the decline in the A rating was greater than the decline in the w rating. This is explained by inspection of the profiles in Fig. 6.1.15 which shows a declining adiposity, relatively stable bone breadths, and probable increased muscularity as inferred from the girths, particularly the skinfold corrected arm and chest girths. The individual profiles were printed by on a dot matrix printer in a microcomputer program which accessed each, and displayed them as a profile on a fourth, 50th and 96th percentile grid for the appropriate age and sex category of the subject. (For instance, raw score and z-values of 20–25-year-old males and females are shown in Table 6.1.2.)

Skinfold caliper formulae to predict percent fat are site and sample specific. This is illustrated by differences obtained on the same subject. Pre- and post-training values were assessed at 26.8 to 18.4% (Yuhasz, 1974); 27.1 to 20.7% (Sloan *et al.*, 1962); and 34.1 to 28.8% (Durnin & Womersley, 1974).

New instrumentation   Any method which has demonstrable precision can be useful in assessing changing physique status, particularly if used in concert with comprehensive anthropometric assessment and sophisticated regional tissue fractionation models. The claim of being able to predict percent fat or LBM in individuals has not been satisfactorily demonstrated nor have

Table 6.1.3   O-scale adiposity ratings for females and males.

Age	1	2	3	4	5	6	7	8	9
Females									
6	46.8	56.1	61.7	69.5	77.9	96.7	128.6	144.0	
7	44.3	47.4	60.2	68.3	76.1	91.8	113.2	140.0	
8	43.7	49.2	63.9	69.8	81.4	94.5	111.7	143.2	
9	45.5	53.4	66.1	73.2	87.7	98.6	111.7	143.3	
10	49.2	59.6	67.6	78.6	98.3	109.7	143.2	173.5	
11	51.9	56.4	66.5	75.6	96.4	108.8	150.0	173.4	
12	53.0	59.3	66.5	77.8	98.7	111.4	153.0	175.6	
13	46.7	56.9	67.9	77.4	97.7	114.9	153.0	165.5	
14	46.7	60.9	69.0	81.9	99.6	113.4	147.4	164.8	
15	49.4	62.6	72.4	85.4	99.6	113.2	145.3	162.1	
16	53.8	65.0	76.2	90.3	101.1	112.0	142.4	158.1	
17	62.1	69.4	78.3	92.8	106.5	117.6	141.4	156.4	
18–19	63.4	70.5	78.5	90.2	103.4	118.2	135.9	155.7	
20–24	64.0	72.5	81.2	92.0	104.2	118.9	138.0	164.0	
25–29	65.2	74.1	82.2	93.0	107.9	122.9	141.0	169.2	
30–34	64.1	72.0	81.9	94.6	108.0	126.0	144.3	172.2	
35–39	64.5	73.9	85.5	97.9	112.1	131.7	148.0	178.4	
40–44	69.5	80.5	90.3	102.4	120.7	140.9	161.1	187.3	
45–49	72.5	83.2	97.7	110.5	125.7	141.8	165.1	194.0	
50–54	70.0	84.5	96.2	112.5	127.8	144.8	168.3	196.5	
55–59	76.9	90.1	102.6	115.7	130.5	152.8	169.9	198.2	
60–64	78.3	85.3	96.8	114.6	130.6	146.4	166.0	194.0	
65–69	74.3	84.8	97.0	110.4	130.7	140.7	153.4	164.6	
Males									
6	43.0	47.4	57.4	63.0	70.0	80.9	92.7	121.0	
7	40.2	44.6	51.2	59.0	70.9	83.0	99.5	131.0	
8	41.2	45.7	50.7	56.8	65.4	77.6	99.5	137.9	
9	43.6	47.1	50.9	55.9	64.2	77.7	105.2	172.4	
10	45.1	47.1	53.7	59.1	65.4	83.7	129.1	183.2	
11	41.5	45.1	50.8	58.4	68.3	90.9	154.7	193.2	
12	37.6	43.1	47.0	53.4	65.7	89.3	126.6	188.9	
13	34.8	40.2	44.9	51.7	62.7	86.1	116.4	166.5	
14	34.7	37.2	43.4	49.3	57.3	70.9	103.5	146.1	
15	33.5	35.7	42.1	47.0	55.9	69.0	100.8	146.1	
16	32.3	35.4	40.4	44.6	53.3	63.1	79.4	126.7	
17	32.3	35.4	39.5	44.7	53.3	62.4	79.4	107.8	
18–19	31.5	34.3	41.7	47.6	57.0	70.3	87.3	109.3	
20–24	35.0	40.9	48.1	57.8	71.5	89.0	109.0	130.0	
25–29	38.3	45.5	54.5	66.8	81.8	99.5	119.3	144.0	
30–34	41.9	49.8	60.3	72.2	87.3	103.9	121.3	145.5	
35–39	43.9	53.0	62.3	73.9	88.1	102.5	121.9	143.0	
40–44	46.0	53.9	64.2	74.6	87.5	102.5	121.0	142.5	
45–49	44.7	55.2	64.8	76.3	90.5	106.8	123.4	147.0	
50–54	47.2	56.3	66.3	75.7	87.8	105.0	121.0	140.0	
55–59	46.9	56.8	65.8	76.4	87.5	101.1	115.9	136.0	
60–64	47.3	53.9	64.8	74.5	87.2	98.3	116.8	134.3	
65–69	43.0	53.0	60.5	71.6	84.3	92.9	104.8	121.5	

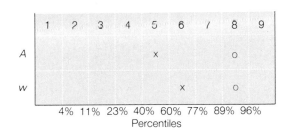

Date = March 1986 ×
       June 1985 ○

Female 30.871 years of age   Height = 170.2 cm
       30.170   170.2

Weight = 67.5 kg   Proportional weight = 67.5 kg
         76.0   76.0

Sum of 6 skinfolds (Slim Guide) = 95.5 mm
                                  150.1

Height corrected sum of 6 skinfolds = 95.5 mm
                                      127.7

	1	2	3	4	5	6	7	8	9
A						×		○	
w						×		○	

4% 11% 23% 40% 60% 77% 89% 96%
Percentiles

Fig. 6.1.14 O-scale computer report showing pre- (○) and post- (×) physique status of woman undergoing an exercise and dietary constraint programme. The decline in A (adiposity) was greater than the decline in w (proportonal weight) as shown by stanine values based on size-adjusted values for her own stature, age and sex norm category.

any of the implicit assumptions been validated. Laboratories on limited budgets should invest in microcomputers with comprehensive data resolution power rather than limited purpose impedance devices and other instruments with dubious value for individual assessment. The inescapable fact of individual differences defies assumptions of biological constancy of anatomical entities. The need is for relatively inexpensive, practical tools which can be made in non-specialized machine shops. A second generation of instruments will probably involve computer inter-facing and perhaps applications of ultrasound technology to assess tissue thickness and estimate bone mineral content at different foci.

Maturation

While some sports physicians will be concerned mainly with élite class competitors, most will be involved with young athletes of varying capabilities and age levels, some as young as 3 years old. Thus, much as exercise physiology was framed in a paediatric setting for the practitioner by Bar-Or (1983), so too, is it necessary to focus kinanthropometry on growth and maturation of children and youth.

Individual maturity events

There is a normal rhythm of human growth and development from birth to demise, the tempo, however, varies. Thus, a mean indicator of developmental status is only a general reference. An elementary account of normal growth and assessment techniques can be found in Tanner (1978) and a more advanced treatment in a three-volume handbook by Faulkner and Tanner (1986). A summary paper written for paediatric endocrinologists with a discussion of normal events and the prediction of adult stature is also a useful reference for sports physicians (Tanner, 1986).

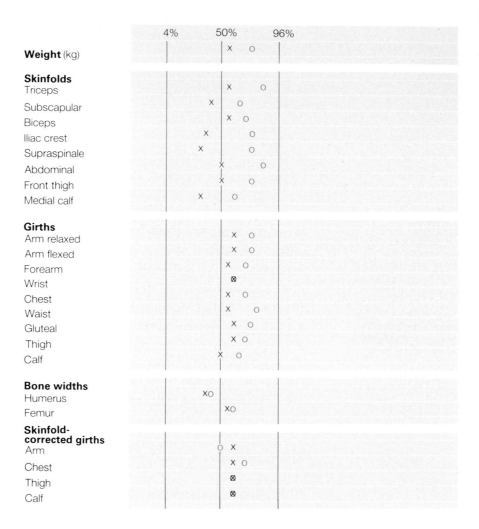

Fig. 6.1.15 O-scale computer profile on normative grid showing pre- (o) and post- (x) training values illustrating loss in adiposity, relative stability of bone breadths, and probable increase in muscularity inferred from girth values, particularly the skinfold-corrected arm and chest girths.

Characteristic adolescent stature velocity curves derived from the Saskatchewan Boys and Girls Growth Study by Bailey and Mirwald are shown in Figs 6.1.16 and 6.1.17. The superimposed genitalia standards are redrawn from *Growth Diagrams 1965* by Van Wieringen *et al.* (1971) and Roede and Van Wieringen (1985) with curve parameters from Mirwald and Bailey (1986).

In order to emphasize that maturation rates vary for each sex and that there is a systematic difference in maturity events, such as the occurrence of peak height velocity in girls at age 12 and boys at age 14, one can ask the rhetorical question 'How old is a 12-year-old child?' From the historical fact of birth to the present time the child may be chronologically 12 years, but may be developmentally younger than 10 or older than 14 years. The earliest maturing 12-year-old girl in elementary school is

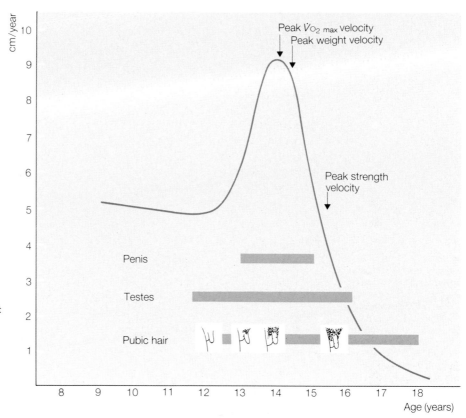

Fig. 6.1.16 Typical maturity events for boys showing stature velocity curve with indication of peak aerobic power, weight and strength velocities (Mirwald & Bailey, 1986), with illustrative secondary sex characteristics from redrawn standards by Van Wieringen *et al.* (1971) and Roede & Van Wieringen (1985).

developmentally as old as the latest maturing 18-year-old male university student.

Variability in maturation rates is illustrated in Fig. 6.1.18 which shows three-dimensional stature velocity curves of 100 boys in the Saskatchewan study (Leahy *et al.*, 1980). The reordering of subjects according to curve characteristics and the use of similar three-dimensional graphic techniques for studying team growth, training intensities and performance is an important new perspective for kinanthropometry and has many potential applications in sports medicine.

Growth curve resolution

Generally the monitoring of growth can be managed with stature measures taken every 3 months, such as the first weekday of September, December, March and June. In the overall appraisal of growth, even annual measurements are useful. Occasionally, daily or twice daily weight records in closely monitored training are required. However, these may be as infrequent as monthly or quarterly, as for stature.

Ideally, the records should have regular time intervals between measurement occasions. These should coincide with changes in the

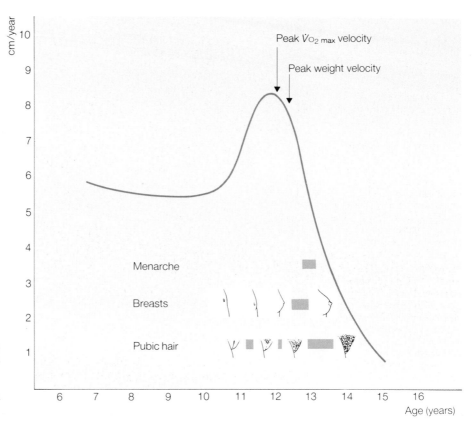

Fig. 6.1.17 Typical maturity events for girls showing stature velocity curve with indication of peak aerobic power and weight velocities and age of menarche (Mirwald & Bailey, 1986), with illustrative secondary sex characteristics from redrawn standards by Van Wieringen *et al.* (1971) and Roede & Van Wieringen (1985).

training programmes, complement all physiological testing and accommodate the schedule of the client or patient and laboratory. Practically, it is impossible to adhere exactly to a regular schedule of measurement and thus distance curves must be fitted to irregular measurement occasions and velocities derived from the fitted curve. There are a variety of computer-based curve fitting programs including those evolved from the proposed procedures by Preece and Baines (1978). In the fast-evolving microcomputer field, today's solutions are only precursors to better solutions tomorrow. A recent version of the Preece–Baines procedure has been developed for the IBM personal computer for height, weight, sitting height, leg length, and maximal oxygen uptake, with five initial parameters each for boys and girls, as reported by Mirwald and Bailey (1986).

Early and late maturation

In some sports, early maturation is a distinct advantage in age-restricted programmes. An early-maturing boy may be a precocious performer largely because he has proportionally greater muscle mass, greater cross-sectional areas of muscle, greater strength, more ATP, greater blood

Fig. 6.1.18 Variability in maturation rates illustrated by individual stature velocity curves displayed three-dimensionally with 100 boys' longitudinal curves arrayed on the y axis (cm/year), time of measurement on the x axis (ages from 7 to 16 years), and stature velocity on the z axis. (a) The display is arranged according to subject number, and shows an unordered pattern. (b) The display is ordered from late to early maturity according to peak height values and curve characteristics; there is an ordered early peak velocity point in the background, which becomes later in the foreground. (Leahy *et al.*, 1980.)

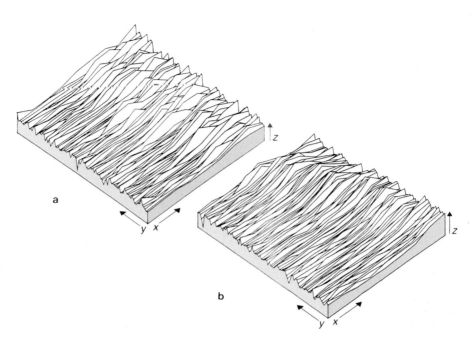

volume and greater storage space for lactates than his normal and later maturing peers. When, inevitably, they catch up, the early maturer's advantage is lost and he may not excel or live up to expectation. This has emotional and behavioural ramifications. Conversely, the late maturer, typically ectomesomorphic, may not perform up to expectation and either gets discouraged from lack of early success or is 'deselected' in the innovative ways that boys find to become sport drop-outs.

In girls, late maturation is associated with success in sport which emphasize centripetal forces where the limbs propel the body mass. The pre-adolescent physique typifies female gymnasts, divers, figure skaters, runners and jumpers. Without the compensatory muscularity associated with the male growth spurt, smallness and leanness may be a necessary condition for minimization of ballast weight in females.

Menarche The age of menarche or the onset of the first menstrual flow (even though subsequently irregular) is a recognized biological benchmark. As illustrated in Fig. 6.1.18, menarche comes after the age of peak height velocity and signals the approaching adult stature. Athletes, coaches and parents should be alerted that menarche is a maturation indicator and a routine reporting procedure should be adopted.

In *A History of the Study of Human Growth*, Tanner (1981) documents a secular trend to earlier maturation with the age of menarche somewhere around 17 years at the end of the 18th century to somewhere between 12.5 and 13.0 years reported in the 1980s. There are vast individual differences with systematic effects. For example, urban girls tend to be earlier than rural girls and plump girls tend to be earlier than lean girls.

Delayed maturation has been associated with specific sports. In general, the greater the dependence on centripetal force to propel the body, the later the age of menarche. Malina (1983, 1984) has found that female athletes, with the exception of swimmers, are delayed in biological maturity status; Alpine skiers also appear to not be delayed (Ross *et al.*, 1977a). Marker (1981) reported a mean age of menarche values of 15 years for international and national class gymnasts and figure skaters and reported that these and other late-maturing athletes did not appear to have a greater incidence of subsequent gynaecological or parturition problems. Longitudinal studies of athletes subsequent to their competitive period is the responsibility of research-granting agencies and the sports physician since long-term effects are of major concern.

Skeletal age

Clearly a child's chronological age is an unreliable estimate of his or her developmental status. Assessment of skeletal age by either the atlas method of Gruelich and Pyle (1959) or the bone-specific method by Tanner *et al.* (1983) provides one of the best estimates of developmental status. Apart from limited clinical applications, the use of X-rays for routine monitoring of maturation is clearly inappropriate.

Developmental age

Individual differences in maturation is a biological fact which cannot be ignored by the sports physician. Some of the variation can be assessed by shape characteristics of the child. A primary area of research is to use anthropometric modelling to predict skeletal age from available data and then apply the method in longitudinal series using the reduction of variance of maturity events in other longitudinal samples as a validity criterion (stature and body mass velocity curve characteristics, genitalia stages, menarche).

Gross function

Theoretical basis for scaling for size

The assumption of morphological constancy at each stage is also assumed in the use of age category percentile scoring of performance tests. Those who construct such norms and promote their use obviously do not share the conceptual insight about centripetal and centrifugal applications of force and the dominant role of size and proportion at every chronological age level (Tittel, 1978).

Another way of interpreting performance test data is to express values as percent predicted for the subject or client's own sex, age, and size of relevant structures and masses. One such approach is illustrated in the formula shown below which use longitudinal data assembled by Mirwald and Bailey (1986) to ascribe index values, with 100 being the normal expectancy for age, size and sex based on the Saskatchewan samples.

$$\mathrm{rel}\dot{V}_{O_2}\text{ boys }(8\text{–}16) = \frac{V \times h^{-2.6316} \times 24123881}{V \times w^{-0.9513} \times 1523}$$

$$\mathrm{rel}\dot{V}_{O_2}\text{ girls }(8\text{–}13) = \frac{V \times h^{-2.5713} \times 20272251}{V \times w^{-0.8966} \times 1423}$$

where $\mathrm{rel}\dot{V}_{O_2}$ is relative maximal oxygen uptake in percent expected, V is maximal oxygen uptake in l/min, and h and w are height (cm) and weight (kg).

From the above, a 12-year-old girl, 151.2 cm, 41.0 kg, $\dot{V}_{O_2\ max}$ of 1.97 l/min would have a $\mathrm{rel}\dot{V}_{O_2}$ of 99.6 and 99.3 for height and weight—roughly 100, as expected for mean performance. A $\dot{V}_{O_2\ max}$ of 2.33 l/min for the same height and weight would yield aerobic power indices of 117.6 and 121.4 for her height- and weight-adjusted indices.

Rather than assuming that maximal aerobic power is a simple function of bodyweight across the age range, the aerobic power index is a rough scaling to the expectancy for a longitudinal series of 75 boys and 22 girls studied by Mirwald and Bailey (1986). This provides an alternative way of dissociating size from that of dividing by bodyweight, which has different metabolic relevance with the changing composition of the growing child.

Age, sex and size dissociation in performance tests

The simple question of how good a performance test score is for a boy or girl of a given age and size, is not readily answerable. Despite large expenditures for assembling cross-sectional physical performance test data, the resultant tables for age and sex are no more sophisticated than those developed by physical educators in the 1940s who used rotary hand calculators to produce them. The need is to develop norms for age and sex with projections of expectancy for size.

The use of spread sheet assemblies of raw data makes all modelling less hazardous since one can quickly recall individual data and examine the differential effects in the model.

Anthropometry and sports medicine

Scientists and physicians should be aware of the danger of extrapolating simplistic relationships to individual predictions. They should recognize that precision and accuracy in measurements sufficient for group comparisons and experimental designs is often inadequate for individual assessment. Moreover, they must accept that comprehensive data can and should be collected serially and that it can be managed by evolving microcomputer technology and creative use of iconometrographic techniques. For some, this means a basic re-orientation and deployment in a clinical setting.

According to De Rose (1973), in addition to a professional competence in internal medicine, a sports physician also needs to be identified with basic areas related to performance such as: (a) anthropometry; (b) applied physiology; (c) biomechanics; and (d) sports psychology. Education of the physician in anthropometry applied to sports performance has been less rigorous than in the other three areas. This will have to change if sports physicians intend to establish effective collegial relationships with scientifically, rather than medically, trained personnel. An understanding of the interactions of many anthropometrical and functional factors for the analysis of sports performance is difficult, complex and important. Obviously, if one is to make use of comprehensive data assemblies and iconometrographic techniques in medical counselling and guidance, it cannot be done without conceptual, theoretical and methodological insight.

Acknowledgements

The authors acknowledge the Brazilian National Council of Research for an enabling grant received by Professor Eduardo Henrique De Rose; members of the International Society for the Advancement of Kinanthropometry working group on scholarship, awards and curriculum for their counsel; Dr John Dickinson and Ms M. V. Savage of the School of Kinesiology at Simon Fraser University for encouraging innovation in graduate studies; and Dr Michael Hawes of the University of Calgary and other participants for their contributions during the 1987 summer session seminar programme in kinanthropometry which served as a pilot for future ventures.

References

Adams, J., Motolla, M., Bagnall, K. M. & McFadden, K. D. (1982) Total body fat content in a group of professional football players. *Can. J. Appl. Sport Sci.* 7, 36.

Bailey, D. A., Carter, J. E. L. & Mirwald, R. L. (1982) Somatotypes of Canadian men and women. *Hum. Biol.* 54, 813.

Bar-Or, O. (1983) *Pediatric Sports Medicine for the Practitioner: From Physiologic Principles to Clinical Applications.* Springer-Verlag, New York.

Behnke, A. R. (1942) Physiological studies pertaining to deep sea diving and aviation, especially in relation to the fat content and composition of the body. *Harvey Lect.* **1941-1942**, 198.

Borms, J., Hebbelinck, M., Carter, J. E. L., Ross, W. D. & Lariviere, G. (1979) Standardization of basic anthropometry in Olympic athletes: the MOGAP procedure. In U. Novotny & S. Titlbachova (eds) *Methods of Functional Anthropology*, pp. 31–39. Charles University, Prague.

Cameron, N. (1986) Methods of auxological anthropometry. In F. Faulkner & J. M. Tanner (eds) *Human Growth*, 2nd edn, pp. 3–46. Plenum, New York.

Carter, J. E. L. (1980) *The Heath Carter Somatotype Method.* San Diego State Syllabus Service, San Diego.

Carter, J. E. L. (1982) Body composition of Montreal Olympic athletes. In J. E. L. Carter (ed) *Physical Structure of Olympic Athletes. Pt. I, Montreal Olympic Games Anthropological Project*, pp. 107–116. Karger, Basel.

Carter, J. E. L. (1984) *Physical Structure of Olympic Athletes. Pt. 2, Kinanthropometry of Olympic Athletes.* Karger, Basel.

Carter, J. E. L., Ross, W. D., Aubry, S. P., Hebbelinck, M. & Borms, J. (1982) Anthropometry of Olympic athletes. In J. E. L. Carter (ed) *Physical Structure of Olympic Athletes. Pt. I, Montreal Olympic Games Anthropological Project*, pp. 25–52. Karger, Basel.

Carter, J. E. L., Ross, W. D., Duquet, W., Aubry, S. P. (1983) Advances in somatotype methodology and analyses. *Yearbook Phys. Anthrop.* 26, 193.

Chovanova, E. & Zrubak, E. (1972) Somatotypes of prominent Czechoslovak ice hockey and football players. *Acta FRN Univ. Comen., Anteropologia* 21, 59.

Clarys, J. P., Martin, A. D. & Drinkwater, D. T. (1984) Gross tissue masses in adult humans: data from 25 dissections. *Hum. Biol.* 56, 459.

Copley, B. B. (1979) *An anthropometric, somatotypological and physiological study of tennis players with special reference to training.* Ph.D. Thesis, Wiwatersrand University.

Day, J. A. P. (1984) Bilateral symmetry and reliability of upper limb measurements. In J. A. P. Day (ed) *Perspectives in Kinanthropometry*, pp. 257–262. Human Kinetics, Champaign.

Day, J. A. P. (1986) Reliability and bilateral symmetry of upper limb measurements: the last word. In T. Reilly, J. Watson & J. Borms (eds) *Kinanthropometry II*, pp. 109–114. University Park Press, Baltimore.

DeGaray, A. L., Levine, L. & Carter, J. E. L. (1974) *Genetic and Anthropological Studies of Olympic Athletes.* Academic Press, New York.

De Rose, E. H. (1973) O exame médico do jogador de futebol. *Med. Esporte* 1, 15.

De Rose, E. H., Pigatto, E. & De Rose, R. C. F. (1984) *Cineantropometria, Educação Física e Treinamento Desportivo.* Editora do Brasil, Rio de Janeiro.

Drinkwater, D. T. (1984) *An anatomically derived method for the anthropometric estimation of human body composition.* Ph.D. Thesis, Simon Fraser University.

Drinkwater, D. T. & Ross, W. D. (1980) The anthropometric fractionation of body mass. In M. Ostyn, G. Beunen & J. Simmons (eds) *Kinanthropometry II*, pp. 177–189. University Park Press, Baltimore.

Durnin, J. V. G. A. & Womersley, J. (1974) Body fat assessed from total body density and its estimation from skinfold thickness measurements on 481 men and women age 16 to 72 years. *Br. J. Nutr.* 32, 77.

Eiben, O. G. (1972) *The Physique of Women Athletes.* Hungarian Scientific Council for Physical Education, Budapest.

Faulhaber, J. (1978) Algunos cambios morfologicos durante el crecimiento. *An. Antropologia* 15, 323.

Faulkner, F. & Tanner, J. M. (1986) *Human Growth*, 2nd edn, 3 vols. Plenum, New York.

Garn, S. M. (1986) Who are the obese? *Currents* 2, 26.

Garn, S. M., Leonard, W. R. & Hawthorne, V. M. (1986) Three limitations of the body mass index. *Am. J. Clin. Nutr.* 44, 996.

Greulich, W. W. & Pyle, S. I. (1959) *Radiographic Atlas of Skeletal Development of the Hand and Wrist*, 2nd edn. Stanford University Press, Stanford.

Johnston, F. E. (1982) Relationships between body composition and anthropometry. *Hum. Biol.* 54, 221.

Leahy, R. M., Drinkwater, D. T., Martin, G. R., Ross, W. D. & Vajda, A. S. (1980) Computer solutions for longitudinal data: tridimensional computer graphing in the resolution of growth curves. In M. Ostyn, G.

Beunen, J. Simons (eds) *Kinanthropometry II*, pp. 443–449. University Park Press, Baltimore.

Lohman, T., Roche, A. S. & Martorell, R. (eds) (1987) *Anthropometric Standardization Reference Manual.* Human Kinetics, Champaign, (in press).

Malina, R. M. (1983) Menarche in athletes: a synthesis and hypothesis. *Hum. Biol.* **10**, 1.

Malina, R. M. (1984) Maturational considerations in elite young athletes. In J. P. P. Day (ed) *Perspectives in Kinanthropometry*, pp. 29–43. Human Kinetics, Champaign.

Marker, K. (1981) Influence of athletic training in the maturity process in girls. In J. Borms, M. Hebbelinck & A. Venerando (eds) *The Female Athlete*, pp. 117–126. Karger, Basel.

Martin, A. D. (1984) *An anatomical basis for assessing human body composition: evidence from 25 cadavers.* Ph.D. Thesis, Simon Fraser University.

Martin, A. D., Drinkwater, D. T., Clarys, J. P. & Ross, W. D. (1986) The inconsistancy of the fat-free mass: a reappraisal with implications for densitometry. In T. Reilly, J. Watson & J. Borms (eds) *Kinanthropometry III*, pp. 92–97. Spon, London.

Martin, A. D., Ross, W. D., Drinkwater, D. T. & Clarys, J. P. (1984) Prediction of body fat by skinfold calipers: assumptions and cadaver evidence. *Int. J. Obes.* **7**, 17.

Martin, R. (1928) *Lehrbuch der Anthropologie.* Gustav Fischer, Stuttgart.

Martin, R. & Saller, K. (1966) *Lehrbuch der Anthropologie*, 3rd edn. Gustav Fischer, Stuttgart.

Matiegka, J. (1921) The testing of physical efficiency. *Am. J. Phys. Anthropol.* **4**, 223.

Mazess, R. B., Peppler, W. W., Chesney, R. W., Lange, T. A., Lindgren, W. & Smith jr, E. (1984) Total body and regional bone mineral by dual-photon absorbtiometry. *Calcif. Tissue Int.* **36**, 8.

Mirwald, R. L. & Bailey, D. A. (1986) *Maximal Aerobic Power: A Longitudinal Analysis.* Sports Dynamics, London, Ontario.

Perez, B. M. de (1981) *Los Atletas Venezolanos su tipo Fisico.* Universidad Central de Venezula, Caracas.

Pollock, M. L., Gettman, L. R., Jackson, A., Ayres, J., Ward, A. & Linnerud, A. C. (1977) Body composition of elite class distance runners. *Ann. NY Acad. Sci.* **301**, 361.

Preece, M. A. & Baines, M. J. (1978) A new family of mathematical models describing the human growth curve. *Ann. Hum. Biol.* **5**, 1.

Roede, M. J. & Van Wieringen, J. C. (1985) Growth diagrams 1980. *Tijds. Soc. Gezond.* (Suppl.) **63**, 1.

Ross, W. D. (1985a) Phantom stratagem for pro-

portional growth assessment: questions and answers. *Hum. Biol. Budap.* **16**, 153.

Ross, W. D. (1985b) The design of a parallax-correcting anthropometer for replication in non-specialized machine shops. *Am. J. Phys. Anthropol.* **66**, 93.

Ross, W. D., Brown, S. R., Faulkner, R. A. & Savage, M. V. (1977a) Age of menarche in Canadian skaters and skiers. *Can. J. Appl. Sport Sci.* **1**, 163.

Ross, W. D., Brown, S. R., Hebbelinck, M. & Faulkner, R. A. (1978) Kinanthropometry terminology and landmarks. In R. J. Shephard & H. Lavallée (eds) *Physical Fitness Assessment*, pp. 44–50. Charles C. Thomas, Springfield.

Ross, W. D., Brown, S. R., Yu, W. & Faulkner, R. A. (1977b) Somatotype of Canadian figure skaters. *J. Sports Med. Phys. Fitness* **17**, 195.

Ross, W. D., Drinkwater, D. T., Bailey, D. A., Marshall, G. R. & Leahy, R. M. (1980a) Kinanthropometry: traditions and new perspectives. In M. Ostyn, G. Beunen, J. Simons (eds) *Kinanthropometry II*, pp. 3–27. University Park Press, Baltimore.

Ross, W. D., Drinkwater, D. T., Whittingham, N. O. & Faulkner, R. A. (1980b) Anthropometric prototypes; age 6 to 18 years. In K. Berg & B. O. Eriksson (eds) *Children and Exercise IX*, pp. 3–12. University Park Press, Baltimore.

Ross, W. D., Eiben, O. G., Ward, R., Martin, A. D., Drinkwater, D. T. & Clarys, J. P. (1984) Alternatives for the conventional methods of human body composition and physique assessment. In J. A. P. Day (ed) *Perspectives in Kinanthropometry*, pp. 203–220. Human Kinetics, Champaign.

Ross, W. D. & Marfell-Jones, M. J. (1982) Kinanthropometry. In J. D. MacDougall, H. A. Wenger & H. J. Green (eds) *Physiological Testing of the Elite Athlete*, pp. 75–117. Mutual, Ottawa.

Ross, W. D., Martin, A. D. & Ward, R. (1987) Body composition and aging: theoretical and methodological implications. *Coll. Antropol.* **11**, 15.

Ross, W. D. & Ward, R. (1982a) Sexual dimorphism and human proportionality. In R. Hall (ed) *Sexual Dimorphism in Homo Sapiens*, pp. 317–361. Praeger, New York.

Ross, W. D. & Ward, R. (1982b) Proportionality of Montreal athletes. In J. E. L. Carter (ed) *Physical Structure of Olympic Athletes. Pt. I, Montreal Olympic Games Anthropological Project*, pp. 81–106. Karger, Basel.

Ross, W. D. & Ward, R. (1984) Proportionality of Olympic athletes. In J. E. L. Carter (ed) *Physical Structure of Olympic Athletes. Pt. II, Kinanthropometry of Olympic Athletes*, pp. 110–145. Karger, Basel.

Ross, W. D. & Ward, R. (1986) Scaling anthropometric data for size and proportionality. In T. Reilly, J. Watson & J. Borms (eds) *Kinanthropometry III*, pp. 85–91. Spon, London.

Ross, W. D., Ward, R., Sigmon, B. A. & Leahy, R. H. (1983) Anthropometric concomitants of X-chromosome aneuploidies. In A. V. Sandberg (ed) *The Cytogenetics of the Mammalian X-chromosome*, pp. 127–157. Alan R. Liss, New York.

Ross, W. D. & Wilson, N. C. (1974) A stratagem for proportional growth assessment. In J. Borms & M. Hebbelinck (eds) *Children in Exercise*, pp. 169–182. (*Acta Paed. Belgica* **28**.)

Sheldon, W. H., Dupertuis, C. W. & McDermott, E. (1954) *Atlas of Men*. Harper, New York.

Sloan, A. W. (1967) Estimation of body fat in young men. *J. Appl. Physiol.* **23**, 311.

Sloan, A. W., Burt, J. J. & Blyth, C. S. (1962) Estimating body fat in young women. *J. Appl. Physiol.* **17**, 967.

Stewart, T. D. (ed) (1952) *Hrdlička's Practical Anthropometry*. Wistar Inst. Anat. Biol., Philadelphia.

Tanner, J. M. (1976) Population differences in size, shape and growth rate: a 1976 review. *Arch. Dis. Child.* **51**, 1.

Tanner, J. M. (1978) Physical growth and development. In J. O. Forfar & G. C. Arneil (eds) *Textbook of Paediatrics*, 2nd edn. Churchill Livingstone, London.

Tanner, J. M. (1981) *A History of the Study of Human Growth*. Cambridge University Press, Cambridge.

Tanner, J. M. (1986) Normal growth and techniques of growth assessment. *Clin. Endocrinol. Metab.* **15**, 411.

Tanner, J. M., Whitehouse, R. H. & Cameron, N. (1983) *Assessment of Skeletal Maturity and the Prediction of Height*, 2nd edn. Academic Press, London.

Tittel, K. & Wutscherk, H. (1973) *Sportanthropometrie*. Barth, Leipzig.

Tittel, K. (1978) Tasks and tendencies of sport anthropometry's development. In F. Landry & W. A. R. Orban (eds) *Biomechanics of Sport and Kinanthropometry*, pp. 283–296. Symposia Specialists, Miami.

Van Wieringen, J. C., Waffelbakker, F., Verbrugge, H. P., De Haas, D. H. (1971) *Growth Diagrams 1965*. Wolters-Noordhoff, Groningen.

Weiner, J. S. & Lourie, J. A. (1981) *Practical Human Biology*. Academic Press, London.

Yuhasz, M. S. (1974) *Physical Fitness Manual*. University of Western Ontario, London, Ontario.

PART 7

TRAINING CHILDREN AND ADOLESCENTS

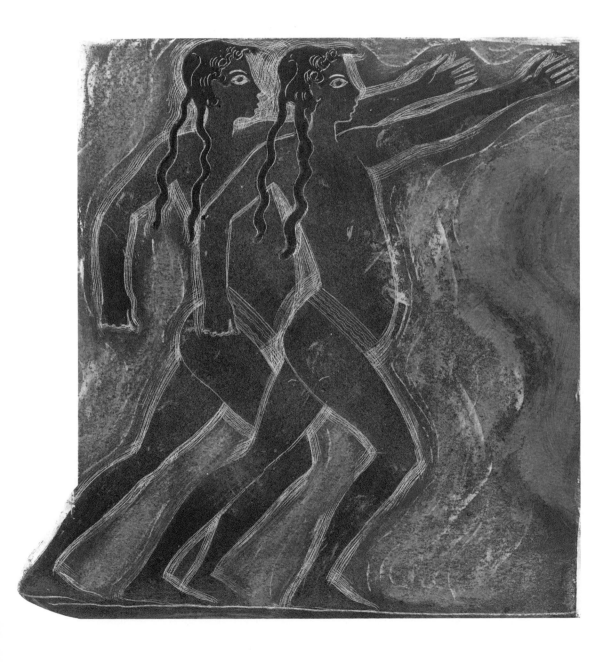

7.1 Adaptability of the musculoskeletal, cardiovascular and respiratory systems

O. BAR-OR

While children's physiological responses to training are qualitatively similar to those of adolescents and adults, there are several age- and development-related quantitative differences in trainability. These differences are overviewed in this chapter. For some detailed reviews, see Bar-Or (1983), Rowland (1985) and Weltman (1988).

Of special interest to the clinician are the effects of training on the child with disease or illness. An outline of such relationships will be given, as well as a discussion of the possible uses of exercise and sports in paediatric treatment and rehabilitation.

Trainability of healthy children and adolescents

There are major methodological constraints in designing studies to compare trainability in children, adolescents and adults. First, it is important to realize that physiological changes induced by training are often identical to those that accompany growth and maturation. Examples are the decrease in submaximal heart rate and oxygen uptake per kg bodyweight, and the increase in muscular power, maximal blood lactate and athletic performance. To isolate the training effect, one must select, therefore, a control group that does not train. One problem, however, is that the habitual activity of children, even when not in a training programme, is often quite high. Another problem is how to select controls who are sufficiently similar in their developmental stage to those in the training group; chronological age *per se* may not be an adequate criterion for matching.

An additional challenge is to match the training dosage across age groups. Can one assume that a certain running velocity presents an identical stimulus to a child and to a young adult? Would a given submaximal heart rate denote the same cardiovascular strain in various ages? Should the metabolic load be equated by a certain percentage of maximal oxygen uptake? By a certain multiple of resting metabolic rate?

Is the strain at anaerobic threshold similar across ages? These and other questions need answering before one can launch definitive comparative studies about the trainability of different age groups. Conclusions based on the following data, therefore, should be taken as tentative.

Muscular strength

Very few controlled studies are available on the trainability of muscular strength at different ages. It seems, however, that prepubescent, pubescent and postpubescent girls (Nielsen *et al.*, 1980) and boys (Pfeiffer *et al.*, 1986; Weltman *et al.*, 1986) can all respond to appropriate resistance training with an increase in muscular strength. While some authors (Vrijens, 1978) have suggested that the degree of muscle strength trainability is lower before puberty, others (Nielsen *et al.*, 1980) have shown that prepubescents may have a greater strength trainability than older age groups. A recent study (Pfeiffer *et al.*, 1986), found no development-related difference in strength trainability. This is notwithstanding the fact that the natural development of muscle strength in boys reaches its peak only about a year following the growth spurt, and in girls during the growth spurt (Beunen, 1988).

A still debated issue is whether resistance training in children is safe, as was recently reviewed by Weltman (1988). While some evidence suggests that resistance training over several weeks causes no damage to muscles or bones of prepubescents (Weltman *et al.*, 1986), precaution should be taken in the conduct of such training. It is particularly important to differentiate between *weight training*, in which the child exercises repeatedly against submaximal resistance, and *weight lifting*, where the resistance is maximal. Unless proven otherwise, the latter should be considered damaging to the growing child (American Academy of Pediatrics, 1983).

Muscular power and endurance

Physical educators and coaches know from experience that training can improve children's performance in activities that require high muscular power (e.g. jumping or throwing) or muscular endurance (e.g. 200–400 m running or rowing). Little laboratory-based information is available, however, on the trainability of muscular power and muscular endurance in children. Children who trained for several weeks with sprint running or with short bouts of supramaximal cycling increased the peak power and muscular endurance of their legs, as measured by the Wingate anaerobic test (Grodjinovsky *et al.*, 1980). This increase, however, was less than 10% of the initial performance.

A combined aerobic–anaerobic training programme in 11- to 15-year-old boys induced an increase in muscle substrates such as creatine phosphate, adenosine triphosphate (ATP) and glycogen, as well as in the activity of the glycolytic enzyme phosphofructokinase (Eriksson, 1972). These biochemical changes lend further support to the notion that anaerobic characteristics of children are trainable. No data are available, however, on the effect of maturation on the *degree* of trainability of muscular power and muscular endurance. Several studies with adults, suggest that trainability of these functions is of the same degree as found in children.

Maximal aerobic power Among adults, aerobic training seems to induce a greater increase in maximal aerobic power in the young than in the old. No such age-related relationship can be found among children. Indeed, several studies (Gilliam & Freedson, 1980; Yoshida *et al.*, 1980) have shown that prepubescents are even less trainable than adolescents or adults. In contrast, based on a review of the literature, Rowland (1985) concluded that, when the training protocols conform to criteria set for adults, prepubescents do increase their maximal aerobic power at a rate similar to other age groups. The aerobic trainability of pubescents and postpubescents has been proven in several studies and does not seem to be different from that of adults (e.g. Ekblom, 1969). Some authors have suggested that aerobic trainability increases following the age of peak height velocity (i.e. the year during which height growth is at its maximal rate) (Kobayashi *et al.*, 1978). More research, with appropriate design, is needed to confirm this claim.

Running economy Even when aerobic training fails to increase maximal oxygen uptake, the running performance of children can markedly improve. One explanation is a decrease in the oxygen uptake at any given submaximal running speed, which increases the 'metabolic reserve' of the child. Such an improvement in running economy, which occurs during growth and maturation, even without training, is further enhanced by training (Daniels & Oldridge, 1971; Burkett *et al.*, 1985). It is interesting to find out whether improvement in running economy can be achieved in children by improving their running style, even without aerobic training.

Trainability of children with common diseases

Does disease affect a child's ability to improve her or his physical fitness? Numerous studies are available to show that, in most cases, a child is trainable, whether healthy or ill. Table 7.1.1 is a summary of some of the

Table 7.1.1 Paediatric diseases in which physical fitness was found to improve through training.

Disease	Improved fitness component	Selected reference
Bronchial asthma	Max. aerobic power, strength	Fitch *et al.* (1976)
Cerebral palsy	Max. aerobic power, strength, muscular power and endurance	Lundberg *et al.* (1967) Bar-Or unpubl. data
Cystic fibrosis	Max. aerobic power	Orenstein *et al.* (1981)
Diabetes mellitus	Max. aerobic power, skills	Larsson *et al.* (1962)
Muscular dystrophy	Strength, muscle power and endurance	Vignos & Watkins (1966) Bar-Or unpubl. data
Obesity	Max. aerobic power, gait economy	Parizkova *et al.* (1962)
Scoliosis	Max. aerobic power	Bjure *et al.* (1969)
Undernutrition	Muscular endurance (rats)	Raju (1977)

more common paediatric diseases in which a training programme was found to improve the patient's fitness. It should be realized, however, that only few of the quoted studies were conducted with a proper random allocation and controlled design (Bar-Or, 1985).

The compatibility of some paediatric diseases with athletic excellence is a testimony to the trainability of the young athletes afflicted by them. Examples are numerous athletes with insulin-dependent diabetes mellitus and bronchial asthma, who have broken world records and gained Olympic medals.

Exercise in paediatric treatment and rehabilitation

In addition to its effect on fitness, physical training can induce *specific* beneficial changes in the child with a disease. Such changes, as summarized in Table 7.1.2, provide the rationale for the use of exercise prescription as a means of treatment and rehabilitation in paediatrics. Some of these benefits, such as reduced intensity of exercise-induced bronchoconstriction in asthma, enhanced respiratory mucus clearance in cystic fibrosis, better metabolic control in diabetes mellitus and increased appetite in chronic renal failure, require further proof by research.

Many young patients are physically hypoactive because they have low self confidence and self esteem. Others are socially isolated by their peers (e.g. those with obesity or kyphoscoliosis). An extremely important benefit of exercise in such children is, therefore, the psychosocial effect. Training, with or without improvement in fitness, can increase self confidence, self esteem and happiness of the patient and allow for better sociability.

Table 7.1.2 Specific beneficial effects of exercise in paediatric treatment and rehabilitation. Adapted from Bar-Or (1983).

Disease	Specific benefits
Anorexia nervosa	Means for behaviour modification
Bronchial asthma	Reduced rate and intensity of EIB(?)
Cerebral palsy	Ambulation, increased range of motion, weight control
Chronic renal failure	Increased appetite(?)
Cystic fibrosis	Increased ventilatory endurance, enhanced respiratory mucus drainage(?)
Diabetes mellitus	Improved metabolic control(?)
Haemophilia	Mobilization, increased range of motion
Hypertension	Mild decrease in resting blood pressure
Mental retardation	Socialization, increased environmental stimuli
Muscular dystrophy	Ambulation, strengthening of residual muscle, weight control
Obesity	Weight control, improved self esteem
Rheumatoid arthritis	Mobilization, increased range of motion

EIB = exercise-induced bronchoconstriction; (?) = non-definitive information.

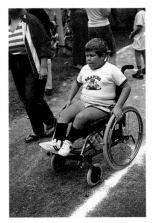

Fig. 7.1.1 The prescription of exercise for disabled children and encouragement for competitive sport must be considered with respect to the specific problem and the psychosocial and physiologicl effects. Courtesy of O. Bar-Or.

For an exercise prescription to be effective, it should be specific to the problem at hand. For example, a training regimen for the increase of strength in muscular dystrophy will be entirely different from one prescribed for weight control in obesity, or for the increase of aerobic fitness in bronchial asthma. Sometimes, two children with the same disease may require an entirely different training regimen. If a child with spina bifida, for example, is lean, much attention should be given to strengthening of the upper body in order to attempt walking. In contrast, a child with spina bifida who is also obese, must first be given a wheelchair-based programme with a high metabolic cost (i.e. wheeling for long distances) and nutritional modifications, and only once bodyweight has decreased sufficiently should emphasis be shifted to strengthening of specific muscle groups.

One should further realize that some activities may cause damage to the child (e.g. exercise-induced bronchoconstriction in asthma, hypoglycaemia in diabetes mellitus, or arterial oxygen desaturation in cystic fibrosis). Such detrimental effects are usually preventable by modifying the exercise regimen or by proper medication. A diagnostic exercise test, given prior to the start of the therapeutic programme, will help identify those children at risk.

References

American Academy of Pediatrics (1983) Weight training and weight lifting: information for the pediatrician. *Physician Sportsmed.* **11**, 157.

Bar-Or, O. (1983) *Pediatric Sports Medicine for the Practitioner.* Springer Verlag, New York.

Bar-Or, O. (1985) Physical conditioning in children with cardiorespiratory disease. *Exerc. Sport Sci. Rev.* **13**, 305.

Beunen, G. (1988) Biological age in pediatric exercise research. In O. Bar-Or (ed) *Advance in Pediatric Sports Sciences*, Vol. 3. Human Kinetics, Champaign, (in press).

Bjure, J., Grimby, G. & Nachemson, A. (1969) The effect of physical training on girls with idiopathic scoliosis. *Acta Orthop. Scand.* **40**, 325.

Burkett, L. N., Fernhall, B. & Walters, S. C. (1985) Physiological effects of distance running training on teenage females. *Res. Quart. Exerc. Sports* **56**, 215.

Daniels, J. & Oldridge, N. (1971) Changes in oxygen consumption of young boys during growth and running training. *Med. Sci. Sports* **3**, 161.

Ekblom, B. (1969) Effects of physical training in adolescent boys. *J. Appl. Physiol.* **27**, 350.

Eriksson, B. O. (1972) Physical training, oxygen supply and muscle metabolism in 11- to 15-year old boys. *Acta Physiol. Scand.* (Suppl.) **384**, 1.

Fitch, K. D., Morton, A. R. & Blanksby, B. A. (1976) Effects of swimming training on children with asthma. *Arch. Dis. Child.* **51**, 190.

Gilliam, T. B. & Freedson, P. S. (1980) Effects of a 12-week school physical education program on peak VO$_2$ body composition and blood lipids in 7 to 9 year old children. *Int. J. Sports Med.* **1**, 73.

Grodjinovsky, A., Bar-Or, O., Dotan, R. & Inbar, O. (1980) Training effect on the anaerobic performance of children as measured by the Wingate anaerobic test. In K. Berg & B. O. Eriksson (eds) *Children and Exercise IX*, pp. 139–145. University Park Press, Baltimore.

Kobayashi, K., Kitamura, K., Miura M., Sodeyama, H., Murase, Y., Miyashita, M. & Matsui, H. (1978) Aerobic power as related to body growth and training in Japanese boys: a longitudinal study. *J. Appl. Physiol.* **44**, 666.

Larsson, Y. A. A., Sterky, G. C. G., Ekegren, K. E. K. & Moller, T. G. H. O. (1962) Physical fitness and the influence of training in diabetic adolescent girls. *Diabetes* **11**, 109.

Lundberg, A., Ovenfors, C. O. & Saltin, B. (1967) Effect of physical training on schoolchildren with cerebral palsy. *Acta Paediatr. Scand.* **56**, 182.

Nielsen, B., Nielsen, K., Behrendt-Hansen, M. & Asmussen, E. (1980) Training of 'functional' muscular strength in girls 7–19 years old. In K. Berg & B. Eriksson (eds) *Children and Exercise IX*, pp. 68–69. University Park Press, Baltimore.

Orenstein, D. M., Franklin, B. A., Doershuk, C. F., Hellerstein, H. K., Germann, K. J., Horowitz, J. G. & Stern, R. G. (1981) Exercise conditioning in cystic fibrosis. The effects of a supervised running program. *Chest* **80**, 392.

Parizkova, J., Vaneckova, M. & Vamberova, M. (1962) A study of changes in some functional indicators following reduction of excessive fat in obese children. *Physiol. Bohemoslov.* **11**, 351.

Pfeiffer, R. & Francis, R. S. (1986) Effects of strength training on muscle development in prepubescent, pubescent, and postpubescent males. *Physician Sportsmed.* **14**, 134.

Raju, N. V. (1977) Effect of exercise during rehabilitation on swimming performance metabolism and function of muscle in rats. *Br. J. Nutr.* **38**, 157.

Rowland, T. W. (1985) Aerobic response to endurance training in prepubescent children: a critical analysis. *Med. Sci. Sports Exerc.* **17**, 493.

Vignos, P. J. & Watkins, M. P. (1966) The effect of exercise in muscular dystrophy. *J. Am. Med. Assoc.* **197**, 843.

Vrijens, J. (1978) Muscle strength development in the pre- and post-pubescent age. *Med. Sports (Basel)* **11**, 152.

Weltman, A. (1988) Weight training in prepubertal children. Physiologic benefit and potential damage. In O. Bar-Or (ed) *Advances in Pediatric Sports Sciences*, Vol. 3. Human Kinetics, Champaign, (in press).

Weltman, A., Janney, C., Rians, C. B., Strand, K., Berg, B., Tippit, S., Wise, J., Cahill, B. & Katch, F. I. (1986) The effect of hydraulic resistance strength training in pre-pubertal males. *Med. Sci. Sports Exerc.* **18**, 629.

Yoshida, T., Ishiko, I. & Muraoka, I. (1980) Effect of endurance training on cardiorespiratory functions of 5-year-old children. *Int. J. Sports Med.* **1**, 91.

7.2 The identification of performance potential

L. KOMADEL

The identification and selection of future élite athletes in childhood or adolescence has become a necessity. It takes many years of intensive regular training until an international sports performance level is achieved. The children selected for élite sport activities require suitable conditions and sports facilities, equipment of high quality, a rational style of life, and the service of experts including a sports physician, a well educated and experienced coach, etc. Such conditions can be created for selected children only. Therefore, the correct identification and selection of young talent is becoming important everywhere.

From the medical point of view, when young sports talent is identified and selected it is useful, in each case, to take into consideration:

1 State of health.
2 Somatotype.
3 Functional capabilities.
4 Psychologic abilities.

Genetic influence on sports efficiency

It is generally believed that genetic predispositions are of great importance for a successful sports career. Each sports performance is a very complex phenomenon involving many different factors: an equal performance can be achieved by various combinations of participating factors. It is therefore very difficult to identify the genetic influence on sports efficiency. The examination of young athletes and their parents has not produced any definite results. There are many successful athletes with parents who were also very good at sports, but there are also many with parents who have never competed in any sports.

In our examination of 680 young élite athletes, the results indicated that in comparison with a random sample the fathers of athletes were involved in some kind of sports activities in a relationship of 70 to 54% and the mothers in a relationship of 57 to 37%. In the majority, the children were engaged in a different kind of sports to their parents. The comparison of the achieved performance level of the children and their parents did not give any useful results. This study showed some influence of parents' sports activities upon the sports success of their children, although it is difficult to say which mechanisms were, in fact, in play. It could be the somatotype, the functional capabilities, the psychological dispositions or other factors, but it may be only a general atmosphere in the family, favouring and supporting regular sports activity.

Šimková *et al.* (1982) studied the genetic influence on particular motor capabilities. They examined a group of 7-year-old children and their parents, looking for capabilities of both groups in endurance, speed and strength exercises. The preliminary results proved that the motor performance of boys is more determined by the father in reaction time, in the 12 min run and in the forward bend. The motor performance of girls was more determined by the mother in the 50 m run, in the 12 min run and in the strength of the back muscles.

The genetic dependence of maximum oxygen uptake is the functional parameter most often studied. Klissouras (1971) found in a group of monozygous twins, that the coefficient of heredity was 93.8, i.e. a high genetic dependence. Taylor and Rowell (1974) stressed that 98.6% of adult young men had a $\dot{V}_{O_2 max}$ of 31.5 to 58.5 ml/min/kg. Only 0.13% of the male population achieved values of 61.5 to 67 ml/min/kg. According to them only one boy in 1000 has a genetic disposition for an endurance performance of international level. Shephard (1980) estimated the probability of the incidence of supranormal values of $\dot{V}_{O_2 max}$ in the male population; he estimated a probability of 1 : 2000 for a $\dot{V}_{O_2 max}$ of 86 ml/min/kg. Higher values seem to be even more rare.

It is considered as proved that there is a high genetic influence on the $\dot{V}_{O_2 max}$. Persons with genetically higher $\dot{V}_{O_2 max}$ have preconditions for a higher performance in endurance exercises. Similar results for the capabilities of speed, strength, power, coordination and balance are not yet available, but it is generally supposed that the genetic dependence of these parameters is also a high one.

Health preconditions for participation in élite sports

A good state of health is one of the most important preconditions for participation of children and adolescents in élite sports. Based on long experience and expertise a list of diseases considered as absolute and/or relative contraindications for participation in élite sports was drawn up (Komadel *et al.*, 1985a). This list was later approved by the Ministry of

Table 7.2.1 Factors considered by the Czechoslovak Ministry of Health to be absolute contraindications to playing sports.

1. Psychoses and psychopathies of any kind	18. Anaemia and other haemopathies
2. Poliomyelitis and consequent illnesses	19. Hepatitis epidermica—sports forbidden for 6 to 12 months
3. Encephalitis epidemica	20. Cholecystopathy
4. Meningitis acuta	21. Diabetes mellitus
5. Epilepsy	22. Nephritis acuta—sports forbidden for 12 months
6. Radiculitis with hernia disci intervertebrales	
7. Chronic diseases of the brain and spinal cord	23. Cystopyelitis acuta
8. Myopia of more than 4.5 dioptres	24. Chronic diseases of the kidneys and urinal ways
9. Blindness, even of one side	25. Scoliosis (identified by X-ray)
10. Pleuritis exudativa	26. Scheuermann's disease and other osteochondropathies, spondylolisthesis and other serious anomalies of the spine
11. Bronchitic asthma	
12. Congenital and acquired heart disease	
13. Myocarditis—sports forbidden for 18 months	27. Luxatio coxae congenita treated in early childhood with special apparatus
14. Carditis rheumatica—sports forbidden for 24 months	28. Arthrosis of any joint, even if incipiens
15. Rheumatic fever—sports forbidden for 24 months	29. Pes equinovarus
	30. Osteomyelitis
16. Hypertension	31. Any other diseases causing permanent, serious dysfunctions
17. Haemophilia	

Health and declared as a rule binding all Czechoslovak physicians to consider the state of health of children and adolescents before their inclusion in competitive élite sports.

The absolute contraindications are listed in Table 7.2.1. The time periods indicated where sports are forbidden, is measured from the end of the acute state of the relevant disease according to the usual clinical development as well as individual biochemical parameters.

There are some very successful international athletes who suffer from some of the diseases listed in Table 7.2.1. These are principally: bronchial asthma, diabetes mellitus, the condition after poliomyelitis with some handicaps, etc. In the past, in exceptional cases, it was possible to be successful in international sports even with some handicaps. Nowadays, the volume and intensity of training in all sports has become much higher — and this trend will probably continue in the future. When considering potential sports talent in a child or adolescent it is therefore important to bear the contraindications in mind. For a child with asthma, diabetes and some other diseases, regular exercise and mass sports activities are recommended, but not competitive sports at top levels.

The relative contraindications (Table 7.2.2) to be considered in individual cases depend on the stage and extent of the disease, the kind of sport, the sports performance level already achieved, the discipline of the specialization, the individual conditions, etc. Some of the indicated diseases can be effectively treated, and therefore the relative contraindications are limited by the time period of the treatment.

Table 7.2.2 Factors considered by the Czechoslovak Ministry of Health to be relative contraindications to playing sports.

1. Retardation of somatic development	16. Joint inflammations
2. Sight disorders	17. Coxa vara, coxa valga, genus vara, genus valga
3. Deafness	
4. Dumbness	18. Luxatio coxae congenita treated in early childhood without special apparatus
5. Juvenile hypertension	
6. Bronchiectases	19. Pedes plani
7. Recidivant infections of the upper and lower respiratory ways	20. Disorders and handicaps caused by injuries
8. Dysfunctions of endocrine glands	21. All other diseases mentioned in personal anamnesias should be individually considered
9. Chronic gastritis	
10. Gastric (duodenal) ulcers	
11. Anomalies and dysfunctions of the genital system	22. Diseases mentioned in personal anamnesias with high familial disposition should be considered
12. Nephrolithiasis	
13. Chronic dermatological diseases	23. All diseases listed in Table 7.2.1 for a certain period of time; for particular individuals they may be considered as relative, not absolute, contraindications
14. Anomalies of the carriage (but not fixed scoliosis, etc.)	
15. Organogenical disorders of movements	

Čermák (1983) has summarized 4 years of study of the state of health of 459 athletes (average age 15.1 years) who were examined as candidates for a centre of élite sports in Prague. For health reasons, 78 could not be recommended, i.e. 17% of them; from these about 70% were because of anomalies of the skeletal system. The rating of particular diseases and disorders was as follows: Scheuermann's disease 32 cases, scoliosis 14, Legg–Calvé–Perthes disease 6, valvular cardiopathies 4, spondylolisthesis 3, hypertension 3, sight disorders 3, chronic infections of urinal ways 2, and one case each from the following: state after a glomerulonephritis, kyphosis, ankylosis digiti manus posttraumatica, state after a ganglioneuroma mediastinum, Charcot–Marie–Tooth disease, duodenal ulcer, recidivant sprains, shortening of one leg, retarded physical development, deformity of the chest, spondyloarthrosis, and epilepsy.

All the examined children and adolescents were considered as talented, because all achieved a good level of sports performance. This experience is clear proof of an absolute necessity to carefully examine the state of health of all children and adolescents before they start the high training load of élite athletes.

Prediction of somatotype

Certain somatotypes may become limiting factors of performance in many sports. It is only in exceptional cases that individuals are able to compensate for an unfavourable somatotype with other excellent capabilities.

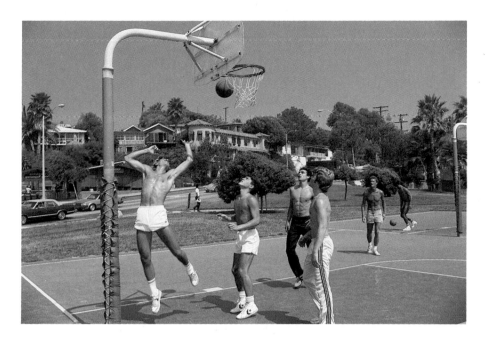

Fig. 7.2.1 Basketball is an example of a sport where, other factors being essentially equal, supranormal height provides an athlete with a distinct advantage. Courtesy of Bob Thomas Sports Photography.

Heredity exercises a crucial influence on each component of the somatotype, as well as on the somatotype as a whole. Šimková *et al.* (1982) demonstrated that in boys the mesomorphic component is the more genetically determined, while in girls it is the ectomorphic one. In boys, the variance of the somatotype is mainly explained by the father; the highest values were found in arm circumference and body height. Girls are more influenced by their fathers in the body height, bodyweight and biacromial distance; all other somatotype features are more influenced by the mother. Mothers have somatotypes more similiar to their children than do fathers, and this is expressed more clearly in daughters than in sons. This has been confirmed in other studies. Chovanová *et al.* (1982) found indices of heritability for each somatotypological component, markedly higher in boys than in girls.

The most often requested prediction concerns the adult stature. There are many kinds of sports in which supranormal body height is one of the most important limiting factors of sports performance, e.g. basketball, volleyball, water polo, high jump, rowing and recently also swimming, tennis, etc. Contrarily, in some sports a subnormal body height is still preferred, e.g. gymnastics, water jumping, figure skating, etc.

There are several possibilities for the prediction of adult stature. The authors have extensively used equations and nomograms elaborated by Šimková *et al.* (1982). Large groups of children and their parents were

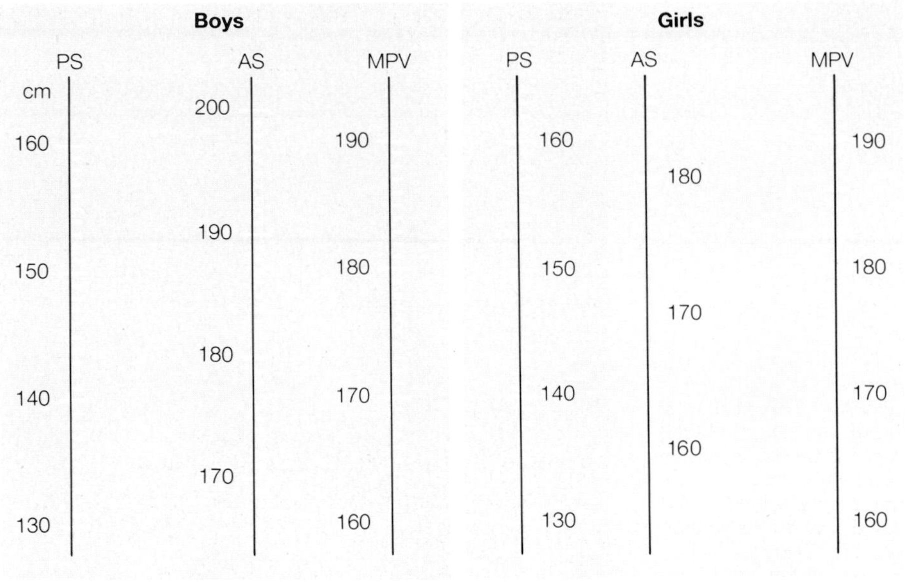

Boys

PS	AS	MPV
cm	200	
160		190
	190	
150		180
	180	
140		170
	170	
130		160

Girls

PS	AS	MPV
160	180	190
150	170	180
140	160	170
130		160

Fig. 7.2.2 Nomograms for the prediction of adult stature in 11-year-old boys and girls. From Šimková *et al.* (1982). PS = present stature, AS = predicted adult stature, MPV = mid-parents value. All measurements are in centimetres.

examined, and the following multiple regression equations for the ages of 6 and 11 years were calculated:

$$\left. \begin{aligned} y &= 48.5085 + 0.7173x_1 + 0.2584x_3 \\ y &= 34.8579 + 0.7360x_2 + 0.2230x_3 \end{aligned} \right\} \text{Boys}$$

$$\left. \begin{aligned} y &= 38.9075 + 0.3718x_1 + 0.4856x_3 \\ y &= 37.8652 + 0.3887x_2 + 0.4250x_3 \end{aligned} \right\} \text{Girls}$$

where y = adult stature in cm, x_1 = stature at the age of 6 years, x_2 = stature at the age of 11 years, x_3 = mid parents value ([body height of the father + body height of the mother]/2).

Prediction of the adult body height can in this way be ascertained with a standard error of ± 4 cm. Nomograms are even easier to use and an example is presented in Fig. 7.2.2.

Assessment of functional capacity by laboratory examination and motor field tests

Sports performance of children depends very much on previous training, principally on the mastering of the technique of the relevant sports discipline. Talent can only be realized at an adequate level of skill; a child with poor talent with a longer training period can perform more than a talented child after a shorter period of training. Therefore, in beginners,

Table 7.2.3 Average values of the $\dot{V}_{O_2\,max}$ in the Czechoslovak population. After Seliger *et al.* (1975).

Age (years)	$\dot{V}_{O_2\,max}$, l/min		$\dot{V}_{O_2\,max}$, ml(kg × min)	
	Male	Female	Male	Female
12	1.694	1.457	44.2	37.0
15	2.514	1.892	44.9	35.2
18	3.088	2.049	45.7	35.1
25	2.922	1.933	39.0	32.0
35	2.856	1.907	36.8	29.4
45	2.790	1.922	35.3	27.7
55	2.484	1.723	32.7	25.2

sports performance is not sufficient to assess level of talent. More information on talent can be gained by functional examinations in well-controlled laboratory conditions and by using field motor tests.

The most important functional parameter is the $\dot{V}_{O_2\,max}$. A genetically high value of $\dot{V}_{O_2\,max}$ is a favourable prerequisite for a high efficiency in endurance sports events. Values can be compared to the norms or average values of the population, according to sex and age. An example of average values of the Czechoslovak population, based on an examination of 2186 male and 1572 female subjects by Seliger *et al.* (1975), is presented in Table 7.2.3. Higher average values were found in Sweden, the German Federal Republic and Canada.

Many children who are good at sports have advanced physical development, so their biological age is higher than their chronological one. The $\dot{V}_{O_2\,max}$ values should be considered in relation to bodyweight, which corresponds better with biological age. For example, in a group of 21 swimmers (average age 12.6 years) the average $\dot{V}_{O_2\,max}$ value was 2.3 l/min, and this value was 36% above the population average. However, if the value was compared to bodyweight, it only exceeded the population average by 6% (Komadel *et al.*, 1985b).

Endurance athletes of international standard have $\dot{V}_{O_2\,max}$ levels about two times higher than the average population. Figure 7.2.3 shows average $\dot{V}_{O_2\,max}$ values of 339 young athletes engaged in competitive sports for 3 to 5 years, in comparison with average values of the Czechoslovak population and with world class endurance athletes. The Czechoslovak athletes had $\dot{V}_{O_2\,max}$ levels about 10–40% greater than the average population, but were well below the top athletes. This could be due to a lack of talent or to a less than optimal system of training. Longitudinal follow-up studies of young athletes have often shown an initial increase of the absolute value of the $\dot{V}_{O_2\,max}$ followed by a

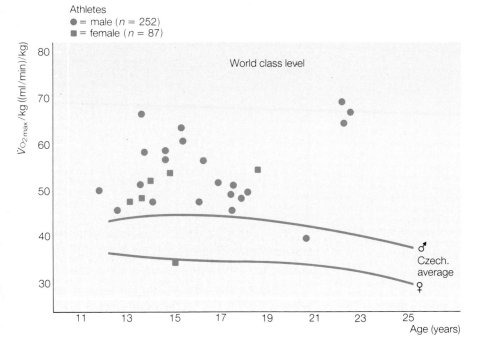

Fig. 7.2.3 Average $\dot{V}_{O_2\,max}$ values for a group of 339 young athletes, in comparison with the average for the Czechoslovak population and with world class endurance athletes. From Komadel *et al.* (1985b).

stagnation, or even a decrease, of the value related to bodyweight, even in the case of an intensive endurance training programme and increasing sports efficiency.

Examination of the anaerobic threshold, half-time oxygen uptake at the onset of exercise, and of other functional parameters, can give more precise information on the aerobic power of a child or adolescent. However, the anaerobic capacity of children does not seem to be useful for the identification of young talent in anaerobic types of sports. Muscle biopsies to determine the muscle fibre types predominant in particular muscles do not help ascertain potential talent either, although it seems hopeful from a theoretical point of view.

Motor tests reflect better the basic predisposition for particular kinds of sports. Based on a large amount of research work with numerous motor tests, the authors decided to use the following six tests (as having the highest discriminatory powers) to identify different capabilities: (a) 50 m run; (b) 12 min run (Cooper's test); (c) shuttle run; (d) standing long jump; (e) medicine ball throwing; and (f) motor reaction time.

A high reliability was confirmed for these tests, and the methods and procedure of testing was standardized (Havlíček *et al.*, 1982). Norms for the test results according to age and sex were established and are given in Tables 7.2.4 and 7.2.5 (Šemetka, 1982). Physicians and trainers are able to use such tables to compare individuals to performance norms. It was

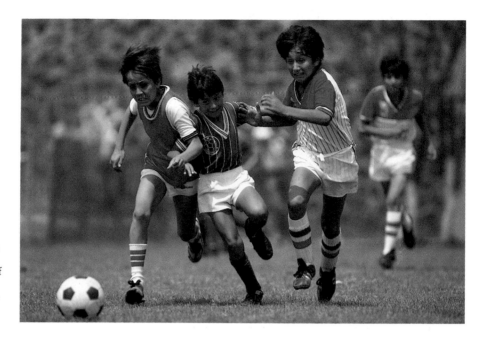

Fig. 7.2.4 Because of the many factors involved, information such as the fibre-type population of the leg musculature of children has not been shown to be of use in predicting eventual success in élite competition. Courtesy of Bob Thomas Sports Photography.

considered to be useful to differentiate the starting value as high, middle or low, in order to make clearer the changes due to applied training systems. Performance in particular motor tests can also be expressed numerically, making it possible to get one final value summarizing the results of all the tests applied.

Table 7.2.4 Performance norms in motor tests for boys aged 7 to 14 years.

Test	Starting level	7	8	9	10	11	12	13	14
50 m run (s)	High	9.3	8.2	7.9	7.7	7.1	6.8	6.5	6.3
	Middle	10.3	9.2	8.8	8.6	8.0	7.7	7.4	7.2
	Low	11.3	10.2	9.8	9.6	9.0	8.7	8.4	8.2
12 min run (m)	High	2450	2648	2818	2865	2969	3044	3135	3257
	Middle	2098	2295	2466	2513	2617	2692	2783	3257
	Low	1746	1943	2114	2161	2265	2340	2431	2552
Shuttle run (s)	High	12.4	11.8	11.5	11.1	10.6	10.5	10.1	9.9
	Middle	13.5	12.8	12.5	12.1	11.6	11.5	11.1	11.0
	Low	14.5	13.8	13.5	13.2	12.7	12.6	12.2	12.0
Standing long jump (cm)	High	169	185	195	204	208	214	223	233
	Middle	147	163	173	182	186	192	201	211
	Low	126	141	151	160	164	170	179	189
Medicine ball throw (m)	High	4.3	4.8	5.3	5.8	6.2	6.8	7.6	8.5
	Middle	3.4	3.9	4.4	4.9	5.3	5.9	6.7	7.6
	Low	2.5	3.0	3.5	4.0	4.4	5.0	5.8	6.6

Table 7.2.5 Performance norms in motor tests for girls aged 7 to 14 years.

Test	Starting level	Age (years)							
		7	8	9	10	11	12	13	14
50 m run (s)	High	9.4	8.5	8.2	7.9	7.2	6.9	6.7	6.7
	Middle	10.5	9.6	9.3	9.0	8.3	8.0	7.8	7.7
	Low	11.6	10.6	10.3	10.1	9.4	9.0	8.9	8.8
12 min run (m)	High	2158	2297	2508	2407	2600	2666	2615	2671
	Middle	1848	1988	2199	2177	2290	2357	2305	2362
	Low	1538	1678	1890	1867	1980	2047	1995	2052
Shuttle run (s)	High	13.0	11.8	11.6	11.4	10.9	10.7	10.5	10.3
	Middle	14.1	13.0	12.7	12.5	12.1	11.9	11.6	11.5
	Low	15.3	14.1	13.9	13.7	13.2	13.0	12.8	12.6
Standing long jump (cm)	High	163	171	187	193	199	205	216	238
	Middle	141	149	165	171	177	183	194	216
	Low	119	126	143	149	154	161	172	177
Medicine ball throw (m)	High	3.6	4.0	4.4	5.0	5.5	6.0	6.7	7.1
	Middle	2.8	3.2	3.6	4.2	4.7	5.2	5.9	6.3
	Low	2.0	2.4	2.8	3.4	3.9	4.4	5.1	5.5

Psychological abilities

Psychological abilities are also important prerequisites for the achievement of top level sports performances. Among these, the personality characteristics, namely emotional stability, are of prime importance. Emotional stability combined with a low anxiety level contribute substantially to a good tolerance of a high level of training. Of a similar importance, is a low level of neuroticism which increases frustration tolerance and decreases the risk of overtraining, and in this way guarantees a more stable sports efficiency.

The next most important factor represents a need for some achievement, or an ambition to excel in a competitive situation. A motivation for the particular sport, coming from an internal need and subjective interest, is necessary to cope with long term and often monotonous training and to prevent premature burnout. Sensomotoric abilities are important in the learning of motor skills.

Intellectual abilities are a prerequisite for fast and correct interpretation of information, decision making, and to make original solutions in new situations; these also contribute to a good sports performance. Social skills, influencing social relationships in a team or group of athletes, should also be taken into account.

From the above mentioned psychological abilities, those which should preferably be tested when assessing potential talent are: emotional stability, motivation for the particular sports discipline and intellectual capabilities.

Conclusion

Talent identification and the selection of future athletes in their childhood is a very complex problem. There are many factors involved which are not yet well known. The physician plays a very important role in this procedure, because he or she has at their disposal enough knowledge and experience concerning the health and physique (including the prediction of adult stature) of the child to measure some important functional values, e.g. $\dot{V}_{O_2 \, max}$. The physician's duty to protect the health of the child should also be carefully applied in this procedure. In this way, risks of later health damage can be minimized and a stable sports efficiency guaranteed.

References

Čermák, V. (1983) Health aspects in selection of young athletes for centers of elite sports. In I. Havlíček (ed) *Selection and Preparation of Talented Youth in Sports* (in Czech), pp. 47–49. Šport, Bratislava.

Chovanová, E., Bergman, P. & Štukovský, R. (1982) Genetic aspects of somatotypes in twins. *Anthropos* **22**, 5.

Havlíček, I. (1982) *Scientific Base of Sports Training in Youth* (in Slovak). Šport, Bratislava.

Klissouras, V. (1971) Heritability of adaptive variation. *J. Appl. Physiol.* **31**, 338.

Komadel, L., Hamar, D., Nápravník, Č. & Tintěra, J. (1985a) *Sports Medicine* (in Slovak). Slovenské pedagogické nakladatel'stvo, Bratislava.

Komadel, L., Hamar, D. & Marček, T. (1985b) *Assessment of the Training State* (in Slovak). Šport, Bratislava.

Seliger, V., Máček, M., Škranc, O., Pirič, J., Handzo, P., Horák, J., Rouš, J. & Jirka, Z. (1975) *Methods and Results of Examination of the Physical Fitness of the Population* (in Czech). Charles University, Prague.

Šemetka, M. (1982) Physical development and motor efficiency of 7 to 14 year old Slovak population (in Slovak). *Tréner* **26**, 1.

Shephard, R. (1980) *The Fit Athlete*. Oxford University Press, Oxford.

Šimková, N., Havlíček, I. & Ramacsay, L. (1982) Prediction of some anthropological data with use of correlation and regression analysis. *Anthropos* **22**, 65.

Taylor, H. L. & Rowell, L. B. (1974) Exercise and metabolism. In W. R. Johnson & E. R. Buskirk (eds) *Science and Medicine of Exercise and Sport*, 2nd edn. Harper & Row, New York.

7.3 Somatic development in children (aged 7 to 18 years)

W. CRASSELT

Introduction

In this chapter, average courses of development of bodily structure are presented which were obtained in a 12-year longitudinal study on the development of physique and sports performance of students between the ages of 7 and 18 years (Crasselt *et al.*, 1985). This investigation was started with more than 5700 girls and boys, and 1000 children at the age of 9 years were added later. The outlined results represent the essence of basic knowledge on the laws of somatic development in the selected age group.

Growth of body height and bodyweight

Body height The average growth in body height (Fig. 7.3.1) illustrates that girls and boys show similar values between the seventh and 13th year of age. The largest difference in the mean values of this age group (1.6 cm) are observed at the age of 12 years 2 months. After this period, body height growth of girls increasingly stays behind that of boys. The average total body height growth at school age from 7 to 18 years is 40.6 cm for girls and 53.1 cm for boys.

The growth dynamics are illustrated by the annual body height growth (Fig. 7.3.1). Between the seventh and ninth year of age, there is almost no difference in the annual growth rates of both sexes. The regression of annual body height growth beginning at preschool age lasts until this age. In the following years, growth in both sexes is accelerated again, even more for girls than for boys. At the age of 11 to 12 years, girls reach the strongest school-age body height growth with 6.5 cm. This growth corresponds to the pubertal growth explosion which often begins 1.5 years before the menarche (cf. Scholz, 1957). If the menarche is assumed to occur at an average age of 12 years (and 3

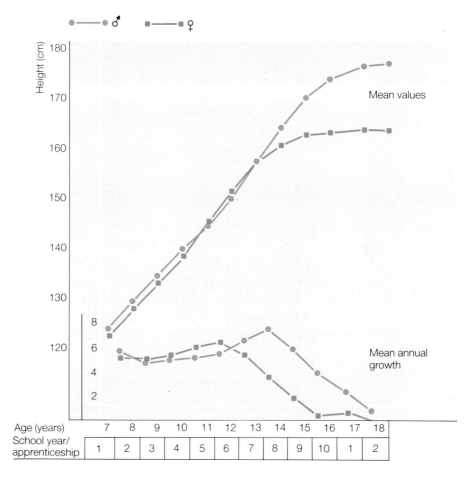

Fig. 7.3.1 Body height (girls and boys), 7 to 18 years, mean values and mean annual growth.

months), the investigation reveals the beginning of the pubertal growth explosion to be situated about 3 years before menarche. However, it must be remembered that puberty is characterized by considerable individual differences in biological age among children of the same chronological age. The growth increase in those aged 9 and 10 years is certainly due to premature development.

At the age of 13, the absolute body height growth in girls is reduced by 1 cm as compared with the previous year. Here begins the girls' body height growth regression which becomes even stronger in subsequent years. At the age of 16, the average growth is reduced to only a few millimetres. In the 17th and 18th years, an average body height growth is no longer found. When observing the individual body height development, it was found that a certain proportion of the girls do not grow in height any more after the 14th year of age.

In boys, the annual growth rates between 9 and 12 years are only half of those of the girls. At the age of 13, where the girls' body height growth

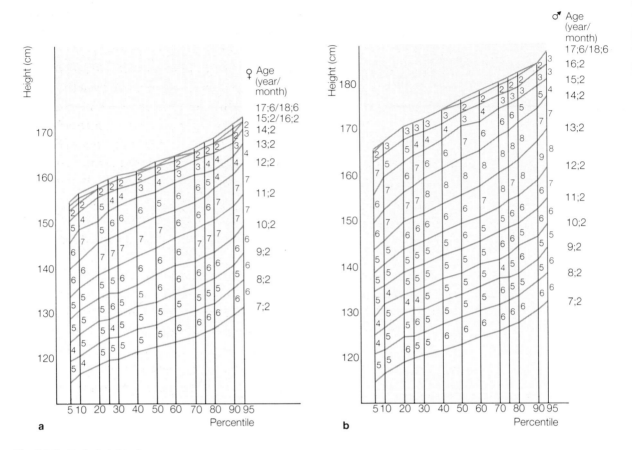

Fig. 7.3.2 Body height of girls (a) and boys (b), percentile values, 7 to 18 years (longitudinal section 1968 to 1979).

is already in regression, the boys grow quickly. Two years later, the boys do not reach the growth rates of the previous year. Their growth regression is then parallel to the girls.

The differences in growth dynamics lead to the well-known phenomenon that, in a certain period of school age, the girls are on the average taller than the boys. At present, this period is delimited from 10 years 6 months to 13 years 4 months. The percentile values account for the growth dynamics studies within the variation of single age classes.

In Fig. 7.3.2, the abscissa represents the percentiles and the ordinate the body height scale. The body heights obtained in the single percentiles of one age class are connected by a line. The overlaying lines characterize the body height development in the subsequent years of study. The 'ribbons' limited by lines account for the annual average body height growth in the single percentiles. This growth is also indicated in figures (cm) on the diagram.

The existence of periods of higher and lower growth rates for all percentile areas is obvious. Furthermore, we find that the 'ribbons' have a different range. This means that the upper, medium, and lower percentile areas have partly different body height growths.

In the eighth year, girls whose body height is situated above the percentile 50, show a somewhat greater body height growth. In the following year, the annual growth within the variation is mostly balanced. Thereafter, a stronger body height growth of the upper percentile areas at the age of 10 years and especially 11 years occurs. One year later, the strongest growth has shifted to the medium position. At the age of 13 and 14 years, the growth in the lower percentiles prevails. Between the average age of 14 years 2 months and 15 years 2 months, the body height growth within the whole variation is still 2 cm. Thereafter, the differences between the single lines are so small that they cannot be unambiguously distinguished any more.

The total growth in the single percentiles from 7 to 18 years ranges from 40 to 42 cm with absolute body height differences of 20 cm at the age of 18 years (P5 153.5 cm, P95 173.5 cm). This means that the total growth during school time is nearly balanced, although the annual growth of the single percentiles is different. The absolute body height differences when coming into school are only slightly exaggerated, if at all, by the approximately equal growth rates during the school period.

Boys show a growth rhythm similar to that of the girls. From age 7 to 10 years, the annual body height growth within the range of variation is almost equal. In the subsequent age period up to 13 years, the body height growth of the tallest boys shows a stronger increase. After the 13th year of age, it is first the boys with medium, later with smallest, body heights who show the strongest increase. From the 17th year onwards, growth cannot be observed in all the percentile areas any more.

The total growth in these 12 years increases from P5 to P50 from 50 to 55 cm. Hence, the absolute body height difference between P5 and P95 increases from 18 cm at the age of 7 years to 22 cm at the age of 18 years. Prior to the pubertal length explosion (in those aged 11), the body height difference increases to 22 cm, so that the body height growth after the 11th year in the single percentile areas takes a different course with regard to time, but finds a balance by the 19th year of age.

Bodyweight The development of bodyweight is presented in Fig. 7.3.3. From the seventh to the tenth year of age, the girls' and boys' bodyweight mean increases almost to the same extent. As a rule, the girls' values are somewhat lower than those of the boys. At the age of 11, the girls' bodyweight increases more than the boys. At the age of 12 to 13 years, there is a difference of 2 kg between the sexes on average, but at the end of the 14th year, the boys have caught up with the girls. This means that by mid school age, the girls exceed the boys not only in terms of average body height, but also average bodyweight. For the latter, the boys reach the girls' values almost 1 year after they catch up with body height. After the 14th year, there is a stronger divergence of bodyweight means between the sexes. The average total bodyweight increase from the seventh to the 18th year of age is 33.5 kg for girls, and 43.8 kg for boys.

Figure 7.3.3 also shows the annual bodyweight increase of both sexes. Although the body height growth declines as compared with the previous year at the age of 9 years, the bodyweight increase rises for girls and boys. The differences in the bodyweight development of both sexes become obvious from the 11th year onwards. While the girls show an almost linear body height growth increase in the tenth to 12th year, the bodyweight increase rises faster at the age of 11, and remains consistent for approximately 2 years, i.e. 1 year longer than the greatest body height growth. After the 14th year, the annual bodyweight increase declines

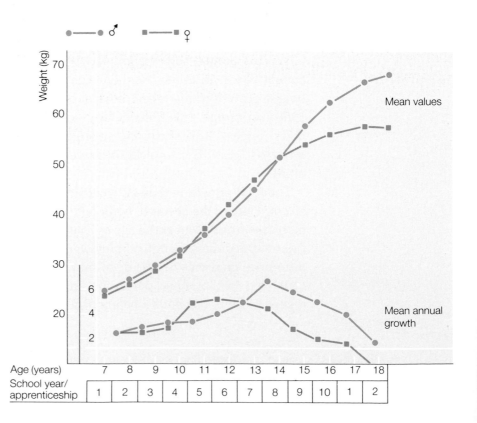

Fig. 7.3.3 Bodyweight (girls and boys), 7 to 18 years, mean values and mean annual growth.

quickly. Boys show a stronger relationship between bodyweight increase and body height growth. The 14th year shows a particular increase in both; thereafter, the decline of the annual body height growth is accompanied by a declining bodyweight increase.

The annual bodyweight development in the single percentiles shows a similar pattern to that of body height. With growing age, the greatest bodyweight increase for girls and boys shifts from the upper to the lower percentiles—although not as significantly as for body height. The total bodyweight increase is much stronger in the upper percentiles than in the lower ones (contrary to body height development), so that a too large bodyweight development in some young people may be deduced.

Growth of the body and extremities

Sitting height The average development course of sitting height for both sexes is presented in Fig. 7.3.4a. Up to the 11th year of age, the girls' sitting height is less than that of the boys. Simultaneously with body height (10 years 6 months), they reach the boys' mean sitting height and show higher values up to an average age of 14 years 2 months. Thereafter, the girls' values remain below that of the boys, and the difference between the sexes increases up to the 18th year of age.

The annual sitting height growth (Fig. 7.3.4b) shows even more distinct sex-specific development courses. Until the ninth year, the growth declines slightly for both sexes. In the following 2 years, the girls' sitting height growth increases rapidly and reaches an annual growth of

Fig. 7.3.4 (a) Sitting height (girls and boys), mean values, 7 to 18 years. (b) Mean annual growth.

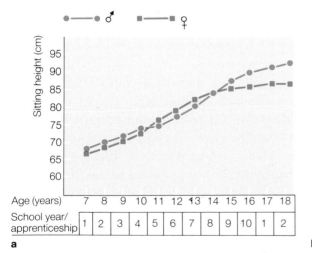

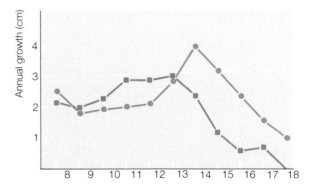

a   b

up to 3 cm between the 11th and 13th year of age. Hence, the greater body growth lasts 1 year longer than the spurt in the growth of the whole body (standing height). After the 13th year, the annual growth declines and comes to an end at the age of 17 years.

The boys' annual growth between 10 and 12 years is somewhat smaller than that of the girls. In the 13th and 14th years, the boys' sitting height growth increases strongly, and afterwards declines parallel to the decline of the total body height growth, without having come to an end at the age of 18 years. The girls' total sitting height growth during school age is 20.0 cm on average.

This average growth is true not only when the mean values are compared, but also for the different percentiles of the whole range of variation.

The boys' sitting height growth from the seventh to the 18th year of age is 25.4 cm. This is not the end of the growing process. The mean total growth does not apply to all areas of the range of variation (contrary to girls), but only to the percentiles 20 to 60. Below P20, the growth is below average, above P60 it is higher. The question whether this is an expression of sex-specific differences, or of the growing process not yet being completed, can only be answered ambiguously. The latter is supported by the finding that in the upper areas of the range of variation the growth occurs earlier, but that it lasts longer in the lower areas. If this is assumed to be true, the same sitting height growth as the girls could be found within the whole range of variation after the completion of the trunk growth.

Leg length

Figure 7.3.5a shows the leg length* man value course. Similar to the sitting height situation, the girls' values are somewhat below those of the boys up to the 11th year of age. Thereafter, they reach the boys' values for 1 year on average. Contrary to sitting height, a significant overtaking of the boys' values cannot be observed.

In the following years, the girls' leg growth declines rapidly. This confirms the statement that the girls' higher body height values in mid school age are primarily the result of an increased growth of the trunk. The total growth between the seventh and 18th years is 20.6 cm for girls and 27.9 cm for boys. Hence, the girls have on average the same sitting height and leg length growth. The boys have a somewhat greater leg length growth rate.

The average annual growth (Fig. 7.3.5b) suggests further conclusions. After minor annual growth deviations (max. 5 mm) at earlier and mid school age, the girls' leg length growth declines in the 13th year of age

* Leg length is calculated from the difference of the body's standing height and sitting height. Hence, it will be a little below the leg length calculated according to the Martin method.

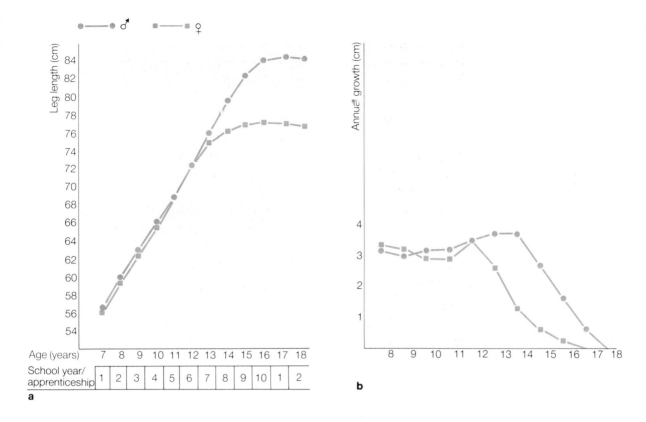

Fig. 7.3.5 (a) Leg length (girls and boys), mean values, 7 to 18 years. (b) Mean annual growth.

and on average comes to an end 1 year before sitting height does. The boys' annual growth deviations, from the seventh to the 14th year, are also relatively small (8 mm). Their increased leg length growth lasts 2 years longer than that of the girls. As found with sitting height, the final values are reached relatively early (by the end of the 18th year).

Upper arm length

Figure 7.3.6a shows the annual upper arm length* mean values for both sexes. From 7 to 13 years, the girls' and boys' values show only minor differences (max. 3.1 mm). However, while the girls have lower average values from 7 to 11 years, they have higher values in the subsequent period up to 13 years 2 months. Hence, the development lines of both sexes will overlap, as is found in sitting height, and contrary to the leg length values. In the following years, the girls' growth rapidly declines. The intersexual differences of the values increase up to the 18th year of age.

The annual growth declines slightly between the seventh and tenth years (Fig. 7.3.6b). In the following 2 years (girls) and 3 years (boys), growth increases and then strongly declines. By the age of 17–18 years, the upper arm growth is almost completed. In the case of upper arm

* Upper arm length was taken to be the distance between the outer upper edge of the shoulder cave (acromion) and the ulnar process (olecranon) when the arm is flexed.

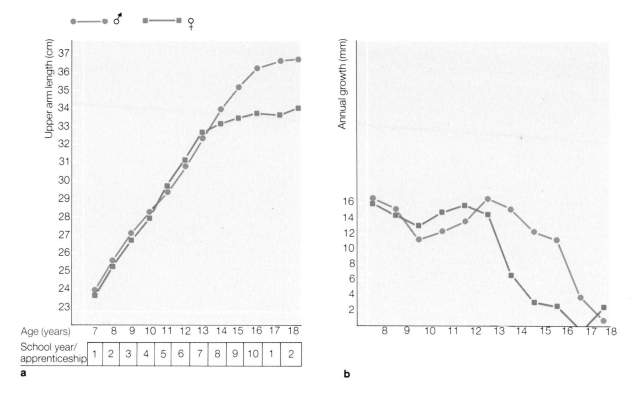

Fig. 7.3.6 (a) Upper arm length (girls and boys), mean values, 7 to 18 years. (b) Mean annual growth.

length, the mean value growth during total school age (girls, 10.3 cm; boys, 12.8 cm) is also realized by the mean value growth of single percentile ranges.

Forearm length   The mean forearm length* growth is illustrated in Fig. 7.3.7a. At early school age, girls have, on average, shorter forearms than boys. At the age of 12 years 2 months, girls reach the boys' mean values. One year later, however, the girls' mean value is again below that of the boys. From the 15th year onwards, scarcely any growth is found. In boys, forearm growth continues until the 18th year of age. The annual average growth (Fig. 7.3.7b) reveals significant differences in the course of upper arm and forearm length growth.

While for upper arm growth, the annual increase declines up to the age of 10 years, the girls' forearm length growth rises until the age of 12, and then declines until the end of the growing process, in a similar way to upper arm length. The boys' forearm length shows an annual growth of 8–9 mm until the age of 11 years. Thereafter, the growth increases and reaches its maximum 1 year later than upper arm length. At the age of 18 years, the average growth is completed in both sexes.

* Forearm length is obtained from the distance from the hind part of the olecranon to the fore-edge of the ulna's styloid process (processus styloideus ulnae) with the arm flexed.

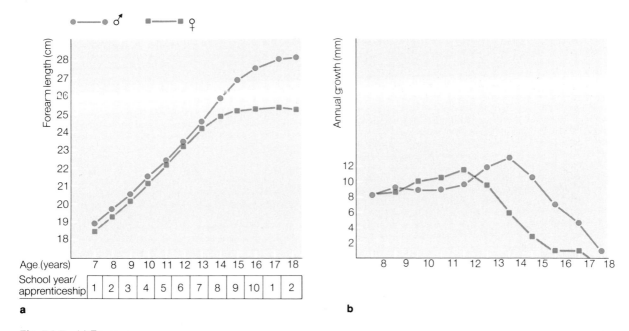

Fig. 7.3.7 (a) Forearm length (girls and boys), mean values, 7 to 18 years. (b) Mean annual growth.

Growth of the trunk and extremities

Shoulder breadth (biacromial breadth)

Figure 7.3.8a shows the mean values for the ages 8 to 18 years. Up to the age of 9, the growth in both sexes is parallel, the girls' values being somewhat lower. Thereafter, the girls' growth is stronger, and from age 12 to 14 years, they show a wider average distance between the acromia than boys do. While the girls' breadth growth starts slowing down at the age of 13 and comes to an end by the age of 17, the boys initially have greater growth rates (Fig. 7.3.8b). The greatest annual growth occurs in the 12th year for girls, and in the 14th to 15th years for boys. The total growth for girls is 80.1 mm, for boys 113.4 mm. Hence, the intersexual shoulder breadth difference increases from an average of 3.5 mm at the age of 9 years to 37.3 mm at the age of 19 years.

Pelvic ridge breadth (bicristal breadth)

The development of the mean pelvic ridge breadth (Fig. 7.3.9a) is relatively greater in girls than in boys at school age. In the first school years, the girls' average values are still below those of the boys, but already by the age of 9 years, girls start a stronger growth than boys. At the age of 10 (approximately 1 year before shoulder breadth and sitting height), they catch up with the boys and show higher average values until the age of 16, contrary to shoulder breadth and sitting height, where by the age of 14, the boys' values are above those of the girls.

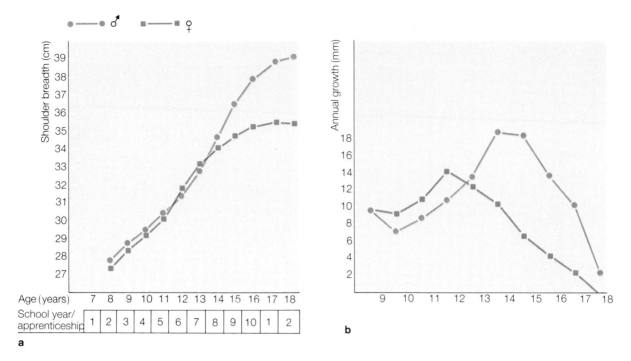

Fig. 7.3.8 (a) Shoulder breadth (girls and boys), mean values, 7 to 18 years. (b) Mean annual growth.

The range of the mean total growth from age 7 to 18 years (Fig. 7.3.9b) is less significant for both sexes (girls, 74.4 mm; boys, 77.8 mm) than those of other anthropometric properties. Up the age of 12 years, the girls' and boys' development tendencies are similar with regard to annual growth, although at different levels. Girls reach their strongest growth at the age of 12, boys at the age of 15. The girls' annual growth deviations after the 13th year cannot yet be interpreted and explained. They may be caused by more or less overlying subcutaneous fat tissue, which affects the accuracy of measurements (growth deviations below 2 mm).

Bicondylar breadth of the right upper arm This breadth parameter indicates the differences in skeleton sturdiness. Contrary to the trunk breadth measurements, the average elbow joint breadth development shows a mostly parallel course in both sexes until the 12th year of age (Fig. 7.3.10a). This breadth growth is only reduced with the regression of the annual body height growth.

Since the bicondylar breadth of the girls' upper arms does not react to the increased upper arm growth after the tenth year with a corresponding growth, the girls have relatively more gracile upper arm bones after puberty (Fig. 7.3.10b). Total growth, too, is rather different in both sexes during school age. For girls, it is only 60% of the boys' growth; while the total upper arm length growth is some 80% of that of the boys. The

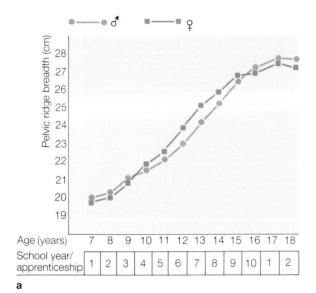

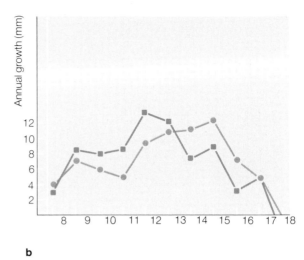

b

Fig. 7.3.9 Pelvic ridge breadth (girls and boys), mean values, 7 to 18 years. (b) Mean annual growth.

average ratio (%) of bicondylar breadth and upper arm length (mean values) changes at school age as indicated:

Girls: 21.0% at 7 years; 18.5% at 18 years.
Boys: 21.5% at 7 years; 19.8% at 18 years.

Bicondylar breadth of the right thigh

Girls' and boys' bicondylar breadth parameters were included in the investigations only from the age of 8 years. Figure 7.3.11a shows the course of development up to the age of 18 years. Both sexes show parallel development between the ages of 8 and 12. The girls' breadth values are somewhat lower than those of the boys. Average growth in boys lasts up to 15 years, and growth appears to be completed by the age of 17; girls, however, reach the average values of those aged 18 years by the age of 13 (Fig. 7.3.11b).

The average ratio (%) of thigh bicondylar breadth and lower leg length (mean values) shows the following changes:

Girls: 19.7% at 8 years; 18.2% at 18 years.
Boys: 20.6% at 8 years; 18.3% at 18 years.

The differences existing between both sexes at the age of 8 are equalized in the course of growth until the 18th year of age.

Conclusion

The description of the courses of development of a large number of anthropometric parameters suggests some general features of physical development. The observation of a sample group of the same age

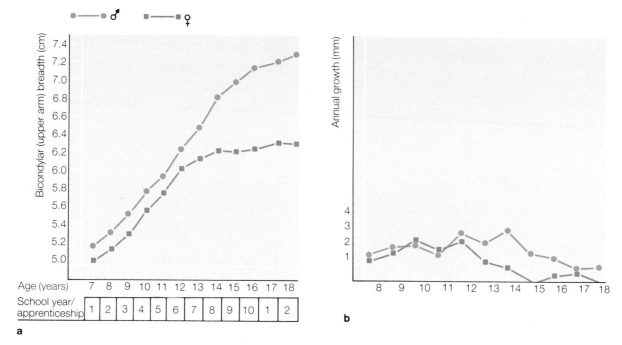

Fig. 7.3.10 (a) Upper arm bicondylar breadth (girls and boys), mean values, 7 to 18 years. (b) Mean annual growth.

throughout the whole school period appears to be appropriate. The complete perfection of physical and mental development of the human being is located in this age period. Three stages may be distinguished in terms of the development of sex-specific features.

The *first stage* occurs between the ages of 7 and 9 years. Here, physical development of girls and boys are parallel to a great extent. The differences in the distinctness of anthropometric parameters (average) are small. In a comparison of the mean values, the girls are situated somewhat below the boys. In this period, the regression in annual body height growth which had already begun at preschool age continues. The annual body-weight increase, which is rising somewhat in this period, indicates an increase in the breadth and size parameters.

The *second stage* comprises the period between the ages of 10 and 13 years. It is characterized by increased growth of the girls (pubertal growth explosion). Increased annual growth is observed for body height (particularly sitting height), bodyweight, and especially for the trunk breadth parameters. The greater limb length growth begins later than that of trunk development. Breadth values of the upper and lower extremities and foot length, however, do not show increased growth. Hence, the girls have developed distinct sex-specific proportions by the age of 13. Thus, the ratio between trunk and limbs, between arm and leg length and breadth, has changed.

At the end of this stage, the girls have—as compared with the previous

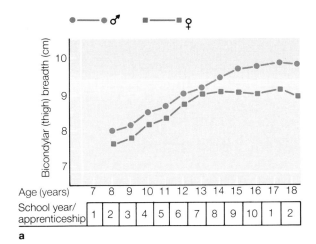

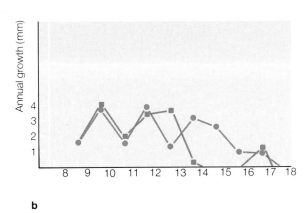

Fig. 7.3.11 (a) Thigh bicondylar breadth (girls and boys), mean values, 7 to 18 years. (b) Mean annual growth.

stage—a relatively bigger trunk, a more slender skeleton, and relatively smaller hands and feet. While at the age of 13, the girls' annual average body height growth declines, increased pubertal growth begins for the boys. Despite the sex-specific development in this period, anthropometric differences between both sexes are still relatively small.

During the *third stage* (ages 14 to 18 years), the girls' annual growth continuously declines and stops during the second half. A certain number reach the parameters characteristic for adult age by the age of 14 years.

For the boys, the pubertal growth explosion has full impact on physical development. From the 16th year of age onwards, the annual average growth rates of the boys, too, are declining. During this stage, however, the process of growth is not yet completed. A divergence in physical development of girls and boys in this period leads to major sex-specific differences which continue through adult life.

References

Crasselt, W., Forchel, I. & Stemmler, R. (1985) *Zur körperlichen Entwicklung der Schuljugend in der Deutschen Demokratischen Republik*. Barth, Leipzig.

Scholz, E. (1957) Das individuelle Sollwachstum von Körpergewicht und Körperlänge im Kleinkind- und Schulalter. *Z. Kinderheilkd*. **79**, 94.

Further reading

Crasselt, W. (1976) Zur körperlichen Entwicklung unserer Schuljugend. *Wiss. Z. Dtsch. Hochsch. Körperkult* **17(2)**, 29.

Hebbelinck, M. & Borms, J. (1978) *Körperliches Wachstum und Leistungsfähigkeit bei Schulkindern*. Barth, Leipzig.

Martin, R. & Saller, K. (1959) *Lehrbuch der Anthropologie*, Vols I & II. Aufl. Fischer, Stuttgart.

Stemmler, R. & Crasselt, W. (1975) Zu differentiellen Erscheinungen von Körperhöhe und Körpergewicht unserer gegenwärtigen Schülerpopulation. *Ärztl. Jugendkd*. **66(2)**, 144.

Tittel, K. & Wutscherk, H. (1972) *Sportanthropometrie*. Barth, Leipzig.

Van Gerven, D. P. & Van Beŭnen, G. (1972) Studie over de physical fitness bij schoolgaande jongens van 12-tot 19-jarige leeftijd. *Hermes* **6(3)**, 151.

7.4 Age and general development

M. MÁČEK

Development of abilities for performance

Endurance   Few studies can be found which deal with the adaptation of young people to prolonged muscular exercise, with the accompanying metabolic and hormonal changes. Prolonged continuous exercise is atypical for children and adolescents, but it is often used in some training methods for some sports.

Endurance, as one of the main abilities needed for exercise, is developed with increasing aerobic fitness in the pubertal and adolescent age groups. In prepubertal children, endurance training programmes improve the running performance without a concomitant increase in maximal oxygen uptake (Bar-Or, 1983; Rowland, 1985). In our study (Máček et al., 1976), ten healthy, prepubertal boys with an average maximal oxygen uptake of 54.1 ml (s.d. 5.4 ml) and without special endurance training, exercised on treadmills and cycle ergometers for 60 min, at 40 and 60% of their $\dot{V}_{O_2 max}$. The heart rate increase was lower in boys than that expected in adults, and the blood lactate increase was negligible in the initial phase of exercise with a subsequent removal from the blood during exercise (Fig. 7.4.1). The changes in oxygen uptake during 60 min of exercise were not statistically significant. No biological handicap could be found for endurance exercise in this group of untrained boys. Similar results were obtained for girls (Máček et al., 1984).

The lack of improvement in aerobic power in endurance training in children could be explained by the high initial values of $\dot{V}_{O_2 max}$ generally observed in this age group. Improvement with endurance training is inversely related to level of aerobic fitness at the onset of the training programme (American College of Sports Medicine, 1978).

Prolonged muscular exercise raises the plasma protein concentration in adults, while haemoconcentration occurs with a decrease of plasma volume (Novosadová, 1977). Our findings in boys under a corresponding relative load, did not reveal any shift of water from the vascular system, on the contrary, a slight haemodilution occurred suggesting that children have a good water balance. This probably contributes to the good physical fitness level of boys (Máček et al., 1976).

300

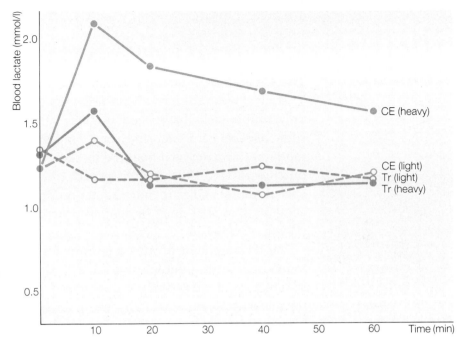

Fig. 7.4.1 Blood lactate levels during prolonged exercise in prepubertal boys. Cycle ergometer (CE)—light exercise at 40% $\dot{V}_{O_2\,max}$, and heavy exercise at 60% $\dot{V}_{O_2\,max}$. Treadmill (Tr)—light exercise at 40% $\dot{V}_{O_2\,max}$, and heavy exercise at 60% $\dot{V}_{O_2\,max}$.

These results indicate that the ability for endurance is present in the prepubertal period, but that it is not possible to recommend specializd endurance training as being beneficial for children. The development, especially of the skeletal and connective system, could be damaged by this type of training for many years.

However, the preference shown by chidren for short-term exercise probably lies in the psychological sphere, as prolonged exercise is regarded as monotonous and motivation is therefore low.

Strength and power Muscle strength increases during the growing period in proportion to the square of the height. This increase is steeper in boys of approximately 13 years, than it is in girls of the same age. Ikai et al. (1967) found that muscular strength and strength endurance increased more in children than in adults for the same relative intensity and frequency of training. These results may be attributed to a larger increase of vascularization and resultant greater muscle blood flow in 13-year-old children. Asmussen (1973) concluded that both fast and slow fibres are susceptible to training stimuli, especially during the growing period.

Isometric strength, as well as being related to size, also varies with sex and age. The sex difference is less pronounced before puberty, but afterwards boys become increasingly stronger especially in the upper extremity in relation to size, whereas girls tend to level off (Asmussen, 1973).

Coordination and balance

The application of strength to various sports activities demands skill. There is a lack of information on the development of skill in children; only simple tasks have been studied, such as jumping, running and some aspects of prehension. In a prepubertal age group the general motor performance is influenced by skeletal maturation, but no distinct differences were found with respect to chronological age. However, specific motor skills are more influenced by chronological age, and this suggests that skill must be seen as a neuromuscular learning process (Vrijens & Van Canter, 1985).

The development of motor performance follows different paths in individuals with different physical activity habits. Generally, it can be said that regular physical training in prepubertal age groups speeds up the rate of development of physical abilities, including coordination and balance (Mészáros et al., 1986). The development is more closely related to the skeletal age than to the chronological age in trained and untrained groups, with no significant changes during puberty. There are important interrelationships in the development of motor performance, between: (a) static strength and aerobic power; (b) aerobic power and basic skills; and (c) general coordination abilities and motor performance. High levels of habitual activity or supervised sports training correlate significantly with strength, aerobic power, basic skills and general coordination. Individual differences in these abilities are strongly related to a lack of physical activity (Schmücker et al., 1984).

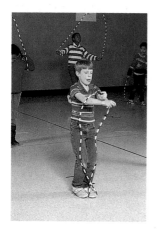

Fig. 7.4.2 It is generally held that development of coordination and balance can be enhanced by organized programmes of physical activity for prepubertal boys and girls. Courtesy of Human Kinetics Publishers.

Flexibility

There is a lack of information on the development of flexibility during childhood. It is known, however, that flexibility is greater during pre-school age and puberty. Flexibility is often confused with hypermobility. Flexibility means the movements over the physiological range of the joints, which could be a predisposition for further pathological development of the skeletal system. Hypermobility as an irreversible prepathological condition, which may cause ischaemic and degenerative changes of the tendons, ligaments and joint capsules, which develop several years after finishing sports activity.

Hypermobility is more frequently found in children engaged in sports, because these children, who have the ability to move over the physiological range of the joints, are welcomed by trainers especially in gymnastics, figure skating, swimming, etc. (Máčková et al., 1985).

Sports activities in the life-style of children and adolescents

Childhood is characterized by a high need for physical activity, which is realized above all by habitual activity. The hypothesis has been proposed that physical activity in childhood determines the level of activity in later life in the same way as eating habits and other factors of life-style. Habitual activity, spontaneous movement activity, or daily physical activity depends on external conditions, inherent abilities and the health or illness of the child. An example of the physiological responses of a child to non-supervised activity during the course of a day is presented in Fig. 7.4.3, where the heart rate of a 4-year-old girl was followed for 11 h.

While habitual activity is predominant in pre-school and early school age, organized activity in the form of class gymnastics or sports training increases after 10 years of age. It is important for the optimal development of every child to maintain a sufficient level of habitual activity; the form, intensity and duration is subconsciously determined by the child itself. The intensity of this kind of activity is mostly higher than in supervised activity and is more necessary for the physiological needs of the growing child.

The child prefers, in play and activity, intermittent exercise with short periods of exercise and short periods of recovery (Máček et al., 1971). The duration of these periods is not longer than 1 min. The high-energy-containing phosphate compounds serve as energy fuels and are completely regenerated during the recovery periods. The accumulation of blood lactate does not occur in this type of activity.

Regular physical training has many beneficial effects on the health and

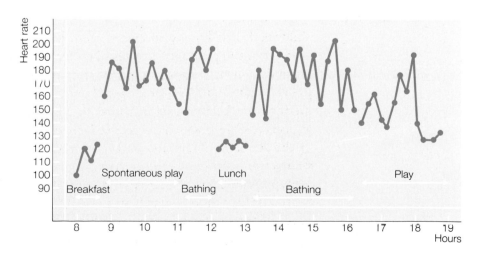

Fig. 7.4.3 A 12 h heart rate recording of a 4-year-old girl during non-supervised activity, each data point represents the mean heart rate for a 10 min interval.

development of the child (Thorén *et al.*, 1973). The important principle to base regular physical training in childhood on is the stimulation and development of all organs and systems by training of a wide variety of functions, such as aerobic and anaerobic, power, strength, endurance and coordination. To train selectively or predominantly one function only, for example stength or endurance, may be inappropriate and harmful during the first years of a sports career. However, the child has an excellent motivation feedback system, so that when the training programme reaches the level of his or her tolerance, the child loses the interest to continue. This system disappears with growth and at the age of adolescence overloading has already become possible (Máček, 1980).

It is very difficult to find any exact statement concerning the age when it is proper to start sports training and competition in various kinds of sports. An attempt has been made in Table 7.4.1, which gives a guide to the optimal ages for the introduction of sports training and competition for different sports. When it is started, however, it is important to maintain the stimulation and development of all systems, and monotonous one-sided training must be avoided. Some organ systems in particular may be damaged by a one-sided training programme. The predominant use of strength techniques and isometric contractions may negatively influence the further development of the skeletal and connective tissue systems. For instance, premature ossification of the epiphysis may occur. The development of the joints and capsular ligaments may be impaired by repeated application of movement over the maximum possible joint range. Examples can be found in gymnastics, figure skating and various ball games. Repeated falls and jumps on hard

Table 7.4.1 Guide to the optimal ages for the beginning of sports training and competition in different sports.

	Age (years)		Age (years)
Athletics (track and field)	11	Rugby	10
Hockey	10	Rowing	10
Basketball	13	Skiing	11
Boxing	15	Swimming	8
Canoeing	11	Table tennis	8
Cycling	14	Tennis	10
Football (soccer)	10	Volleyball	11
Gymnastics	9	Water polo	12
Handball	11	Weight lifting	15
Ice hockey	10	Wrestling	12

surfaces may evoke disturbances of the spinal column such as aseptic necrosis.

Training during childhood and adolescence may result in a high occurrence and accumulation of microtrauma. Myositis ossificans and arthrotic degeneration may follow in later years, if even minor injuries of the muscles, joints and connective tissue are not properly treated.

Another important principle of care in children and adolescents participating in sports training is regular medical supervision. The first task is to identify all children whose health is not perfect. Children with chronic diseases and development disturbances, especially in the skeletal system, may participate in physical recreation but competitive sport should be only permitted for healthy children. This is why the limitation of the intensity of training due to problems of the respiratory, circulatory and other systems is very rare. The growing body displays excellent general adaptability to physical training. Apart from the precaution in respect of the growing skeletal system, the only other important limitation derives from the level of development and maturity of the central nervous system.

Overloading is not very frequent in childhood but it can be found more often in adolescents. Some of the symptoms differ from those in adults. Fatigue, anorexia, and loss of interest are the first to be noted.

Conclusion

The experience of recent years, summarized here, demonstrates that any training programme for a child under the age of 10 years must be directed to the improvement of neuromuscular coordination and to a slight gradual increase of aerobic and anaerobic power. At the age of 12–14 years a successive increase in the endurance component can be added. Strength training presupposes sexual maturity and increased muscle mass. In this type of training respect must be shown to the growing skeletal system.

References

American College of Sports Medicine (1978) Position statement on the recommended quantity and quality of exercise for developing and maintaining fitness in healthy adults. *Med. Sci. Sports Exerc.* **10**, 7.

Asmussen, E. (1973) Growth in muscular strength and power. In: I. Rarick (ed) *Physical Activity*, pp. 60–79. Academic Press, New York.

Bar-Or, O. (1983) *Pediatric Sports Medicine*. Springer, New York.

Ikai, M., Yabe, K. & Ischii, K. (1967) Muskenkraft und muskulare Ermüdung bei willkürlicher Ausspannung und elektrischer Reizung des Muskles. *Sportartz Sportmed.* **18**, 197.

Máček, M. & Vávra, J. (1980) FIMS position statement

on training and competition in children. *J. Sports Med.* **20**, 135.

Máček, M. & Vávra, J. (1981) Prolonged exercise in 14 year old girls. *Int. J. Sports Med.* **2**, 228.

Máček, M., Vávra, J. & Mrzena, B. (1971) Intermittent exercise of supramaximal intensity in children. *Acta Paediatr. Scand.* (Suppl.) **217**, 29.

Máček, M., Vávra, J. & Novosadová, J. (1976) Prolonged exercise in prepubertal boys. *Eur. J. Appl. Physiol.* **35**, 291.

Máčková, J., Javůrek, J., Máček, M. & Vávra, J. (1985) A longitudinal study of the locomotor system in trained children. In R. A. Binghorst, H. C. Kemper & W. H. Saris (eds) *Children and Exercise XI*, pp. 319–322. Human Kinetics, Champaign.

Mészaros, J., Mohácsi, J., Frenkl, R., Szabó, T. & Smodis, J. (1986) In J. Rutenfranz, R. Mocellin & F. Klimt (eds) *Children and Exercise XII*, pp. 347–354. Human Kinetics, Champaign.

Novosadová, J. (1977) The changes in hematocrit, plasma volume and proteins during after different types of exercise. *Eur. J. Appl. Physiol.* **36**, 223.

Rowland, T. W. (1985) Aerobic response to endurance training in prepubescent children. *Med. Sci. Sports Exerc.* **17**, 493.

Schmücker, B., Rigauer, B., Hinrichs, W. & Trawinski, J. (1984) Motor abilities and habitual physical activity in children. In J. Ilmarinen & I. Valimäki (eds) *Children and Sport*, pp. 46–52. Springer, Berlin.

Thorén, C., Seliger, V., Máček, M., Vávra, J. & Rutenfrans, J. (1973) The influence of training on physical fitness in healthy children and children with chronic disease. In S. Linneweh (ed) *Current Aspects of Perinatology and Physiology in Children*. Springer, Berlin.

Vrijens, J. & Van Canter, Ch. (1985) Motor performance as related to somatotype in adolescent boys. In R. A. Binghorst, H. C. Kemper & W. H. Saris (eds) *Children and Exercise XI*. Human Kinetics, Champaign.

PART 8

FEMALE ATHLETES

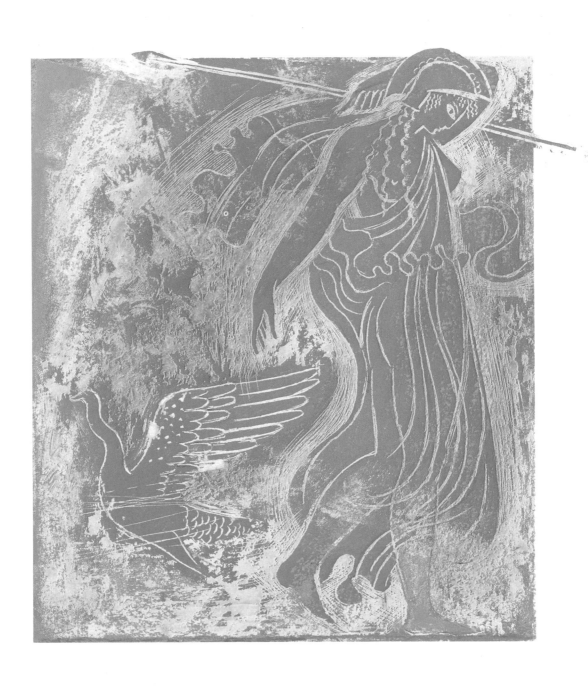

8.1 Training of female athletes

B. DRINKWATER

Introduction

Prior to the early 1970s very few girls and women participated in vigorous competitive sports. Since there were so few female athletes, predictions of women's capacity for endurance-type activities were based on research data obtained from relatively sedentary females. As a result, it was thought that the capacity for strenuous exercise decreased in women after puberty. Rules for many sports reflected this belief and limited the distance women could run, the time they could play, and even the skills they could perform. As the number of female athletes increased, so did the number of studies investigating their physiological response to acute and chronic exercise. The results of this research have forced a re-evaluation of women's potential as athletes and has helped to clarify the role of gender in athletic performance.

Aerobic power

The ability to transport and utilize oxygen is determined more by training and biological potential than by gender. Men and women participating in the same sport will be closer in aerobic power ($\dot{V}_{O_2 \, max}$) than athletes of the same sex in different sports (Table 8.1.1). In Finland's Nordic ski team, for example, men and women had a $\dot{V}_{O_2 \, max}$ of 78.3 and 68.2 (ml/kg)/min respectively (Rusko *et al.*, 1978), while the average values for a male professional basketball team and a woman's collegiate team were 45.8 and 49.6 (ml/kg)/min (Vacarro *et al.*, 1979; Wilmore, 1979). However, in sports where endurance capacity is the primary requisite for success, élite male athletes usually have higher levels of aerobic power than their female counterparts.

The magnitude of the difference depends on how $\dot{V}_{O_2 \, max}$ is expressed, in absolute terms as litres of oxygen per minute or in relative terms by adjusting for differences in body size. When men and women are asked to perform the same work at the same rate, as in some industrial situations, absolute $\dot{V}_{O_2 \, max}$ (l/min) is a meaningful comparison, and the

Table 8.1.1   Aerobic power in (ml/kg)/min of male and female athletes matched for age and sport.

Sport	Female	n	Male	n	References
Nordic skiing	68.2	5	78.3	17	Rusko et al., 1978
Middle-distance running	68.0	4	76.0	7	Ready, 1984
Nordic skiing	61.5	10	73.0	10	Haymes & Dickinson, 1980
Marathon	58.2	9	72.5	13	Davies & Thompson, 1979
Swimming	55.3	11	68.6	12	Holmer et al., 1974
Alpine skiing	52.7	13	66.6	12	Haymes & Dickinson, 1980
Cycling	50.2	7	62.1	22	Burke et al., 1977
Orienteering	46.1	5	61.6	13	Knowlton et al., 1980
Volleyball	50.6	14	56.1	8	Puhl et al., 1982
Speed skating	46.1	13	56.1	10	Maksud et al., 1970
Tennis	44.2	25	50.2	25	Vodak et al., 1980

Reprinted with permission from Drinkwater (1988a). Complete citations can be found in the original article.

male advantage may be as much as 50–60% (Sparling, 1980; Drinkwater, 1984b). However, in most sports the workload is the athlete's bodyweight and $\dot{V}_{O2\ max}$ in (ml/kg)/min is the best measure of sex differences in endurance capacity. Although the difference is much less, the average male value is still 10–25% higher than that of the female. Some of this difference is due to the higher fat content of the female body. When this is removed mathematically by expressing $\dot{V}_{O2\ max}$ relative to lean body mass in (ml/kg)/min, the difference between the sexes ranges from 1 to 10% (Sparling, 1980; Drinkwater, 1984b). Some of this residual difference, which varies from sport to sport, is presumed to represent a basic biological difference between the sexes; the remainder is an actual difference in cardiorespiratory fitness, which may favour one sex or the other, and depends on their training status.

There are several factors that may account for gender differences in the ability to transport and utilize oxygen. The lower haemoglobin levels of women reduce the oxygen-carrying capacity of their blood to about 10% below male levels (Åstrand & Rodahl, 1986). Even though maximal heart rates are the same for males and females, a woman's smaller maximal stroke volume (SV_{max}) results in a lower maximal cardiac output ($\dot{Q}_{max}$) (Wells, 1985). Training diminishes the difference when $\dot{Q}_{max}$ and SV_{max} are related to bodyweight or body surface area (BSA). In reality, there are so few data for élite female athletes describing the dimensions and functional capacity of the cardiovascular system that it is probably premature to cite these variables as basic biological differences once they are normalized for body size. However, there is little doubt that muscle mass, and therefore oxygen utilization, is lower in women. While there

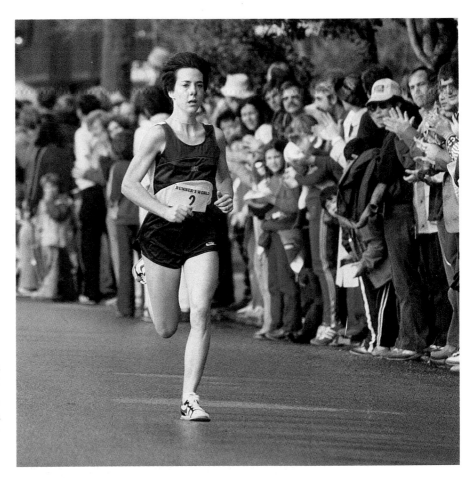

Fig. 8.1.1 A champion woman marathon runner has nearly the same value as a male champion runner for maximal aerobic power when equated for lean body mass but will usually carry a relatively higher proportion of body fat. Courtesy of *Runner's World* magazine. Photo by David Madison.

is general agreement that biological sex differences account for about 5–10% of the male advantage in endurance capacity, it is not yet clear what the respective contribution of each factor may be.

Among female athletes the highest levels of $\dot{V}_{O_2\ max}$ are found in those sports which have a high aerobic component and demand a sustained effort over extended periods of time (Table 8.1.2). To date, the highest $\dot{V}_{O_2\ max}$ reported for a female athlete is 77 (ml/kg)/min; and for a male, 94 (ml/kg)/min. Both of the athletes were Nordic skiers (Åstrand & Rodahl, 1986).

Society's acceptance of women as athletes has encouraged many women to continue active participation in sports beyond their school years. Studies of these masters' athletes show that endurance training is effective in maintaining high levels of aerobic power well into middle age. Female distance runners in their thirties, for example, have a $\dot{V}_{O_2\ max}$ of 56.6 (ml/kg)/min, while young female runners in their twenties average 55.1 (ml/kg)/min (Table 8.1.2).

Table 8.1.2 Physiological responses of female athletes and sedentary women to a maximal exercise stress test. Mean values are presented for selected sports within each age group.

Age (years)	Height (cm)	Weight (kg)	n	$\dot{V}_{O_2\ max}$ ((ml/kg)/min)	HR_{max} (beats/min)	$\dot{V}_{E\ max}$ (l/min)
15–20						
Basketball	173.0	68.3	15	49.6	186	116.9
Runners	163.3	50.7	145	52.6	198	92.8
Swimmers	169.2	60.1	21	51.6	192	121.0
Synchronized swimmers	165.5	54.8	35	43.7	196	92.2
Skiing						
Nordic	165.1	57.2	30	55.5	193	124.8
Alpine	165.1	58.8	13	52.7	198	112.7
Tennis	168.7	58.0	10	48.0	202	101.0
21–30						
Sedentary	164.0	57.9	135	38.7	192	78.3
Cyclers	165.0	55.0	7	50.2	—	—
Lacrosse	164.0	57.4	7	52.9	189	116.9
Orienteers	162.7	58.1	8	51.4	195	99.8
Pentathlon	175.4	65.4	9	45.9	185	106.1
Runners	164.4	52.6	59	55.8	188	101.6
Skaters	175.5	73.9	13	46.1	191	96.5
Swimmers	—	—	10	43.9	179	77.0
Volleyball	177.6	68.9	48	50.0	186	113.9
31–40						
Sedentary	165.2	60.4	136	30.6	183	73.2
Golfers	168.9	61.8	23	34.2	—	—
Runners	165.8	55.2	124	55.9	181	103.4
Swimmers	—	—	10	42.1	178	79.0
Tennis	163.3	55.7	25	44.2	179	82.7
Climbers	167.5	64.7	6	51.9	184	96.4
41–50						
Sedentary	166.0	63.6	117	27.4	180	71.3
Runners	161.5	53.8	10	43.4	177	82.1
Swimmers	—	—	9	38.3	163	74.0
51–60						
Sedentary	165.1	63.6	75	25.6	177	58.6
Swimmers	—	—	7	35.9	163	75.0
61–70						
Sedentary	160.6	61.1	51	25.6	158	55.6
Swimmers	—	—	6	32.1	159	66.0
71–80						
Sedentary	160.9	63.0	67	20.9	136	—
Swimmers	164.2	61.6	2	37.6	162	78.9

Reprinted with permission from Drinkwater (1988b). List of sources can be found in the original article.

Table 8.1.3 Percent improvement in selected maximal and submaximal performance variables for men and women.

Variable	Men	Women	References
$\dot{V}_{O_2\ max}$ ((ml/kg)/min)	15.0	14.2	Eddy *et al.*, 1977
$\dot{V}_{E\ max}$ (l/min)	11.7	11.0	Daniels *et al.*, 1979
Heart volume (ml)	1.3	1.5	Holmgren *et al.*, 1960
Blood volume (l)	6.4	4.9	Holmgren *et al.*, 1960
Strength (lbs)*	20.0	23.0	Wilmore, 1974
Resting heart rate (beats/min)	5.9	~7.9	Holmgren *et al.*, 1960
Submaximal heart rate beats/min	7.4	10.1	Eddy *et al.*, 1977

* Average for curl, leg press and bench press.
Reprinted with permission from Drinkwater (1988a). Complete citations can be found in the original article.

Training The effectiveness of aerobic conditioning programmes is the same for men and women (Table 8.1.3). There are increases in maximal aerobic power, ventilatory volume, oxygen pulse, arterial–venous oxygen difference, and performance time. Maximal heart rate shows little or no change, but increases in maximal stroke volume result in a higher maximal cardiac output.

The functional capacity of the circulatory system is also enhanced by an increase in blood volume and total haemoglobin. Since the increase in plasma is proportionally greater than the increase in red blood cells, both haemoglobin concentration and haematocrit are usually decreased following training. Obviously these decreases should not be interpreted as anaemia, but it is a wise precaution to check young female athletes for iron status prior to the sports season and again if her performance deteriorates for no obvious reason during the season. Women lose approximately 1.5 mg of iron per day, twice as much as men, and frequently fail to meet the recommended daily allowance of 18 mg of iron in their diet (Haymes, 1986). Nutritional counselling rather than oral iron supplements is the best preventive measure unless indicated otherwise by a physician.

The amount of improvement that can be expected in aerobic power depends on the initial fitness level of the women and the characteristics of the training programme. In 28 training studies, those in which women had a $\dot{V}_{O_2\ max}$ above 40 (ml/kg)/min before training reported an increase of 9.1% $\dot{V}_{O_2\ max}$. Women with low levels of fitness initially improved by 19.5% (Table 8.1.4).

For the untrained female, the recommendations of the American College of Sports Medicine (i.e. training 3–5 days a week at 50–85% $V_{O_2\ max}$ or 60–90% HR_{max} for 15–60 min) are as effective as they are for

Table 8.1.4 Effect of training relative to initial fitness level of women, aged 18 to 29 years.

| | Initial fitness level | | | | | | | |
| | <40 (ml O_2/kg)/min | | | | >40 (ml O_2/kg)/min | | | |
	n	Before	After	%	n	Before	After	%
$\dot{V}_{O_2\ max}$ ((ml/kg)/min)	181	35.6	42.5	19.5	105	44.4	48.4	9.1
$\dot{V}_{Emax}$, BTPS (l/min)	146	84.8	92.0	8.5	79	90.0	95.8	6.4
Heart rate (beats/min)	136	192.3	193.1	0.4	74	191.6	189.0	1.3
Weight (kg)	76	59.4	59.4	0	73	58.8	56.2	4.4
Body fat (%)	145	27.1	25.7	5.2	84	22.4	19.3	14.1
Stroke volume (ml)	27	66.0	79.9	21.0				
CaO_2–CvO_2 (ml/l)	27	126.9	132.3	4.2				

Reprinted with permission from Drinkwater (1988b).

males in improving $V_{O_2\ max}$. For the female athlete who starts a sports season with a better than average fitness level, a more intensive programme may be necessary to achieve a substantive gain in aerobic power. The only training study reporting more than a 10% improvement in the $V_{O_2\ max}$ of athletes involved two workouts a day, 6 days a week, for 12 weeks (Withers, 1978).

Strength

A recent innovation in women's sports is the inclusion of weight training as part of an athlete's conditioning programme. The effectiveness of these programmes has demonstrated that women's potential for developing muscular strength has been greatly underestimated. While it is unlikely that female athletes will ever attain the same absolute level of strength as their male counterparts, they can expect close to a 30% improvement in some muscle groups within a few months (Wilmore, 1974).

The male–female difference in strength is due primarily to the anabolic effect of testosterone on the male's musculature. Since strength is proportional to the cross-sectional area of a muscle, the male's larger muscles are a distinct advantage. Although the difference in strength varies from one muscle group to another, the overall strength of women averages about two-thirds that of men (Laubach, 1976). When body size is eliminated as a factor by relating strength to bodyweight or lean body mass, the sex difference in total strength decreases to about 20%.

When strength gains are expressed as percent improvement, the effects of weight training are similar for men and women. In fact, women may have a larger relative gain in strength because their initial levels of strength are lower (Wilmore *et al.*, 1978). However, there is no evidence that weight training can eliminate gender differences in absolute strength (Morrow & Hosler, 1981). Although some female athletes may be stronger than some untrained men, the male athlete will have a definite advantage in those sports where success is determined primarily by strength and/or power.

One of the reasons women were slow to adopt weight training as part of their overall conditioning programme was the cultural bias against large, well-defined muscles on females. Two events within the past 15 years have removed that obstacle. First, many women no longer concern themselves with that particular taboo. If performance is enhanced by larger well-defined muscles, as in power lifting or body-building, women will work to develop those characteristics. Second, it has become apparent that the majority of women gain strength without markedly increasing muscle mass (Wilmore, 1974). The exception would be those women who use anabolic steroids in an effort to enhance their performance, even though the drugs violate the rules of sports organizations and may produce permanent alterations in physique. One young powerlifter who admits to having used both synthetic anabolic steroids and testosterone has facial hair which requires daily shaving, the start of male pattern baldness, clitoral enlargement and a lower voice (Todd, 1987). These side effects are still present 2 years after she stopped taking the drugs.

A strength-training programme for women can use the same equipment and regimen as that used for men (see Part 5). However, women may need special emphasis on upper body strength where their overall strength is 54% that of men, as contrasted to 68% of male strength in the lower body (Heyward *et al.*, 1986). Contrary to popular opinion women can do pull-ups and regular push-ups rather than knee push-ups if encouraged to do so from an early age.

Prevention of injuries is another reason to encourage women to increase muscular strength. Early studies of sports-related injuries reported a higher incidence of overuse injuries among women. It was suggested, for example, that women's wider hips predisposed them to patellofemoral joint problems. Actually, the width of women's hips is similar to that of men but larger in proportion to their other dimensions. A more likely cause of the greater number of injuries was the lack of experience and physical conditioning of the girls and women entering the sport's world for the first time. More recent reports of injury rates show very little difference in the number or location of injuries between men and women in the same sport (Nilson, 1986). Strength training for women, as for male athletes, should be based on an evaluation of their initial status and be directed not only toward improvement of performance but toward avoidance of injury.

Muscle fibres   Histochemical and biochemical analyses of muscle fibres from both sedentary and athletic populations have identified certain similarities and differences between men and women in fibre composition and metabolic potential. However, conclusions drawn from available data must be tentative, since the total number of women athletes who have participated in muscle biopsy studies is relatively small.

Untrained men and women have almost a 50–50 split between slow twitch fibres (STF) and fast twitch fibres (FTF). Among athletes, the percentage of FTF and STF depends more on the sport than on gender. The difference in percentage of STF between sprinters and middle-distance runners, for example, is greater than the difference between any group of men and women. Both male and female endurance athletes typically have 60–70% STF while sprinters may have as few as 25–30%.

It is the fibre area that discriminates between the sexes. The extent of the difference depends upon the activity pattern of the groups and the muscle sampled. In sedentary populations, women have only about two-thirds of the male STF and FTF areas when the sampling site is the

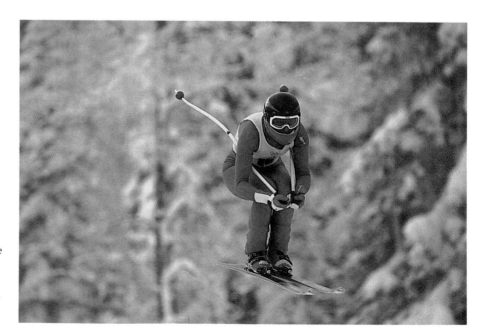

Fig. 8.1.2 The fibre-type pattern of a female Alpine racer will be similar to a male counterpart and both will have much lower slow twitch fibre populations than female and male cross-country skiers. Courtesy of the IOC archives.

gastrocnemius muscle. At the vastus lateralis muscle the STF area is almost equal, while the male FTF area is still about one-third larger.

While female athletes have significantly larger fibre areas than untrained women, male athletes in the same sports retain a size advantage in both STF and FTF. The gender difference is smallest in the endurance sports and most marked in strength and power events. In endurance events where training does not lead to marked muscle hypertrophy, women athletes' STF area is only 10% greater than that of untrained women. The inability of the female to markedly increase muscle bulk becomes apparent in the strength and power sports. Male athletes in these events have a 40% larger FTF area than untrained men, while female athletes have only a 15% advantage over untrained women.

Body composition

College-age females maintain between 20 and 25% of their bodyweight in fat, closer to 20% if they are active and nearer 25% if they are sedentary (Table 8.1.5). For many female athletes this amount of fat is unacceptable because they believe it detracts from their performance. Endurance athletes in particular strive to reduce unessential fat to a minimum, since fat increases the workload without contributing to work capacity. The athlete's conception of a 'minimum' amount of fat depends on the sport and what she perceives as an optimum level for success.

Average values for specific sports and events range from lows of 12% for elite runners to highs near 24% for shot-putters and discus-throwers (Table 8.1.5). At present there is no scientific foundation for claiming a specific percent body fat as the optimal level for any sport. Averages represent a wide range of values within each sport. Some of this variation is due to actual differences among the athletes, but some of it is also due to measurement error. Athletes should be made aware that even the densiometric method, the 'Gold Standard' for assessing body fat, is only an estimate. Two of the basic assumptions underlying this technique are that the density of lean tissue mass is the same for each individual and that the proportion of bone and muscle comprising that lean tissue is a constant. These are questionable when the same formula is used to predict percent body fat (%BF) for trained and untrained women of all ages (Wilmore, 1983).

There have been many attempts to predict %BF from anthropometric measurements such as skinfolds, diameters and circumferences. Most prediction equations are population specific; the same formula cannot be

Table 8.1.5   Percent body fat (%BF) of sedentary, active and athletic women* by age and sport. The sum of five skinfolds (5Sk) with an associated %BF has been added for groups when available. Sample size is given for hydrostatic weighting (n_h) and skinfolds (n_{Sk}) separately.

Age (years)	n_h	%BF	5Sk	%BF	n_{Sk}
15–20					
Sedentary	128	25.1			
Basketball	95	19.8	102.4	19.2	49
Gymnastics	49	15.1	54.8	15.1	49
Distance running	135	15.0			
Swimming	7	18.9	59.1	18.9	7
Tennis	10	23.3			
21–30					
Sedentary	555	26.5	102.2	25.7	385
Active (non-athletic)	36	20.0			
Basketball	10	19.7			
Cycling	27	21.0			
Distance running	110	16.0	42.4	13.3	8
Field events	19	26.5	101.7	24.7	5
Field hockey	53	22.1			
Lacrosse	7	23.1			
Marathon	15	15.2	55.0		
Skiing					
Alpine	20	18.7			
Nordic	25	17.1	63.2	16.1	5
Swimming	20	18.0			
Volleyball	60	19.7			
31–40					
Sedentary	169	26.3	98.0	28.8	64
Active (non-athletic)	17	21.2			
Distance running	20	14.8			
Golf	23	24.0			
Lacrosse	25	20.3			
Marathon	51	15.5	64.0	15.5	42
Swimming	11	18.6			
Tennis	25	20.3			
41–50					
Sedentary	223	30.4	120.0	31.5	87
Active (non-athletic)	23	22.7			
Distance running	10	18.3			
Swimming	10	21.1			
51–60					
Sedentary	65	34.8	120.3	41.9	21
Active (non-athletic)	23	25.0			
Swimming	6	23.8			

* The term athletic includes women who participate in competitive and/or recreational activities. Reprinted with permission from Drinkwater (1988b).

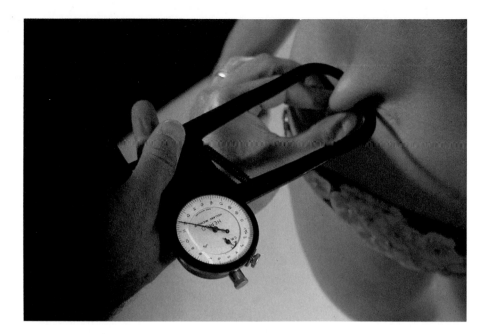

Fig. 8.1.3 Estimation of body fat can be made from skinfold thicknesses (as shown) as well as body diameters and circumferences. Courtesy of J. H. Wilmore.

used for untrained women and athletes or even athletes from different sports (Flint *et al.*, 1977). Even when one uses a prediction equation validated for athletes in the same sport, the error of prediction is usually so large that the formulae are useless for valid estimates of individual %BF. When done carefully, anthropometric measurements may be used to track changes in body composition for individual athletes or for comparison with similar data from other athletes (see Table 8.1.5). It is not necessary to convert them into a %BF.

The use of body composition measures to encourage weight loss in female athletes must be done carefully. The athlete may interpret an unsatisfactory %BF as a rationale for severe dietary restriction which can be detrimental to her health.

Heat tolerance

For many years it was believed that women were unable to tolerate exercise in the heat as well as men. Since the ability to dissipate heat is vital in athletics, particularly endurance sports, women's presumed inability to handle heat stress was used as a rationale for prohibiting their participation in some events. The basis for this belief can be found in studies of sex differences in heat tolerance that were done before it was widely recognized that many indicators of heat strain, such as core temperature and heart rate, are more closely related to relative ($\% \dot{V}_{O_2 \, max}$) rather than absolute exercise intensity (Åstrand, 1960). When men and women were assigned the same absolute exercise intensity in a hot environment, women had higher heart rates, higher core temperatures and lower tolerance times because they were exercising at a higher $\% \dot{V}_{O_2 \, max}$ than the men, not because they had an inferior thermoregulatory system.

More recent studies, which have matched men and women on fitness levels and training regimens and assigned the same relative exercise intensity to both groups, have shown that women tolerate exercise in the heat and acclimatize as well as men (Drinkwater, 1986). Female athletes achieve the same partial heat acclimatization that male athletes do from daily training sessions which cause a sustained elevation of core temperature and activation of the sweating mechanism (Gisolfi & Cohen, 1979). Women marathon runners, for example, have a lower basal core temperature, a larger blood volume and a more efficient sweating response (Drinkwater *et al.*, 1977). They begin sweating sooner than untrained women and also have a lower core temperature, heart rate and skin temperature during exercise in the heat. Endurance training, however, should never be considered a substitute for heat acclimatization.

The procedure for heat acclimatization and the physiological adaptations are the same for men and women. Heart rate and core temperature decrease, tolerance time improves, and both sexes increase sweat sensitivity and capacity. The last point is particularly important, because women's tendency to sweat less than men has been interpreted as an inadequate response to thermal stress. What is frequently overlooked is that sweating, unlike core temperature and heart rate, is related to absolute exercise intensity (Saltin & Gagge, 1968). When a 70 kg man and a 55 kg woman run together, he is producing more metabolic heat than she is even when they are both running at the same $\% \dot{V}_{O_2 \, max}$. To dissipate that extra heat he must also produce more sweat; he may also sweat excessively. At least one study (Frye & Kamon, 1983) has reported that women sweat more efficiently than men. In hot, humid conditions, women's sweat rate matched the need for evaporative heat loss while men produced more than was required. Both were equally efficient in hot, dry conditions.

It has been suggested that a woman's efficient sweating might serve her well in humid conditions where evaporative heat loss is minimal and excessive sweating simply leads to dehydration, but that men would do better in dry heat where a higher sweat rate could be advantageous (Avellini *et al.*, 1980). Two tests of this hypothesis with unacclimatized men and women produced conflicting results (Frye & Kamon, 1981; Horstman & Christensen, 1982). However, once both groups were acclimatized men did no better in dry heat than the women.

The role of oestrogen and progesterone in thermoregulation is still uncertain. A woman's basal body temperature is about 0.5°C higher during the luteal phase of the menstrual cycle. Does this put her more at risk of heat injury during this time? Does oestrogen inhibit sweating as was once believed? Most research suggests that hormonal fluctuations during the menstrual cycle do not markedly affect a woman's ability to exercise in the heat (Wells & Horvath, 1973; Fortney & Senay, 1979; Frye et al., 1982; Horvath & Drinkwater, 1982). Although only a few of these studies confirmed the phase of the cycle by direct measurement of hormone levels and the number of subjects was often small, the replication of results from a number of studies strengthens the conclusion that monthly fluctuations of hormones do not seriously affect women's thermoregulatory control.

There will undoubtedly be more studies comparing the thermoregulatory responses of men and women under a variety of conditions and examining some of the more subtle responses to exercise in the heat, such as fluid dynamics. Unless convincing evidence is presented to the contrary, it appears that fitness level and state of acclimatization are more important than gender in determining heat tolerance. Because the responses of men and women to exercise in the heat are so similar, all of the guidelines for minimizing the risk of heat injury during an athletic event apply equally to male and female athletes.

Menstrual function

There is no doubt that the incidence of menstrual irregularities among women athletes is much greater than among the general female population (Sanborn & Wagner, 1986). The question which concerns the athletes, their coaches and physicians is what are the long-term consequences of these disturbances? Early reports of 'athletic amenorrhoea' caused considerable concern about the future reproductive health of the athlete. As anecdotal reports of former amenorrhoeic athletes giving birth to healthy children became common, concern faded and many athletes welcomed the cessation of the monthly period. However, recent reports of premature bone loss in some amenorrhoeic athletes has rekindled the alarm (Cann et al., 1984; Drinkwater et al., 1984; Marcus et al., 1985; Nelson et al., 1986).

Amenorrhoea is defined as the absence of menses. If menarche has not occurred, the amenorrhoea is primary. When menses has been normal and then ceases, the amenorrhoea is secondary. To be identified as exercise-associated amenorrhoea, the condition must have occurred following the onset of training or some change in the training regimen and have no underlying pathological basis. Another term, oligomenorrhoea, is used when menses has not ceased but is infrequent. One of the difficulties in determining the incidence of these conditions in the athletic population has been defining the point at which infrequent menses becomes cessation of menses. Investigators have differed in their definitions. For example, a woman without menses for 5 months could be classified as oligomenorrhoeic in one study and amenorrhoeic in another. If one combines the two categories, the incidence of interruption in the normal 11–13 cycles/year ranges from about 12% for swimmers and cyclists to more than 40% for distance runners (Drinkwater, 1984a).

Now that more investigators are reporting hormone profiles for athletes, it is becoming obvious that a continuum rather than a dichotomy of menstrual irregularities exists. Women with apparently normal cycles often have a short luteal phase and lower than normal levels of progesterone. Some amenorrhoeic athletes have adequate levels of oestrogen but are anovulatory so that progesterone remains at baseline values throughout the cycle. Finally, there are those women whose oestrogen and progesterone levels remain at the early follicular level continuously. Presumably a woman passes through these various stages during the transition from a normal cycle to the amenorrhoeic state.

A number of theories have been proposed to explain why these menstrual irregularities occur. The four most frequently cited are: (a) a decrease in body fat content; (b) acute and chronic hormonal changes resulting from sustained intense exercise; (c) excessive energy expenditure; and (d) psychological stress. The body fat hypothesis has lost favour as the primary causative factor as more and more studies report no significant difference in %BF between amenorrhoeic and eumenorrhoeic (normal cycling) athletes (Sinning & Little, 1987). There are also reports of women regaining menses with no change in bodyweight and of women with a normal %BF becoming amenorrhoeic.

Relating the neuroendocrine response to acute or chronic exercise with changes in the menstrual cycle is difficult because of the dependence on measuring plasma concentrations of hormones in order to infer biological activity at the tissue level. Changes in plasma concentration may reflect increased secretion, decreased clearance and fluctuations in plasma volume, as well as individual and environmental factors. Since some hormones do not cross the blood–brain barrier, peripheral concentrations cannot be assumed to represent those in the hypothalamic–pituitary area. Considering the technical and procedural problems, it is not surprising that much of the data from this area of research are inconsistent.

Warren (1980) has suggested that athletic amenorrhoea is related to an 'energy drain' but does not define the meaning of the term. One would presume it to mean an excess of energy expenditure, perhaps in relation to caloric intake. Several investigators (Feicht *et al.*, 1978; Dale *et al.*, 1979; Lutter & Cushman, 1982) have reported a higher weekly mileage for amenorrhoeic runners, but others (Baker *et al.*, 1981; Wakat *et al.*, 1982) found no difference in mileage between amenorrhoeic and eumenorrhoeic groups. Evidence regarding the intensity of training for the two groups is not available.

Psychological stress could play a role in the aetiology of menstrual irregularities through the increased production of stress hormones, which in turn may disrupt the finely tuned relationship between the hypothalamus and the pituitary. Unfortunately, stress has proved difficult to quantify in the athletic population. There are self-reports of more stress among amenorrhoeic athletes, but there are no experimental data linking it to menstrual changes in the athletes (Feicht *et al.*, 1978). Presumably the effect on the cycle would be via an increase in the stress hormones such as the catecholamines, endorphins and cortisol, but no one yet has shown such an association.

While the aetiology of changes in menstrual function holds the interest of the scientist, the athlete's concerns are more immediate. Is this a benign and reversible condition? Might there be some adverse effects from the absence of normal levels of ovarian hormones? Athletes should be informed that there are a number of pathological conditions that can result in the cessation of menses. If their amenorrhoea has persisted for more than 1 year, did not coincide with the onset of training or an increase in training intensity, and menses does not resume when training stops, they should consult a physician to be sure there is no pathology.

A prolonged hypo-oestrogenic state may also result in a loss of bone mass. Several studies (Cann *et al.*, 1984; Drinkwater *et al.*, 1984; Marcus *et al.*, 1985; Nelson *et al.*, 1986) have found that amenorrhoeic athletes have a decreased density in the lumbar vertebrae, an area which has a large proportion of trabecular bone. The effect has not been observed as frequently in cortical bone. The decrease in spinal bone mass is similar to that observed in postmenopausal women and is presumed to be related to the decrease in oestrogen levels. While exercise has been shown to assist older women in halting or even reversing bone loss, it apparently does not protect the young athlete from some decrease in bone density. Fortunately, this loss appears to be reversible. Two studies (Lindberg *et al.*, 1987; Drinkwater *et al.*, 1986) have reported an increase in vertebral BMD (bone mineral density) in former amenorrhoeic athletes who resumed menses. Since their BMD was still less than that of regularly cycling athletes, no one knows yet if the original loss can be completely reversed.

Several studies (Lindberg *et al.*, 1984; Marcus *et al.*, 1985; Lloyd *et al.*, 1986) have reported an increased incidence of stress fractures among amenorrhoeic athletes compared with eumenorrhoeic athletes in the same sport. It is still uncertain whether the fractures are a result of decreased bone mass. Many of them occur in areas which are primarily cortical bone, and there is as yet no evidence that amenorrhoeic athletes have a lower BMD in these areas. Nevertheless, there does appear to be a higher incidence of stress fractures among amenorrhoeic athletes. Whether it is a result of a low BMD or some other factor associated with their training programme remains to be seen.

Amenorrhoea may be an indication of overtraining and slight modifications in training and life-style may be enough to bring about regular menses. The women who spontaneously regained menses in the Drinkwater *et al.* (1986) study had decreased their activity level by about 10% and gained an average of 2 kg. This may be a viable option for some athletes, but even modest changes in training regimens and bodyweight may be unacceptable to the professional or highly competitive athlete. If normal menses cannot be regained, the athlete and her physician may want to consider some form of hormone replacement therapy. Opinion regarding the use of this therapy for amenorrhoeic athletes is sharply divided. The athlete herself may resist the use of hormones to regulate her cycle. Some remember the cancer scare in the 1970s and are not aware of the newer oestrogen–progestin combinations. Others are simply not interested in having their monthly period return. However, if the individual athlete does have a markedly decreased bone mass and is experiencing frequent stress fractures, she may be forced to make a choice between present convenience or the possibility of more serious osteoporotic fractures in the future.

It is important to make a distinction between the bone status of eumenorrhoeic and amenorrhoeic women. Exercise has a positive effect on bone when normal oestrogen levels are present and is one of the ways to ensure maximal bone mass within each individual's genetic limits.

PART 9

SPORT AND PHYSICAL ACTIVITIES IN OLDER PEOPLE

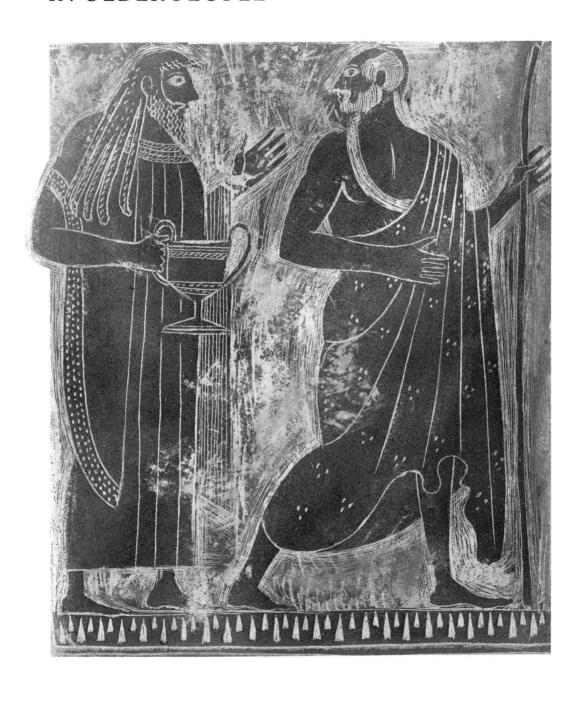

9.1 Maintenance of physical fitness

Y. KURODA

General aspects of the ageing process

With ageing, various functions of a living body gradually deteriorate. Ageing itself is understood as a physiological process which occurs in all living things, not necessarily running parallel to calendar age and showing considerable interindividual variation. All beings become gradually susceptible to disease due to: (a) the decrease in reserve capacity of various functions of the living body; (b) decline of adaptability to changes in external and internal environment; and (c) decreasing resistance to invasion of the living body.

The fundamental organic phenomena which occur in a living body during ageing are as follows:

1   A decrease in number of cells: The number of parenchymal cells decreases and fibrosis occurs. As a result, tissue and organ weights decrease and atrophy occurs. Liver cells decrease gradually in the fifties to sixties and rapidly in the sixties to seventies. The amount of liver cells in the eighties is 30% of that found in young people. In the brain, kidneys, lungs, muscles and other organs a similar decrease of parenchymal cells is found.

2   Changes inside cells: With ageing, increases of glycogen storage, fatty infiltration or fatty degeneration and pigment granules such as lipofuscin are found in many cells. A decrease in number and decomposition of mitochondria is seen. Changes of permeability in cell membranes and failures of the sodium pump process cause a decrease in cellular retention of potassium ions and the exclusion of sodium and water.

3   Changes in connective tissues: Cross-linkage of collagen molecules decreases the compliance of connective tissues. A decrease of elastin lowers elasticity of tissue, flexion and flexibility. Ageing connective tissues show a decrease in their metabolism. As a result of these phenomena, sclerosis of blood vessels and skin wrinkles occur and movement of the joints becomes more and more poor.

The functional changes in the living body resulting from these organic changes are as follows:

1   Decrease in reserve capacity of physiological functions: A decrease in parenchymal cell numbers in tissue and organs and a decline in function of individual cells causes a decline of maximam capacity of functions. Thus, a decrease of reserve capacity results. For example, old people get tired sooner than young people even if they do the same amount of exercise, and old people display less capacity even if they exert themselves to the maximum. With ageing, stress caused by internal and external environmental changes increases, and resistance and preventive power against disease decreases. As a result, old people become ill more easily.

2   Sluggishness of reaction: The living body receives information about environmental changes from its sensory organs. The information is sent to the CNS which sends impulses to a certain organ (effector organ) which alters its function. This is the general system of reaction in the living body. With ageing, the decline in sensory function leads to a decline in information reception, which results in insufficient reception of external and internal information in quality and quantity, which, in turn leads to dullness and inaccuracy of reaction. These phenomena are related not only

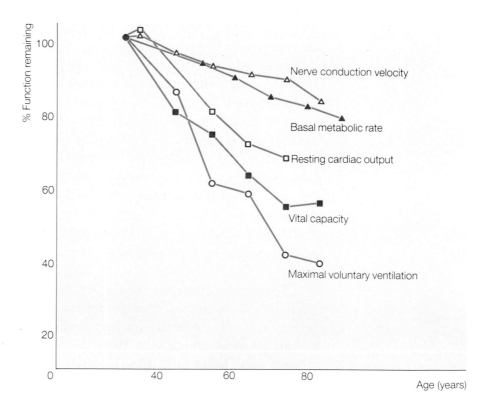

Fig. 9.1.1 Change in selected physiological variables with increasing age. After Shepard (1982); based on the data of Shock (1967).

to a functional decline of the sensory organs but also to a functional decline of the nervous system and effector organs.

Similar phenomena occur in other sensory organs such as baroreceptors and chemoreceptors of blood vessels, which detect changes in blood pressure and chemical components in the blood, leading to a slow adjustment to internal changes. This can be described as a decline in homeostasis.
3 Delay of recovery: Recovery to normal condition is delayed by abnormal conditions which are caused by stress.
4 Decrease of regeneration ability: Decline in proliferation ability of cells causes a delay in regeneration of damaged tissues and organs.

Changes in physical functions

Figure 9.1.1 shows the decline in various physiological functions with ageing (Shephard, 1982). The values for 30-year-olds are set at 100%. Decline in function of the respirocirculatory system is more pronounced than that of the nervous system.

Figure 9.1.2 indicates changes in physical fitness with ageing. The values for 20-year-olds are set at 100%. These indexes are based on average values of physical fitness in the Japanese. Muscular strength such as grip strength which is stimulated fully in daily life declines little, whereas leg muscle strength which is not fully stimulated declines greatly. Decline in balance, which was tested by balancing on one foot with the eyes closed, is

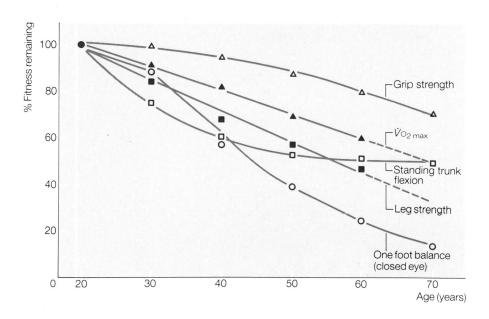

Fig. 9.1.2 Change in selected physical fitness of Japanese males with the ageing process. Based on data from Physical Fitness Laboratory (1982).

remarkable in and over the fifties, but the value for 70-year-olds is just 20% of that for young people.

Maximum heart rate while doing exercise decreases with ageing, and the difference between individuals increases. The rise in blood pressure, however, while exercising shows a tendency to increase with ageing.

Follow-up survey of top athletes at the Tokyo Olympic Games, 1964

Fig. 9.1.3 Twelve years change in back strength (a), vertical jump (b), grip strength (c) and Harvard step test score (d) of 13 Japanese male Olympic athletes who participated in the Tokyo Olympic Games, 1964. Data obtained by follow-up studies by Kuroda (1976).

A follow-up survey on the health and physical fitness of Japanese athletes who participated in the Tokyo Olympic Games in 1964 has been performed every 4 years.

Figure 9.1.3 shows 12 years of change in back strength, grip strength, vertical jump and the Harvard step test for 13 male former athletes who retired from sport after the Tokyo Olympic Games, and have not been doing active physical exercise either for business or recreation (Kuroda *et al.*, 1976). The 13 athletes were aged from 21 to 28 years (average 24.1 years) in 1964.

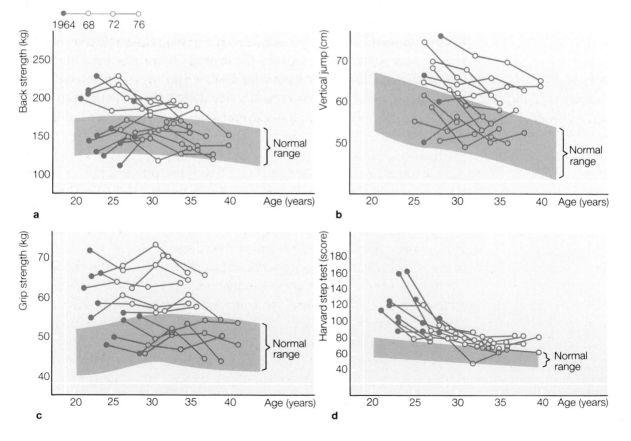

The general tendency of change in grip strength with ageing was found to increase up to 31 or 32 years old, and to decrease slightly thereafter; however back strength was found to peak before 30 years of age and gradually decrease thereafter. Regarding grip strength change of the former Olympic athletes, those who were very strong while competing have shown no remarkable changes over the past 12 years. Contrarily, in back strength, those who were very strong have decreased to the level of the average Japanese male after retirement, and those of average strength in 1964 have shown hardly any change since retirement.

In the vertical jump test, maximum heights achieved generally decrease soon after 20 years of age. The tendency of former Olympic athletes is the same as that of ordinary subjects, i.e. height of vertical jump decreases with ageing. In contrast to back strength, those who were able to make high jumps, although the heights reached fell, were still able to jump higher than ordinary people. Differences in bodyweights while competing and after retirement were not found.

The above facts show that muscle strength, for example grip strength, is retained after retirement; however back strength, which was great during competition, drops to the level of ordinary subjects after retirement. Moreover, in the vertical jump test, the decrease in maximum heights has the same trend as that of ordinary people, although the athletes involved in high-jump competitions retained their superiority. As mentioned above, characteristics of muscles, e.g. different components of fibre types, and ways of using muscles in daily life cause differences in the change of muscle strength with the ageing process after retirement from athletics.

Changes in Harvard step test scores, which tests an index of endurance, were also very characteristic. Almost all former athletes achieved much higher scores than ordinary subjects; although all the athletes showed a tendency to register scores nearer to those of ordinary subjects following retirement. This indicates that respirocirculatory function begins to decline relatively soon after termination of hard training.

In the follow-up survey conducted in 1984, 20 years after the Tokyo Olympic Games, 94 males and 23 females took part in the physical fitness measurement. All of them were retired, however 60% were doing regular physical exercise such as jogging, golf, swimming walking and callisthenics for the improvement of health.

They were divided into three groups: (a) the high-activity group—those doing physical exercise regularly more than three times a week; (b) the medium-activity group—those doing physical exercise once or twice a week; and (c) the low-activity group. The three groups were then

Table 9.1.1   Physical characteristics of three groups of 94 male and 23 female Japanese former Olympic athletes. They were divided by grade of physical activity after their retirement from competition.

Group classification	n	Male Age (years)	Height (cm)	Weight (kg)	n	Female Age (years)	Height (cm)	Weight (kg)
High-activity group (3+ times/week)	25	45.4 4.1	171.2 7.5	72.1 10.2	7	45.1 7.6	160.4 8.6	61.1 10.0
Medium-activity group (1–2 times/week)	32	46.0 5.4	171.5 7.6	72.2 10.7	11	42.0 2.9	162.4 5.9	59.5 6.3
Low-activity group (None/week)	27	44.9 5.4	170.2 7.2	71.1 8.2	5	42.8 4.0	157.8 6.4	53.7 5.2

evaluated. The physical characteristics, seen in Table 9.1.1, show that the three groups of males have very similar average ages, weights and heights. On the other hand, among the females, there are some differences between groups in average age, height and weight; however these differences are not statistically significant.

No significant differences could be found between the three groups of males or females in flexibility (standing trunk flexion), grip strength, arm flexion strength, vertical jump, side-step test scores or forced vital capacity (FEV_1). The high-activity group only showed significantly greater strength ($P < 0.05$) than the low-activity group in back strength. However, in the endurance test (cardiorespiratory endurance) with a gradual loading system by cycle ergometer, performance time and PWC_{170} in males as well as females were significantly higher in the high-activity group than in the low-activity group ($P < 0.05$) (Fig. 9.1.4).

In short, there was no significant difference in muscle strength between recreational exercise performed for 60 min a session done regularly more than three times a week and that done once or twice a week or less. However there was a significant difference in cardiorespiratory function between the high-activity and low-activity groups.

Subjects in their forties and fifties with a low level of physical strength who were university researchers and did not do any regular physical exercise were selected for another investigation (Kuroda *et al.*, 1974). After they had done light physical sports, such as tennis or badminton, for 90 min once a week for 6 months, the effects of such exercise on physical fitness were examined. The results made it clear that the physical capacity of their respirocirculatory system had improved after 6 months of training.

However, in the case of the former Olympic athletes who had possessed much higher physical fitness than the ordinary subjects, in spite of

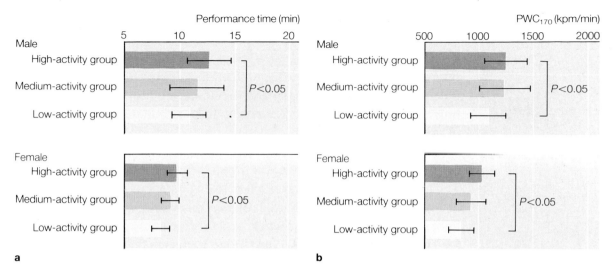

Fig. 9.1.4 Comparison of performance time (a) and PWC$_{170}$ (b) in three groups using endurance tests (Kuroda *et al.*, 1984).

having lower fitness than when they were competing, there were no significant differences unless they did physical exercises more than three times a week.

Conclusion Even people who are physically very fit, once they stop exercising, will find their physical fitness drops to a level no higher than that of ordinary subjects. The tendency is remarkable especially in respirocirculatory functions. Moreover, subjects who are physically very fit, such as the former Olympic athletes, will not show significant differences if they do not do physical exercise more than three times a week. However, ordinary people whose level of physical fitness is low and who have little experience in physical training will obtain higher physical fitness and improvement in respirocirculatory function if they exercise only once a week.

What is important to middle-aged people is not that they used to do physical exercise and used to be physically fit, but whether or not they still exercise. In addition, for the maintenance of good health, apart from strengthening trunk muscles to prevent low back pain, it is not so important for middle-aged and older people to train other local muscles. It is beneficial for them to improve their respirocirculatory function with exercises which train the whole body and improve endurance, such as jogging, walking, swimming, cycling and other light sports, which use large muscle groups.

Finally, in order to prevent and soften stiff connective tissues, it is important to do callisthenics which move all muscles, joints and tendons of the body.

Exercises for the aged

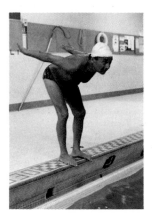

Fig. 9.1.5 It is important for older people to maintain a general level of fitness through exercise and/or sport, such as swimming, which involves movements of the entire body. Courtesy of W. R. Sellers.

In the late sixties, seventies or eighties, the rate of decrease in various physical functions with ageing accelerates. As the reserve capacity of older people decreases greatly and their adaptability also declines, they must take good care to exercise more carefully than middle-aged people in their forties or fifties.

To evaluate physical fitness, the respirocirculatory system and other functions of three groups were compared (Kuroda & Kawahara, 1985). The first group jogged a total of 25 km over 4 days each week, the second group jogged for 10 min, did callisthenics for 40 min, and folk dancing or light sports for 40 min once a week, and the third group played 'gate ball' for 3 hours five times a week. Each group had been doing its activities for more than 8 years.

The average heart rate of the jogging group taken while running was 135 ± 14, which corresponds to about 82% of the estimated maximum heart rate (HR_{max}). The average heart rate of the callisthenics group taken while jogging after 10 min was about 135 ± 12, which corresponds to 78% HR_{max}; while average heart rates during callisthenics or light sports was 99 ± 10 which corresponds to about 20% HR_{max}.

Croquet, or 'gate ball' as it is called in Japan, is the most popular sport of the Japanese aged population. As it is a team game, a great deal of time is spent standing outside the field boundaries, and although 30 min are required to play one game, the average player moves a total distance of only 60 to 100 m. The average heart rate is 98 ± 14 which corresponds to 20% HR_{max}, which qualifies gate ball as a very light sport.

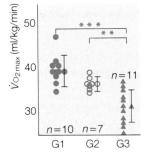

Fig. 9.1.6 Comparison of maximal oxygen uptake in group 1 (●), group 2 (○) and group 3 (▲) (Kuroda *et al.*, 1984). ** = $P < 0.01$; *** = $P < 0.001$.

A comparison of the items measured in the three groups is shown in Table 9.1.2. Group 1 is significantly low in percentage of body fat. The maximum oxygen intake in treadmill running in groups 1 and 2 is significantly higher than in group 3. Although oxygen intake is higher in group 1 than in group 2, the difference is not significant. Maximum ventilation volume ($\dot{V}_{Emax}$) and maximum respiration rate (RR_{max}) are significantly greater in group 1 than in the other two groups.

The most interesting finding of this investigation is that no significant difference in maximum oxygen intake was found between group 1 and group 2, as shown in Fig. 9.1.6.

Conclusion   The conclusion that can be reached from the above results is that, in the case of oxygen intake ability in the aged, exercise with 80% HR_{max} performed for 10 min once a week, and that with 80% HR_{max} performed for 60 min four times a week, have the same overall effect.

Table 9.1.2 Comparison of physical characteristics of three groups (G1, G2 and G3) as described in the text.

	Group 1 (jogging) (n = 10)	Group 2 (callisthenics) (n = 7)	Group 3 (gate ball) (n = 10)	T-test
Age (years)	70.0 ± 7.0	69.0 ± 2.0	70.0 ± 3.0	ns
Height (cm)	161.7 ± 7.6	161.7 ± 3.6	164.7 ± 4.8	ns
Weight (kg)	57.4 ± 6.5	58.3 ± 6.8	58.7 ± 8.9	ns
% Fat	11.5 ± 1.7	14.3 ± 4.2	15.5 ± 4.9	G1 vs G3 $P < 0.05$
$\dot{V}_{O_2max}$ ((ml/kg)/min)	39.0 ± 3.6	36.2 ± 1.6	31.0 ± 3.9	G1 vs G3 $P < 0.001$ G2 vs G3 $P < 0.01$
HR_{max} (beats/min)	165.0 ± 15.0	175.0 ± 7.0	163.0 ± 14.0	ns
SBP after exhaustion (mmHg)	195.0 ± 30.0	206.0 ± 22.0	181.0 ± 24.0	G2 vs G3 $P < 0.05$
$\dot{V}_{Emax}$ (l/min)	85.8 ± 12.5	73.0 ± 8.6	75.2 ± 12.4	G1 vs G2 G3 $P < 0.05$ G1 vs G2 $P < 0.05$
RR_{max} (breaths/min)	49.0 ± 7.0	42.0 ± 4.0	40.0 ± 4.0	G1 vs G3 $P < 0.001$

ns = not significant.

Saltin (1971) has found the training effect on the aged is extremely low, and it is not meaningful to train hard to improve functions since those who are physically fit to some extent cannot obtain much greater levels of fitness as a result. Exercise is considered to be most important for the aged to maintain their health, both mentally and physically. Doing exercises must not cause injury or ill health. Particularly in exercises for the aged, with the increased possibility of their being in pathological states, it is important to instruct them to exercise very carefully under professional sports medical care. Slow, stable and safe are important features of physical exercise for aged people.

References

Kuroda, Y., Kataoka, Y., Oyama, K. & Sawada, M. (1974) Effects of physical training on physical working capacity and body composition for middle aged men. *Proc. Dept. Physic. Educ. Coll. Gen. Educ. Univ. Tokyo* **8**, 1.

Kuroda, Y. & Kawahara, T. (1985) Effects of exercise habits of the aged on the aerobic exercise capacity. *Descente Sports Sci.* **6**, 17.

Kuroda, Y., Tsukagoshi, K., Amemiya, T., Ito, S. & Kaneko, K. (1984) *Fifth Report of the Follow-up Studies on Health and Physical Fitness of Japanese Olympic Athletes.* Annual report no. 7. Sports Science Committee, Japanese Olympic Committee.

Kuroda, Y., Tsukagoshi, K., Amemiya, T., Ito, S., Kitajima, H. & Matsui, M. (1976) *Third Report of the Follow-up Studies on Health and Physical Fitness of Japanese Olympic Athletes for the Tokyo Olympic Games 1964.* Annual report no. 7. Sports Science Committee, Japanese Olympic Committee.

Physical Fitness Laboratory (eds) (1982) *Physical Fitness Standard of Japanese People*, 3rd edn. Tokyo Metropolitan University, Fumaido, Tokyo.

Saltin, B. (1971) Central circulation of the physical conditioning in young and middle aged men. In O. A. Larsen & R. O. Malmborg (eds) *Coronary Heart Disease and Physical Fitness*, pp. 21–26. Symposia Proceedings, Copenhagen, 1970. Munksgaard, Copenhagen.

Shephard, R. J. (1982) *Physiology and Biochemistry of Exercise and Aging*. Praeger, New York.

9.2 Relation to chronic disease

S. ISRAEL

Introduction

All problems connected with chronic diseases are a matter of public concern and of health policy. In former times acute diseases dominated, but for the last few decades chronic diseases have become more and more of a major health problem. Medical progress was very successful in controlling acute diseases, but medicine has been less fortunate in coping with chronic diseases. In addition, life expectancy has been essentially extended, and the number of old and more or less handicapped persons is rising in all countries. Medical care for old people is a high humane and social priority in most societies. Exercise and training can contribute a lot to successful ageing and to the well-being and life satisfaction of old people. A healthy and active old population can also relieve the country's health services to a certain degree.

Ageing, disease and physical immobilization demonstrate many phenomenological analogies; e.g. in all these states the physical working capacity is impaired. It can be proved that habitual physical activity reduces diseases developing with advancing age, and that on the other hand disease promotes the ageing process. The comparison of active and inactive elderly people shows that the active subjects have a relatively lower biological age, a better health status and a higher physical working capacity.

Ageing is accompanied by disease. Because of this fact the scientific problems of ageing are historically a matter of medicine. Indeed, the genetically-controlled ageing processes are closely interrelated to chronic diseases; it is not possible to separate 'natural' and disease-induced ageing events.

Ageing of the human being is governed and determined by the laws of nature. But the time-course and the characteristics of ageing processes depend to a certain degree on environmental influences and on the individual life-style. Diseases also depend to a certain degree on the individual way of life and they exhibit a relationship with ageing, e.g. with advancing age there is a growing physical instability and an enhanced probability for the manifestation of chronic diseases.

340

Exercise-induced adaptations counteract typical changes of ageing, and they also modify the incidence of chronic diseases. The diseases in question are predominantly arteriosclerosis and its complications, emphysema and chronic bronchitis, diabetes mellitus, arthrosis deformans, etc. All these diseases are not confined to old age; they can also occur in young people. But these diseases emerge markedly with advancing age, and they concern many old subjects. Chronic diseases usually have their onset in early periods of the individual's life. Their manifestation takes place decades after the first alterations originated. Because of the very slow development of chronic diseases, there is a good chance for prevention and long-lasting intervention.

Chronic diseases of the cardiovascular system

Arteriosclerosis
Arteriosclerosis, as a degenerative alteration of the wall of arterial vessels, plays a dominating role in the chronic diseases of circulation. Arteriosclerosis is associated with an impairment of perfusion and oxygen supply in all areas of the body, especially the heart, the brain and the lower legs. Angina pectoris and myocardial infarction, stroke and intermittent claudication are the final results of arteriosclerosis in these areas of the body. But prior to these events, hypoxaemia and insufficient oxygen supply to the tissues will have promoted ageing processes and also the progress of other chronic diseases.

The scientific results concerning the problems of physical activity and arteriosclerosis are controversial. It is well known that life-long, hard physical work promotes the manifestation of arteriosclerosis. On the other hand, there is evidence that a sedentary life-style also carries a risk of encouraging its development, while exercise and training undertaken with the aim of improving fitness is a preventative factor. There is evidence that adequate endurance training retards the development of arteriosclerosis, and furthermore the exercise-induced adaptations improve all mechanisms of oxygen supply to the body by an adaptive increase of the capacity of oxygen uptake by respiration, oxygen transport by circulation and oxygen use of the tissues. These adaptations improve the oxygen supply of the tissues even in existing arteriosclerosis. Exercise-induced adaptive properties in the whole oxygen chain of the body is one of the most important factors in maintaining a low biological age, in the prevention of chronic diseases or in postponing them to later periods of life, and for the attenuation of symptoms caused by these diseases.

Training of an appropriate quantity and quality can have a direct contribution in retarding the occurrence of arteriosclerosis and in minimizing its consequences. In addition, regular exercise and training are usually associated with a way of life that further reduces behavioural risk factors such as smoking and overweight.

Hypertension

In industrialized countries arterial hypertension has a prevalence of about 20%; in developing countries the incidence is lower but shows a tendency to increase. Experience and epidemiologic as well as experimental investigations confirm that hypertension is less frequent among subjects who regularly participate in exercise activities. The preventive and therapeutic values of a mild but extensive endurance-accentuated exercise training programme with respect to most kinds of hypertension is well established (Fig. 9.2.1).

The beneficial influence of endurance training on arterial pressure is due to the modification of the tone of the arterial vessels and to an adjustment of the peripheral arterial resistance consistent with the circulatory functions. An endurance-induced reduction of the sympathoadrenal activity and the predominance of a parasympathetic tone of the autonomic nervous system also help maintain low arterial blood pressure.

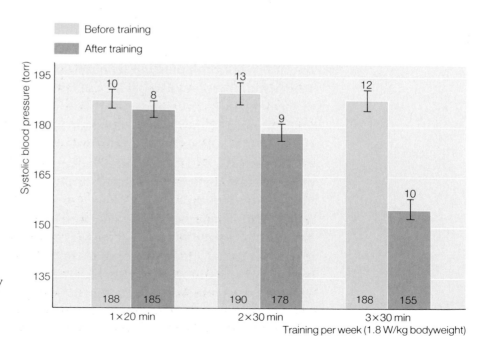

Fig. 9.2.1 Systolic blood pressure (62 males, 35–58 years of age, cycle ergometry with 1.8 W/kg bodyweight) before and after a 6-month period of training (Bringmann, 1982).

Furthermore an arteriosclerotic rigidity of the artery wall may be reduced by metabolic adaptations.

Cardiovascular risks during exercise

Chronic cardiovascular diseases are widespread; their manifestation and progression often starts in middle-age and their occurrence has reached epidemic proportions. Very heavy physical loads, as may be used in some exercise and sports, can be dangerous for people with an impaired cardiovascular system; precautions as outlined below should always be taken. Fatal complications are a very rare event but they do happen (Jokl, 1983, 1985; Israel, 1985).

Even extremely high exertion is not harmful for a heart free from pathological alterations as the peripheral working muscles fail under normal environmental conditions prior to the heart muscle. Death due to exhaustion alone could not be decisively proved. Non-traumatic fatal collapses during or after exercise can always be ascribed to pathological organic findings. In most cases cardiac failure based on myocardial ischaemia has been confirmed; grave rhythmic disorders, hereditary malformations or myocarditis are very rare causes for a fatal collapse in connection with exercise. Men between 35 and 55 years of age, who practice sport intensively in relation to their cardiovascular conditions are those principally at risk; although sometimes such an episode has been found during a game of sport with an untrained person. In most of the subjects in question the (ischaemic) heart disease was asymptomatic, although they frequently exibited organic or behavioural cardiovascular risk factors (e.g. smoking).

An increasing number of elderly or old people have become active in sports and this beneficial development should be supported by those in sports medicine. Endurance training is an effective measure in primary and secondary prevention and in rehabilitation particularly of ischaemic heart disease (Hollmann *et al.*, 1985). Exercise and training must be made more accessible for old subjects but the ethic principle of *primum nil nocere* has always to be regarded. People with cardiac symptoms should train under medical supervision; the endurance training of older people, who are free from symptoms (but certainly not free from pathological alterations) should avoid loads with high intensities. The intensity of the training can be controlled by the heart rate. According to Baum (1971) the target heart rate during training should reach the value of 170 minus the years of age. If this guideline is followed the adaptive threshold of training is reached whilst allowing a sufficient safety margin. A considerable quantity of training without high-intensity levels are, as a rule, well tolerated by subjects with chronic cardiovascular disease.

Sport and risk factors for chronic cardio-vascular diseases

A risk factor is an organic finding or an environmental or behavioural feature that indicates a probabilistic association with the beginning and progress of a disease; the risk factor is not the cause of the disease. The main internal risk factors are:

1 Hypertension.
2 Disorders of fat metabolism.
3 Disorders of carbohydrate metabolism.

The main external risk factors are:

1 Being overweight.
2 Smoking.
3 Psychological stress.
4 Hypokinesia.

It was shown above that a moderate endurance activity has a beneficial influence on an elevated arterial blood pressure. A large number of investigations show that a high concentration of high-density lipoprotein (HDL) in the serum lowers the risk of arteriosclerosis, while a high concentration of low-density lipoprotein (LDL) causes the opposite. It is well established that an endurance training induces a favourable situation, e.g. in active people the HDL concentration and the HDL–LDL relationship is increased. The advantageous effects of physical activity on carbohydrate metabolism are referred to below (under 'Diabetes mellitus').

Excessive weight and obesity as a risk factor for chronic diseases can be controlled by physical activity in two ways: (a) any motor activity increases the energy expenditure, i.e. it causes a negative energy balance; and (b) an endurance training develops particularly those pathways of the fat metabolism that facilitate the mobilization of fat from the depots and that render the deposition of fat more difficult. Furthermore, regular exercise and training are usually combined with personal habits of an efficient nutritional regime.

It is an everyday observation that smoking of cigarettes is less usual among exercisers than among the general population. It is also well documented that a good exercise-induced physical condition is asociated with a high stress tolerance. Exercise and training can lead to a causal elimination of hypokinesia as a risk factor. They can also be a corrective measure for a number of risk factors. The widespread occurrence of chronic disease in old people depends to a certain degree on the long lasting impact of risk factors. These diseases typically originate in early life whilst manifestation occurs in late periods of life. The manifestation frequently takes place after decades of exposition and after long periods without symptoms. The incubation period is extremely long, this provides an opportunity to counteract them over long periods of time. In this field of prevention, exercise and training have an important role through their direct or indirect influence on several major risk factors; preventive measures must begin early in life.

Chronic disorders of the venous system

The veins, which contain almost 90% of the total blood volume, play an increasing role in pathology with advancing age; more than 50% of the middle-aged or old population of an industrialized country suffer from varicosis. The insufficiency of the valves and walls of the veins in the lower body parts is, in many cases, more than a problem of cosmetics. Without doubt, in chronic diseases of the veins genetic properties are essential, but exercise and training can have a substantial effect on tone, pressure, pulse and volume of the veins. The pump mechanisms, which are stimulated by rhythmic muscle activity have a primary and secondary preventive effect on venous pathology. Rhythmic contraction and relaxation of the leg muscles create an anticongestive influence; the consequences of this process are effective to the extent that they act as an additional or second 'heart'. These mechanisms produce up to 50% of the force needed to return the blood to the heart. Old people particularly need to keep the leg muscles active so they can function as a pump and prevent states of congestion. This congestion is a prerequisite for the aggravation of varicosis. Varicosis itself (without thrombosis or phlebitis) does not contraindicate physical activity and sport. Exercise that may involve the possibility of trauma and injury should be avoided (bleeding, thrombosis); in the case of a patient with an extensive varicosis a bandage should be used.

Respiratory disorders

Chronic disease of the respiratory system are very frequent in old people (e.g. emphysema with consecutive loading of the right heart, chronic bronchitis), but successful treatment is difficult. Exercise has a beneficial adaptive impact on respiration and with advancing age these exercise-induced adaptations are of particular value. In trained individuals the breathing capacity and ventilation of the alveoli are increased, and the transition of oxygen from the lungs to the blood is augmented; this leads to an elevation of the saturation rate of blood with oxygen. In this way the first step of oxygen supply of the tissues is improved. Apart from the general benefits, every training session also results in bronchodilatation.

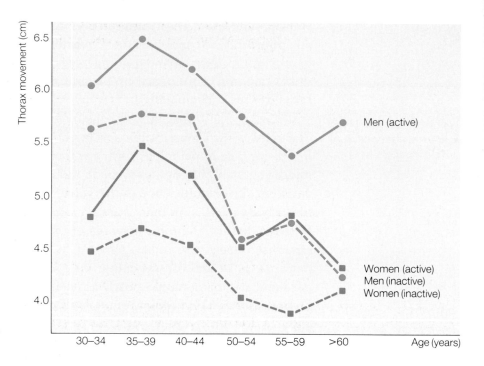

Fig. 9.2.2 Range of thorax movements in trained (2 h exercise per week on average) and untrained subjects (*n* = 864) aged from 30 to 60 years.

With progressive age the training of the respiratory system is particularly important because it makes the lungs more efficient. The typical chronic diseases of the respiratory tract can thus be prevented or their development delayed into later life, and if they do develop their consequences can be attenuated.

Figure 9.2.2 demonstrates the attenuation of the extensibility of the thorax in trained (2 hours sport per week) and untrained persons. The beneficial influence of training is obvious. As the degree of rigidity of the thorax is closely interrelated with the functional capacity of the respiratory system, the findings give evidence that exercise and training only twice per week for 1 hour improve respiratory functions significantly, particularly with advancing age.

Diabetes mellitus

Chronic diseases of metabolism are also widespread in old age. Physical activity has been recommended to diabetics for a long time as an effective measure in modifying the course of this disease. Exercise, undertaken according to medical recommendations, in addition to diet and medication is used in the treatment of diabetes.

Table 9.2.1 Mean values for fasting and 1-hour and 2-hour plasma insulin after an oral glucose tolerance test with 982 Helsinki policemen aged 35–64 years (Pyörälä *et al.*, 1985).

Physical activity class	*n*	Plasma insulin (μU/ml)		
		Fasting	1 hour	2 hour
Inactive	418	8.0	69.7	33.0
Slightly active	225	7.9	62.1	24.6
Active	270	7.0	54.7	23.7
Highly active	68	6.3	48.4	19.2

There is evidence that exercise also plays a role in the prevention of diabetes. Physical activity reduces the concentration of insulin in the serum (Table 9.2.1); trained people have an enhanced sensitivity of body tissues to insulin. Exercise and training stabilize the carbohydrate metabolism and in trained people glucose tolerance is improved (Fig. 9.2.3). Besides these effects, exercise also reduces some risk factors for the occurrence of diabetes (e.g. excessive weight). Of course, exercise-induced adaptations create no absolute protection against diabetes, but they can retard the manifestation, modify the course of the disease in a beneficial way, and moderate typical complications.

Arthrosis

Degeneration of the joints is often found in elderly people, and frequently the spine is markedly concerned. It is well documented that extreme physical loads can accelerate this event, while an adequate use of the joints and the acquisition of a good amount of strength by exercise and training may decelerate it. Adequate power training strengthens the joints and reduces diseases of the joints and the ensuing complaints. An atrophic musculature, typical for most old people, initiates a weakness of the joints. This atrophy is a consequence of disuse and affects the muscles as well as the bones (e.g. osteoporosis), cartilage, ligaments and sinews, and makes them susceptible to chronic disease. Degeneration in these areas of the body also reduces motility and thereby facilitates the progression of the degeneration. It is advisable to strengthen these tissues through adequate power exercise, which preserves and stabilizes the joints and protects them from premature degeneration and chronic

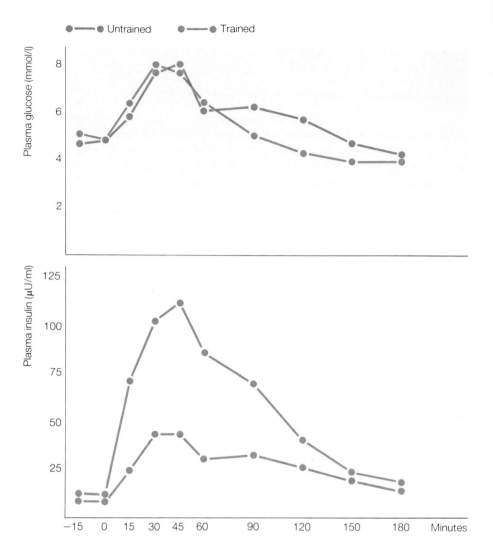

Fig. 9.2.3 Plasma glucose and insulin during an oral glucose tolerance test in trained and untrained subjects (Tremblay *et al.*, 1985).

disease; it is also a preventive measure for accidents and injuries particularly in elderly individuals.

Lower back pain and problems with the feet are frequently complained of by the elderly; spondylarthrosis is a chronic disease common in old age. The spine has more than 100 joints and its complicated construction has to counteract gravity all through one's life. An effective musculature of the body holds the spine and protects it from premature disorders, while a sedentary life-style leads to atrophy and promotes degeneration. It is necessary to improve the quality of the muscles of the trunk through an adequate and regular mild power training. This is a necessary prerequisite to reduce pain, even if there is no marked influence on the occurrence of spondylarthrosis. It is frequently found that alterations

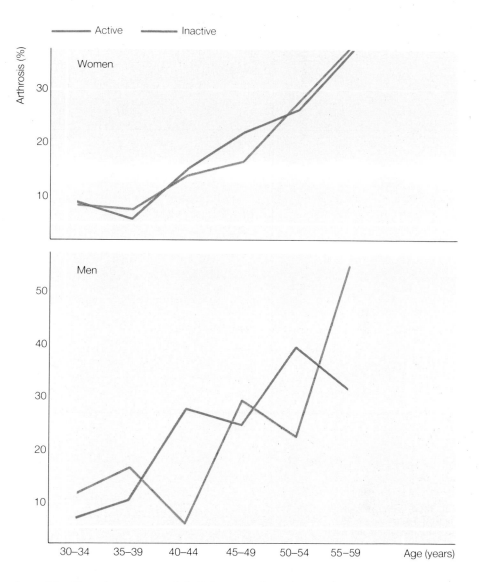

Fig. 9.2.4 Manifest arthrosis in active and inactive women and men aged from 30 to 60 years (*n* = 864).

found by X-raying are not felt if the muscles of the trunk are well adapted and developed.

Figures 9.2.4 and 9.2.5 demonstrate that arthrosis which becomes evident in clinical examinations is equally present in trained and untrained people, but absenteeism (absence from work based on a medical certificate) is significantly reduced in active elderly subjects.

Ageing is associated with a loss of flexibility of the spine; this situation is disadvantageous in everyday life and it impairs well-being. Exercises to promote flexibility are important for all joints, but it is essential not to exaggerate these exercises. It is a principle of training with old people that stability of a joint is more important than its range of flexibility.

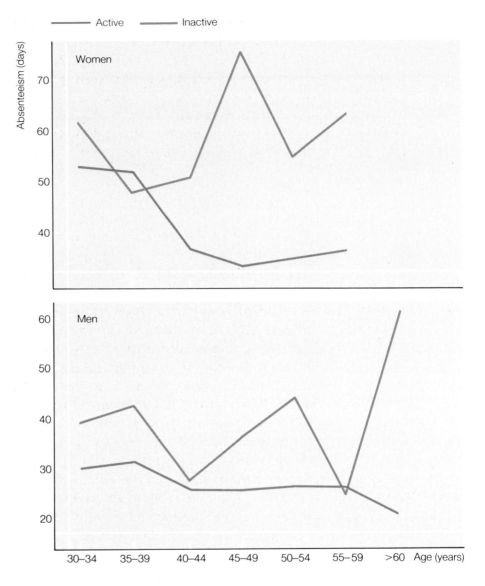

Fig. 9.2.5 Absenteeism (within 3 years before the investigation) in active and inactive women and men aged from 30 to 60 years ($n = 864$).

The feet, another refined construction which is adapted to the upright attitude of the human being, have to carry the weight of the body all through life. The majority of elderly individuals have disorders (deformation and arthrosis) in the skeleton of the feet, and a great part of these disorders cause pain when overloaded. There is also a carryover effect from the feet to the knees, hips and spine, and sometimes back pain has its origin in deformations of the feet. Exercise and training preserve an efficient musculature that protects the shape of the feet or reduces the symptoms associated with foot disorders. Furthermore it is dangerous for elderly people to lose their balance and to fall; strong foot musculature is a good prevention of injuries caused by falling. Short steps, which are typical in old people, are a visible expression of weak feet.

The muscles which determine the capabilities of the feet have an essential impact on the venous system of the lower extremities. Their activity very effectively supports the return of blood to the heart. This mechanism is important as chronic diseases of the veins are frequently found in elderly people. Callisthenics that strengthen the feet should be a medical recommendation to ageing individuals.

Psychological and mental disorders

The topic of ageing and chronic disease has substantial psychological (emotional) aspects. Physical activity elevates the concentration of endogenous opioids in the serum and in definite areas of the nervous system, and this reaction influences important physiological and psychological functions, e.g. alterations in mood, and an elevation of the threshold of pain perception. Physical activity is already used as a treatment for depression. Active people have fewer symptoms, and a high resistance to stress. They are less pessimistic about ageing, are more satisfied with life, tend to be less resigned, and existing chronic diseases are less seriously perceived. There is evidence that active people take significantly less medicines than inactive people do. Exercise-induced adaptations give further motivation for an active life-style and a vigorous age while, on the other hand, the experience of weakness has a contrary effect.

Experience and the results of experiments show that physical activity can improve cognitive functions in the elderly. Hormonal and nerval adaptations, an increased perfusion and oxygen supply to the brain, activation of cerebral metabolism, afferent impulses from the working musculature, etc. may be the causes of the observation that physical activity stimulates mental function.

Recommendations for practising sport

Exercise can be carried out at any age even if the subject suffers from a chronic disease. There are hardly any contraindications against exercise and training; but there are, of course, contraindications against certain methods, types and intensities of exercise. Elderly people with chronic diseases usually need an individual programme which considers their age, state of health, working capacity, tolerance for loads and personal capabilities and impairments. The principle of *primum nil nocere* and a certain safety margin should always be considered. High intensities should be avoided, and exercise should never be continued until a high degree of fatigue or exhaustion is reached. Every training session must begin with a warming-up session.

Exercise and training programmes for old people must take into account certain prerequisities in order to prevent injuries. Exercise must be avoided during acute disease, in extreme climatic conditions, if the patient is in a state of high psychological exitement, or has just eaten. If medicines are being taken, medical advice should be strictly regarded. Exercises should be mild, rhythmic, and short intervals for recovery allowed for. Movements that are common in everyday life are preferable. An elderly person with symptoms of chronic disease reacts slowly, and therefore abrupt movements, quick transitions from a low to high intensity, and sudden changes of position and rapid movements of the head should be avoided. Games which include physical contact with others, and complicated or risky coordinative techniques which demand a high degree of flexibility and jumping are not suitable for old people. The principle is always safety first; health first, then performance!

Exercise with more or less handicapped old people should take place only during daylight hours or in a well-lit room. It should be remembered that sense organs may be impaired, and that clothing should not hamper movements or become a source for accidents and injuries.

Many old people need to improve their technique of breathing, which can be achieved through orderly breathing, and special exercises involving deep in- and exhalation. During exercises which could be associated with a Valsalva manoeuvre, the advice to not stop breathing is necessary. Exercise which is combined with psychological excitation sometimes brings on hyperventilation which may become risky; in such cases it is important to ensure a calm atmosphere. The psychological guidance of old people who have little or no experience of exercise, is of great importance. In some cases it may be necessary to reassure the patient that the performance of the exercise is not dangerous.

Conclusion

The ageing process is often accompanied by chronic diseases; it is a process which favours the occurrence of chronic diseases, which in turn favour the advance of premature ageing. Habitual exercise is an effective means of breaking this interplay to a remarkable degree (Bortz, 1982; Harris, 1986; Sŭominen, 1986).

Evaluation of the ageing processes needs to consider former and present diseases. These are important to find an individual standard for physical performance capacity and physiological properties. Chronic diseases frequently produce scars, defects, instabilities, and disorders which result in premature degeneration in elderly subjects. Habitual exercise has a beneficial influence on the real ageing process by the prevention or correction of disease (and injuries). Exercise-induced adaptations occur predominantly in those areas of the body which determine to a high degree the morbidity of the population.

Weakness and susceptibility in old people are frequently more due to maladaptation and atrophy than ageing. According to the principle 'use it or lose it' the disuse of physiological functions may create more problems than chronic disease or ageing itself. Diseases act synergistically with ageing, and sometimes cause a dysharmonic ageing. Chronic diseases not only limit performance capacity, but often also reduce the range of movements and tolerance for loads. Diseases create atrophy and facilitate the further progress of ageing.

Chronic diseases usually have their onset in the early periods of life, and there is therefore a lot of time for intervention. A sedentary life-style carries a risk of early manifestation of numerous chronic diseases, and hypokinesia has been identified as an independent risk factor for the origin and progression of several widespread chronic diseases (Paffenbarger et al., 1984, 1986; Kannel & Eaker, 1986). Habitual exercise should start early in life, but even late beginners will benefit from regular training. Exercise-induced adaptations and fitness improve physical resistance in all age groups.

Exercise and training not only increase the physical working capacity, but also induce a broad complex of adaptations. Physical activity (catabolism) stimulates regeneration (anabolism) and this ability to make a quick recovery is very important. No doubt this situation also favours conditions which reduce susceptibility to disease. Habitual physical activity acts in two ways. It induces very complex protective adaptations, and usually supports a health-promoting life-style. It is an accepted fact that subjects who practice regular exercise reveal considerable advantages with respect to health stability. With increasing age the beneficial effects of exercise and training become even more evident.

A general explanation for a reduced susceptibility to disorders and diseases amongst active people as compared to inactive people is shown in Fig. 9.2.6. Environmental (or external) factors always interact with internal conditions of the subject, particularly the physical state, which depend to a high degree on the development of exercise-induced

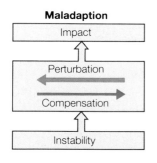

Maladaption

Impact

Perturbation

Compensation

Instability

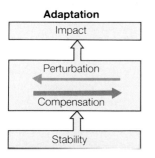

Adaptation

Impact

Perturbation

Compensation

Stability

Fig. 9.2.6 General response of the human body to the states of appropriate exercise-induced adaptation and maladaptation.

adaptations. A trained individual has adaptive reserves and a higher capacity to preserve the homeostasis and to compensate for negative influences.

Habitual exercise and training are no longer a privilege of youth. A good physical capacity, which can be acquired in all age groups, is an essential component of a low biological age and good health. Appropriate training increases physical safety, reduces susceptibility to acute and chronic disease and plays a role in the prevention of premature ageing processes. Exercise and training for elderly subjects are even more important than they are for young people. Ageing not only means degeneration, but also adaptation; regular exercise and training are an essential component in slowing premature ageing, they encourage an active improvement in health status, and on the basis of the mental and psychological adaptive effects provide a relatively optimistic experience of ageing. In old age people are frequently more impaired by immobility and maladaptation than by chronic disease.

The importance of health in the ageing process and the protective effects of exercise and training are no longer in doubt. The notion of 'being trained' has, particularly in connection with elderly subjects, a positive meaning. It leads not only to strength, efficiency and capability, but also to health and resistance.

References

Baum, K. V. (1971) Trainings-Pulsfrequenz: 170–Lebensalter. *Sportarzt Sportmed.* **22**, 20.

Bringmann, W. (1982) Die Beeinflussung der Borderline-Hypertonie mit unterschiedlichen sportlichen Belastungsprogrammen. *Med. Sport* **22**, 170.

Bortz, W. M. (1982) Disuse and ageing. *JAMA* **10**, 1203.

Harris, R. (1986) Aging, exercise and longevity. *Rev. Int. Council Sport Sci. Phys. Educ.* **9**, 56.

Hollmann, W., Rost, R. & Liesen, H. (1985) Die Bedeutung des Sports für das Herz des älteren Menschen. *Z. Kardiol.* **74**, 39.

Israel, S. (1985) Gesundheitsrisiko Sporttreibender mit chronisch-degenerativen Herz-Kreislauf-Erkrankungen. *Wiss. Z. DHfK.* **26**, 93.

Jokl, E. (1983) Physical activity and aging. *Ann. Sports Med.* **1**, 43.

Jokl, E. (1985) *Sudden Death of Athletes.* C. C. Thomas, Springfield.

Kannel, W. B. & Eaker, E. D. (1986) Psychosocial and other features of coronary heart disease: insights from the Framingham study. *Am. Heart J.* **112**, 1066.

Paffenbarger, R. S., Hyde, R. T., Wing, A. L. & Hsieh, C. C. (1986) Physical activity, all cause mortality, and longevity of college alumni. *New Engl. J. Med.* **314**, 605.

Paffenbarger, R. S., Hyde, R. T., Wing, A. L. & Steinmetz, Ch. H. (1984) A natural history of athleticism and cardiovascular health. *JAMA* **252**, 491.

Pyörälä, K., Savolainen, E., Kaukola, S. & Haapakoski, J. (1985) Plasma insulin as coronary heart disease risk factor: relationship to other risk factors and predictive value during 9½-year follow-up of the Helsinki policemen study population. *Acta Med. Scand.* (Suppl.) **701**, 38.

Sŭominen, H. (1986) Research problems in the relationship between physical activity and ageing. *Rev. Int. Council Sport Sci. Phys. Educ.* **9**, 25.

Tremblay, A., Fontaine, E. & Nadeau, A. (1985) Contribution of the exercise-induced increment in glucose storage to the increased insulin sensitivity of endurance athletes. *Eur. J. Appl. Physiol.* **54**, 231.

9.3 Osteoporosis in the elderly

Y. HAYASHI

Physical exercise and bone strengthening

It is well known that physical activities or sports are efficient in the prevention and treatment of osteoporosis. In studies done of astronauts, lack of mechanical stress against bone for only 4 days of flight increased the excretion of urinary calcium and decreased the density of their calcaneal bone on X-ray films (Mack & LaChance, 1967). However, it was also observed that systematic dynamic and isometric exercises done four times daily during 14 days of space flight inhibited the urinary calcium loss. Dalén and Olsson (1974) reported that the mineral content of various bones of cross-country runners (mean age 56.4 years) were higher than those of age- and body size-matched control subjects. Mean bone mineral content of cross-country runners, who had been practising the sport for at least 25 years, was 20% higher than found among the control subjects. This finding covered calcaneal bone as well as the humeral, distal radial, and ulnal bones. In the study of necropsies, ash weight of the third lumbar vertebral body was significantly correlated to the weight of the left psoas muscle; from this study it was proposed that the weight of muscles is an important determinant of bone mass (Doyle *et al.*, 1970).

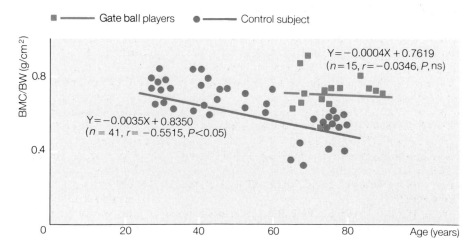

Fig. 9.3.1 Relationship between bone mineral content (BMC) of the left radius in 15 male gate ball players and 41 male control subjects.

Although numerous studies have confirmed that physical activities or mechanical stress against bone is efficient for the maintenance of bone mass, most studies have been performed on healthy middle-aged individuals. Recent studies have, however, confirmed that exercise or sports are also beneficial for the bones of old subjects with senile osteoporosis.

Physical exercise and bone mineral content

Figure 9.3.1 demonstrates the bone mineral content of gate ball (croquet) players in advanced age compared with a sedentary control group. The bone mineral contents of the gate ball players were significantly higher than those of the control subjects. Their values were not different from those of younger adult control subjects (ranging in age from 25 to 50 years). Changes in bone mineral content of eight players over 4 years are shown in Fig. 9.3.2. Although two inactive participants showed a decrease in their bone mineral contents during the 4 years, six players continuing regular exercise demonstrated a clear-cut efficacy in their bone mineral content, even in the elderly.

Several studies have indicated that regular exercise and training are an efficient means of increasing bone mineral content in every age group and particularly in the elderly. From these results, mild low-stress

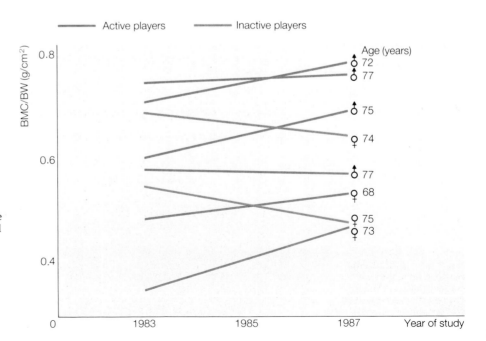

Fig. 9.3.2 Changes in bone mineral content of the distal third of the left radius in eight gate ball players during 4 years. Participants consisted of two inactive people without daily exercise and six active players involved in exercise on a regular basis.

exercise or sports which increase the mean heart rate to only 65% of the maximum heart rate (Miyake, 1987), are suitable to maintain or increase the bone mass without remarkable risks.

Habitual walking and osteoporosis

The beneficial effects of physical activity on the bone mineral content among old subjects can be demonstrated by the results of a study concerning 141 residents of a geriatric institution (mean age 76.8 ± 6.8 years). Participants were individually interviewed to establish their walking habits. Degree of curve and apex height of each participant's rounded back were estimated by projecting the upright posture on a large sheet of paper. The time taken to walk 10 m and the muscular strength of the quadriceps femoris muscle (measured by a spring scale) were evaluated as the parameters of physical capacity of the participants.

A summary of the relationships found between the various parameters are shown in Fig. 9.3.3. Habitual walking was negatively related to the degree of rounded back, which was indirectly related to the degree of osteoporosis through apex height of the rounded back or range of knee motion. Regular walking was also related to walking ability and muscular strength of the quadriceps femoris muscle. According to the scheme, the habit of walking was efficient in maintaining bone thickness, functions of the lower extremities and walking ability of the elderly.

Factors affecting femoral neck fracture

Several studies (e.g. Katsuno et al., 1986) have revealed the relationships between the degree of osteoporosis, data from medical examinations, physical performance capacity and personal information obtained by

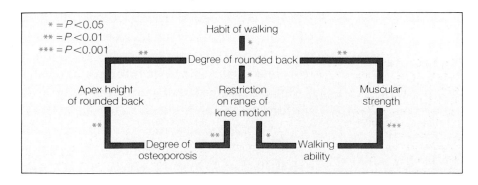

Fig. 9.3.3 Schematic presentation of the relationships between habit of walking, walking ability, functions of lower extremities and degree of osteoporosis in 141 aged residents of a geriatric institution.

Table 9.3.1 Comparison of various data of patients having an episode of femoral neck fracture with those of control subjects.

	Patients (n = 42)	Controls (n = 57)	X² or t-test
Background			
Age (years)	79.5 ± 9.8	79.8 ± 9.7	ns
Bodyweight (kg)	42.3 ± 6.4	45.9 ± 8.5	$P < 0.05$
Degree of osteoporosis			
Metacarpal index (%)	3.53 ± 0.43	3.78 ± 0.81	ns
Max. bone density	2.60 ± 0.35	2.75 ± 0.57	ns
Laboratory data			
Serum albumin (g/dl)	4.04 ± 0.94	4.65 ± 0.57	$P < 0.001$
Serum calcium (mg/dl)	8.51 ± 0.90	8.87 ± 1.00	$P < 0.1$
Physical assessment			
Standing on one leg:			
> 4 s	10	21	$P < 0.1$
≤ 4 s	4	11	
Personal information			
Milk intake (ml/day):			
≤ 200	20	36	$P < 0.1$
> 200	21	21	
Frequent falls:			
Yes	16	33	$P < 0.1$
No	23	24	

ns = not significant.

interviews. Physical capacity, for example, was obtained from the balance test of standing on one leg. Personal information included habits of meat and milk consumption and frequency of episodes of fall. The data of patients who had had an episode of femoral neck fracture within the past 3 years were compared with the data obtained from age- and sex-matched control subjects (Table 9.3.1).

Although no statistically significant differences were seen between the degree of osteoporosis (assessed by X-ray) of patients having an episode of femoral neck fracture compared to control subjects, there was a tendency for lower cortical thickness and lower bone density in the patients. According to medical records, bodyweight and serum albumin concentration of the patients were significantly lower than those of the control subjects. Higher tendencies of poor balance, smaller amounts of daily milk intake, and frequent episodes of fall were seen in the patients. It can be assumed that patients having an episode of femoral neck fracture tend to have a lower physical activity, lower ability of balance and poorer physical condition compared to control subjects.

Aloia *et al.* (1978) ascertained that postmenopausal women who exercised for 1 h three times weekly increased their total body calcium from 781 ± 95 g to 801 ± 118 g (s.d.). Their mean age was 53 ± 5.6 years. In contrast, control women who did not perform any regular exercises decreased their total body calcium from 824 ± 121 g to 804 ± 116 g in the same time period. Based on the literature, mild but regular physical activity of only a few hours per week increased the whole bone level of calcium.

It can therefore be considered as definite that habitual walking or mild exercise are effective in increasing or maintaining the bone quality of the elderly. Vigorous exercise or sports are not necessary to improve the bone strength, and these sports may even increase the chance of accidents and promote chronic degeneration of joints. Another benefit of habitual exercise for the elderly is the general improvement in quality of life. Furthermore, mild exercises can play an important role in the prevention and treatment of many problems common to the elderly, such as hypertension, obesity, coronary diseases, diabetes mellitus and depression (Israel *et al.*, 1982; Prokop & Bachl, 1984; Harris, 1986).

References

Aloia, J. F., Cohn, S. H., Ostuni, J. A., Cane, R. & Ellis, K. (1978) Prevention of involutional bone loss by exercise. *Ann. Int. Med.* **89**, 356.

Dalén, N. & Olsson, K. E. (1974) Bone mineral content and physical activity. *Acta Orthop. Scand.* **45**, 170.

Doyle, F., Brown, J. & Lachance, C. (1970) Relation between bone mass and muscle weight. *Lancet* **1**, 391.

Harris, R. (1986) Diagnostic and therapeutic aspects of physical exercise and sport in clinical health care of the aging. In B. D. McPherson (ed) *Sports and Aging*. Human Kinetics, Champaign.

Israel, S., Köhler, E., Ehrler, W. & Buhl, B. (1982) Die Trainierbarkeit in späteren Lebensabschnitten. *Med. Sport* **22**, 367.

Katsuno, M., Kanamori, M., Sato, R., Takaoka, M., Shinkai, S., Kondo, T., Kato, H., Satomi, H., Kubo, N., Hatano, S., Shitida, K. & Hayashi, Y. (1986) A case-control study of femoral neck fracture in aged Japanese women. *Jpn. J. Geriat.* **23**, 552.

Mack, P. B. & LaChance, P. A. (1967) Effect of recumbency and space flight on bone density. *Am. J. Clin. Nutr.* **20**, 1194.

Miyake, Y. (1987) Proper physical exercises of the elderly from the aspect of internal medicine. *J. Clin. Sports Med.* **4**, 1367.

Prokop, L. & Bachl, N. (1984) *Alterssportmedizin*. Springer, New York.

PART 10

PREVENTION AND MANAGEMENT OF SPORTS INJURIES

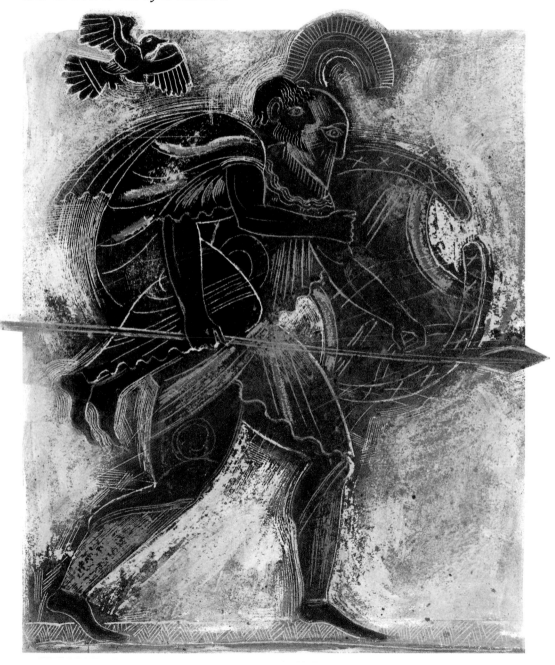

10.1 Causes of injuries

Extrinsic factors

B. NIGG

Introduction

Injury frequency has increased drastically over the last 100 years in parallel with the development of sports activities. Studies have been published analysing the occurrence of sports injuries (Krahl & Steinbrueck, 1980) and speculations have been made about possible factors that may influence the occurrence of these injuries (Segesser, 1970; Cavanagh, 1980; Roesler, 1980; Marcus, 1983; Falsetti *et al.*, 1983; Nigg, 1986; Kristoff & Ferris, 1987). When analysing these factors a model can be used, as illustrated in Fig. 10.1.1.

There are basically two main groups of factors that influence the occurrence and frequency of load and therefore the frequency of injuries: the movement and the boundary conditions. Movement includes external factors such as type of movement and velocity of movement, and internal factors such as muscle activity. The boundary conditions include external factors such as shoes, surfaces and equipment, and internal factors such as anthropometric factors, fitness levels and others. In this section the emphasis lies on the extrinsic factors, i.e. the factors acting externally to the human body.

If an athlete is jumping, running or performing any sports activity, he or she is subject to the forces listed in Fig. 10.1.1, which are possible sources of injuries and pain. The purpose of this section is to show how changes in these factors can influence the forces acting on the athlete's body and therefore can be the reason for possible injuries.

General points
Load
Load can be defined as the sum of all the forces and moments acting on a body. In this section the expression *external force* is used for forces which are acting externally to the athlete's body. The expression *internal force* is used for forces acting on an internal structure in the athlete's body. An internal structure can be a tendon, ligament, muscle, etc.

363

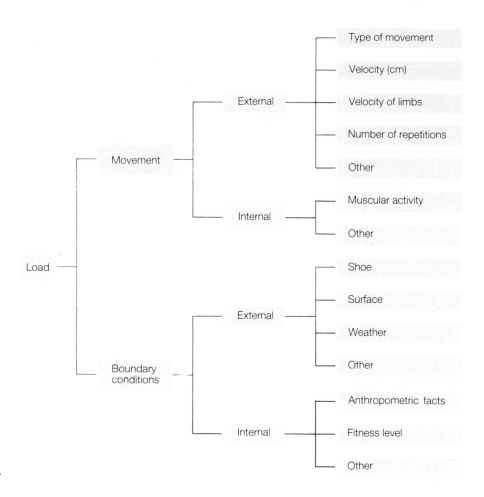

Fig. 10.1.1 Factors influencing load and stress.

Moment   If a force is acting with a certain lever arm this force may produce a rotation. The multiplication of the force times the lever arm is defined as moment. A diver who wants to jump a double somersault must therefore jump in a way that a moment acts at the initial stage of the jump in order to produce a rotation of the body with respect to the transversal axis.

Types of force   Depending on the loading rate, two types of forces are distinguished. *Impact forces* are forces which reach their maximum value earlier than 50 ms after first contact. Impact forces typically occur during landing (Cavanagh & Lafortune, 1980; Nigg & Denoth, 1980; Frederick *et al.*, 1984). Impact forces occur, for instance, when a car crashes into a concrete wall or when a foot lands on the take-off board in long jump. The foot is on the take-off board for about 100 ms and during the first 20–30 ms the force is an impact force. Impact forces occur immediately on landing in gymnastics, when two bodies crash in ice hockey during a

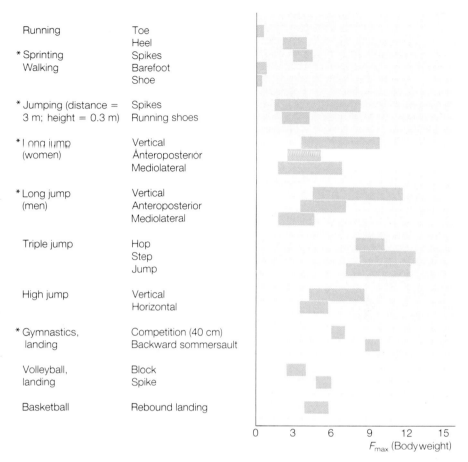

Fig. 10.1.2 Summary of experimentally determined maximum external impact forces at the ground. If nothing else is mentioned, the forces are measured in the vertical direction. Values with an asterisk are calculated from absolute force values reported in the literature with the assumption of a body mass of 70 kg for men and 60 kg for women. The results are summarized from data published by Nigg (1974); Ramey (1976); Baumann & Stucke (1980); Cavanagh & Lafortune (1980); Nigg et al. (1981); Frederick et al. (1984); Nigg (1985); Ramey (1985); Valiant & Cavanagh (1985); Wielki & Dangre (1985); Nigg et al. (1986); and B. M. Nigg (unpublished results).

check, in running, jumping and basically in all the movements where one part of the human body impacts the ground, equipment, partners, opponents or solid objects.

Active forces are forces which reach their maximum later than 50 ms after first contact (Clarke *et al.*, 1982, 1983; Nigg, 1983). Typical active forces occur during walking, during take-off for jumps and during most movements that are not connected with landing. They are forces which are produced by muscle activity together with gravity forces. If an athlete, for instance, stands on both feet, bends his or her knees and goes back into the upright position then all the forces that were responsible for these movements were active forces.

Magnitude of force   Load on the athlete's body is usually quantified by using force platforms (instruments that measure the forces exerted by an athlete), high speed video or film, instruments that allow the quantification of muscle

Fig. 10.1.3 Summary of maximum external active forces from experimental measurements. Values with an asterisk are calculated from absolute force values with the assumption of a body mass of 70 kg for men and 60 kg for women. Values with a triangle are values for which the expression 'active force' can only be used in a very loose sense. The results are summarized from data published by Miller & Nelson (1976); Sim & Chao (1978); Cavanagh & Lafortune (1980); Lafortune & Cavanagh (1980); Nigg (1980); Dessureault & Lafortune (1981); Saegesser *et al.* (1981); Adrian & Laughlin (1983); Asami & Nolte (1983); Clarke *et al.* (1983); Nigg (1983); Nissinen (1983); Frederick *et al.* (1984); Ekstrom (1985); and B. M. Nigg (unpublished data).

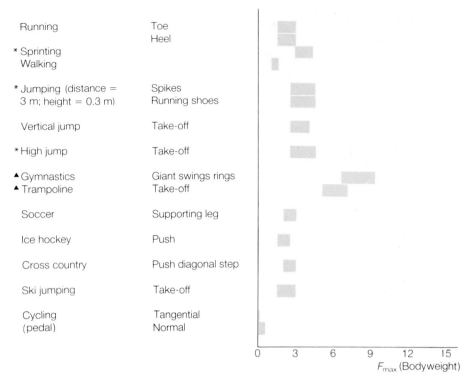

activity (EMG), accelerometers that allow the quantification of acceleration of a part of the human body and many other highly technological methods.

Figures 10.1.2–10.1.5 give an indication of the order of magnitude reported in the literature for external and internal impact and/or active forces. Different units are used in the literature to describe the magnitude of forces, in this example the unit 'bodyweight' is used. It is interesting to see that external, as well as internal forces, can easily reach ten times bodyweight, and it is surprising that some internal forces are commonly in that range. For instance, the forces in the ankle joint and the forces in tendon and muscles during running are reported to be about ten times bodyweight. However, external active forces are commonly lower than about five times bodyweight. The forces indicated for gymnastics and trampolining are forces produced due to centrifugal effects and in this sense different to active forces produced by muscle activity.

Once it is realized how large forces can be, it is not surprising that they may be the reason for injuries; it is possible that a reduction of forces may be connected to a reduction in injuries.

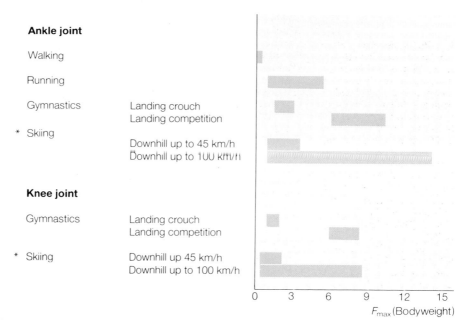

Fig. 10.1.4 Summary of maximum internal impact forces at an idealized ankle and knee joint. Values with two asterisks are calculated assuming an effective mass of 5 kg and a lower leg mass of 2 kg for the determination of internal impact forces (Nigg, 1980). The results are summarized from data published by Nigg (1980); Denoth & Nigg (1981); and B. M. Nigg (unpublished data).

Factors influencing forces

Type of movement

In order to understand the influence that movement may have on the magnitude of forces and the occurrence of injuries, movement can be subdivided into two categories: (a) a general category describing the overall movement; and (b) a category describing specific aspects of certain elements of the human body during movement.

In the general category, it is easily understood that different movements, such as standing, walking, running and sprinting, produce different forces on and in the human body. However, if a person wants to run at a particular time, the question is not whether to walk or to run; he or she wants to run at a certain speed for a particular reason. Another athlete may want to practice on the high bar in gymnastics, or another to play tennis. This means that the movement in a general sense is predetermined. However, there are other possibilities to change movement. In a specific sense, one can concentrate, for instance, on the foot. Again, taking the example of running one can run by landing on the heel or landing on the forefoot. In landing on the heel, the point of application of the ground reaction force and the line of action of the force are both behind the ankle joint. Therefore, the structures on the anterior part of the leg are loaded on first contact and the Achilles tendon is unloaded. Heel landing, therefore, can be used to unload the Achilles tendon. If a subject is running with toe landing, the point of application of the

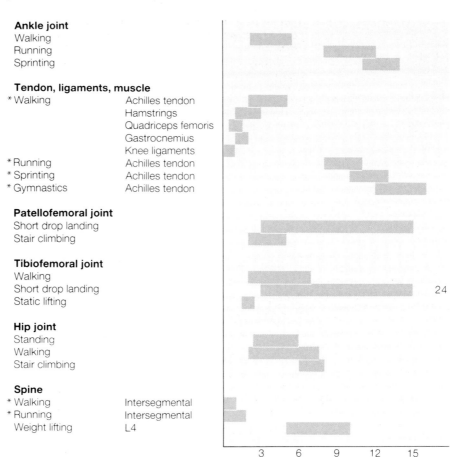

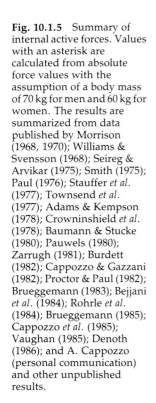

Fig. 10.1.5 Summary of internal active forces. Values with an asterisk are calculated from absolute force values with the assumption of a body mass of 70 kg for men and 60 kg for women. The results are summarized from data published by Morrison (1968, 1970); Williams & Svensson (1968); Seireg & Arvikar (1975); Smith (1975); Paul (1976); Stauffer et al. (1977); Townsend et al. (1977); Adams & Kempson (1978); Crowninshield et al. (1978); Baumann & Stucke (1980); Pauwels (1980); Zarrugh (1981); Burdett (1982); Cappozzo & Gazzani (1982); Proctor & Paul (1982); Brueggemann (1983); Bejjani et al. (1984); Rohrle et al. (1984); Brueggemann (1985); Cappozzo et al. (1985); Vaughan (1985); Denoth (1986); and A. Cappozzo (personal communication) and other unpublished results.

ground reaction force is on the forefoot. The line of action of the force is on the anterior part of the ankle joint which means that the posterior structures are loaded (Achilles tendon, gastrocnemius and soleus). Toe landing therefore unloads anterior structures and loads the posterior structures of the lower leg.

This example illustrates that in changing the movement, even in a relatively small way as illustrated with heel or toe landing, load and load distribution will be influenced and certain structures of the human body can be unloaded while other structures will be loaded. Movement in a general sense and technique of movement in a specific sense, can therefore be used to influence load acting on the locomotor system.

Velocity of movement   The velocity of movement is extremely important for the forces acting on the human body. Table 10.1.1 illustrates this in running; the data shows mean averages for 14 subjects running at different speeds landing on the

Table 10.1.1 Summary of vertical impact force peak values and vertical active force peak values for different running speeds in heel–toe running (mean and standard deviation for 14 subjects). Forces are measured in newtons (N).

Speed (m/s)	Impact force F_{zi} (N)	Active force F_{za} (N)
3	1.39 (0.20)	1.87 (0.16)
4	1.66 (0.29)	2.00 (0.21)
5	2.03 (0.43)	2.22 (0.31)
6	2.27 (0.48)	2.32 (0.43)

heel of the foot (heel–toe running). As the results in Table 10.1.1 show, the impact forces increase drastically from 3 to 6 m/s of running speed. The increase is about 64% from the lowest value at 3 m/s to the highest value at 6 m/s. At the same time the maximum vertical active forces, the ones that are responsible for the push-off phase, increase by about 24%. This example illustrates that the velocity of movement is important in increasing or decreasing the forces acting on the athlete's body.

Velocity of limbs
The influence of the velocity of movement is certainly connected with the influence of the velocity of limbs. If a person runs faster then that person probably lands differently with different parts of the body. As an example the vertical and the anteroposterior landing velocity of the heel in heel–toe running are illustrated in Table 10.1.2. The results show a significant increase in the vertical heel landing velocity between 3 and 6 m/s. However, there is no significant difference in the anteroposterior direction. This example illustrates that the human athlete tries to adjust his or her specific movement, in this case the movement of the heel just before landing, to the new situation. It also illustrates that change in the speed of movement may also change the speed of certain limbs and therefore have an influence on the forces acting on the athlete's body.

Number of repetitions
The influence of amount and rate of repetition of movement in various sports activities is well known from a cardiovascular point of view. The literature offers many suggestions for training: one, for instance, could be that an athlete should do about 10 min of activity at a heart rate frequency of 180 minus his or her age each day, another one may suggest 20 min at the same rate every second day. However, little is known about the number of repetitions and their effects with respect to load on the

Table 10.1.2 Summary of vertical and anteroposterior landing velocities of the heel for heel–toe running at different running speeds (mean and standard deviation for 42 subjects).

Speed (m/s)	Velocity, vertical v_{oz} (m/s)	Velocity, A–P v_{oy} (m/s)
3	0.8 (0.5)	2.0 (1.0)
4	1.1 (0.4)	2.6 (1.0)
5	1.6 (0.6)	2.8 (1.4)
6	1.9 (0.5)	2.3 (1.6)

athlete's body. Since this information is not available, some theoretical considerations are offered here.

In material science, the influence of repeated stress on a specific material is known. Steel, for instance, loses its particular resistance against bending during a repeated loading process. Dead human material may react in a similar way. However, in studying the effect of loading on the critical limits of living biological material there are two aspects to be discussed. One aspect is the direct mechanical influence on the structure, the second is the *in vivo* response of the biological material to the applied stress. It is the *in vivo* response mechanism which is of interest in this context; it may be positive or negative for the material. If the response effect is bigger than the mechanical fatigue effect the tissue is strengthened. However, if the response effect is smaller than the fatigue effect then bionegative results must be expected. It is known that cartilage and tendon material show a small and slow response to a stimulus because of low nutrition flow. Bone and muscles, however, show a higher and faster response. In order to estimate biopositive or bionegative effects of sports activities one should know more about the material properties of biomaterials. However, the impact of repetitive loading and fatigue problems with respect to load on the athlete's body is only in a very rudimentary stage of development. Despite this fact, every athlete and every coach knows that fatigue injuries occur frequently—which underlines the importance of this problem.

Surface One important factor with respect to load on the athlete's body and with respect to overload and injury problems, is the playing surface. During each contact of the foot with the ground, the ground acts on the foot with a ground reaction force and the foot acts on the ground with a force of the same magnitude but in an opposite direction. These forces during landing and take-off can be quite different on different surfaces. Playing volleyball on a sandy beach produces a different ground reaction force compared to playing volleyball on an asphalt court. Running on grass produces forces which look different to forces running on asphalt. The impact force (the force at first contact) is much higher for running on asphalt than for running on grass or sand. As a matter of fact, on sand those impact forces disappear completely. However, the active part of the ground reaction force remains about the same when comparing running on grass with running on asphalt. It is speculated that these high impact forces are one of the causes of many injuries in running as well as in other sports (Segesser, 1970; Hess & Hort, 1973; Hort, 1976; Light *et al.*, 1980; Segesser & Nigg, 1980).

Surfaces therefore can be selected specifically in order to reduce forces acting on the athlete's body. In many cases the athlete does not have a choice in the selection of the surface; it is therefore very important that people who are responsible in the development of sports facilities know the possibilities of reducing forces through the appropriate selection of sports surfaces.

An example of the influence of surfaces on the percentage of pain and injuries is illustrated in Fig. 10.1.6. The results are based on a study with subjects playing on different tennis surfaces. The surfaces used were: (a) clay-type surfaces; (b) synthetic surfaces with loose synthetic granules on top producing a similar effect to the clay surfaces in allowing some sliding; (c) synthetic surfaces; (d) a surface group including concrete and asphalt; (e) felt carpet surfaces mainly used for indoor tennis; and (f) synthetic grill surfaces used to cover concrete surfaces. More than

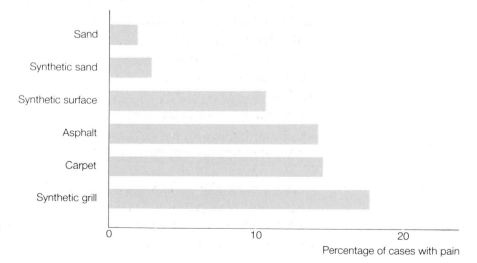

Fig. 10.1.6 Relative frequency of pain and injuries in tennis depending on the tennis surface. From Nigg & Denoth (1980).

Percentage of cases with pain

2000 cases were analysed, one case being a subject playing during a period of 6 months on one particular surface. The result illustrated in Fig. 10.1.6 shows that the frequency of cases with pain is significantly lower for the clay-type surfaces and the synthetic sand surfaces. These two surfaces have injury frequencies of about 2–3% while the other surfaces all have injury frequencies of more than 10%. Statistically there is a difference between the first two and the latter four surfaces. This example illustrates that the type of a surface used for sports activities has a dominant influence on the occurrence of injury, pain and discomfort. It is obvious in this case that a certain construction of a surface may drastically reduce the injury frequency by a factor of 4, 5 or 6.

Shoes If an athlete wants to train, the question is not whether he or she wants to walk or to run; the movement is usually given for the workout. The places available for such a workout are usually restricted to a limited number of possible surfaces. Movement and surface, therefore, can only be changed or adapted in a very limited way for an athlete in daily workout activities. It is therefore important to study the possibilities a sports shoe has to influence or to reduce load on the athlete's body.

Most research has been done in the last 15 years in the field of running shoes, and this has yielded three main conclusions: (a) a running shoe should absorb and/or reduce impact forces; (b) a running shoe should provide mediolateral stability avoiding excessive pronation; and (c) a running shoe should provide guidance at take-off avoiding oversupination of the foot. These conclusions are widely supported in the literature (Nigg et al., 1986), and can be applied and expanded to cover all sports activities.

In general, a sports shoe may influence and reduce load on the athlete's body if the aspect of *cushioning* is well under control. Furthermore, the shoe should provide *support* during stance and take-off, and finally the *friction* aspect of the shoe is of great importance. While these general aspects are widely acceptable, it is difficult to have detailed instructions for shoe requirements for specific sports. What cushioning is appropriate, for instance, in basketball? Is cushioning for basketball the same as cushioning for running? This will probably involve differences in shoe construction, but little research has been done for many sports. The same is true for friction and support aspects of the shoe. Friction is a particularly difficult consideration as, from a performance point of view, the athlete wants to have a lot of friction to make movement faster, but from an injury point of view friction should be reduced to reduce the forces acting on the athlete's body.

It is generally accepted that the shoe is one of the most important means to reduce forces acting on the athlete's body. More research has to be done to understand exactly how shoes should be constructed to really provide a reduction of forces and therefore adequate protection of the athlete.

Weather It seems obvious, but it should be mentioned in this context that the weather has an effect on injury frequency during sports activities. However, as before, we cannot usually influence this aspect and have to take it as a given factor. It is speculated that injury frequency is higher in cooler temperatures than in warmer temperatures, which means that an athlete should protect him or herself better in colder temperatures.

Conclusion

Various extrinsic factors can influence the load on the athlete's body. The most important are: movement, speed, number of repetitions, shoe and surface. It has been shown that the appropriate use of these factors can reduce the load and the injury frequency significantly.

References

Adams, D. & Kempson, G. E. (1978) Direct measurement of local pressures in the cadaveric human hip joint. *Med. Biol. Eng. Comput.* **16**, 113.

Adrian, M. J. & Laughlin, C. K. (1983) Magnitude of ground reaction forces while performing volleyball skills. In H. Matsui & K. Kobayashi (eds) *Biomechanics VIII-B*, pp. 903–914. Human Kinetics, Champaign.

Asami, T. & Nolte, V. (1983) Analysis of powerful ball kicking. In H. Matsui & K. Kobayashi (eds) *Biomechanics VIII-B*, pp. 695–700. Human Kinetics, Champaign.

Baumann, W. & Stucke, H. (1980) Sportspezifische Belastungen aus der Sicht der Biomechanik (Sport specific load from a biomechanical point of view). In H. Cotta, H. Krahl & K Steinbrueck (eds) *Die Belastungstoleranz des Bewegungsapparates*, pp. 55–64. Thieme-Verlag, Stuttgart.

Brueggemann, P. (1983) Kinematics and kinetics of the backward somersault take off from floor. In H. Matsui & K. Kobayashi (eds) *Biomechanics VIII-B*, pp. 793–800. Human Kinetics, Champaign.

Brueggemann, P. (1985) Mechanical load on the achilles tendon during rapid dynamic sport movements. In S. M. Perren & E. Schneider (eds) *Biomechanics: Current Interdisciplinary Research*, pp. 669–674. Martinus Nijhoff, The Hague.

Burdett, R. G. (1982) Forces predicted at the ankle during running. *Med. Sci. Sports Exerc.* **14**, 308.

Cappozzo, A., Felici, F., Figura, F. & Gazzani, F. (1985) Lumbar spine loading during half-squat exercises. *Med. Sci. Sports Exerc.* **17**, 613.

Cappozzo, A. & Gazzani, F. (1982) Spinal loading during abnormal walking. In R. Huiskes, D. Van Campen & J. de Wign (eds) *Biomechanics: Principles and Applications*, pp. 141–148. Martinus Nijhoff, The Hague.

Cavanagh, P. R. (1980) *The Running Shoe Book*. Anderson World Inc., Mountain View.

Cavanagh, P. R. & Lafortune, M. A. (1980) Ground reaction forces in distance running. *J. Biomech.* **13**, 397.

Clarke, T. E., Frederick, E. C. & Cooper, L. B. (1982)

The effects of shoe cushioning upon selected force and temporal parameters in running. *Med. Sci. Sports Exerc.* **14**, 144.

Clarke, T. E., Frederick, E. C. & Cooper, L. B. (1983) Biomechanical measurement of running shoe cushioning properties. In B. M. Nigg & B. A. Kerr (eds) *Biomechanical Aspects of Sport Shoes and Playing Surfaces*, pp. 25–33. University Printing, Calgary.

Crowninshield, R. D., Brand, R. A. & Johnston, R. C. (1978) The effects of walking velocity and age on hip kinematics and kinetics. *Clin. Orthop.* **132**, 140.

Denoth, J. (1986) Load on the locomotor system and modelling. In B. M. Nigg (ed) *Biomechanics of Running Shoes*, pp. 63–116. Human Kinetics, Champaign.

Denoth, J. & Nigg, B. M. (1981) The influence of various sport floors on the load on the lower extremities. In A. Morecki, K. Fidelus, K. Kedzior & A. Wit (eds) *Biomechanics VII-B*, pp. 100–105. University Park Press, Baltimore.

Dessureault, J. & Lafortune, M. A. (1981) Biomechanical features of two styles of highjumping. In A. Morecki, K. Fidelus, K. Kedzior & A. Wit (eds) *Biomechanics VII-B*, pp. 264–270. Human Kinetics, Champaign.

Ekstrom, H. (1985) The force interplay foot-binding-ski in X-country skiing. In *Proceedings of the 6th International Symposium on Ski Trauma and Skiing Safety, Naeba, Japan.*

Falsetti, H. L., Burke, E. R., Feld, R., Frederick, E. C. & Ratering, C. (1983) Hematological variations after endurance running with hard and soft soled running shoes. *Physician Sportsmed.* **11(8)**, 118.

Frederick, E. C., Clarke, T. E. & Hamill, C. L. (1984) The effect of running shoe design on shock attenuation. In E. C. Frederick (ed) *Sport Shoes and Playing Surfaces*, pp. 190–198. Human Kinetics, Champaign.

Hess, H. & Hort, W. (1973) Erhoehte Verletzungsgefahr beim Leichtathletiktraining auf Kunststoffboeden (Increased danger of injuries on artificial surfaces during training in track and field). *Sportarzt Sportmed.* **12**, 282.

Hort, W. (1976) Ursachen, Klinik, Therapie und Prophylaxe der Schaeden auf Leichtathletik Kunststoffbahnen (Origin, clinical treatment, therapy and prevention of injuries on artificial track and field surfaces). *Leistungssport* **1**, 48.

Krahl, H. & Steinbrueck, K. (1980) Traumatologie des sports. In H. Cotta, H. Krahl & K. Steinbrueck (eds) *Die Belastungstoleranz des Bewegungsapparates*, pp. 166–74. Thieme-Verlag, Stuttgart.

Krissoff, W. B. & Ferris, W. D. (1979) Runner's injuries. *Physician Sportsmed.* **7(12)**, 55.

Lafortune, M. A. & Cavanagh, P. R. (1980) Effectiveness and efficiency during bicycle riding. In H. Matsui & K. Kobayashi (eds) *Biomechanics VIII-B*, pp. 928–36. Human Kinetics, Champaign.

Light, L. H., McLellan, G. E. & Klenerman, L. (1980) Skeletal transients on heel strike in normal walking with different footwear. *J. Biomech.* **13**, 477.

Marcus, B. (1983) *The influence of footwear and surfaces on performance and injury potential in running.* Ph.D. Thesis, Imperial College, University of London.

Miller, D. I. & Nelson, R. C. (1976). *Biomechanics of Sport.* Lea & Febiger, Philadelphia.

Morrison, J. B. (1968) Bioengineering analysis of force actions transmitted by the knee joint. *Biomed. Eng.* **4**, 164.

Morrison, J. B. (1970) The mechanics of the knee joint in relation to normal walking. *J. Biomech.* **3**, 51.

Nigg, B. M. (1974) *Sprung, Springen, Spruenge* (Jump, jumping, jumps). Juris-Verlag, Zurich.

Nigg, B. M. (1980) Biomechanische Ueberlegungen zur Belastung des Bewegungsapparates (Biomechanical considerations on the loading of the musculo-skeletal system). In H. Cotta, H. Krahl & K. Steinbrueck (eds) *Die Belastungstoleranz des Bewegungsapparates*, pp. 44–54. Thieme-Verlag, Stuttgart.

Nigg, B. M. (1983) External force measurement with sport shoes and playing surfaces. In B. M. Nigg & B. A. Kerr (eds) *Biomechanical Aspects of Sport Shoes and Playing Surfaces*, pp. 11–23. University Printing, Calgary.

Nigg, B. M. (1985) Loads in selected sports activities. In D. Winter, R. Norman, R. Wells, K. Hayes & A. Patla (eds) *Biomechanics IX-B*, pp. 91–6. Human Kinetics, Champaign.

Nigg, B. M. (1986) Biomechanical aspects of running. In B. M. Nigg (ed) *Biomechanics of Running Shoes*, pp. 1–26. Human Kinetics, Champaign.

Nigg, B. M., Bahlsen, A. H., Denoth, J., Luethi, S. M. & Stacoff, A. (1986) Factors influencing kinetic and kinematic variables in running. In B. M. Nigg (ed) *Biomechanics of Running Shoes*, pp. 139–59. Human Kinetics, Champaign.

Nigg, B. M. & Denoth, J. (1980) *Sportplatzbelaege* (Playing surfaces). Juris-Verlag, Zurich.

Nigg, B. M., Denoth, J. & Unold, E. (1981) Die Belastung des menschlichen Bewegungsapparates bei ausgewaehlten Bewegungen im Kunstturnen (Load on the locomotor system in selected movements in gymnastics). *Leistungssport* **2**, 93.

Nissinen, M. A. (1983) Kinematic and kinetic analysis of giant swing on rings. In H. Matsui & K. Kobayashi (eds) *Biomechanics VIII-B*, pp. 781–6. Human Kinetics, Champaign.

Paul, J. P. (1976) Approaches to design: force actions transmitted by joints in the human body. *Proc. R. Soc. Lond. B.* **192**, 163.

Pauwels, F. (1980) *Biomechanics of the Locomotor Apparatus*. Springer-Verlag, Berlin

Procter, P. & Paul, J. P. (1982) Ankle joint biomechanics. *J. Biomech.* **15(9)**, 627.

Ramey, M. R. (1976) Analysis of the somersault long jump. *Res. Quart.* **47**, 167.

Ramey, M. R. (1985) Ground reaction forces in the triple jump. *Int. J. Sport Biomech.* **1(3)**, 233.

Roesler, H. (1980) Biomechanische Abschaetzung der Belastung von Achillessehnen bei Spruengen (Biomechanical estimation of the forces in the achilles tendon during jumps). In H. Cotta, H. Krahl & K. Steinbrueck (eds) *Die Belastungstoleranz des Bewegungsapparates*, pp. 72–80. Thieme-Verlag, Stuttgart.

Saegesser, A., Neukomm, P., Nigg, B. M., Ruegg, P. & Troxler, G. (1981) Forces measuring system for the take off in ski jumping. In A. Morecki, K. Fidelus, K. Kedzior & A. Wit (eds) *Biomechanics VII-B*, pp. 478–82. University Park Press, Baltimore.

Segesser, B. (1970) Sportschaeden durch ungeeignete Boeden in Sportanlagen (Sport injuries as a consequence of unsuitable surfaces). *Arztdienst.* ETS Magglingen.

Segesser, B. & Nigg, B. M. (1980) Insertionstendinosen am Schienbein, Achillodynie und Ueberlastungsfolgen am Fuss-Aetiologie, Biomechanik, therapeutische Moeglichkeiten (Tibial insertion tendinoses, achillodynia and damage to overuse of the foot-etiology, biomechanics, therapy). *Orthopaede* **9**, 207.

Seireg, A. & Arvikar, R. J. (1975) The prediction of muscular load sharing and joint forces in the lower extremities during walking. *J. Biomech.* **8**, 89.

Sim, F. H. & Chao, E. Y. (1978) Injury potential in modern ice hockey. *Am. J. Sports Med.* **6(6)**, 378.

Smith, A. J. (1975) Estimates of muscle and joint forces at the knee and ankle during a jumping activity. *J. Movement Studies* **1**, 78.

Stauffer, R. N., Chao, E. Y. S. & Brewster, R. C. (1977) Force and motion analysis of the normal, diseased and prosthetic ankle joint. *Clin. Orthop. Rel. Res.* **127**, 189.

Townsend, P. R., Rose, R. M., Radin, E. L. & Raux, P. (1977) The biomechanics of the human patella and its implications for chondromalacia. *J. Biomech.* **10**, 403.

Valiant, G. A. & Cavanagh, P. R. (1985) A study of landing from a jump. In D. Winter, R. Norman, R. Wells, K. Hayes & A. Patla (eds) *Biomechanics XI-B*, pp. 117–22. Human Kinetics, Champaign.

Vaughan, A. L. (1985) Biomechanics of running gait. *CRC Crit. Rev. Biomed. Eng.* **6**, 1.

Wielki, Cz. & Dangre, M. (1985) Analysis of jump during the spike of volleyball. In D. Winter, R. Norman, R. Wells, K. Hayes & A. Patla (eds) *Biomechanics IX-B*, pp. 438–42. Human Kinetics, Champaign.

Williams, J. F. & Svensson, N. L. (1968) A force analysis of the hip joint. *Biomed. Eng.* **4**, 265.

Zarrugh, M. Y. (1981) Kinematic prediction of intersegment loads and power at the joints of the leg in walking. *J. Biomech.* **14(10)**, 713.

Further reading

Bejjani, F. J., Gross, C. M. & Pugh, J. W. (1984) Model for static lifting: relationship of loads on the spine and the knee. *J. Biomech.* **17(4)**, 281.

Rohrle, H., Scholten, R., Sigolotto, C., Sollbach, W. & Kellner, H. (1984) Joint forces in the human pelvis-leg skeleton during walking. *J. Biomech.* **17(6)**, 409.

Intrinsic factors

R. LORENZTON

Introduction

Table 10.1.3 Intrinsic factors in overuse injuries in sports.

Malalignment
  Foot hyperpronation
  Pes planus
  Pes cavus
  Forefoot varus
  Hindfoot varus
  Tibia vara
  Genu valgum
  Genu varum
  Patella alta
  Femoral neck anteversion
Leg length discrepancy
Muscle weakness/imbalance
Decreased flexibility
Sex, body size and body composition

Any injury can be caused by intrinsic or extrinsic factors, either alone or in combination. In overuse injuries an interplay between the two categories is probable. In a recent study of injuries in runners, intrinsic factors were found to be involved in 40% of cases, being the only demonstrable factor in 10% (Lysholm & Wiklander, 1987). Important intrinsic factors that have been proposed to be involved in the development of overuse injuries include alignment abnormalities, leg length discrepancy, muscle weakness, muscle imbalance and decreased flexibility (Table 10.1.3). In general, it should be stressed that this area is highly conjectural and that many plausible hypotheses at present lack substantiating evidence. Prospective, controlled studies are certainly warranted to allow more definite conclusions about the relative importance of intrinsic factors, if any, in the development of different overuse injuries in athletes. These general remarks should be kept in mind when reading the following text.

Malalignment

Abnormalities of the foot

Conditions associated with hyperpronation

Frank biomechanical alterations of the foot may be present which, in combination with intense training, create excessive or unusual stress on various structures of the entire lower extremity. In running, one of the most critical biomechanical points is the amount and timing of

Hyperpronation   Normal

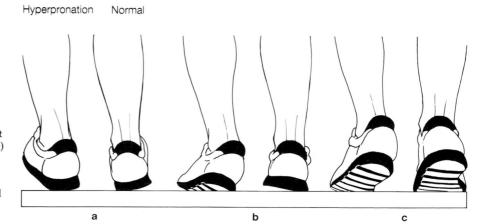

Fig. 10.1.7 The normal left foot (right part of the figure) during heel strike (a), support phase (b) and heel rise (c). The left part of the figure, shows excessive and prolonged pronation of the left foot.

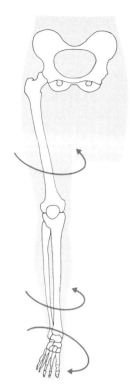

Fig. 10.1.8 Pronation of the foot is associated with an obligatory internal rotation of the tibia and femur.

Table 10.1.4 Situations where increased or prolonged pronation occurs.

Pes planus

Forefoot varus

Weakness of the gastrocnemius–soleus musculature

Tightness of triceps surae (functional ankle joint equinus)

Leg length discrepancy

inversion and eversion of the subtalar joint during a stride (Marshall, 1978).

Running biomechanics has been studied extensively: at foot strike, initial contact is made with the lateral aspect of the shoe and the foot is in a supinated position with the tibia externally rotated (Fig. 10.1.7). Immediately after foot strike, the foot is loaded, pronation of the subtalar joint occurs, being maximal at about 40% of the support (stance) phase. Pronation is a normal occurrence allowing adaptation to the running surface by unlocking the midtarsal joint and making the foot more flexible. The amount of pronation of the foot during the early support phase is subject to extreme individual variation (Mann, 1986). At pronation of the subtalar joint there is an obligatory internal rotation of the tibia and the femur (Fig. 10.1.8). Just after the swinging leg passes the stance leg, the femur and tibia rotate externally causing a return to supination of the subtalar joint and locking (stabilization) of the transverse tarsal joint. This results in a fairly rigid forefoot. The foot must not remain pronated during heel rise, when normally an almost instantaneous inversion of the heel should occur (Mann, 1986). The constraints of pronation are the shape of the subtalar joint and the ligamentous support, and to a lesser degree the support of intrinsic and extrinsic muscles (Mann *et al.*, 1981).

Excessive or prolonged pronation during the support phase creates increased or unusual stress on the structures of the foot, and also on the extrinsic muscles.

Excessive or prolonged pronation may occur due to anatomic reasons (pes planus, forefoot varus) or weakness of the gastrocnemius–soleus musculature or tightness of the triceps surae muscle with a functional ankle joint equinus (Table 10.1.4). It may also occur as a compensatory mechanism in leg length discrepancy. In a group of athletes with lower extremity problems, pronation of the foot in a static weight bearing position was found in 58% of the cases (James *et al.*, 1978), but no single anatomical variation correlated with any specific diagnosis. In clinical practice, it is often not easy to determine the amount of pronation—and it requires a lot of experience to do so. Treadmill running with bare feet and high-velocity filming are accurate but seldom accessible methods for correct diagnosis. In practice, valuable information is gathered by inspecting the wear pattern of the shoe (Fig. 10.1.9). Wear of the medial side of the outsole strongly suggests hyperpronation, but wear on the outer (lateral) side of the heel may occasionally also be seen in overpronation.

Normal biomechanical events in the foot during the running cycle require proper alignment of the forefoot–heel as well as the leg–heel.

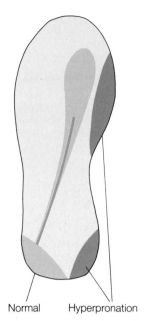

Normal   Hyperpronation

Fig. 10.1.9 In hyper-pronation, the wear of the shoe is most pronounced on the medial side of the outsole, while the normal wear is concentrated in the lateral aspect of the heel.

With the subtalar joint in the neutral position, the plane of the forefoot parallel to the metatarsals is perpendicular to the long axis of the calcaneus (Torg *et al.*, 1987). Leg–heel alignment is present when the subtalar joint is in the neutral position and the heel is parallel to the distal third of the leg (Torg *et al.*, 1987). Determination of the relationship of the hindfoot to the forefoot can be carried out either with the patient sitting on the examining table with the knee flexed at 90° and the foot in the air, or with the patient prone on the table and the knee flexed at 90° (Mann, 1986). The talonavicular is manipulated to its neutral position and the plane of the forefoot in relation to the long axis of the calcaneus is determined. Forefoot varus is present when the plane of the metatarsals is supinated, i.e. the medial side of the forefoot is above the neutral plane (Fig. 10.1.10). In forefoot valgus, the plane of the metatarsals is pronated, i.e. the medial side of the forefoot is below the neutral plane.

In an individual with a marked forefoot varus and a neutral position of the hindfoot, there is a compensatory hyperpronation and rotation of the calcaneus into an everted position during the early stance phase. In runners, this may cause pain along the medial side of the foot or ankle (Mann, 1986). The eversion of the heel may also constitute the underlying cause in other clinical problems of the lower extremity in runners (see below).

By configuration of the longitudinal arch, the foot can be classified into normal, pes planus (flat foot), and pes cavus (high arched) (Fig. 10.1.11).

According to Mann (1986) there are at least two categories of pes planus, one of which is characterized only by a depressed longitudinal arch without eversion of the heel. This complicating factor is also seen in the other category of pes planus (Fig. 10.1.12) in which there is angulation

Fig. 10.1.10 In forefoot varus, the plane of the metatarsals is supinated (b). In forefoot valgus it is pronated (c) compared to the neutral position (a).

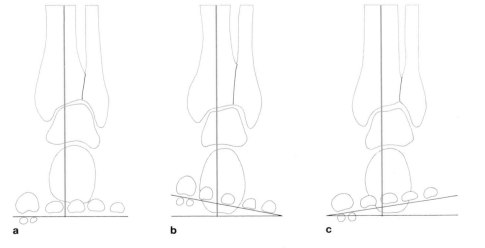

a   b   c

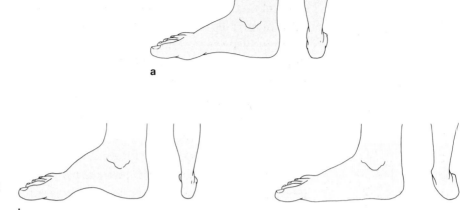

Fig. 10.1.11 By configuration of the longitudinal arch, the foot can be classified into normal (a), pes cavus (b) and pes planus (c).

Table 10.1.5 Increased or prolonged pronation—proposed overuse injuries.

Medial tibial stress syndrome (shin splints)

Posterior tibialis tendinitis

Achilles tendinitis

Iliotibial band friction syndrome

Patellofemoral pain syndrome

Plantar fasciitis

Stress fractures

of the Achilles tendon on weight bearing. Runners with pes planus feet suffer from injuries attributed to excessive motion at the subtalar joint, i.e. hyperpronation (McKenzie *et al.*, 1985).

A number of common running injuries that have been proposed to be associated with increased pronation are listed in Table 10.1.5.

In 35 male athletes with medial tibial stress syndrome, Viitasalo and Kvist (1983) found significantly greater passive mobility values of the subtalar joint in inversion, eversion, and their sum than in the control group of 13 male athletes without known foot problems. While running, the Achilles tendon angle in the medial tibial stress syndrome was significantly greater at heel strike, most probably suggesting greater pronation of the subtalar joint. There were also indications of prolonged pronation time. Their results suggested structural and functional

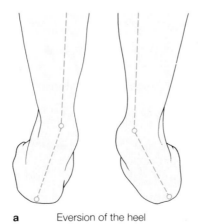

Fig. 10.1.12 Eversion of the heel is seen as a complicating factor in one category of pes planus (a). There is also another category without heel eversion (b).

a Eversion of the heel

b Normal

differences in the foot and ankles between healthy athletes and those with medial tibial stress syndrome.

It has recently been proposed that the medial tibial stress syndrome is not secondary to posterior tibial muscle pathology, but a result of stress changes at the origin of the soleus muscle and its enveloping fascia (Michael & Holder, 1985), particularly when the heel is in the pronated position. In this study, the torsion of the Achilles tendon (White, 1943) and also the medial insertion of the soleus on the calcaneus (Cummins *et al.*, 1946) were confirmed (Fig. 10.1.13). Biomechanically, this twisted course of the soleus muscle should make it vulnerable to excessive elongation associated with pronation of the foot (Michael & Holder, 1985). This concept of the aetiology of the medial tibial stress syndrome is also in line with the previously cited study by Viitasalo and Kvist (1983) in which athletes with medial tibial stress syndrome were found to have greater pronation of the subtalar joint.

From a biomechanical standpoint, the soleus part of the Achilles tendon is, of course, subjected to the same stress mechanisms during hyperpronation as described above for the soleus muscle in the medial tibial stress syndrome. The whipping action or bowstring effect of the Achilles tendon during hyperpronation (Fig. 10.1.13) has been suggested as a causative factor in the development of Achilles tendinitis (Clement *et al.*, 1984) by contributing to microtears in the tendon. In that study, 56% of 109 runners with Achilles tendinitis displayed functional overpronation. Some anatomic abnormalities proposed to be associated with Achilles tendinitis are listed in Table 10.1.6.

Excessive pronation is associated with increased and prolonged internal rotation of the tibia which causes the insertion site of the iliotibial tract to be drawn anteromedially, and therefore tighter across the lateral femoral epicondyle. In this way, excessive frictional irritation of the tract, the underlying bursa and the periosteum is suggested to occur, i.e. the iliotibial band friction syndrome develops (Taunton & Clement, 1981). Abnormal pronation with excessive internal rotation of the entire leg has also been proposed as a contributing factor to the development of patellofemoral pain syndrome by causing lateral displacement of the patella (Andrews, 1983).

Plantar fasciitis can be caused either by abnormal pronation or supination (Torg *et al.*, 1987). In pes planus with excessive pronation, the plantar aponeurosis is subjected to repetitive stretch resulting in fascial strain.

Biomechanical alterations may also constitute contributory factors in the development of stress reactions and stress fractures (Torg *et al.*,

Table 10.1.6 Anatomic factors contributing to Achilles tendon disease (Singer & Jones, 1986).

Excessive pronation

Hindfoot varus

Forefoot varus

Tight heel cords

Tibia vara

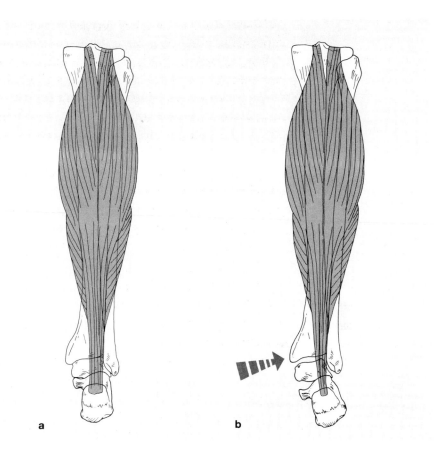

Fig. 10.1.13 There is a torsion of the Achilles tendon with a medial insertion of the soleus on the calcaneus (a). During hyperpronation (b), a whipping action of the tendon occurs.

a   b

1987). Supination is said to be involved in tibial stress fractures and pronation in fibular stress fractures.

Cavus foot Athletes with a cavus foot (Fig. 10.1.11) constitute a minority in the running population. These individuals have a rigid foot with decreased motion of the subtalar joint with subsequent decreased internal rotation of the tibia. After foot strike, the heel remains in varus, the longitudinal arch is maintained, and the midtarsal joint does not unlock (Lutter, 1981). During the midstance phase of running, the foot remains rigid resulting in a decreased ability to adapt to the underlying surface and it therefore absorbs the force of ground contact. The cavus foot is often combined with a tight triceps surae muscle.

The decreased or absent internal rotation of the tibia has been proposed to result in tightening of the structures of the lateral aspect of the knee (Lutter, 1981). In pes cavus, the plantar aponeurosis is tight. The

windlass effect is therefore pronounced and there is strain on the calcaneal insertion (Torg *et al.*, 1987), possibly resulting in plantar fasciitis.

The decreased ability of the cavus foot to absorb the force of ground
contact, and the relatively frequent occurrence of concomitant tightness
of the triceps surae have associated cavus feet with the development of
Achilles tendinitis. In the study by Clement *et al.* (1984), only six out of
109 runners with Achilles tendinitis had cavus feet. The decreased
shock-absorbing ability has also imputed it in the development of stress
fractures (McKenzie *et al.*, 1985), although without presenting any
substantiating data.

Abnormalities of the knee, tibia and femur

Malalignment of the lower extremity may cause altered knee mechanics
and is a common cause of anterior and peripatellar knee pain, particularly in the athletically active individual (Carson, 1985). The Q-angle is a
clinical measure obtained by connecting the central point of the patella
with the anterior superior iliac spine above and the tibial tuberosity
below (Fig. 10.1.14). When measured with relaxed quadriceps, normal
values of the angle are less than 15° in men and less than 20° in women
(Insall *et al.*, 1976). Smaller angles are obtained when measuring with
contracted quadriceps (Hughston *et al.*, 1984). The standing alignment of
the extremity is such that the width of the pelvis creates a valgus vector
(Fig. 10.1.14) resulting in a tendency for the patella to shift laterally (Fox,

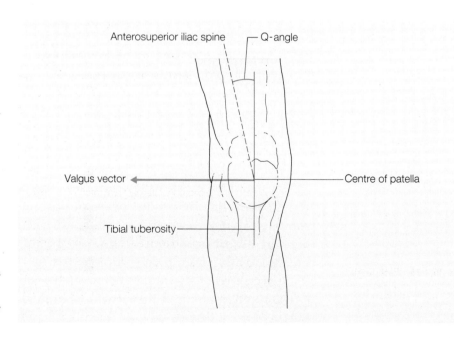

Fig. 10.1.14 An increase in the Q-angle will result in excessive lateral tracking of the patella by increasing the valgus vector.

Table 10.1.7 Cavus foot—proposed overuse injuries.

Achilles tendinitis
Plantar fasciitis
Stress fractures

1975). Disorders of the patellofemoral joint are more often present in females. Some women may show a wide pelvis and a high Q-angle and there may also be excessive internal rotation of the femur with secondary external tibial torsion and hyperpronation of the feet. In runners this was previously described as the miserable malalignment syndrome (James *et al.*, 1978), often being associated with patellofemoral problems.

A genu valgum deformity will effectively increase the Q-angle, and thereby the lateral tracking (valgus) vector of the patella which predisposes the patella to lateral displacement, particularly when a forceful quadriceps contraction occurs (Table 10.1.7). This may be associated with patellofemoral arthalgia, excess lateral pressure syndrome (Ficat & Hungerford, 1977) or subluxation–dislocation of the patella (Larson, 1979) (Table 10.1.8). However, it should be noted that the resultant effect of such malalignment may be evident only over a period of time or following an injury (Ficat & Hungerford, 1977). Therefore, an alignment abnormality alone may not produce lateral tracking symptoms (Grana & Kriegshauser, 1985).

Rotational malalignment can be detected by noting the position of the patella with the feet straight ahead. In 'squinting' patellae, both patellae point inwards in a medial fashion. This can be due to excessive femoral anteversion or increased femoral torsion (Larson, 1979) leading to a compensatory outward rotation of the tibia resulting in an increased Q-angle and patellofemoral disorders.

Table 10.1.8 Alignment abnormalities associated with increased Q-angle of the knee.

Genu valgum
Femoral neck anteversion
External tibial torsion

Genu varum or tibia vara may be associated with peripatellar pain due

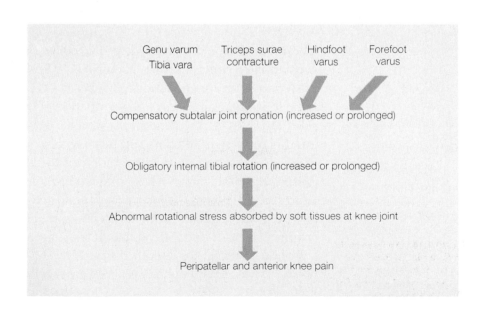

Fig. 10.1.15 Pathologic conditions frequently associated with patello-femoral disorders (Henry, 1986).

Table 10.1.9 Alignment abnormalities associated with patellofemoral arthalgia.

Genu valgum

Femoral neck anteversion

Genu varum

Tibia vara

Patella alta

to excessive subtalar pronation and obligatory internal rotation of the tibia that is required to produce a plantigrade foot (Larson, 1979) (Table 10.1.9). The increased amount of rotatory stress during hyperpronation is absorbed through the peripatellar soft tissues at the knee joint (James *et al.*, 1978) (Fig. 10.1.15). Accordingly, in patients with patellofemoral pain it is important to examine the entire lower extremity in the standing position, and not only concentrate on the knee (Carson, 1985). Genu varum is also considered as a predisposing factor in the development of iliotibial band friction syndrome (Jones & James, 1987).

In high-riding patella, patella alta, there is lateral tracking of the patella since the patella does not seat in the trochlear groove of the femur during early flexion and then continues to ride over the lateral femoral condyle (Grana & Kriegshauser, 1985). The presence of patella alta has been linked to recurrent dislocation of the patella (Insall *et al.*, 1972) and to patellofemoral arthalgia, but may be present without symptoms.

Leg length discrepancies

The detrimental effect of smaller leg length discrepancies has been a matter of controversy for decades. The traditional orthopaedic view is that discrepancies of less than 20 mm are mostly cosmetic (Friberg, 1983).

Many biomechanical alterations have been proposed to occur as a result of leg length discrepancy (Table 10.1.10). The leg length inequality is accompanied by a pelvic tilt to the short side, which in turn is associated with a compensatory lumbar scoliosis with the convexity toward the short leg side (Fig. 10.1.16) and compression of the intervertebral disc on the concave side of the curve (Friberg, 1983). Other less substantiated compensatory changes include: (a) increased abduction of the femur of the longer leg side; (b) smaller weight bearing surface of the same hip joint; and (c) increased pronation of the foot (on the long *or* the short leg side) during running, associated with an obligatory excessive internal rotation of the tibia and possibly also secondary increased knee valgus. In addition, outward rotation of the shorter leg has been suggested as another compensatory mechanism which might detrimentally affect the function of the hip rotator or adductor muscles. On the whole, however, there seems to be no definite consistency in the adaptive changes of the body to inequality of leg length.

In non-athletes, leg length discrepancy has been associated with a normal (Hult, 1954; Bevins *et al.*, 1985), as well as an increased (Nichols, 1960; Friberg, 1983), incidence of low back pain (Table 10.1.11). Leg

Table 10.1.10 Leg length discrepancy—proposed compensatory alterations.

Pelvic tilt to the short side

Functional lumbar scoliosis

Increased abduction of the hip (longer leg)

Excessive pronation of the foot (longer *or* shorter side)

Secondary increased knee valgus

Outward rotation of the leg

Table 10.1.11 Leg length discrepancy—proposed clinical significance.

Low back pain

Osteoarthritis of hip

Trochanteric bursitis

Iliotibial tract friction syndrome

Stress fractures

length discrepancy has also been proposed to be a causative factor in the development of osteoarthritis of the hip on the longer side (Gofton & Trueman, 1971). In athletes subjected to increased force loads and stresses by repetitive loading in running, smaller amounts (even 0.5 cm) of leg length discrepancy are considered more significant and possibly cause pain of the hip, back or leg (Brody, 1980). It has occasionally been stated that runners with discrepancies cannot successfully tolerate marathon training and competition. No substantiating evidence for this statement was found in a recent study of 35 male marathon runners of whom 18 were found to have a length difference of less than 5 mm, ten a difference of 5–9 mm, and seven a difference of 1.0 cm or greater (Gross, 1983). This indicated that the incidence and amount of leg length discrepancy in marathon runners was comparable to the population at large. It was concluded that discrepancies of 5–25 mm are not necessarily a functional detriment to marathon runners (Gross, 1983).

The widely different opinions on the clinical impact of leg inequalities are probably partly explained by unreliable results of conventional clinical examinations (observer error ± 10 mm) and the lack of reliable radiological methods. Supine orthoroentgenograms suffer from the potential shortcoming of not including any difference in height of the feet (Gross, 1983). Therefore, a standing radiological method which is simple and causes low exposure to radiation is recommended in screening studies (Friberg, 1983).

Leg length discrepancy causing an abnormal pelvic tilt has been proposed to be a contributing factor in the development of trochanteric bursitis (Reilly & Nicholas, 1987) and iliotibial band friction syndrome (Taunton & Clement, 1981) (Table 10.1.10), because of the accompanying stretching of the tract over the lateral femoral condyle of the longer leg. In contrast, no such correlation between leg length inequality and iliotibial band friction syndrome could be demonstrated in another study (Lindenberg *et al.*, 1984). A predisposing role of leg length discrepancy in the aetiology of stress fractures has also been suggested (Friberg, 1980).

Obviously, leg length discrepancy might be involved in the development of a number of overuse injuries in the lower extremities. It should be stressed that the real occurrence of these proposed biomechanical alterations, their magnitude, and above all their clinical significance are not well known. Further investigations in athletes providing substantiating data are certainly needed before any firm conclusions can be drawn.

In general, small leg length discrepancies should usually not be used as the only explanatory factor in hard-training athletes with problems. Correction of training errors is certainly warranted more often.

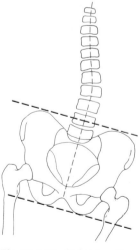

Fig. 10.1.16 In leg length discrepancy there is a pelvic tilt and a compensatory lumbar scoliosis.

Muscle weakness and imbalance

Muscle imbalance means that there is either an asymmetry between the extremities or a differential with an anticipated normal value (Grace, 1985).

It is well known that athletes with previous joint injuries which have required surgery have persistent and very long-lasting muscle strength deficits of the affected leg, despite their own belief of being fully rehabilitated (Grimby *et al.*, 1980; Arvidsson *et al.*, 1981). In such athletes, muscle weakness has been proposed to be associated with a high rate of re-injury. There is support for the proposition that proper rehabilitation and conditioning programmes can lessen the re-injury rate (Heiser *et al.*, 1984). In a prospective study, Ekstrand (1982) showed that non-contact knee injuries in soccer players affected those who had had inadequate rehabilitation after previous knee injuries. However, it is not clear whether muscle imbalance *per se* is the most important causative factor for re-injury in these athletes. Persistent knee instability, effects of previous operations and impairment of neuromuscular coordination may also be involved (Table 10.1.12).

In athletes without previous injuries, it is also commonly believed that the weaker or more imbalanced a muscle group is, compared to normal, the more prone it is to joint or soft tissue injury (cf. Grace, 1985). There is some evidence that multifactorial conditioning programmes can lessen injury rate (Heiser *et al.*, 1984). However, apart from muscle strength there are many interacting factors in the development of athletic injuries (see below). In a prospective study, it was found that soccer players sustaining contact knee injuries did not differ in muscle strength from other players (Ekstrand, 1982). Nor was there any muscle imbalance in players with hamstring strains. A prospective study in American football players also questions whether a direct relationship exists between muscle imbalance and injury (Grace *et al.*, 1984).

As a matter of fact, the question of a relationship between muscle imbalance and injury constitutes a highly conjectural area between muscle physiology and pragmatic sports medicine. The actual magnitude of what constitutes balance and imbalance has never been accurately defined (Grace, 1985) but a 10–20% discrepancy is used in clinical practice as a guide for an athlete to return to sports participation following knee injury. However, what constitutes a significant discrepancy may depend on the anatomic region involved, the sport, and the subject's age, size and gender (Grace, 1985) (Table 10.1.12). Furthermore, since a difference exists between the dominant and non-dominant limb

Table 10.1.12 Athletic injuries and muscle imbalance—interacting factors.

Athletes with previous injury
  Persistent knee instability
  Effects of previous operations
  Impairment of neuromuscular coordination
Athletes without previous injury
  Anatomic region
  Sex
  Age
  Size
  Sport

strength, pre-injury evaluation is important (Stafford & Grana, 1984) and comparison of the injured limb with the uninjured may be inaccurate. Bilateral agonist–antagonist muscle strength ratios also need to be compared at different speeds of isokinetic velocities (Stafford & Grana, 1984). In addition, evaluation of strength should be carried out at a velocity of motion comparable to the athlete's functional activities.

It is presently obvious that the question of any relationship between imbalance and injury remains open. Only future prospective and blind studies can definitely answer the question.

Flexibility

Flexibility may be defined as the range of motion available in a joint or group of joints, i.e. mobility. In sports, muscle flexibility is an important factor for physical performance (Corbin, 1984). It is probably also important in the prevention of certain sports injuries (Ekstrand, 1982). Thus, it has been proposed that muscle tightness may predispose to muscle rupture and tendinitis (Glick, 1980; Ekstrand, 1982). Examples of articles in which muscle tightness has been imputed as a potential predisposing factor in different lower extremity injuries are listed in Table 10.1.13. It has also been proposed that the growth process itself is involved in the development of traction apophysitis by causing increased muscle–tendon tightness about the joints during growth spurts (Micheli *et al.*, 1986; Micheli, 1987). In rapidly growing athletes with decreased flexibility, the repetitive stress applied to the apophysis is the final factor causing the overuse injury. The strong pull of a well-developed (and tight?) quadriceps muscle in athletic adolescent boys is probably the most important

Table 10.1.13 Muscle tightness—potential predisposing factor to lower extremity injury.

Injury	Tight muscle	Authors
Hamstring strain/tendinitis	Hamstrings	Nicholas, 1976
Achilles tendinitis	Gastrocnemius/ soleus	Clement *et al.*, 1984
Patellofemoral disorders	Hamstrings	Grana & Kriegshauser, 1985
Excess lateral pressure syndrome of the patella	Vastus lateralis	Ficat & Hungerford, 1977
Patellar tendinitis	Hamstrings Quadriceps	Hunter & Poole, 1987
Iliotibial band friction syndrome	Iliotibial band	Henry *et al.*, 1982; Jones & James, 1987

aetiological factor in patella alta associated with Osgood–Schlatter disease (Jakob *et al.*, 1981).

The retrospective studies cited above do not allow any conclusion on whether muscle tightness is the result or the cause of injuries to the musculotendinous unit. In prospective studies, muscle strains have been found to be more common in soccer players with muscle tightness of the adductors of the hip (Ekstrand, 1982). However, in that prospective study, no significant difference in range of motion was found between soccer players with hamstring strains and those without. In other categories of athletes, no relation between muscle tightness and the frequency of muscle strain has been found (Jackson *et al.*, 1978). Furthermore, all cited studies illustrate that the risk for certain injuries in a particular sport is certainly also influenced by the specific performance demands of the sport as well as the predisposing conditions that may lead to injury (Nicholas, 1976). Prospective studies of different sports are urgently needed in order to definitely determine whether muscle tightness is a common primary causative factor in certain athletic injuries (cf. Table 10.1.13).

When discussing flexibility training it should be stressed that a steady-state value of the stretched tissue will ultimately be arrived at, i.e. there is an optimum length of the tissue over which further stretch is of little or no anatomical or physiological value (Jenkins & Little, 1974; Wallin *et al.*, 1985).

Sex, stature and body composition

Runners with high stature and, accordingly, high bodyweight put a greater stress on their musculoskeletal system, which does not increase in strength in direct proportion to the bodyweight (Stipe, 1982). Of course, tall runners have larger feet but the impact force per unit area of the foot is comparatively higher in the tall runner (Stipe, 1982).

In studies analysing body fat in conditioned athletes, there is a great variability among athletes from different sports. In track athletes, the average percent of fat in conditioned women is 10–15% of bodyweight while conditioned men generally have less than 7% (Hunter, 1986). Women have less muscle mass per bodyweight (23%) than equally trained men (40%) (Klafs & Lyon, 1978). Men also have greater bone mass than women. This means that in running the repetitive impact loads of bodyweight will be taken up by a weaker musculoskeletal system in women compared to men of equal bodyweight. Theoretically,

Table 10.1.14 General factors—stress-related injuries.

Sex
Percent body fat
Bone mass
Muscle mass

these factors might predispose to overuse injuries of the lower extremity in women.

Whether stature and/or body fat, or bone mass and muscle mass, are important factors in the development of overuse injuries of the lower extremity (Table 10.1.14) is presently speculative and further studies providing substantiating data are needed.

References

Andrews, J. R. (1983) Overuse syndromes of the lower extremity. *Clin. Sports Med.* **2**, 137.

Arvidsson, J., Eriksson, E., Häggmark, T. & Johnsson, R. J. (1981) Isokinetic thigh muscle strength after ligament reconstruction in the knee joint. *Int. J. Sports Med.* **1**, 7.

Bevins, T., Wilder, D. G. & Frymoyer, J. W. (1985) The relationship between anthropometric, postural, muscular, and mobility characteristics of males ages 18–55. *Spine* **10**, 644.

Brody, D. (1980). Running injuries. *Ciba Found. Symp.* **32**, 4.

Carson jr, W. G. (1985) Diagnosis of extensor mechanism disorders. *Clin. Sports Med.* **4**, 231.

Clement, D. B., Taunton, J. E. & Smart, G. W. (1984) Achilles tendinitis and peritendinitis: etiology and treatment. *Am. J. Sports Med.* **12**, 179.

Corbin, C. B. (1984) Flexibility. *Clin. Sports Med.* **3**, 101.

Cummins, E. J., Anson, B. J., Carr, B. W. *et al.* (1946) The structure of the calcaneal tendon (of Achilles) in relation to orthopaedic surgery. *Surg. Gynecol. Obstet.* **83**, 107.

Ekstrand, J. (1982) *Soccer injuries and their prevention.* Ph.D. Thesis, Linköping University. Medical Dissertation No. 130.

Ficat, P. & Hungerford, D. (1977) Disorders of the patellofemoral joint. Williams & Wilkins, Baltimore.

Fox, T. (1975) Dysplasia of the quadriceps mechanism: hypoplasia of the vastus medialis muscle as related to the hypermobile patella syndrome. *Surg. Clin. North Am.* **55**, 199.

Friberg, O. (1980) Leg length asymmetry of lower extremities—an etiological factor of stress and fractures. *Ann. Med. Milit. Fenn.* **55**, 149.

Friberg, O. (1983) Clinical symptoms and biomechanics of lumbar spine and hip joint in leg length inequality. *Spine* **8**, 643.

Glick, J. M. (1980) Muscle strains. Prevention and treatment. *Physician Sportsmed.* **11**, 73.

Gofton, J. P. & Trueman, G. E. (1971) Studies in osteoarthritis. Part II, osteoarthritis of the hip and leg length discrepancy. *Can. Med. Assoc. J.* **104**, 791.

Grace, T. G. (1985) Muscle imbalance and extremity injury. A perplexing relationship. *Sports Med.* **2**, 77.

Grace, T. G., Sweetser, E. R., Nelson, M. A., Ydens, L. R. & Skipper, B. J. (1984) Isokinetic muscle imbalance and knee-joint injuries. *J. Bone Joint Surg. (Am)* **66**, 734.

Grana, W. A. & Kriegshauser, L. A. (1985) Scientific basis of extensor mechanism disorders. *Clin. Sports Med.* **4**, 247.

Grimby, G., Gustavsson, E., Peterson, L. & Renström, P. (1980) Quadriceps function and training after knee ligament surgery. *Med. Sci. Sports* **12**, 70.

Gross, R. A. (1983) Leg length discrepancy in marathon runners. *Am. J. Sports Med.* **11**, 121.

Heiser, T. M., Weber, J., Sullivan, G., Clare, P. & Jacobs, R. R. (1984) Prophylaxis and management of hamstring muscle injuries in intercollegiate football players. *Am. J. Sports Med.* **12**, 368.

Henry, J. A. (1986) The patellofemoral joint. In J. A. Nicholas & E. B. Hershman (eds) *The Lower Extremity and Spine in Sports Medicine*, p. 1013. C. V. Mosby, St Louis.

Henry, J., Lareau, B. & Neigut, D. (1982) The injury rate in professional basketball. *Am. J. Sports Med.* **10**, 16.

Hughston, J. C., Walsh, W. M. & Puddu, G. (1984) Patellar subluxation and dislocation. W. B. Saunders, Philadelphia.

Hult, L. (1954) The Munkfors investigation. *Acta Orthop. Scand.* (Suppl. 16) **24**, 30.

Hunter, L. Y. (1986) Aspects of injuries to the lower extremity unique to the female athlete. In J. A. Nicholas & E. B. Hershman (eds) *The Lower Extremity and Spine in Sports Medicine*, p. 90. C. V. Mosby, St Louis.

Hunter, S. C. & Poole, R. M. (1987) The chronically inflamed tendon. *Clin. Sports Med.* **6**, 371.

Insall, J. N., Flavo, K. & Wise, D. W. (1976) Chondromalacia patellae—a prospective study. *J. Bone Joint Surg. (Am)* **58**, 1.

Insall, J. N., Goldberg, V. & Salvatti, E. (1972) Recurrent dislocation and the high-riding patella. *Clin. Orthop.* **88**, 67.

Jackson, D. W., Jarrett, H., Bailey, D., Kausek, J., Swanson, J. & Powell, J. W. (1978) Injury prediction in the young athlete. A preliminary report. *Am. J. Sports Med.* **6**, 6.

Jakob, R. P., von Gumppenberg, S. & Engelhardt, P. (1981) Does Osgood–Schlatter disease influence the position of the patella. *J. Bone Joint Surg. (Br)* **63**, 579.

James, S. L., Bates, B. T. & Osternig, L. R. (1978) Injuries to runners. *Am. J. Sports Med.* **6**, 40.

Jenkins, R. B. & Little, R. W. (1974) A constitutive equation for parallel-fibered elastic tissue. *J. Biomech.* **7**, 397.

Jones, D. C. & James, S. L. (1984) Overuse injuries of the lower extremity. *Clin. Sports Med.* **6**, 273.

Klafs, C. E. & Lyon, M. J. (1978) *The Female Athlete.* C. V. Mosby, St Louis.

Larson, R. L. (1979) Subluxation—dislocation of the patella. In J. C. Kennedy (ed) *The Injured Adolescent Knee.* Williams & Wilkins, Baltimore.

Lindenberg, G., Pinshaw, R. & Noakes, T. D. (1984) Iliotibial band friction syndrome in runners. *Phys. Sports Med.* **12**, 118.

Lutter, L. D. (1981) Cavus foot in runners. *Foot Ankle* **1**, 225.

Lysholm, J. & Wiklander, J. (1987) Injuries in runners. *Am. J. Sports Med.* **15**, 168.

McKenzie, D. C., Clement, D. B. & Taunton, J. E. (1985) Running shoes, orthotics, and injuries. *Sports Med.* **2**, 334.

Mann, R. A. (1986) Principles of examination of the foot and ankle. In R. A. Mann (ed) *Surgery of the Foot*, 5th edn. C. V. Mosby, St Louis.

Mann, R. A., Baxter, D. B. & Lutter, L. D. (1981) Running symposium. *Foot Ankle* **1**, 190.

Marshall, R. N. (1978) Foot mechanics and jogger's injuries. *NZ Med. J.* **88**, 288.

Michael, R. A. & Holder, L. E. (1985) The soleus syndrome. A cause of medial tibial stress (shin splints). *Am. J. Sports Med.* **13**, 87.

Micheli, L. J. (1987) The traction apophysitises. *Clin. Sports Med.* **6**, 389.

Micheli, L. J., Slater, J. A., Woods, E. & Gerbino, P. G. (1986) Patella alta and the adolescent growth spurt. *Clin. Orthop.* **213**, 159.

Nicholas, J. (1976) Risk factors, sports medicine and the orthopaedic system. An overview. *Am. J. Sports Med.* **3**, 243.

Nichols, P. J. R. (1960) Short leg syndrome. *Br. Med. J.* **1**, 1863.

Reilly, J. P. & Nicholas, J. A. (1987) The chronically inflamed bursa. *Clin. Sports Med.* **6**, 352.

Singer, K. M. & Jones, D. C. (1986) Soft tissue conditions of the ankle and foot. In J. A. Nicholas & E. B. Hershman (eds) *The Lower Extremity and Spine in Sports Medicine*, p. 498. C. V. Mosby, St Louis.

Stafford, M. G. & Grana, W. A. (1984) Hamstring/quadriceps ratios in college football players. A high velocity evaluation. *Am. J. Sports Med.* **12**, 209.

Stipe, P. (1982) The prediction of vertical impact force during running. *Nike Res. Newslett.* **2**, 1.

Taunton, J. E. & Clement, D. B. (1981) Iliotibial tract friction syndrome in athletes. *Can. J. Appl. Sports Sci.* **6**, 76.

Torg, J. S., Pavlov, H. & Torg, E. (1987) Overuse injuries in sport. The foot. *Clin. Sports Med.* **6**, 291.

Viitasalo, J. T. & Kvist, M. (1983) Some biomechanical aspects of the foot and ankle in athletes with and without shin splints. *Am. J. Sports Med.* **11**, 125.

Wallin, D., Ekblom, B., Grahn, R. & Nordenborg, T. (1985) Improvement of muscle flexibility. A comparison between two techniques. *Am. J. Sports Med.* **13**, 263.

White, J. W. (1943) Torsion of the Achilles tendon—its surgical significance. *Arch. Surg.* **47**, 784.

10.2 Diagnostic principles

F. A. COMMANDRÉ, C. ABOULKER, A. CHOUCHANE, F. DENIS,
A. ROGOPOULOUS, P. VANUXEM & H. ZAKARIAN

Basic principles

The basic principles of the diagnosis of sports injuries are complex. The situations found are very different; acute injuries on the field or chronic soft tissue diseases do not act in the same way. The athlete must be able to return to a good state of health as quickly as possible—avoiding any risks—and accurate diagnosis is therefore essential.

Figure 10.2.1 summarizes briefly the different steps needed to make a diagnosis in sports injuries, but reality is, of course, more complex. Diagnosis must consider acute or chronic injuries, the sports activity and practice, and the mechanism of injury.

Acute injuries   It is not uncommon to see an athlete fall to the ground in great pain, receive rapid attention consisting of rubbing or kneading the injured part, and jump up to resume play. The crowd roars at the seemingly 'magic' treatment which has instantly restored damaged bones and ligaments. The public is impressed by what it perceives as treatment and appreciates the continued performance of the athlete. First aid treatment is important on the field—at the place of injury. The initial step should be a carefully performed physical examination and determination of the mechanism of injury. An accurate diagnosis is imperative for successful treatment, and the physician should know all possible associated injuries, e.g. underlying tissue injuries, and other bone and fracture sites.

On the field, the immediate examination should reveal:

1 A haemorrhage and its spread; it should be stopped as soon as possible.
2 Shock and its symptoms. Treatment is important to enable transportation.
3 Open wounds, with the risk of tetanus and other infections.
4 Principal sites of injured parts: sprains, dislocations and fractures, especially spine fractures. Immobilization is important.

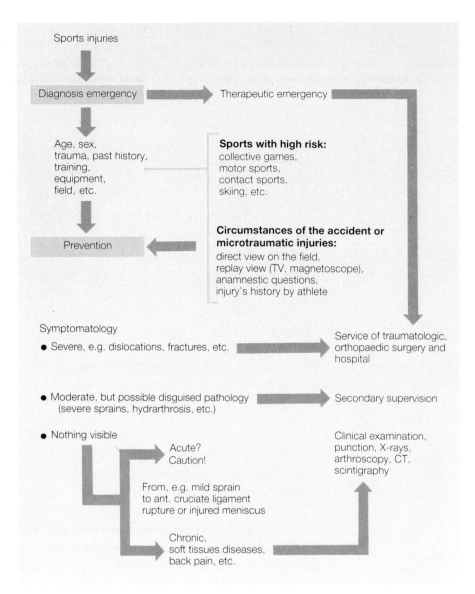

Fig. 10.2.1 Management for diagnosis and treatment in sports injuries.

In the hospital or medical centre, if the injured athlete is better and the trauma history is accurate, a new clinical and X-ray examination can be performed immediately. The X-ray analysis should evaluate the injuries and look for the causes and mechanism of injury. All diagnostic tools should be used as needed—computerized tomography (CT), nuclear magnetic resonance (NMR), etc. This results in an accurate diagnosis which permits suitable treatment for a quick rehabilitation and return to the sports field.

Chronic injuries   Chronic injuries are very frequent, e.g. tennis elbow, Achilles tendinitis, lumbar pain. Overuse and overload are responsible for muscle and tendon tears and degenerative arthropathies.

The diagnosis is often easily made, based on clinical signs only. But the physician must also investigate:

1   The anatomical disabilities (genu valgum or varum, hyperpression syndrome of the patella, sacralization, spondylolysis, etc.) which may worsen the injury.

2   Defects of the equipment (shoes, helmet, etc.) and materials (rackets, artificial fields, etc.).

3   A general interview (doping, drinks, foods, etc.) in coordination with the athlete's own physician if possible.

Diagnostic tools can be used to evaluate the degree of injury ('pulled' or 'ruptured' muscles), the number of attacks (three partial muscle tears may indicate the need for surgery), the evolution (ultrasound scan, scintigraphy) and future development of injury. Each athlete will have a unique injury and history.

Conclusion   A good diagnosis is dependent on the application of multidisciplinary medical knowledge. The identification of the injury, the treatment and rehabilitation, and future preventive measures must be completed before the athlete can return to the sports field.

Diagnostic tools

Trauma can occur to anyone at anytime in sports activities, but, in sports medicine, the microtraumatic injuries are particularly important. All too often, trauma to the skeleton and its soft tissues is incorrectly diagnosed and serious complications frequently result.

X-ray techniques and new diagnostic tools allow a precise diagnosis giving complete details. This accurate interpretation is of paramount importance in providing appropriate preventive care and treatment of athletes, who have trained for many years to achieve high levels of excellence. All the best techniques should be used for diagnosis and treatment, although, of course, the cost must be borne in mind.

X-ray examination and its different techniques   The first step in the care of an injured athlete, and before an X-ray examination, should be a carefully performed physical examination and determination of the mechanism of the injury whenever possible.

An X-ray examination is often indicated and can detect numerous problems (fracture, dislocation, dysplasia). X-rays of two planes at different angles are often necessary, sometimes with oblique views for joints or heads of bone. This static image gives an excellent representation in one plane, but other significant soft tissue components or small bone defects are badly observed. Enlarging or magnification radiology, light X-rays, xeroradiography, dynamic negatives, etc. are able to show the finer points needed for diagnosis (linear and fine fractures, diastasis in sprains, etc.).

Bone tomography evaluates a structure or object obscured by overlapping shadows in the plain radiograph (e.g. depression fracture of lateral tibia plateau); trabecular bone tissue also shows the fine details (undetected scaphoid fracture of the wrist, or a fracture of the hook of the hamate).

Numerous techniques use contrast products, which have better tolerance and resorption. They are often used in sports injuries: arthrography, saccoradiculography, computed angiography, etc. Meniscus injuries or glenoid rim tears in soccer-, tennis- or golfplayers can be detected. The ligamentous tears or ruptures of the shoulder or ankle are shown. Arthroscopy permits a visual diagnosis and may indicate immediate surgical treatment.

Xeroradiography is a photoelectric process, whereas conventional radiography using photographic film is a photochemical process (Roach, 1970; Roach & Hilleboe, 1975). It produces superior images of wood or plastic foreign bodies in soft tissues. This complex technique is not used frequently.

X-ray techniques are numerous, cheap and frequently used in bone injuries resulting from sports practices. They are also used for aptitude examination and detection (lungs, heart, dysplasia, scoliosis, spondylolysis and spondylolisthesis).

Computerized tomography

Computerized tomography (CT) provides excellent visualization of the spatial relationship in the transverse plane, and also the sagittal or coronal plane in some scanners. A scan of the opposite joint may be helpful for interpretation.

Techniques using contrast products (arthro-CT) give a very good view of bone (measurements of angle), muscles and soft tissues in the hips, shoulders, knees and spine, and ruptures can be detected (Fig. 10.2.2). Acetabular fractures, dislocations, cartilaginous fragments, myositis ossificans, discal nucleus and stress fractures can also be observed, and

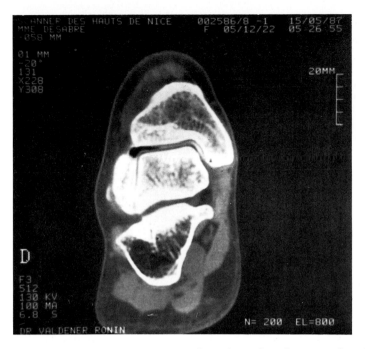

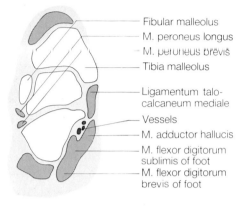

Fibular malleolus
M. peroneus longus
M. peroneus brevis
Tibia malleolus

Ligamentum talo-
calcaneum mediale
Vessels
M. adductor hallucis
M. flexor digitorum
sublimis of foot
M. flexor digitorum
brevis of foot

Fig. 10.2.2 Arthro-CT of an ankle sprain. Rupture of the anterior talofibular ligament and the calcaneofibular ligament.

are often found to be complex. This technique, however, is expensive and is reserved for use in specialized centres, where it supercedes tomographies, etc.

Scintigraphy
(⁹⁹mTc bone scan)

Bone scanning, 3 hours after the radionuclide technitium ^{99}m complexed with a diphosphonate derivative intravenous injection, shows an uptake in certain sports injuries.

Stress fractures In stress fractures, the bone scans give an early, intense and stable hyperfixation, when the scanning is quantitative and timed. In many cases, an increased radionuclide uptake is the prodromal state to an overt fracture. Three phases are observed:

1 During the first pains a light and boundless area is observed in the painful zone and, sometimes, in other unpainful areas.
2 After a few days the uptake is intensive. Sometimes, in the trabecular bones (talus, calcaneus), a special and specific aspect is observed: parallel, hyperfixed lines, perpendicular to the direction for the bony rows.
3 In the third phase, which occurs after some months, the uptake returns to normal.

Bone scanning can give a precocious diagnosis of stress fractures, which can then be prevented, as well as detecting numerous unpainful and rare fracture localizations (Garrick, 1976; Greaney *et al.*, 1983). The

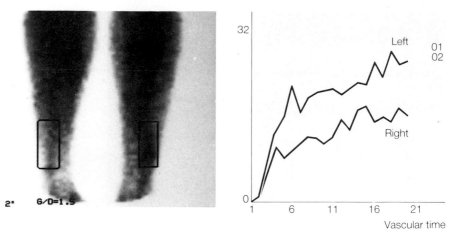

Fig. 10.2.3 Scintigraphy of a fibular stress fracture in a 24-year-old jogger.

radionuclide uptake is positive in the early and late periods (angioscintigraphic and vascular) (Fig. 10.2.3); no uptake means there is no stress fracture.

Periostitis   In periostitis (shin splints), scintigraphy may be positive in the late period and the periosteum is not affected. Scintigraphy in combination with CT and NMR is very useful for detecting the inflammatory reaction.

Soft tissue lesions   In soft tissue lesions (tendinitis, fasciitis, myositis, bursitis), the uptake is positive during the early period and is normal in the late period.

Small trauma   In small trauma (haematoma, ligamentous rupture with little bone fragmentation), biomechanical support problems and pathological diseases, some confusion may be possible, but consideration of the clinical context usually helps diagnosis. A new bone scan is made on the third day; if it is negative the diagnosis of a stress fracture can be excluded.

Algodystrophy   In algodystrophy, the same intense uptake is detected immediately and the differential diagnosis with stress fracture is sometimes very difficult. The linear isotopic uptake permits confirmation of the diagnosis of stress fractures in certain cases.

Other bone diseases (inflammatory, infectious, tumoral, metabolic, etc.) show an uptake which will be discussed in the clinical, biological and radiological contexts.

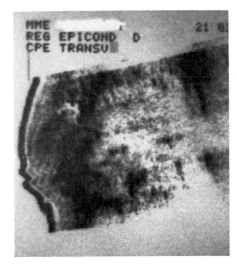 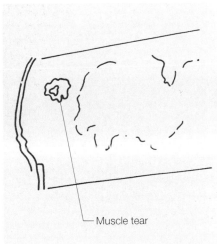

Muscle tear

Fig. 10.2.4 Ultrasound scan of a partial muscle tear, triad aspect 'small round bell', in tennis arm.

Ultrasound scan A digitalized echotomograph equipped with a transducer or probe pulsed to a rate of 7 mHz or more, focalized to 3 cm, is generally used. Serial views in different spatial planes are obtained with a gelatinized skin-probe connection ('water' pouch) and by automatic or manual scanning, with the examined muscle or tendon in an attitude of passive or active function (testing by real time), with a possible tape or video recording.

Muscles Myopathy can be subdivided into four areas:

1 Extrinsic injuries: contusions. The cause of injury and its force, with or without simultaneous muscle contraction, and the direction of impact give variable problems (superficial or intramuscular haematoma). These injuries can include twisted areas, unstructured and blurred areas caused by oedemas, and hypoechogenic areas.

2 Intrinsic traumatology (Fig. 10.2.4). These injuries are genuine lesions, resulting from the limits of elastic and physiological properties of a muscle being exceeded. This is often due to a lack of coordination (fatigue, faulty training). Some muscles (e.g. biceps femoris muscle) are difficult to examine. Table 10.2.1 summarizes aspects of examining intrinsic traumas with ultrasound scanning. A muscular hernia is a hyperechogenic aspect through the muscle aponeurosis which ripples during muscle contraction.

3 Cicatricial aspects. The clinical presentation is uniform: chronic muscle pain, fatigability, repeated relapses and therapeutic failures without manifest symptomatology. Five aspects are described:

(a) Cicatricial granuloma—oval or round hyperechogenic flashes.

Table 10.2.1 Aspects of ultrasound scanning of intrinsic strains.

	Degree of strain	Ultrasound scan aspects
0	Histological rupture of tropho- or collagen fibres, cramps, spasms	0
1st	Pulled muscles (some)	Flake aspect (40%)
2nd	Partial muscle tear (a few or more)	Triad aspects: flap of bell small round bell
3rd	Complete tear or rupture	Large triad aspect or anechogenic cavity

(b) Calcification—hyperechogenic area with an echoless (posterior silence) zone.

(c) Residual cyst—hyper or echoless aspects, with a fine hyperechogenic border, is a sequela to acute inflammatory attacks ('accordion' picture).

(d) Fibrous degeneration (old athlete, long immobilization in a cast, or a spastic invalid).

(e) Myositis ossificans—a diffuse hyperechogenic area is detected early (7–10 days after trauma).

4   Muscle diseases. Lipoma, rhabdomyosarcoma, neurinoma, etc. can be identified.

Ligaments   An anechogenic aspect sometimes showing a total or partial rupture of a ligament (anterior cruciate or lateral ligaments of the ankles).

Tendons   The ultrasound scan provides good information on tendons and the static view shows an iconographic aspect which is useful. The scan of tendon pathology is different in the joint and its tendons. The following are examples:

1   Shoulder: rupture of the rotator cuff in an older person does not need arthrography, but in an athlete the scan allows the decision to be made whether to use arthrography, before surgery, to quantify the degree of the rupture.

2   Elbow: an anechogenic or hypoechogenic aspect indicates tennis arm in 5–10% of cases of epicondyle pain.

3   Wrist and fingers: the tenosynovitis or nodular tendinitis are distinguished in an anechogenic cavity. However, the important feature is the ability of the active ultrasound scan to visualize the rupture of the sheath or palmar aponeurosis (real testing).

4   Patellar and Achilles tendons, and other tendons: hyperechogenic aspects (nodular tendinitis) and anechogenic areas (bursitis, partial or

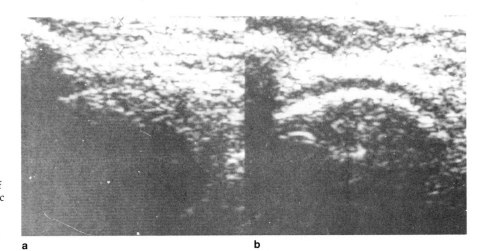

Fig. 10.2.5 Ultrasound scan of patellar tendinitis of the left knee: hypoechogenic aspect by the inflammation on the longitudinal plane. (a) Normal knee. (b) Patella tendinitis.

a   b

total ruptures) are observed. The ultrasound scan testing in real time shows the normal aponeurosis; in Fig. 10.2.5 the rupture is partial.

The ultrasound scan is a useful and reliable diagnostic tool for examining muscles and tendons in athletes if it is considered in a clinical context. It is also not invasive. The scan can make an accurate diagnosis, which orientates the therapeutic management (surgery), follows the evolution and prognosis, and the eventual resumption of sports practice. It can be used as a medicolegal document and is cheap. However, in the examination of tendons, the ultrasound scan can often have defects and NMR may be better although more expensive.

Teletalermography   The use of infrared computerized equipment measures the thermal emissions from the skin and subcutaneous tissues. Four processes condition these variations: inflammation, vasomotricity, tissue trophicity and peripheral ischaemia.

Its advantage in identifying the pathology of the locomotor apparatus is limited to:

1 Locate the juxta- and osteoarticular areas with inflammation.
2 Judge the degree of inflammation and its evolutionary possibilities.
3 Control the action of anti-inflammatory drugs.
4 Provide a repeatable medicolegal document.

In *muscular pathology*:

1 A partial muscular tear gives a hot area.
2 A haematoma gives a cold area which masks the hot area. Teletherm-ography identifies the future development of the muscular defect and

can detect an undesireable evolution (risk of myositis ossificans if the hot area persists after 3–6 weeks).

3 However, a deep injury is not detected and the examination of certain muscles is difficult.

In *osteoarticular injuries*:

1 The sprain produces a hot area, which decreases in 10–20 days in non-surgical cases.

2 The lesions of soft tissues (tendinitis, entrapment syndromes) are characterized by a hot, variable area (variations of inflammation).

In *vascular pathology*, two diseases of athletes may be detected:

1 Frostbite of fingers or toes of mountaineers (Foray *et al.*, 1980). Telethermography identifies the hyperthermal area upstream, which characterizes the vascular participation in the freezing action and the evolution of frostbite.

2 Microtraumatic arteriopathy of pilotaris' fingers (Laporte, 1980) with a cold area in one or several fingers.

Nuclear magnetic resonance (NMR) imaging

NMR imaging uses the properties of certain nuclei (hydrogen) and their capacity, after magnetic excitation, to return a detection signal. The result gives a better quality of imaging than standard radiography and even CT scan images of the anatomy of joints. Investigation of tumours, osteonecrosis, soft tissue diseases and compound fractures are all markedly facilitated by the use of NMR imaging which allows a precise diagnosis with complete details to be made and an appropriate therapy to be applied.

Stress fractures; myositis ossificans The possible confusion of the periosteal and reconstructive reaction of stress fracture with osteogenic sarcoma, especially in young athletes, means an accurate diagnosis is needed. NMR imaging can be used for this (Stafford *et al.*, 1986). The NMR image demonstrates the extent of the marrow or cortical abnormalities, because of low proton density and extremely short T_2 relaxation times; cortical bone produces a weak NMR signal and soft tissues a poor NMR image. The ability of NMR imaging to detect stress fractures is unexpected, but confirmed by Stafford *et al.* (1986).

The NMR imaging can detect marrow and soft tissue abnormalities early on, and the finding of a cortical rupture can be interpreted as suggesting malignancy. This is also the case for myositis ossificans.

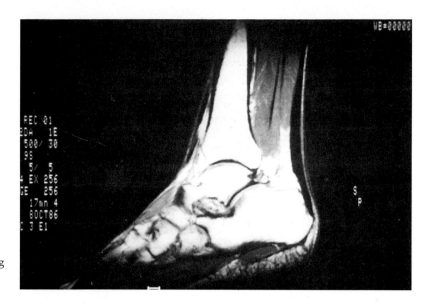

Fig. 10.2.6 Nuclear magnetic resonance imaging of Achilles rupture in a professional soccer player.

Soft tissue abnormalities (tendinitis, ruptures) Different anatomical structures and some pathologies can be visualized, for instance:

1 Structures of aponeurosis (Achilles tendon, plantar aponeurosis) with its pathology in jogging or marathon athletes (Fig. 10.2.6).
2 Certain forms of tendinitis with a hypersignal T_1 in the oedematous area.
3 Low signals on the bony cortical; good bony signals are received in other cases.
4 Some low vascular areas (decrease of the signal) and high vascular areas (inflammation).

Doppler effect and its application in sports medicine

Ultrasonography with a Doppler effect is used in physiological studies of the vascular flow of muscular contractions and pulmonary ventilation (Harichaux & Viel, 1982).

Neuromuscular electrodiagnosis

Several techniques are used to examine neuromuscular functions:

1 Neuromuscular electrodiagnosis examines the degree of excitability of the nerve or muscle by measuring the chronaxie, the time taken for the nerve or muscle to reply. The measured intensity (mA) equals double the threshold of normal excitability in ms. This technique is simple and cheap. The supervision of muscular recovery after injury (for example, sprain of knee with hypotrophy) is facilitated.
2 Electromyography studies muscle activity, step by step or by muscular group. The measurement of speed of the motor or sensitive nervous conduction gives a better diagnosis when the nervous system is injured.

This sophisticated equipment, used by a qualified person, only has an application in nervous and muscular pathology in a diagnostic and prognostic way.

3 Evoked potential responses study the times of the central and medullar conductions (visual, auditory). These techniques can help in the detection of sensory reactions in some sports (car or motor racing, skiing, shooting, etc.).

References

Foray, J., Cahen, C. & Mont, J. P. (1980) Les accidents de haute montagne. *Concours Medical* **102–5**, 375.

Garrick, J. (1976) Presentation at the 43rd American Academy of Orthopedic Surgeons Meeting, New Orleans, February 1976.

Greaney, R. B., Gerber, F. H., Laughlin, R. L., Kmet, J. P., Metz, C. D., Kilcheski, T. S., Rao, B. R. & Silverman, E. D. (1983) Distribution and natural history of stress fractures in US Marine recruits. *Radiology* **146**, 339.

Harichaux, P. & Viel, E. (1982) Application de l'ultrasonographie à effet Doppler à la physiologie et médecine du sport. In F. A. Commandré & Y. R. Bence *Explorations Fonctionnelles Neuromusculaires*, pp. 96–108. Masson, Paris.

Laporte, C. (1980) Arteriopathies digitales traumatiques des pilotaris à main nue. *Med. Sport* **54(6)**, 357.

Roach, J. F. (1970) Xeroradiography. *Radiol. Clin. North. Am.* **8**, 271.

Roach, J. F. & Hilleboe, H. F. (1975) Xeroradiography. *Am. J. Roentgenol.* **73**, 5.

Stafford, S. A., Rosenthal, D. I., Gebhardt, M. C., Brady, T. J. & Scott, J. A. (1986) MRI in stress fracture. *Am. J. Roentgenol.* **147**, 553.

Further reading

Bowerman, J. (1977) *Radiology and Injuries in Sports*. Appleton-Century Crofts, New York.

Commandre, F. A. (1984) La ecotomografia en el diagnostico de las lesiones musculares. *Arch. Med. Deporte* **1**, 7.

Commandré, F. A. & Bence, Y. R. (1982) *Explorations Fonctionnelles Neuromusculaires*. Masson, Paris.

Commandré, F. A. *et al.* (1977) Intérêt en pathologie para- et juxta- articulaire d'origine sportive de la xéroradiographie. *L. M. M. Med. Sud-Est* **13(3)**, 183.

Commandré, F. A., Dumoulin, J., Scholem, M., Valdener, V., Bence, Y. R. & Occelli, G. (1984) Place de la thermographie dans les affections de l'appareil locomoteur. *L. M. M. Med. Sud-Est* **20**, 9297.

Geslien, G. E., Thrall, J. H. & Espinosa, J. L. (1976) Early detection of stress fracture using 99 mTc polyphosphate. *Radiology* **121**, 683.

Pera, D. (1985) *Evolution échotomographique des lésions musculaires traumatiques. A propos de 16 observations*. Thèse Médecine, Montpellier.

Roub, L. W., Gumerman, L. W., Hanley, E. W., Clark, N. W., Goodman, M. & Herbert, D. L. (1979) Bone stresses: a radionuclid imaging perspective. *Radiology* **132**, 431.

Schweitzer, Y. (1984) *L'apport de l'échotomographie dans l'étude du tendon d'Achille*. Thèse Médecine, Nice.

Zuinen, C. & Commandré, F. A. (1981) *Les Urgences du Stade*. Masson, Paris.

10.3 Principles of diagnosis and management of traumatic injuries

Bone injuries

F. A. COMMANDRÉ, C. ARGENSON, A. BOUZAYEN,
P. VANUXEM & H. ZAKARIAN

All types of human activity can cause a traumatic injury to bones. Sports activities can result in fractures, but they are relatively rare and usually occur in violent sports (rugby, US football, skiing) or if the athlete is tired. These fractures are often sustained during great muscular contraction and may worsen if not treated.

Two aspects of injured bones must be considered in sports activities:

1 In childhood and adolescence, training must show a respect for the growing skeletal system. Strength training and repetitive competition can create a lesion on sensitive growth areas, resulting in, for instance, Osgood–Schlatter or Sever's disease.

2 In young adults (untrained army recruits, joggers) or trained athletes, repetitive actions of running or jumping, can cause, most commonly, stress fractures of the bones of the lower limbs.

Microtraumatic and traumatic actions on joints sometimes result in sports-related degenerative arthropathies (jumper's knee, soccer's hip).

Diseases of the growing epiphyses

A tremendous cellular activity takes place at the epiphyses during the growth phase in childhood, particularly during two peaks (7–9 and 12–16 years), which is a time of great sports activity. Stresses and strains on the sensitive growth areas can cause irregular fragmentation of the ossification centres and, sometimes, an acute trauma or an abnormal stress (jumping hurdles, etc.). This may provoke avulsion fractures of the apophysis, with the possibility of a cartilage fracture of the tibial plate in an avulsion fracture of the anterior tibial tuberosity (Fig. 10.3.1).

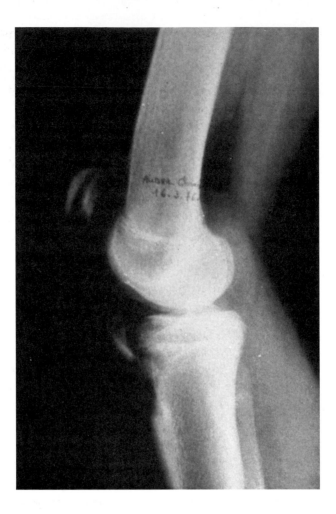

Fig. 10.3.1 Avulsion fracture of the tibia tubercle (female hurdler, 14 years old).

Table 10.3.1 names some of the eponyms given to various epiphyses. Clinical symptoms commonly found are painful, local discomfort and tender swelling, with some inflammation. Rest from 2 to 12 months is sometimes needed, with a short period of cast immobilization or, better still, an infrapatellar strap. Restriction of jumping or bounding activities is necessary, this is particularly important in adolescents.

Local ice friction, quadriceps stretching and, rarely, non-steroidal anti-inflammatory drugs are used (but not for adolescents). The approach with growing adolescents is to restrict activities. An ossific loose body of the ossification centre can detach and climb in the patellar tendon. An irritation results in tendinitis and ablation is necessary. Avulsion fractures (more than 4 mm) are fixed by wires or nails. Return to activity is allowed as symptoms dictate, but it will usually take another 6–12 weeks or more.

Table 10.3.1 Epiphyses and their eponyms resulting from different sports activities.

Epiphysis ossification centres	Eponyms	Responsible sports
Elbow humeral condyle, elbow olecranon	Palmer	Gymnastics, baseball, tennis, javelin, and other throwing sports
Spine vertebral plates	Scheuermann	Numerous sports: judo, cycling, etc.
Femoral capital epiphysis	Legg–Calvé–Perthes	Soccer, US football, jumping, running
Tibial tubercle	Osgood–Schlatter–Lannelongue	Soccer, jumping, running, etc.
Patella	Sinding–Larsen–Johansen	Soccer, jumping, running, etc.
Tarsal navicular	Köhler I	400 m running
Apophysis of calcaneus	Sever	Fencing, soccer, running
Second metatarsal head	Freiberg–Köhler II	Dancing, cold?

Stress fractures (fatigue or exhaustion fracture)

In 1855, Breithaupt described the first localization in Prussian soldiers, with persistent painful feet found among the new recruits after long marches. In 1877, Pauzat gave a good clinical description of this march fracture. In 1897, Strewchow identified, using radiographic examination, this as a fracture of the metatarsal shaft and called it a fatigue fracture.

These occur in the normal bone of healthy soldiers or athletes without history of injury or disease, in response to the stress of repeated and intense activities. The type and the site varies with the military activity or sports training. The bony ^{99}mTc (technetium) scintigraphy can identify fractures in all bones, especially trabecular bones (talus, calcaneus), before spontaneous and provoked local pain is felt.

Most stress fractures have been reported in military recruits, men or women (15 to 30 years old), during basic training and particularly in the first days (commonly of the metatarsal shaft and tibia), before 1960–1966. After the modification of military training (commandos) and, more recently, the increased numbers of professional or amateur athletes and joggers, the sites of stress fractures have changed (calcaneus, talus, femur, tibia, ramus of pubis). Table 10.3.2 summarizes fracture sites and the activities responsible.

Repetitive tensile, compressive or bending loads are responsible. Cyclical stresses (loading and unloading) on viscoelastic bone material can result in a fatigue fracture, similar to those found in metal or crystalline substances.

The treatment is simple—rest for 6 to 12 weeks. A continuation of activities can displace fragments, resulting in a true fracture and its consequences.

Table 10.3.2 Sites of fractures and the responsible activities.

Locality	Responsible activity	Sports/military activities
Coracoid process, teres minor insertion	Vibrations, strength, carrying	Ball-trap, body building, lifting
Clavicle		Ball-trap, body building, lifting
Humerus	Throwing	Baseball, tennis
Cubitus	Vibrations, throwing	Throwing, tennis, cricket, ball games
Radius	Throwing, falling	
Hook of hamate	Vibrations	Tennis, golf, racket-ball
Ribs	Action of pectoralis major m., contusion	Golf, baseball, water skiiing
Vertebra		
D11–L1	Clipping	Golf,
L4–S1	Vibrations, carrying, clipping	Water skiiing, judo, lifting
Ramus of pubis	Adduction of inferior limbs	Jogging, marathon, hurdler, fencing, jumping, gymnastics
Femoral neck	Jumping, contusion	
Femur	Jumping	
Patella	Motion of knee ligaments, contusion	Hockey, baseball, basketball, long-distance running, skiing
Tibia		
tibial plateau	Running	
third middle	Jumping, twisting	
third inferior	Carrying	Dancing
Fibula		
superior	Running	Jogging, ice skating, ball games, cycling
inferior	Jumping	Ice skating, parachuting, ball games, gymnastics
Talus	Jumping	Commandos, parachuting
Calcaneus	Jumping	Commandos, parachuting, indoor ball games, tennis
Navicular	Running	400 m running
Cuneiforms cuboid	Running, jumping	Commandos
Metatarsal bones	Running, marching	Marching, jogging, skiing, track and field games

Fractures

Practically every sport has a defined risk for accidental fracture injury, but certain sports are more dangerous, for instance downhill skiing, climbing, rugby, US football.

On the field, the initial step is a careful physical examination and determination of the mechanism of injury as exactly as possible. Immediate care is important in order to stop haemorrhaging and to protect open wounds; measures should be taken against shock, to immobilize the injured part and to avoid further injury from lifting and transportation. An accurate diagnosis is important, and the physician should know all the associated possible skeletal injuries: underlying visceral injury, other fracture sites, etc. A radiographic examination should be performed immediately after arriving at the hospital.

Causes Two main causes of bone injuries in sports are found:

1 Direct: violent contact between two players or an accident in cycling, skiing or a car race.

2 Indirect: the force causing the break is not applied directly to the injured bone but at a distance, for instance a fall on an outstretched hand which might break the head of the radius.

The nature of the force determines the type of injury, and its gravity increases if it is exposed to the external environment (open wounds, risk of tetanus, etc.).

Sites and types Fractures of the ribs are frequent in falls (skiing, bob-sleighing, cycling,
Ribs and thorax motor sports, riding, collective games) and from direct blows to the chest (ice hockey, soccer, rugby, wrestling, judo, boxing, gymnastics). Lesions of the pleura and lung are found simultaneously in 50% of cases. Sternal, vertebral, scapular and clavicular fractures are observed in 3 to 8% of cases.

If two or more ribs are injured a special strapping and 3–4 weeks rest are necessary before the injured person is fit again. Thoracic pulmonary or mediastinal traumatism should always be suspected before rib fractures are diagnosed.

Clavicle Fracture of the clavicle (10–15% of all accidents) is the most common fracture found in childhood, resulting from direct violence (combat sports, cycling, sledging, bob-sleighing) or indirect trauma from falls on outstretched hands (riding, gymnastics, collective games). Blood vessels or the brachial nerve plexus can be compressed, often with acromio-clavicular dislocation in adolescents. An exostosis impingement of the inferior side of the glenoid cavity may be found in baseball pitchers.

Upper limbs **1** Humerus: the Neer classification describes the possible types of fractures of the proximal humerus (surgical and anatomical necks, greater and lesser tuberosities). They can result from direct blows or indirect falls (cycling, skiing, gymnastics). The plexus brachial nerve and axillary artery can be compressed, and an aseptic necrosis is possible. Avulsion fractures of the proximal humeral epiphysis in adolescent baseball pitchers or of the tuberosities in throwers, gymnasts or fencers, are observed due to the effort of throwing or contraction.

2 Elbow: approximately 7% of all fractures and dislocations occur in the elbow resulting from indirect trauma transmitted through the forearm bones or a direct blow to the radius and ulna against the distal humerus. Diagnosis is sometimes difficult, especially in children where 60% are supracondylar fractures. This type of fracture is called a gymnastic's fracture, it results from extension or flexion, and may be associated with injuries of the brachial artery or the ulna nerve.

In adults, under 50% of all fractures of the elbow involve the radial head or neck, nearly 20% are breaks of the olecranon, and in other cases fractures of the capitellum and coronoid process may be observed. Throwing, with its violent contraction of the flexor pronator muscles, may result in avulsions (baseball pitchers, javelin throwers), but elbow fractures are often also a result of high-speed sports (motor sports, ice skating, skiing, ski jumping, cycling, riding) and an exostosis impingement may be observed of the olecranon (cycling, boxing, baseball). Fractures of the shaft of the radius and ulna are possible by direct or indirect trauma (high-speed sports); they can be isolated, combined or comminutive.

Treatment is very cautious—casting if there is no displacement, otherwise open reduction, with supervision to avoid Volkmann's syndrome, injuries of the ulnar nerve or myositis ossificans (Fig. 10.3.2) in immediate post-injury manipulation of the elbow.

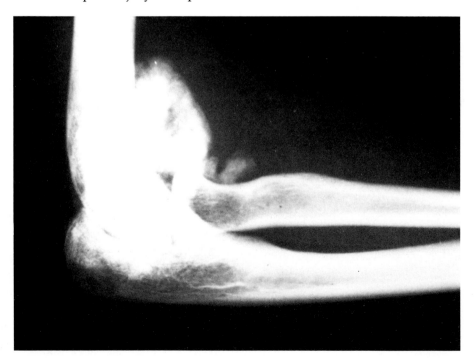

Fig. 10.3.2 Boxer's elbow (33 years old) showing osteoarthrosis, myositis ossificans and loose bodies.

Distal forearm, wrist and hand   Age alone gives a good prediction of the likely area of fracture: from 4 to 10 years old, transverse fractures of the lower end of the radius and ulna; from 11 to 16 years, separation of the distal epiphysis; from 17 to 40 years, navicular fracture; and after 40 years, Pouteau–Colles fracture. Reduction and casting are used during treatment.

1   Injuries of the carpus are rather frequent.

(a) The scaphoid navicular is vulnerable. The identification of injury is important to avoid aseptic necrosis or pseudarthrosis. Repeated X–rays or CT scans are necessary after crushing injuries. Casting and surgery are used in treatment.

(b) The lunate fracture, especially the hook, is uncommon. Pain is localized, and identification with scintigraphy and CT scans is possible. It is found as a result of injuries in racketball, golf, tennis, baseball and trauma. The lunate is sometimes a site of a vascular disturbance (Kienböck's disease), for instance an aseptic necrosis after an unknown initial injury.

(c) Other rare fractures of the outstretched hand, e.g. of the triquetrum, pisiform bone, trapezium, trapezoid.

2   The metacarpals and phalanges are the most common sites of injury in sports, as in normal life. It is important for function to be restored as fully as possible. Mallet or baseball finger is frequently found, with an avulsion fracture of the extension tendon at its insertion in 25% of cases; it is found in all handball players (basketball, volleyball, handball, rugby, US football). Buttonhole deformities or dislocation fractures (50% of the thumb, 25% of the index fingers) are observed; more specifically, Boxer's fracture of the fifth metacarpal head, Bennett's fracture of the first metacarpal base, goalkeeper's or gamekeeper's thumb by chronic repeated ligamentous stress of the first metacarpal phalangeal joint.

Pelvis   The pelvis ring is only usually traumatized in motor sports, cycling, skiing and riding, with possible severe damage to the bladder or bowels.

Femur   Fractures of the hip, the intertrochanteric area, and the femoral neck and shaft are not common but are seen, for instance in skiing. They are common in the aged population where a small trauma can create a lesion of an osteoporotic bone. Myositis ossificans is noted in the thigh after muscular trauma (Charley horse). Avulsion fractures of the apophysis of the lesser trochanter, like the ischial tuberosity or anterior, superior or inferior iliac spines, can be observed during a violent contraction in a soccer player, fencer, sprinter, skier, jumper or weightlifter.

Knee joint   This complex and important joint is particularly vulnerable. Its anatomical, functional and mechanical characteristics, however, make it a stable joint. The forces resulting in injury (directly by impact or indirectly by twisting or angulation movements) are usually great. The fractures are not characteristic and result from direct violence, falling or a blow during contact sports (US football, soccer, etc.), motor cycling, cycling or skiing. The ligamentous injuries are, however, the most frequent and severe.

Impingement exostoses are seen on the patella (horned patella of the cyclist or soccer player) (Fig. 10.3.3).

Tibia and fibula   Fractures of the tibia are common, e.g. skiing. Longitudinal fractures heal well; whilst high-energy transverse fractures take longer to heal.

Ankle and foot   These complex, interdependent joints may be injured independently or in various combinations, with the ligaments playing an important role. Bimalleolar or supramalleolar fractures of the ankle are seldom found in young athletes. Safety standards and high skiboots have also reduced their occurrence in skiing; instead the injuries are transferred to the knee (ligament injuries). In numerous sports, only avulsion fractures of the malleoles are found associated with a sprain.

Tarsal and metatarsal bones of the toes are rarely injured, except in cases of severe stress (bad landing of a parachutist, jumping, motor sports). In soccer, unsuitable shoes may facilitate a fracture of the big toe.

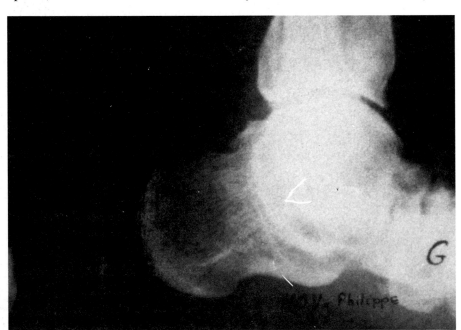

Fig. 10.3.3 Soccer player's ankle (male, 28 years old) showing the trigonium bone, talus–navicular arthropathy and osteo-arthrosis.

Treatment The treatment of fractures is undertaken by orthopaedic surgeons using immobilization by casts or strapping, and surgery (wires, nails, etc.). Afterwards, physiotherapy, rehabilitation exercises in swimming pools, stretching, and progressive training must be undertaken to achieve perfect function and a come-back to the sportsfield.

Arthropathies

Arthropathies are easily recognized by their uniform clinical and radiological signs. Their mechanism in sports is usually related to the technique of racket gesture or motion. It can be:

1 Acute (single trauma): Bennett's fracture in boxing.

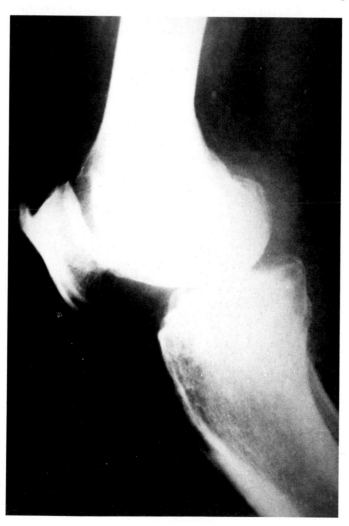

Fig. 10.3.4 'Horned' patella with impingement exostosis of the tibial tubercle (male squash player, 40 years old).

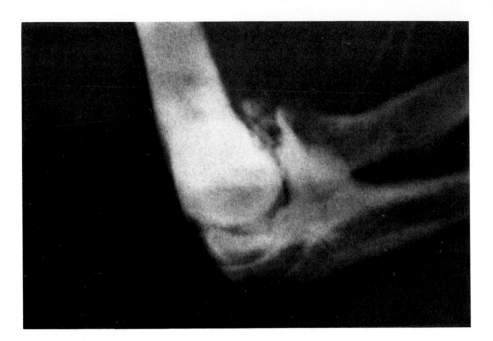

Fig. 10.3.5 Javelin thrower's elbow (male, 25 years old) showing osteo-arthrosis and loose bodies.

2 Microtraumatic with cumulative effect on a precise point of the bone and joint: enthesitis, exostosis impingement (glenoid and olecranon in baseball pitcher) or overuse arthropathy (jumper's or soccer player's knee, javelin thrower's or boxer's elbow) with degenerative and constructive aspects (Figs 10.3.4 and 10.3.5). These sometimes occur with Pellegrini–Stieda disease (ossification of insertion of the medial collateral ligament), loose bodies, osteo-enthesophytis (soccer player's ankle, sportsman's hip). However, the uninjured well-trained muscles reduce pain and function is often quite good.

3 Hyperbaric professional injury (Caisson's disease of heads of femur, humerus, shaft or tibia) or osteocondensation points (in submarine divers) are also known.

Further reading

Commandré, F. A. (1982) Aspects radiologiques de l'appareil locomoteur d'origine sportive. In R. Trial, M. C. Plainfosse, M. Blery & A. Chevrot (eds) *Traité de Radiodiagnostic*, Vol. XII, pp. 112–125. Ed. Masson, Paris.

Greaney, R. B., Gerber, F. H., Laughlin, R. L., Kmet, J. P., Metz, C. D., Kilcheskit, T. S., Rao, B. R. &

Silverman, E. D. (1983) Distribution and natural history of stress fractures in US Marine recruits. *Radiology* **146**, 339.

Resnick, D. & Niwayama, G. (1981) *Diagnosis of Bone and Joints Disorders*. W. B. Saunders, Philadelphia.

Rogers, L. F. (1982) *Radiology of Skeletal Trauma*, 2 vols. Churchill Livingstone, New York.

Muscle injuries

P. RENSTRÖM

Muscle injuries are often misunderstood and maltreated. These injuries have not been a subject of great interest among surgeons since most patients suffering from muscle injuries are able to return to work. Athletes, however, require 100% restitution after a muscle injury and, therefore, these types of injuries have attracted greater attention in recent years.

Muscle injuries are common in sports. Different studies have shown that muscle tears and strains comprise 4–15% of all injuries. When contusion strains or muscle bruising are taken into account these injuries account for about 10–30% of all injuries in sport (Friedrich & Biener, 1973; Kvist & Järvinen, 1980). In veteran athletes, 15% of the injured athletes during the World Master Championships (1977) in track and field, had sustained their injuries in the thigh muscle and 13% in the gastrocnemius (Peterson & Renström, 1980a). Thirty percent of all injuries in soccer are muscle strains and haematomas (Renström & Peterson, 1977).

Functional anatomy of muscles

A muscle comprises 10 000–500 000 fibres, e.g. the vastus lateralis in normal, younger individuals has 450 000 fibres; with increasing age the number of fibres will decrease. The muscle fibres consist of myofibrils, which in turn form an organization of myofilaments organized into units called sarcomeres. In these units there are dark bands of thick filaments made up of myosin and light bands of thin filaments made up of actin.

There are different classes of fibre types: type II fibres are physiologically faster than type I fibres, i.e. in response to a nerve stimulus they generate peak tension quicker than type I fibres. The slower type I fibres are more resistant to fatigue compared to type II fibres. The type II fibres are divided into type IIA and IIB fibres, where type IIA fibres are intermediate between type I and type II fibres.

The muscle tendon unit can pass across one, two or more joints. Muscles expanding over two joints, e.g. quadriceps, hamstrings and gastrocnemius muscles, are less effective in producing tension over a full range of motion. These muscles are often superficially located and more involved in phasic activity. Muscles over one joint are often broad and flat in shape and are usually located deeper and are more involved in postural or tonic activity.

The force produced by the muscles is proportional to their cross-sectional area and orientation of the fibres. Muscle activity controls the motion of the joints and can prevent subluxation and protect the ligaments of the joint being stretched.

Muscles are considered to be a major factor in reducing bending stress in bone. They act like guide-wires supporting a telephone pole; by converting bending stress to compressive stress, they lower the tension on the convex side of the bone when it is subjected to loading (Radin, 1986).

Location of muscle strains

Muscles tear after a stretch of approximately 25% of the resting length (Garret, 1986). A muscle injury may occur in the muscle itself or where the muscle inserts into bone or at the muscle–tendon junction. According to 'Radin's rule' structures will tear at their weakest place (Radin, 1986). The tears most commonly occur at the distal muscle–tendon junction with a remnant of muscle fibres of less than 1 mm remaining with the avulsed tendon.

The most frequently injured muscles are muscles expanding over two or more joints, e.g. hamstrings, triceps surae and quadriceps femoris muscles. These muscles are all subject to stretch and force over two joints, but the muscle fibre orientation may not be able to cope with this. The most powerful phasic muscles of the lower extremity are the most likely to be strained (Garret, 1986).

Activated muscles absorb more energy before failure than relaxed muscles. It is therefore possible that stronger muscles might absorb more energy than weak muscles before failure, and thereby reduce the likelihood of strain. Weakness of a specific muscle or a strength imbalance might be a factor related to the occurrence of muscle strain (Heiser et al., 1984). Strength training is therefore part of the prevention of muscle injuries as well conditioned athletes suffer less often from strains than those that are untrained.

Muscle tears can be partial or complete, even though complete muscle tears are not common. Muscle injuries can be divided into muscle tears or strains and muscle haematomas. Damage to any part of the muscle tendon unit should be called a strain or tear.

Acute muscle strains and tears

Acute muscle strains and tears may be divided into distraction and contusion injuries. The principles for diagnosis and treatment follow those described by Peterson and Renström (1986).

Distraction strain   A distraction strain often occurs in a muscle which works across two joints, e.g. the quadriceps muscles, which extends in the knee joint and flexes in the hip joint. As both these functions cannot occur at the same time, one function, governed by the sensitive neuromuscular unit, is active while the other is inactive.

A strain most commonly occurs in a muscle which is not well warmed up or which is fatigued. Fatigued muscles may not adequately respond to the protective neuromuscular reflex. When a muscle accidentally contracts and is pulled simultaneously, it will tear, e.g. a discus thrower who slips while throwing, a runner who steps in a hole while running. The pulling or tensile strain results from bending and rotation (Radin, 1986). Tension in rotation occurs internally in the material being rotated as the ends of the structure are twisted away from each other.

Distraction strains usually occur in explosive sports like sprinting, jumping and football. This type of distraction strain is often located in the superficially lying muscles, i.e. rectus femoris, semitendinosus and gastrocnemius muscles.

The symptoms of a distraction muscle strain depend on the severity of the strain. Strains are, therefore, divided into first, second and third degree strains.

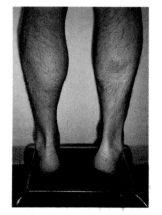

Fig. 10.3.6 An example of a second degree strain in the left gastrocnemius muscle.

First degree strain   In a first degree strain there is no appreciable tear. There is a low level of inflammation with swelling and some discomfort during movement. There is no great loss of strength or restriction of motion. Early examination will indicate pain during the early motion of a passive stretch, but this pain is usually localized in the area of damage. Even a mild strain can, however, often be very distressing for the athlete.

Second degree strain   In a second degree strain (Fig. 10.3.6) there has been actual damage to the muscle but there is not a complete tear. At the time of injury there is a sharp pain in the muscle. The pain is aggravated by attempts to contract the muscle, i.e. to continue the sports activity. It might even be impossible for the muscle to contract because of pain. There is a definite loss of strength and the muscle is likely to be tender on palpation. There might be swelling, discoloration, spasm, etc. within 24 h.

Third degree strain　A third degree strain or tear usually includes a complete tear of the muscle tendon unit. Diagnosis may, however, be quite deceptive. Complete tears often result in a lack of functional capacity. Pain is often sharp at the time of injury, but gradually the pain decreases. The pain is then milder compared to the sharp pain experienced when using a muscle with a partial tear. In the completely torn muscle there is frequently an obvious defect of the whole muscle belly and the muscle may also bunch up and form a tumour. There is usually localized tenderness over the defect itself and the muscle is unable to contract. Other symptoms may be swelling and muscle spasm.

Clinical examination is initially carried out with an analysis of the cause of the injury. Thereafter, a close inspection and careful palpation can be carried out. The most important test is often a functional test with and without resistance. In large muscle injuries the risk for compartment syndromes must always be anticipated especially in the lower leg. A functional test of the circulation and neurological functions should be carried out distally to a muscle injury in the lower leg.

Contusion strain or bruising　A contusion strain or bruising is the result of an injury to the muscle, e.g. a knee knocked against the thigh muscle in soccer. The anatomical topography will indicate the location and severity of the strain. Severe external damage to the limb will cause the muscle to be compressed against the underlying bone. The muscles closest to the bone will be injured. A contusion strain or bruising is therefore often located in the deeper lying muscles, but they may also be located superficially. If the compression strain is located in a deeper part and the resulting haematoma is large, the strain symptoms may be disguised and dominated by the haematoma symptoms. Muscle haematomas are often a symptom of muscle strain.

The symptoms and diagnosis are similar to those described for the first and second degree muscle tears.

Muscle haematomas

During physical activity there is a redistribution of the cardiac output. During rest, the blood flow to the active muscles is 0.8 l/min (15% of cardiac output) compared with approximately 18 l/min (72% of cardiac output) after 12 min of physical exercise. This means that the muscles are well vascularized after a good warm-up and during physical activity. The degree of haemorrhage and haematoma formation is directly propor-

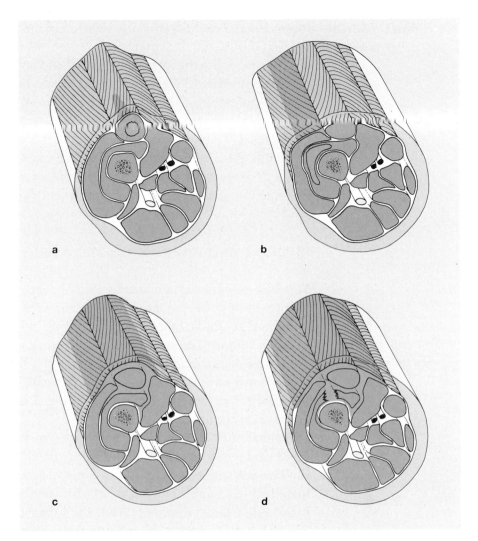

Fig. 10.3.7 Different types of muscle haematomas. (a) Superficial intramuscular haematoma. (b) Deep intramuscular haematoma. (c) Intermuscular haematoma. (d) Deep intramuscular haematoma with an intermuscular spread. Redrawn with permission from Peterson & Renström (1986).

tional to the vascularity of muscle and inversely proportional to the degree of general muscle tone. Two different types of haematomas can be identified because of the different principles of treatment and prognosis: intramuscular and intermuscular haematomas (Fig. 10.3.7).

Intramuscular haematomas

Intramuscular haematomas may be caused by a muscle strain or bruise. The haematoma formation is limited by the intact muscle fascia, the epimysium. If the epimysium is intact the blood flow is retained within the muscle which leads to an increase in the intramuscular pressure, this compresses and limits the haematoma. There is typically long-lasting pain and a loss of function. These haematomas can cause problems for a long time.

Intermuscular haematomas

Intermuscular haematomas may develop in the interfacial and interstitial spaces when the muscle and fascia vessels are injured. The haematoma might spread into the interstitial spaces and an increase in pressure will thereby be avoided. The haematoma will spread distally. A combination of intra- and intermuscular haematomas are common and this is associated with an injured fascia allowing an intermuscular spreading of the haematoma. The symptoms are the same as described in muscle tears. A thorough clinical examination should be made and in cases of haematomas it is especially important to carry out a test of the functions distal to the injury as there is a risk of compartment syndrome.

Healing of damaged muscle tissue

There are different opinions as to whether early mobilization or immobilization should be the preferred choice of treatment. It is therefore important to study what happens during the recovery and repair of damaged tissue. The repair of muscle injury includes two competitive processes: regeneration of muscle fibres and the simultaneous production of connective tissue scar. Such scar tissue may inhibit the complete regeneration of muscle fibres by forming a granulation tissue barrier (Järvinen et al., unpublished data).

Skeletal muscle possesses a high capacity for regeneration (Carlson, 1968), and recovery begins almost immediately. Morphological changes can be seen within 2–3 days with the appearance of myoblasts around the edges of the affected tissue. In contusion injuries where myofibres have been totally or partially torn, the repair process is more complex, consisting of necrosis, inflammation, regeneration and re-innervation and simultaneous production of connective scar tissue (Reznik, 1973).

Seven to 8 days after the injury, the contractile properties of the muscle gradually return. Although functional re-innervation of the regenerating muscle occurs, complete recovery in terms of strength is not achieved (Carlson, 1968). Each of the new fibres possesses almost normal functional characteristics, but the new muscle contains relatively few fibres and large amounts of connective tissue. The total tension which the muscle is capable of producing is therefore less than that of normal muscles.

The repair of the muscle injury also includes production of granulation tissue and formation of non-contractile collagenous fibres. After an injury, the tissue is infiltrated by macrophages which are converted to fibroblasts which proliferate rapidly in the damaged area. There is an increase in the number of fibroblasts within 24 h of the injury and these fibroblasts secrete a soluble protein precursor of collagen; these cells remain in the tissue as fibrocytes. The process of maturation is accompanied by irreversible shortening of the fibrocytes which induces the muscle wounds to heal. The strength of this scar tissue progressively increases, reaching a maximum some months after its initial formation.

Muscles do not regenerate across the scar, and functional continuity is not restored (Garret, 1986). The part of the muscle which is isolated from the motor unit loses its innervation, and the muscle then loses a significant proportion of its ability to produce tension. In a muscle with a partial strain there is a decrease in the ability to produce tension. This means that the active function of the muscle only remains in the portion of the muscle with the intact nerve supply.

The maximum working capacity and force of the muscles depend not only on the performance of the contracted component and the capacity of the vascular system to transport metabolism and supply oxygen, but also upon the elasticity of the muscle. Since shortening of the muscle induces healing, the tensile properties of the healing muscle are important in evaluating the results of different methods of treatment.

Rest vs. early activity Some authors (Järvinen, 1976) believe that early mobilization should be the chosen treatment, but others (O'Donoghue, 1980) suggest that immobilization is preferable (Table 10.3.3). Järvinen (1976), studied the healing of muscle tissue in 600 rats, and found that after thorough morphological, microangiographical and tensiometrical studies, that healing of partial contusion strain of the skeletal muscle can be accelerated by mobilization treatment rather than by immobilization.

In an experimental study with rats, Lehto (1983; Lehto & Järvinen, 1985) found that immobilization following injury accelerates granulation

Table 10.3.3 Benefits of mobilization and immobilization in the treatment of muscle injuries.

Mobilization	Immobilization
Increases tensile strength	Accelerates formation of granulation tissue matrix
Improves orientation of regenerating muscle fibres	Limits size of scar
Stimulates resorption of connective tissue scar	Improves penetration of fibres through connective tissue
Improves recapillarization	
Decreases atrophy of muscles	

tissue production, but if continued too long, it leads to the concentration of scar tissue and poor structural organization of the regenerated muscle fibres and scar-tissue components. Yet a sufficient period of immobilization of about 5 days for rat muscle is needed to reach the stage when newly formed granulation tissue covers the entire injured area and possesses tensile strength great enough to resist the forces caused by mobilization treatment, which might lead to further ruptures. However, mobilization seems to be essential for more rapid resorption of scar tissue and a better structural organization of the reparative elements. Mobilization is also important in order to avoid atrophy.

Rerupturing is often caused by physical activity after prolonged immobilization. Rerupturing may also occur when mobilization is too vigorous and intense (Jackson & Feagin, 1973).

Principles of treatment

Treatment in first 2–3 days

All acute injuries should be treated in the same way as other acute soft tissue injuries: with ice, compression, immobilization, protection, unloading, elevation and rest. The treatment should aim to stop the bleeding, minimize the oedema, prevent further injury, minimize loss of function and promote healing.

During this phase, repeated trauma should be avoided. Although it will take only a few hours for the blood to clot, it will remain friable for 2–3 days, therefore bleeding may be induced by further trauma. During the first 2–3 days after injury, there should be no massage, heat, ultrasound, cortisone injections or active stretching.

Repeated examinations are necessary in order to differentiate between inter- and intramuscular haematomas. A decrease in swelling and a rapid recovery of the muscle function indicates an intermuscular haematoma. An increased swelling and an impaired muscle function indicates an intramuscular haematoma. Initially it might be difficult to distinguish precisely between the types of haematomas. During the first 2–3 days the following questions should therefore be asked (Peterson & Renström, 1986).

1   Has the swelling decreased? If this is not the case there is probably an intramuscular haematoma.

2   Has the haematoma spread into the surrounding areas leading to discoloration of the skin distal to the injury (Fig. 10.3.8)? If this is not the case there might be an intramuscular haematoma.

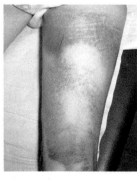

Fig. 10.3.8 The haematoma has spread out into the surrounding areas leading to discoloration of the skin, and indicating an intermuscular haematoma.

3 Has the ability for muscle contraction returned? If this is not the case there might be an intramuscular haematoma.

4 Is the haematoma a symptom of a complete or incomplete muscle tear?

Mobilization treatment

After 2–3 days the diagnosis is usually clear. Careful, active treatment may be carried out after the acute treatment on first and second degree strains, intermuscular haematomas and smaller intramuscular haematomas. This conservative treatment usually consists of early mobilization, as mentioned above, with muscle exercises specifically for the injured muscle. The muscle training should be carried out as follows:

1 Isometric training without load within the limits of pain. Voluntary pain-free contraction tends to aid absorption. Isometric training can be used soon after an injury.

2 Dynamic training without load.

3 Flexibility training, including stretching, is an important part in the rehabilitation after muscle injuries. In first and second degree strains, flexibility training can be started early; but when a third degree strain is sustained, flexibility training should be delayed.

4 Dynamic training with increasing load including both concentric and eccentric contractions. This type of training is an essential part of all training programmes and should be used some time after the injury.

5 Dynamic isokinetic training and training with varying resistance can be used some time after the injury; it is part of common strength training programmes.

6 Training of proprioception can be started soon after the injury is sustained, and should continue for several months.

7 Specialized training, ie. training in the athlete's particular event.

Warming up before strength training after injury is important. Initially, the training should be carried out without load and there should be an increase in the frequency before there is an increase in load. The training should be wide ranging, and strength training should be combined with flexibility training.

Heat treatment

Biomechanically, localized heat in combination with stretching will result in stretching of the collagen fibres to maximal length. Heat retainers are often used in order to produce and maintain heat between the retainer and the skin. Myrhage *et al.* (1981) have shown that heat is generated under the retainer and is maintained for much longer than without any protection. These heat retainers have been produced in

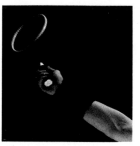

Fig. 10.3.9 Example of a wrist heat retainer.

various forms in order to fit the active parts of the body during sports (Fig. 10.3.9). They may be used in prevention, and also in rehabilitation before muscle exercises are carried out. This increase in heat will lead to an increase in the elasticity of the collagen fibres which is of value in the training procedure.

High-voltage galvanic stimulation can reduce oedema without aggravating the condition (Grana & Schelberg-Kornes, 1983). The mechanical and chemical effects of pulsed ultrasound may also reduce oedema without resulting in significant heat production.

Surgical treatment   Muscle tissue usually heals well, although there is a tendency for a fibrous scar to result. There are, however, a few instances when surgical treatment may be considered (Peterson & Renström, 1986):

1 Large intramuscular haematomas with lasting serious symptoms should be treated surgically by removal of the haematoma. This procedure is usually very successful as the haematoma is larger than may be imagined preoperatively. It is probably important to remove these haematomas, which might otherwise cause a mechanical delay in the joining of the fibres.

2 Third degree strains or tears in muscles which have few or no agonists, i.e. muscles with the same function. One example of this type of injury is a tear of the pectoralis major which can separate from the muscle insertion on the humerus during weight lifting, wrestling, etc.

3 Second degree strains with more than 50% of the muscle belly torn may be treated surgically by removal of the haematoma and joining of the muscle fibres. The degree of the tear may be difficult to evaluate. Franke (1980) considers that if more than 25% of the muscle is torn, surgery should be carried out.

A suture of the torn muscle should be carried out within the first few days after the injury. The musculotendinous unit is normally under continuous tension as the muscle is ready for contraction. When the muscle is torn, the fibres will separate and within a short time a contracture is formed, and it will be difficult to unite the fibre ends to each other. Careful haemostasis and suction drainage are important during surgery. Immobilization may be used for 3–10 days in order to avoid surgical complications with haematoma formation, etc. After removal of the splint, muscle training can begin according to the principles mentioned above.

It should be pointed out that the athletes should carry out specific training of the injured muscle for years to come. Preliminary results from a follow-up of athletes who have been treated for muscle tears have shown that many of them suffered a loss of 20–25% strength, both isometrically and isokinetically at low and high speeds (Renstöm & Konradsen, unpublished data).

Return to sports   The athlete may return to competitive sport when there is no pain during muscle exercises. Ideally, the athlete should have the same power, strength, endurance and flexibility of the muscle groups of both extremities. This is, however, difficult to achieve and therefore the return to sports activities should be gradual. This can be done through, for example, swimming, cycling and cross-country skiing, and thereafter, running followed by increasingly specialized training.

Evaluation of the prognosis   The prognosis depends on the type of injury, treatment and healing time. A clinical evaluation of the severity of, for example, a quadriceps injury can be made by studying the athlete's ability to flex his/her knee. If, for example, the knee can only be bent to 20–50° there is potentially a severe injury in the quadriceps muscles with 1–4 months healing time needed; if the knee flexion is 80–110° the injury may be assessed as mild with 1–3 weeks healing time; and if the knee can be flexed more than 120° only a few days healing is indicated.

Laboratory tests are also useful. Serum enzymes taken after a muscle strain may show an increase in the creatine phosphokinase level (CPK) compared to levels of GOT (glutamic oxalo-acetic transaminase) and GPT (glutamic pyruvic transaminase) (Heiss, 1977). A relationship of 9 : 1, compared to a normal relationship of 5 : 1 indicates a serious injury.

Similar studies have been made by Thorblad *et al.* (1983). They measured CPK levels in a study of 31 soccer players with muscle injuries. The players without an increase in CPK returned to soccer training within 14 days, while players with an increased CPK had longer absences from sport.

Complications to muscle injuries

Myositis ossificans   A single missed severe haematoma or repeated injury may contribute to the formation of myositis ossificans. Repeated wounding may cause new injuries to occur over the initial repair. The result may be an ossification which is caused by the invasion of osteoblasts, probably derived from the damaged periosteum. There might be a partial separation of the muscle fibres from the periosteum or simple bruising of the bone, causing a subperiostal haematoma. Maturation of osteoblasts will form an open network of bone in the muscle. The ossification will continue as long as the healing is disturbed.

The heterotropic bone formation is usually possible to visualize on X-ray 2–4 weeks after a severe contusion. It often starts as a contusion strain and a haematoma close to the bone. In order to make a correct diagnosis it is important to associate the bone mass and the radiographic changes with the history of a contusion, because this condition can mimic an osteogenic sarcoma.

The early treatment of myositis ossificans is traditionally preventive and not surgical. The treatment consists of an extremely conservative approach, as exercise of the affected limb should be strictly avoided (Ellis & Frank, 1966). Rehabilitation should be carried out well within the limits of pain, at least for the first months. With rest, anti-inflammatory medication and heat treatment the ossification will cease, and in many cases the bone will resorb after a couple of years.

According to O'Donoghue (1980) there is no place for surgical treatment in the early stages of myositis ossificans. Groh (1962) recommends that surgery should be postponed for 2 years until the ossification is complete. Beck (1980) has, however, stated that surgery is possible when sharp limitations of the ossification are found on X-ray.

Peterson and Renström (1980b) have reported on 5 athletes with myositis ossificans after severe intramuscular haematoma. These athletes had sustained contusion injuries to their thigh muscles. After 6–8 weeks, calcifications were found on X-rays of the thigh muscles. The athletes could not return to sport, and after 6 weeks they still had severe extension and flexion problems of their knee joints. Because of the significant decrease in function, the athletes were operated on 6–8 weeks after injury. The ossification could easily be removed. Microscopic investigation showed heterotropic ossification following muscle haematoma. Six weeks after the operation, the athletes had recovered full range of motion in their knee joints, good contraction ability of the muscles, and could return to full sports activity. They were re-examined 1 year after surgery, and there were no signs of recurrence on X-ray. The explanation for the success of this early active surgery, could be that this type of myositis ossificans matures more rapidly. Sharp limitations of the ossificans were present in these cases. These results should initiate further studies on this problem.

Old muscle tears   Old muscle tears may sometimes cause problems at a late stage, mainly because of the fibrous and scar tissue formed. They are sometimes mistaken for being malignant tumours. Sometimes it may be difficult to diagnose old ruptures. The diagnosis is usually obvious when carrying out a functional examination during muscular relaxation and contraction. In relaxation there is little or no evidence of a tear or tumour, but during contraction a tumour and a rupture are easily recognized (Fig. 10.3.10).

One example of this is a muscle tear of the semitendinous muscle, one of the hamstrings. In the proximal and middle third of this muscle there is a tendinous insertion running proximal and medial in the distal and lateral directions. Seven misdiagnosed cases of semitendinous muscle ruptures have been studied (Peterson & Renström, 1980b). These were misdiagnosed because of persisting problems or a suspicion of a tumour; and they all involved ruptures through the tendinous insertion of the muscle. After isokinetic training for 4–6 weeks, five of these athletes could return to sports, but two had to be operated on with excision of scar tissue.

Another example is a complete tear of the adductor longus muscle which may occur without causing undue problems to the athlete. It is possible for complete muscle tears to occur without causing the athlete noticeable pain. In one report, seven cases were examined with suspicion of a soft tissue tumour (Peterson & Stener, 1976). These patients had noticed a growing mass. The increase in size was probably due to a compensatory hypertrophy of several muscles, resulting from extra work because of the shortened distance between its origin and new insertion.

Fig. 10.3.10 Old rupture of one of the hamstring muscles (semitendinous): (a) The muscle without contraction. (b) The muscle during contraction.

Muscle tears may be misinterpreted as tumours because of other factors. A haematoma may, after an acute muscle tear, be suspected to be

a

b

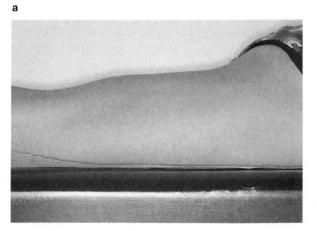
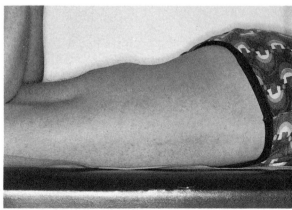

a malignant tumour during its angiographic organization phase, depending on the vascular granulation tissue formed around the haematoma. The scar tissue, after a muscle tear, can also cause a palpable mass which has the character of a tumour.

In these cases, diagnostic methods such as soft tissue X-ray, computed tomography, arteriography, ultrasound, etc. may be helpful. Old muscle tears do not usually cause the athlete great problems, although there may be some weakness in the muscle region. The scar formation may, however, cause an inflammatory reaction if a continuous moderate level of muscle exercise is not maintained.

Chronic muscle and tendon strain

Chronic muscle strain is the result of overloading of the tissues causing microruptures and an inflammatory reaction, and often localized in the muscle origin, e.g. tennis elbow. Pain and impaired function occur, and the athlete may sometimes suffer muscle spasm and ischaemia.

These conditions can always be prevented as they are usually a result of repetitive injuries. If a chronic strain condition occurs, the treatment is usually rest, localized heat, sometimes local anaesthetics, and protection against additional stress. Specialized muscle exercise should be carried out; heat protectors are also helpful.

Chronic strains are most likely to occur at the origin of the muscle and tendon and at the muscle–tendon junction. They are not very common in the muscle itself.

Conclusion

Muscle injuries are very common in sports, but knowledge about these injuries is limited. They cause a significant reduction in the athlete's capacity for full performance, and because of this, as well as consideration of the athlete's health, they have to be treated seriously.

Most muscle injuries can be prevented by a thorough warming up of the body which increases the vascularity, and by strength training combined with stretching and flexibility training. The athlete should not just consider body building, but also body function. If, in spite of all precautions, a muscle injury occurs, it should be treated immediately, and repeated examinations should be carried out in order to obtain a correct diagnosis.

The effects of common treatment methods on the healing of muscle injuries is poorly understood (Lehto, 1983). During the healing process of a muscle injury two competitive events take place simultaneously: the regeneration of muscle tissue and the production of a connective tissue scar. Intensive, gentle therapy with early mobilization is usually the preferred treatment, but a short time of immobilization or early surgical treatment should sometimes be considered. Muscle injuries should be treated with care and thoughtfulness.

References

Beck, E. (1980) Muskel-, Sehnen- und Bandverletzungen beim Sport. *Z. Allg. Med.* **56**, 228.

Carlson, B. M. (1968) Regeneration of the completely excised gastrocnemius muscle in the frog and rat from muscle fragments. *J. Morph.* **125**, 447.

Ellis, M. & Frank, H. (1966) Myositis ossificans traumatica with special reference to the quadriceps femoris muscle. *J. Trauma* **6**, 724.

Franke, K. (1980) *Traumatologie des Sports*. Georg thiem-Verlag, Stuttgart.

Friedrich, H. & Biener, K. (1973) Handballsportunfälle. *Sportartz Sportmed.* **24**, 236.

Garret, W. E. (1986) Basic science of musculo-tendinous injuries. In J. Nicholas & E. G. Hershman (eds) *The Lower Extremity and Spine in Sports Medicine*. Mosby, St Louis.

Grana, W. & Schelberg-Kornes, E. (1983) How I manage deep muscle bruises. *Phys. Med.* **11(6)**, 123.

Groh, H. (1962) Sportverletzungen. In H. Groh (ed) *Sportmedizin*. Ferdinand Enke-Verlag, Stuttgart.

Heiser, T. M., Weber, J., Sullivan, G., Clare, P. & Jacobs, P. R. (1984) Prophylaxis and management of hamstring muscle injuries in intercollegiate football players. *Am. J. Sports Med.* **12**, 368.

Heiss, F. (1977) *Unfallverhutung und Nothilfe beim Sport* (Trauma prevention and first aid in sport). Karl Hoffmann, Schorndorf.

Jackson, D. W. & Feagin, J. A. (1973) Quadriceps contusions in young athletes. Relation of severity of injury to treatment and prognosis. *J. Bone Joint Surg. (Am.)* **55**, 95.

Järvinen, M. (1976) *Healing of a crash injury in rat striated muscle*. Ph. D. Thesis, University of Turku, Finland.

Kvist, M. & Järvinen, M. J. (1980) Zur epidemiologie von Sportverletzungen und Fehlbelastungstolgen. *Med. Sport* **20**, 373.

Lehto, M. (1983) *Collagen and fibronectin in a healing skeletal muscle injury. An experimental study in rats under variable states of physical activity*. Ph. D. Thesis, University of Turku, Finland.

Lehto, M. & Järvinen, M. (1985) Collagen and glycosaminoglycans synthesis of injured gastrocnemius muscle in rat. *Eur. Surg. Res.* **17**, 179.

Lehto, M., Sims, T. J. & Bailey, A. J. (1985) Skeletal muscle injury — molecular changes in the collagen during healing. *Res. Exp. Med.* **185,** 95.

Myrhage, R., Peterson, L. & Renström P. (1981) *Effect of heat protectors*. Paper presented in Stockholm at the Medical Report, December 1981.

O'Donoghue, H. (ed) (1980) *Treatment of Injuries to Athletes*. W. B. Saunders, Philadelphia.

Peterson, L. & Stener, B. (1976) Old total rupture of the adductor longus muscle. *Acta Orthop. Scand.* **47**, 653.

Peterson, L. & Renström, P. (1980a) Världsmästerskap för veteraner (World Master championships in track and field). *Läkartidningen* **77(41)**, 3618.

Peterson, L. & Renström, P. (1980b) Muskelskador inom idrotten (Muscle injuries in sport). *Ronden* **22**.

Peterson, L. & Renström, P. (1986) *Sports Injuries: Their Prevention and Treatment*. Martin Dunitz, London.

Radin, E. L. (1986) Role of muscles in protecting athletes from injury. In P.-O. Åstrand & G. Grimby (eds) *Physical Activity in Health and Disease*, p. 143. Acta Med. Scand. Symposium Series **2**.

Renström, P. & Peterson, L. (1977) *Fotbollsplan med konstgräs* (Soccer on artificial fields). Valhalla idrottsplats i Göteborg. Naturvardsverket SNV PM 846, Solna, Sweden.

Reznik, M. (1973) Current concepts of skeletal muscle regeneration. In C. M. Pearson & F. K. Mostofi (eds) *The Striated Muscle*. Williams & Wilkins, Baltimore.

Thorblad, J., Gillqvist, J. & Ekstrand, J. (1983) *Serumenzymer vid muskeltrauma* (Serum enzymes in muscle trauma). Swedish Sports Medicine Society, May, 1983.

Further reading

Thorndike, A. (1956) *Athletic Injuries*, 4th edn. Lea & Febiger, Philadelphia.

Tendon ruptures

P. RENSTRÖM

Tendon injuries constitute some of the most common injuries in sport. There is great controversy concerning the treatment of both traumatic and overuse injuries of the tendons.

Human motion is governed by an ingenious interaction between joints, muscles, tendons and nerves. A nerve impulse will activate the muscle, which will contract and make the tendon carry out the work over the joints and bones. A typical example of the interplay between the muscles and tendons is the anatomy of the posterior part of the lower extremity, i.e. the interplay between the gastrocnemius and soleus muscles with the Achilles tendon. Leonardo da Vinci (b.1452) labelled the tendons as 'mechanical instruments' because they transmitted tension to bone.

There are basically five risk factors for injury in the musculotendinous system: (a) where the muscle inserts into bone, e.g. tennis elbow; (b) in the muscle itself, e.g. muscle haematomas; (c) in the musculotendinous junction, e.g. tennis leg; (d) in the tendon itself, e.g. Achilles tendon ruptures; and (e) in the insertion of the tendon into bone, e.g. Osgood–Schlatter disease.

The type and location of injury depends on many factors such as age, degree of degeneration in the connective tissue, type of trauma, etc. To clarify the principles and the problems in musculotendinous injuries, the musculotendinous complex on the posterior side of the lower leg will be used as an example as it is a location frequently encountered in common sports medicine problems.

Functional anatomy of tendons

The tendons consist of collagen fibres orientated in parallel in the longitudinal direction. The tendons are strong with a tensile strength of 49–98 N/mm². Maximum concentric and isometric tensions are well below the tensile strength of the tendon (Stanish *et al.*, 1985). Therefore, neither concentric nor isometric contractions are likely to cause tendon breakdown. Tendons effectively withstand tensile longitudinal forces, resist shear forces less well and provide little resistance to compressive forces.

The collagen fibres are bound together with cross-links. In a stress

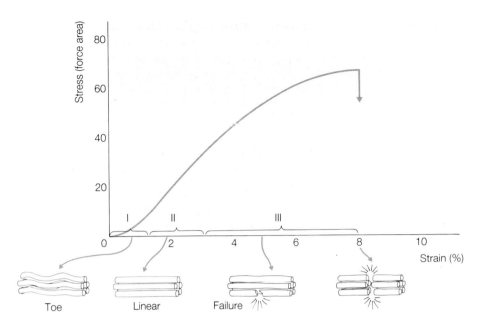

Fig. 10.3.11 A typical stress strain curve for tendons. From Curwin & Stanish (1984).

situation the cross-links will rupture depending on the degree of stress. Normally a tendon has a wavy configuration up to 2% of strain (Fig. 10.3.11). Between 2 and 4% of strain there is a physiological load on the tendon. Between 4 and 8% strain the cross-links start to rupture and there may be an inflammatory reaction and a partial rupture. Above 8% strain there may be a total rupture of the tendon.

The blood supply to the tendons is usually poor. Studies of the Achilles tendon have shown that the area of lowest vascularity is 2–6 cm above the insertion of the tendon. The blood supply consists mostly of longitudinal arterioles that course the length of the tendon, supplemented by vessels from the mesotendon. The area of lowest vascularity is the area where most of the injuries to the Achilles tendon occur.

In the posterior musculotendinous complex of the lower leg, the soleus and gastrocnemius muscles contribute separately to the formation of the Achilles tendon. The tendon fibres themselves rotate laterally as they descend. This rotation plays an important role in the aetiology of Achilles tendon injuries.

Causes and aetiology

Injuries in tendons may be divided into overuse injuries and traumatic injuries, e.g. ruptures. The most important factors contributing to tendon injuries are presented in Chapter 10.1. The most common extrinsic factors are training errors, e.g. increase in training mileage, increase and changes in training intensity, running up- and downhill or on uneven or slippery terrain, etc. Intrinsic factors include anatomical malalignment such as excessive pronation, cavus foot, hindfoot or forefoot varus, tibia vara, tight heel cords, etc.

Causes   There are some potential causes for tendon injuries (Clancy, 1982):

1   Repetitive trauma or changes in loading of the musculotendinous unit leading to collagen failure. This fatigue or stress failure of the tendon can be considered as analogous to stress fractures of bones.

2   Shortening and decreased flexibility may result in passive increased loading of the tendon during relaxation. Tight muscles may transmit a peak load to the tendon or may alter the biomechanics of the foot during stance and thereby alter the stress on the tendon.

3   Malalignment is a factor in the production of, for example, Achilles tendinitis, with the most common malalignment being excessive pronation. This results in a compensatory rotation of the tibia. Hyperpronation results in an angled traction resulting in an increased stretch of the Achilles tendon. Fatigue of the muscles may give the same result. Causes of traumatic injuries, e.g. tendon ruptures, are sudden overload strains or direct blows to the tendon during a contraction.

Aetiology   Aetiologic factors may be chronic degenerative changes. In tendons like the Achilles or supraspinatus tendons, the poor blood supply a few centimetres proximal to the insertion is probably an important aetiological factor. Old injuries can possibly also contribute as they decrease the strength of the tendon thereby forming a weak area. Factors like poor training, poor warm-up, fatigue, inactivity, etc. may also be of importance.

Galen (AD 130–200) accepted the concept that tendons will develop to the extent they are used, because they would waste away if they were idle.

Diagnosis

Tendon injuries and pathological changes can be divided into partial and total ruptures, peri- or paratendinitis, tenoperiostitis, bursitis and tendinosus. A correct diagnosis depends on a thorough clinical history and examination. Total rupture will be discussed below, other tendon injuries are considered in Chapter 10.4.

Ruptures   The history when a rupture occurs is classic. As an example, a 30–40-year-old athlete may describe a sudden pain in the Achilles tendon during, for example, landing after heading in soccer, jumping in badminton, or running downhill. Deceleration and eccentric contractions are often involved. The athlete will experience a sharp pain or discomfort at the time of injury. It is usually impossible for him or her to continue with sports activities.

Partial ruptures   In a partial rupture the pain will be consistent and there will, after a while, be some swelling and tenderness over the injured area. These symptoms are often experienced in connection with physical activity. At physical examination there is a distinct tenderness and swelling, usually only over the injured area, distinguishing it from tendinitis in which there usually are more general findings (see Chapter 10.4).

Total ruptures   If the tendon is totally ruptured there is an initial, sudden, intensive pain and the athlete will hear something 'pop'. There will be impaired motion of the joint involved. In a total injury the pain will, however, often subside. Total ruptures of tendons, muscles and ligaments will therefore often be missed, because the pain after the injury is not as substantial as in partial ruptures.

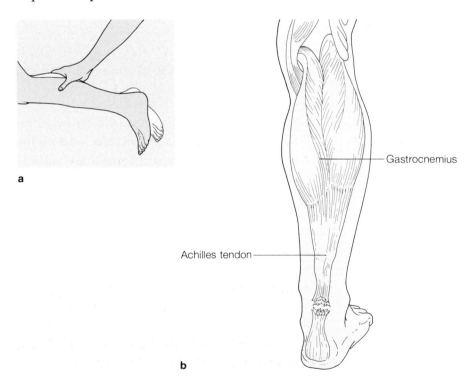

a

Gastrocnemius

Achilles tendon

Fig. 10.3.12 Thompsen's test (a) for total Achilles tendon rupture (b).

b

Tests　　If an athlete has a total Achilles tendon rupture he or she can often not plantar flex the foot in a non-weight bearing situation. Sometimes, however, the tibialis posterior, the toe flexors and the peroneal tendons can contribute to the ability to plantar flex making the diagnosis more difficult. The Thompsen's test (Fig. 10.3.12) is, however, reliable. The examiner firmly squeezes the major bulk of the muscle belly and the normal foot will then plantar flex. If plantar flexion does not occur the test is positive and the Achilles tendon is totally disrupted. There is almost always a palpable defect in the acutely disrupted tendon as well (Fig. 10.3.13).

In ruptures of the supraspinatus tendon the ability to abduct and elevate the arm from 60° to 120° is impaired. If the athlete has a total rupture he or she can lower the arm from 180° down to 120° and then the arm suddenly drops down because of a total rupture or because of pain. This test indicates some kind of tear of the supraspinatus muscle.

The diagnosis of tendon ruptures is based on a thorough clinical examination. There are, however, some diagnostic adjuncts to identify tendon ruptures and partial tears, such as soft tissue X-ray, bursography, ultrasound, electromyography (EMG), nuclear magnetic resonance (NMR) imaging. These diagnostic methods are discussed in Chapter 10.2.

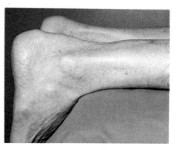

Fig. 10.3.13 A total untreated rupture of the Achilles tendon.

Treatment

The main objective of the treatment of tendon injuries is to restore pain-free function and motion.

Total ruptures　　The main object of treatment should be to restore normal length and strength as closely as possible. Great controversy exists, however, concerning the treatment of some total tendon injuries, especially in the Achilles tendon. The principles of treatment will therefore be discussed by using a total rupture of the Achilles tendon as an example.

Some advocate non-operative treatment of total Achilles tendon ruptures (Lea & Smith, 1972; Nistor, 1981). This treatment includes immobilization in a cast for 8–10 weeks and thereafter very careful rehabilitation. A heel wedge should be worn for 4–6 months, and no sports activities are allowed for 1 year. The main risk with this treatment is a re-rupture. Some report a high incidence of re-ruptures in the non-surgical group combined with a decrease in strength and a more pronounced muscle atrophy (Inglis & Sculco, 1976). Nistor (1981) found, however, in his randomized prospective study virtually no difference between surgically and non-surgically treated patients. The great importance of a careful and long-term follow-up of the non-surgically treated patients must be emphasized. Experience has shown, that as soon as the patients are left without adequate instructions, the incidence of re-ruptures will quickly increase. Inactive people, especially the elderly, can successfully be treated non-surgically.

Most centres prefer to repair the tendons in most individuals, especially those that are active in some kind of sports. The repair procedures vary, but basically a suture is made, often with some kind of reinforcement. Percutaneous repair with good results has been presented. A cast is used postoperatively for a varying period of time. Six weeks in a lower leg cast with the foot in a neutral position is often used as the tendon heals better if there is some tension involved. Partial weight bearing is allowed after 2–3 weeks. A heel wedge is used for 1–2 months after the cast is taken away. Early mobilization is important; if active mobilization is considered potentially dangerous, it is often possible to start with passive mobilization.

When a tendon is injured, the repair includes the formation of collagen. The proliferating fibrous scar lacks inherent elasticity, which is a problem for athletes. A graduated early mobilization programme which includes stretching techniques is of importance. This training should be combined with progressive strength training and muscle rebalancing. It should be remembered that repaired tissue will require a long time, at least 6 months or longer, for the recovery to be complete. Return to sports is often possible after a repair with augmentation within 4–8 months.

Other tendon injuries

Most other tendon injuries, like overuse injuries and partial tears, can be treated conservatively. Acute partial tears in tendons may, however, need immobilization over a short period of time. This should be carried out with tension of the tendon in order to minimize the scar and granulation tissue formed. Immobilization of some kind may be of great value in the initial treatment of acute partial tendon tears. Rehabilitation should start as early as possible as immobilization in itself has a deleterious effect. Passive mobilization procedures will facilitate the repair process of tendons; but rehabilitation should include a well planned progressive exercise programme.

Total tendon ruptures are often missed as they usually do not cause much pain and because the loss of motion and strength can often, to some extent, be compensated for. The aim of treatment in active people and athletes should be to restore full functioning of the body.

References

Clancy, W. G. (1982) Tendinitis and plantar fasciitis in runners. In R. D'Ambrosia & D. Drez jr (eds) *Prevention and Treatment of Running Injuries*, pp. 77–88. Charles Slack, Thorofare.

Curwin, S. & Stanish, W. D. (1984) *Tendinitis: Its Etiology and Treatment*. The Collamore Press, Lexington.

Inglis, A. E. & Sculco, T. P. (1981) Surgical repair of rupture of the tendo Achilles. *Clin. Orthop.* **156**, 160.

Lea, R. B. & Smith, L. (1972) Non surgical treatment of tendo Achilles rupture. *J. Bone Joint Surg. (Am)* **54**, 1398.

Nistor, L. (1981) Surgical and non-surgical treatment of achilles-tendon rupture. *J. Bone Joint Surg. (Am)* **63**, 394.

Stanish, D. S., Curwin, S. & Rubinovich, M. (1985) *Tendinitis: The Analysis and Treatment for Running Clinics in Sports Medicine*, p. 593. Saunders Co., Toronto.

Joint injuries

G. P. H. HERMANS & S. MIRONOV

Anatomically, a joint is comprised of the articular surfaces (i.e. the cartilage-lined extremities of the bones that articulate in the joint), the subchondral layer of the bone, directly beneath the cartilage, the fibrous capsule with the ligamentous apparatus, the synovial capsule and the appertaining musculature. Together, the anatomical components of a joint constitute a functional unit. This basic principle is of great importance for the diagnosis of injuries and of the resulting functional disorders, as well as for rehabilitation. The concept of the functional unit can be defined in two ways:

1 The joint as a biomechanical functional unit.
2 The joint as a biological functional unit.

The joint as a biomechanical functional unit

The integrated functioning of parts of a joint can be regarded as a compromise between mobility and stability. The mobility of a joint is determined by the shape of the articular surfaces, the ligamentous apparatus and the fibrous capsule, and the musculature appertaining to the joint. These structures, and the shape of the articular surfaces, capsule and musculature also determine the stability.

In the stability of a joint the following can be distinguished:

1 Osseous stability (static stability).
2 Ligamentous–capsular stability (partly of a static, partly of a dynamic character).
3 Muscular stability (which has a wholly dynamic character).

The proportions of the various forms of stability differ in different joints. The hip joint, for instance, has very high osseous stability, while the knee joint has very low osseous stability but highly developed capsulogenous, ligamentous and muscular stability. The functional adjustment of a joint to the stability and mobility required for a particular movement is governed by a neurophysiological connection of the receptors in the capsular and ligamentous systems and the appertaining musculature. This makes possible rapid and effective functional stabilization of a joint depending on the strain exerted on the joint and its posture at the moment.

Because of the functional interdependence of the components of a joint, an injury to one of the components will affect all other elements of the functional unit. For instance, a contusion of the fibrous articular capsule will lead to interruption of a number of proprioceptive circuits to the adjacent musculature, rapidly followed by atrophy of these muscles.

The joint as a biological functional unit

Cartilage The articular cartilage is avascular, the calcified deep layers of the cartilage form the 'tidemark' between the vascularized bone of the metaphysis and the avascular cartilage. The principal functions of the cartilage are: guidance of movements, absorption of shocks and distribution of forces. For the performance of these functions, articular cartilage has a specific structure.

Articular cartilage consists of a network of collagen bundles which are continuous with the collagen of the underlying bone, and which at the surface of the cartilaginous layer curve back again towards the deep layers. The resulting network fills with cellular material, the chondrocytes or cartilage cells. These produce proteoglycans, large complexes of protein–sugar molecules that have a high water-binding capacity enabling them to keep the collagenous network of the cartilage at the required tension. For its nourishment the avascular articular cartilage is dependent upon the synovial fluid. Owing to the variable strains during motion and weight bearing of a joint, this synovial fluid is forced into the articular cartilage, and at negative pressures part of it is sucked out again. The synovial fluid has another, mechanical function, i.e. lubrication of the joint which permits a low-energy movement between the articular surfaces and greatly reduces the frictional resistance.

The synovial fluid is produced by the synovial membrane which lines the inside of the articular cavity and consists of a loose-meshed stroma in which capillaries are embedded. This loose-meshed stroma is delimited on the articular side by a single layer of cells in which there are two types of cells, the so-called a-cells with a predominantly phagocytic function and the b-cells that have a predominantly secretory function. A characteristic aspect of the synovial membrane is that, unlike, for instance, vascular endothelium, it lacks the basal membrane. Thus, there is an 'open' connection between the capillaries in the loose-meshed stroma and the articular cavity. The synovial fluid is an ultrafiltrate of blood plasma to which the b-cells add hyaluronic acid. As a result, the synovial fluid becomes a biological link between the avascular cartilage and the capillaries in the loose-meshed stroma of the synovial membrane.

For the synovial fluid to reach the cells in the deeper layers of the articular cartilage, mechanical strain is required. The mechanical strain forces the synovial fluid into the cartilage, resulting *inter alia* in transport of glucose. When the pressure decreases or shifts to a different part of the joint, the hyaluronic acid molecules in the relieved part of the cartilage expand and the colloid–osmotic gradient between cartilage and synovial fluid is inverted, permitting rediffusion of the fluid from the cartilage into the joint. This explains why movement, i.e. strain, is necessary for physiological nourishment of the articular cartilage. In this way, the biological and the biomechanical functions are linked together.

Diagnosis and treatment of knee joint injuries

The knee joint is an articulation characterized by a very low osseous stability and a high dynamic stability provided by ligaments and the large muscle groups of the lower leg and thigh.

The low osseous stability between the flat tibial surface and the concave condyles is increased slightly by the presence of the menisci which lie on the tibial surface and transform it into a cup-shaped structure providing the joint with at least some static stability. To sustain the complex movements at the knee joint, an intricate ligamentous apparatus is required. Its dorsal part (Fig. 10.3.14) comprises the fibrous capsule which contains the expansions of the five different divisions of the semimembranous and popliteus muscles and the two heads of the

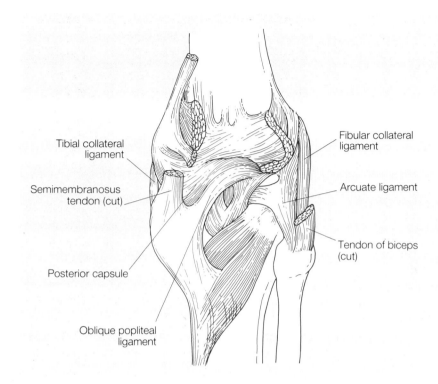

Tibial collateral
ligament

Semimembranosus
tendon (cut)

Posterior capsule

Oblique popliteal
ligament

Fibular collateral
ligament

Arcuate ligament

Tendon of biceps
(cut)

Fig. 10.3.14 Ligamentous structures of the dorsal side of the knee, with the gastrocnemius head cut. Redrawn from Larson (1975).

gastrocnemius muscle that cross the joint on the dorsal side. On the ventral side, the dynamic stability is provided by the patella and the patellar ligament inserting on it, and the quadriceps tendon on the cranial side. As well as this, the patella, like a sesamoid bone, lies caught between the medial and lateral retinacula.

The collateral–lateral stability is ensured by the lateral–collateral ligament, the iliotibial tract and the lateral fibrous capsule (Fig. 10.3.15). Medially, the superficial medial collateral ligament can be distinguished which runs from the medial condyle to fairly far distally on the tibia, the meniscofemoral and meniscotibial ligaments which have a very short tract and, on the dorsomedial side, the posterior oblique ligament. As a dynamic stabilizer on the medial side, there is also the pes anserinus which contains the tendinous expansions of the semitendinosus, gracilis and sartorius muscles (Fig. 10.3.16).

Other characteristic components of the knee joint are the very important 'central pillars' of the stability, i.e. the anterior and posterior cruciate ligaments. These bands, situated inside the knee joint but outside the synovia, are essential for the functioning of the joint. They contribute not only to the stability in the sagittal plane but also to the physiological realization of the rotating movement in the knee joint.

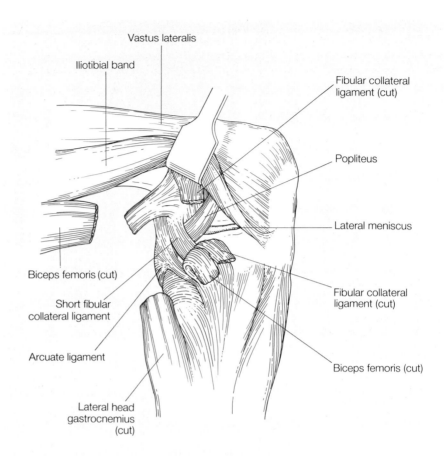

Fig. 10.3.15 Lateral supporting structures of the knee. Redrawn from Larson (1975).

Biomechanical function of the knee joint

This consists of a flexion movement which in its turn is comprised of a complex sliding–rolling movement and a rotating movement that occurs largely during the last part of extension.

Injuries to the ligamentous apparatus

If an injury occurs in the complex system described above, the interlinking of the various structures and functions lead to a complex set of symptoms in which it is frequently difficult to reduce a particular symptom to a traumatic lesion in a circumscribed part of the knee joint. For instance, presence of swelling in the knee joint due to hydrops is just an indication of synovial hyperactivity, the cause of which still remains to be traced. Also, swelling due to extravasation of blood into the joint (haemarthrosis) may be caused by a number of intra-articular lesions such as ruptures of cruciate ligaments, meniscal avulsions or osteochondral fractures of the articular surfaces. All injuries of this nature that are accompanied by haemarthrosis constitute a serious threat to the knee joint and there is an urgent indication for arthroscopic examination.

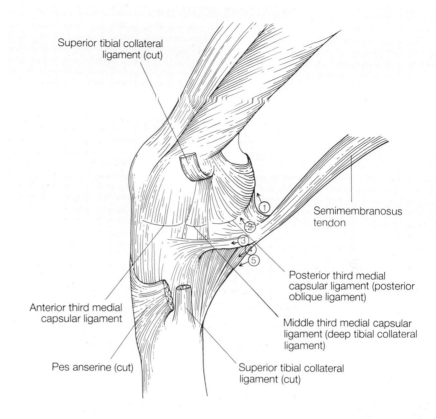

Superior tibial collateral
ligament (cut)

Semimembranosus
tendon

Posterior third medial
capsular ligament (posterior
oblique ligament)

Anterior third medial
capsular ligament

Middle third medial capsular
ligament (deep tibial collateral
ligament)

Pes anserine (cut)

Superior tibial collateral
ligament (cut)

Fig. 10.3.16 Medial supporting structures of the knee. 1, Oblique popliteal ligament; 2, posterior capsule and posterior horn of the medial meniscus; 3, anterior or medial tendon of the semimembranosus; 4, direct head of the semimembranosus; 5, distal portion of the semimembranosus tendon. Redrawn from Larson (1975).

Lock-like phenomena, finally, are often attributed exclusively to meniscal lesions but they may also occur in post-traumatic cartilaginous damage, in severe chondromalacia, in the presence of free bodies and, sometimes, in the presence of a plica parapatellaris medialis.

Anamnesis The violence of an impact has a certain predicting value with respect to the consequences of the accident. The consequences of a heavy impact on a joint in a weight bearing position in which an opponent may have been involved are completely different from those of a mild torsion injury to a joint in a non-weight bearing position.

Owing to the frequency in sports of situations in which the body-weight is all on one leg, the other leg being used to play, the two more or less classical accident mechanisms are the flexion–valgus–endorotation trauma and the flexion–varus–exorotation trauma. Accordingly, the nature and gravity of the accident may provide information for the diagnosis of the consequences of the accident.

The anamnesis is of great importance in knee injuries because the knee joint itself allows little access for physical diagnostics, particularly after a recent injury.

Direct consequences of the accident In serious ligamentous injury to the knee the weight bearing capacity of the leg often remains surprisingly good for several hours after the accident. Development of swelling immediately after an accident, i.e. during the first few hours, is strongly suggestive of haemarthrosis. Haemarthrosis in its turn always signifies a severe internal knee injury, often with damage to an anterior cruciate ligament or avulsion of the meniscus in the vascularized, peripheral portion, or an osteochondral fracture in one of the articular surfaces. A puncture may then be useful for the differential diagnosis between haemarthrosis and hydrops.

Pain localization In recent injuries, the pain localization is difficult to interpret because the presence of blood in the joint and the reactive synovitis render the pain distribution round the joint diffuse. As early as a few hours after the accident, the joint is inaccessible for exact pain point diagnostics, owing to the presence of oedema of the various structures in the capsule of the knee joint.

Impairment of movement A true lock phenomenon, i.e. impairment of the mobility of a joint due to a mechanical cause, occurs virtually exclusively as the consequence of a bucket-handle lesion of the meniscus or of a so-called interposing flap tear. A lock phenomenon should not be confused with an antalgesic flexion position of the joint or with a relieving 'Bonnet' position in the presence of haemarthrosis or hydrops. Severe retropatellar chondromalacia and the presence of a plica para-patellaris may also bring about lock-like phenomena.

Instability symptoms A patient with an extensive, new ligamentous knee injury often notices little instability at first because he or she is forced to adopt a very cautious gait and cannot rest weight on the joint. Inveterate ligament ruptures, on the other hand, frequently bring about progressive instability symptoms, often with the pivot shift phenomenon, a form of instability which the patient is unable to control and which can be very alarming. This type of instability is characteristic of an inveterate rupture of the anterior cruciate ligament; it is caused by the tibia being dislocated from below the femur in extension and repositioned in flexion.

Patients themselves frequently mistake instability symptoms for momentary sensations of giving way due to brief episodes of muscular insufficiency of the quadriceps. The latter should be interpreted as a disorder of the coordination of the quadriceps function rather than as a consequence of ligamentous instability.

Physical diagnosis *Inspection* Sometimes a local haematoma is visible after a few days, especially in medial ligamentous lesions, in which there is either deep avulsion of the superficial collateral ligament at the tibial insertion or avulsion of the posterior oblique ligament on the dorsal side of the medial femoral condyle. Also, swelling of the joint may be visible in the form of an obliterated patellar outline, as the consequence of either haemarthrosis or hydrops. Atrophy of the musculature of the thigh, and particularly of the vastus medialis obliquus muscle is an early feature in intra-articular injuries to the knee joint. It is particularly clearly notice-able when it is compared with the normal side with tensed musculature.

Palpation Hypotony of the quadriceps can easily be established by palpation.

Pain point diagnostics This diagnostic method is of limited value; the best information can be obtained near the articular cleft at the origin and insertion of the ligamentous apparatus. Pressure pain points in the region of the posterior oblique ligament, in the region of the menisco-femoral and meniscotibial ligaments and in the region of the lateral capsule at the origin on the tibia, may direct the examiner to any severe ligamentous lesions.

Stability examination In recent knee joint injuries the stability examina-tion is often difficult to perform because of the pain and the defensive tension and impaired function it causes in the patient. Especially in new lesions of the anterior cruciate ligament, the anterior drawer phenomenon is often still negative or difficult to assess.

The same holds true of the combined instabilities in which sagittal instability and damage of the posteromedial and/or posterolateral structures lead to rotatory instability components in which the tibia, either in exorotation or in endorotation at 90° of flexion in relation to the femur, can be subluxated in the ventral direction.

A stability examination shortly after a recent ligamentous injury to the knee is difficult to carry out reliably and offers little certainty. In particular, the absence of an anterior drawer phenomenon at 90° flexion of the knee does not guarantee that the anterior cruciate ligament is intact. A more reliable method of testing the sagittal, ventral instability is the Lachman test, in which with the knee in 20° of flexion the tibia can be subluxated in the ventral direction in relation to the femur. Owing to the absence of muscular defence of the hamstrings, the reliability of this manoeuvre is better. The collateral instability can as a rule be established better, at any rate with the knee in 20° of flexion, because here the muscular defence factor plays a less important role.

The fact remains, however, that a reliable stability examination is difficult to carry out immediately after a fresh injury to a knee ligament and during the next few days, and that if offers little diagnostic certainty. Sometimes, other lesions of the same extremity are so impressive that ruptured ligaments are overlooked. This often occurs with ruptures of the posterior cruciate ligament caused by ventral impact on the tibia, a frequent phenomenon in traffic accidents.

Radiological examination   Skeletal X-rays are of little informative value in lesions of the menisci and ligaments. Stress X-rays are often difficult to assess because of the pain and the muscular defence. In regard to meniscal lesions, it should further be kept in mind that the predictive value of arthrography is limited; the literature gives reliability rates of 60–80%. This means that a negative arthrogram does not definitely exclude meniscal pathology, nor does a negative stress X-ray exclude the presence of ligamentous lesions. This holds particularly true of a lesion of an anterior or posterior cruciate ligament.

Articular puncture   Puncture of a joint is mainly useful if haemarthrosis is suspected. Such a suspicion is justified if swelling of a joint occurs soon, i.e. a few hours, after the accident. If the swelling takes 24 h or longer to appear, it usually indicates hydrops rather than haemarthrosis. If haemarthrosis is demonstrated, this means that a serious internal injury of the knee is almost certainly present. The most common injuries, in the order of frequency, are: a ruptured anterior cruciate ligament, an avulsion of the meniscus in the vascularized part, an osteochondral fracture or a combination of these three lesions.

Demonstration of haemarthrosis constitutes an indication for further examination in the form of arthroscopy.

Arthroscopy   Arthroscopic examination of the knee joint considerably improves the clinical diagnostic possibilities, especially in injuries to the anterior cruciate ligament, meniscal lesions and osteochondral fractures. Further examination of the knee by arthroscopy may be regarded as definitely indicated in all cases in which haemarthrosis is established or seriously suspected.

Diagnosis and treatment of ankle joint injuries

Diagnosis
Anamnesis

The anamnesis offers a starting point for the diagnosis and also helps in the choice of subsequent treatment.

1 Age: The age is relevant in that generally conservative treatment is indicated in young children and elderly patients.

? Primary injury or habitual distortion?: In the case of a primary injury, surgical treatment may be considered; for habitual distortion, primary conservative treatment is indicated in any case, if necessary to be followed by plastic ligamentous reconstruction at a later stage.

3 Occupation and hobbies: The demands on the ankle joint that arise from the patient's occupation and hobbies will be considered in the choice of treatment. If none of these activities require maximal ankle stability, there is little reason to consider surgery.

Inspection

Fresh injuries, particularly in the area of the anterior talofibular ligament, are often followed by very rapid circumscribed swelling of the joint on the anterolateral side. With more extensive rupturing the swelling is more diffuse, but the subsequently developing haematoma may be an important aid in the diagnosis of the extension of ruptures.

Palpation

Over ruptured ligaments there is often intense pressure pain; if oedema is not too copious, a capsular defect may be felt, and often crepitations as well when the ankle is moved slightly during palpation.

Stability examination

Inversion movements will not give a reliable idea of lateral instability of the ankle. More reliable is the anterior drawer phenomenon, i.e. the tarsus in the tibiotarsal joint can be subluxated in the anteriomedial direction. This examination is carried out most easily when the patient is sitting with the lower leg dangling.

Radiological examination

Standard X-rays are, as a rule, used to exclude fractures; a stress examination may be carried out in addition to establish instability. This stress examination may be performed by means of manual or mechanical inversion stress. Frequently, supplementary examination by means of arthrography and tenography is desirable. Using these techniques, a higher level of reliability may be achieved.

Treatment
Conservative

Immobilization is a condition of conservative treatment. It may be produced by means of a plaster cast or by taping. The latter offers the advantage that it permits functional rehabilitation. This exerts a positive effect on wound healing in the ligamentous apparatus and is undeniably better for the joint.

In general, the results of conservative treatment of injuries to ankle ligaments are so favourable that surgical treatment is only indicated to a limited extent. Accordingly, optimal conservative treatment consists in functional immobilization by taping, combating pain and oedema with ice and, if necessary, drugs. Swelling and pain permitting, functional exercise therapy may be started, possibly in combination with physio-technical applications.

Surgery   When surgical treatment is opted for, the periods of choice are either within a few hours after the accident, or several days later, depending on swelling and oedema. At operation, the ruptured ligaments, which are often caught between articular bones or, in the case of the calcaneofibular ligament, dislocated from behind the peroneal fossa, are repositioned and adapted by means of sutures.

Surgical treatment also requires functional after-treatment using braces or bandages. Emphasis in the after-treatment phase should be on restoration of muscular strength and coordination by means of training of the peroneal muscles, the anterior tibial muscle and the anterior muscles of the leg. In a later phase of the after-treatment, attention should also be particularly paid to restoring the articular mobility of the

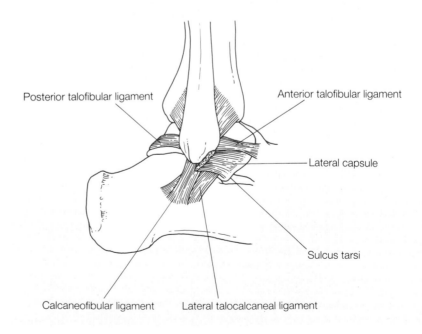

Posterior talofibular ligament

Anterior talofibular ligament

Lateral capsule

Sulcus tarsi

Calcaneofibular ligament   Lateral talocalcaneal ligament

Fig. 10.3.17 Lateral ligaments of the ankle. Redrawn from Anderson *et al*. (1952).

tibiotarsal joint, the subtalar joint and the articulations of Chopart and Lisfranc.

Prevention Many primary distortions of the ankle joint become habitual distortions owing to inadequate after-treatment of the primary injury. A sufficient amount of adequate and functional after-treatment is an elementary condition of the prevention of recurrences. Preventive bandages and braces have proved of great value in the early phases of resumed athletic activity.

References

Anderson, K. J., LeCocq, J. F. & LeCocq, E. A. (1952) Recurrent anterior subluxation of the ankle joint. A report of two cases and an experimental study. *J. Bone Joint Surg. (Am)* **34**, 853.

Larson, R. L. (1975) Dislocations and ligamentous injuries of the knee. In C. A. Rockwood & D. P. Green (eds) *Fractures*, Vol. 2. J. B. Lippincott, Philadelphia.

10.4 Diagnosis and management of overuse injuries

P. RENSTRÖM

The diagnosis and treatment of overuse injuries are of increasing importance in sports medicine. These injuries increase in number not only because of the increasing participation in sports, but also because the duration and intensity of athletes' training are increasing.

These injuries have received early recognition. As early as 1855, Breithaupt reported on stress fractures of the metatarsal bones. Runge described the tennis elbow syndrome in 1873, and Albert described Achilles tendinitis in 1893. Little research has, however, been performed regarding the aetiology, diagnosis, treatment and rehabilitation of these injuries. There remains remarkable ignorance not only in the general medical community, but also among many sports medicine practitioners about the management of these injuries. Today's theoretical knowledge is based on clinical experience, which, however, is limited for most physicians. Overuse injuries do not usually prevent athletes from carrying out their daily activities.

Aetiology

There are two basic mechanisms behind tissue trauma: single impact macrotrauma or repetitive microtrauma. The macrotrauma can be a blow to a leg resulting in a fracture or a rotational injury of a joint resulting in a ligament sprain, or a direct blow to the muscle resulting in a muscle strain. Repetitive microtrauma, which is basically repeated exposure of the tissue to low magnitude forces, result in injury at the microscopic level. These latter injuries are what we call overuse injuries.

Many factors are potential causes of these overuse injuries. Repeated overload in, for example, running and jumping are often associated with overuse injuries. In the running gait a force in the range of three to five times the bodyweight ascends up the lower extremity at heel strike. This force behaves like a sound wave with a short duration (20–40 ms) with rapid dissipation. Considering an impact of 250% of bodyweight, a

Table 10.4.1 Intrinsic and extrinsic factors relating to overuse injuries in sport. From Renström & Johnson (1985).

Intrinsic	Extrinsic
Malalignment:	Training errors:
Excessive pronation	Over distance
Femoral neck anteversion	Intensity
Orthopaedic disorders	Hill work
Leg length discrepancy	Technique
	Fatigue
Muscular imbalance	
Quadriceps and hamstring insufficiency	Surfaces
	Environmental conditions
	Footwear and equipment

runner absorbs at ground contact 110 Mg (110 tons) on each foot per 1.6 km (1 mile) (Mann, 1982). The forces for longer distances can be imagined, considering that a long-distance runner, who runs 160 km (100 miles) per week plants each foot about 3 million times a year (Subotnick, 1975).

Overuse injuries are basically heterogenous injuries caused by repetitive microtrauma. There are, however, many factors which in combination result in overuse injuries. These factors are divided into extrinsic and intrinsic factors (Table 10.4.1).

Intrinsic factors

Intrinsic factors including malalignment and muscle imbalance are common causes of overuse injuries. Increased pronation was present in more than 60% of a group of injured runners (James *et al.*, 1978). It was, however, not reported what percentage of uninjured runners have increased pronation. With excessive pronation of the foot during midstance there is increased medial stress and a compensatory increased internal rotation of the entire leg. This may result in increased twisting forces within the Achilles tendon (Fig. 10.4.1), cause abnormal concentration of stress on the patellofemoral joint because of lateral displacement of the patella, change the muscle contraction mechanism of the thigh muscles causing trochanteric problems, etc.

In a group of injured runners, cavus feet were present in about 20% (James *et al.*, 1978). In cavus feet with a rigid middle foot, there is an increased stress concentration on the forefoot and the heel. Cavus feet are often associated with plantar fasciitis and Achilles tendinitis.

Anatomical factors such as leg length discrepancy, femoral neck anteversion and quadriceps and hamstring insufficiency are also associated with overuse injuries. The lower extremity should be looked upon

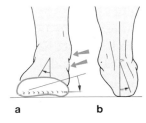

a   b

Fig. 10.4.1 Increased pronation will result in increased medial stress and angulated traction of the Achilles tendon.

as a complete functional unit. This means that an overuse syndrome involving the knee should be examined by making an anatomical functional examination of the entire lower extremity.

Extrinsic factors

Extrinsic factors are mainly training errors which are present in 60–80% of reported injuries to runners (James *et al.*, 1978). The most common causes are too much distance, too great intensity and too much hill work. Even minor technique faults, which are continually repeated, can cause overuse problems. Training techniques which are improper can also lead to muscular imbalance.

Fatigued muscles have a decreased ability to absorb repetitive shock or stress and may result in overuse injuries such as stress fractures, tennis elbow and medial tibial stress syndromes. Inadequate or worn-out shoes may cause increased stress and overuse. Slippery roads and uneven surfaces may cause overuse injuries. Running too much on the pitch of the road, which often leans 4–9°, may cause a short/long leg syndrome and thereby overuse problems.

There has been a rapid rise in the rate of occurrence of overuse injuries in children during the last decade. This is due to the fact that training is more intense and harder, and can occur in even younger age groups. This may turn out to be a great problem and should be closely observed by sports medicine physicians.

Location of injuries

All major tissues in the muscular–skeletal system are subject to overuse injuries.

Musculotendinous system

The musculotendinous unit is composed of a muscle, which is a contractile element, attached to bone either by an elastic tendon or by direct insertion. Injuries may occur at any point along this unit: within the muscle belly, within the tendon at the musculotendinous junction or at the origin or insertion of the muscle or tendon into the bone. Failure will occur at the weakest point within the unit (Fig. 10.4.2).

The major overuse injury in this system is tendinitis but there may also be paratendinitis, partial to total ruptures, bursitis or tenoperiostitis. Muscle strains are common and these can also be the result of microtrauma of muscle tissue or supporting tissues.

The location and severity of the injury are influenced by the athlete's age. In young athletes and adolescents, avulsion fractures through the

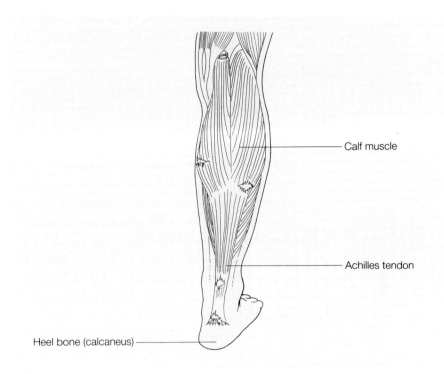

Fig. 10.4.2 Locations of injuries in a musculotendinous unit in the posterior aspect of the lower leg. From Peterson & Renström (1986).

Calf muscle

Achilles tendon

Heel bone (calcaneus)

apophyseal plate or traction and fragmentation of the bone at the attachment site (e.g. Osgood–Schlatter disease, Sever's disease) are most likely to occur. After 25–30 years of age there is a progressive degeneration of the collagen fibres, especially within the tendon, making the tendon itself a weak area and more susceptible to both traumatic and overuse injuries.

Around ligaments and tendons there are often bursae located in order to unload a pressure or protect the area. When ligaments and tendons are injured or subjected to an inflammatory reaction a bursitis may be present. Bursitis is a common overuse injury around the Achilles tendon, around the knee joint, at the trochanteric region and in the shoulder and elbow regions.

Skeletal system   Overuse injuries of bones include stress fractures which are most commonly seen in the long bones of the lower leg, fibula and tibia and in the foot but also around the hip and knee. In the joints repetitive microtrauma may injure the articular cartilage. There is initially a softening of the cartilage which can progress to shredding and thinning of the articular surface down to the underlying bone. The most common location for this involves the articular cartilage of the patella.

The foot is often involved as a location of pain or as a contributor to overuse injuries because of malalignment. Problems of the foot are, for example, Morton's neuroma, stress fractures of the metatarsal bones and plantar fasciitis.

Lower leg problems include compartment syndromes, medial tibial stress syndrome or medial tibialis posterior syndrome. Stress fractures of the tibia or fibula should be suspected if pain occurs during exercise. Achilles tendon injuries are some of the most common overuse injuries in sports. The knee is also a common location for overuse injuries. Patellofemoral stress syndrome or so-called chondromalacia, is very common in adolescent girls particularly. Lateral knee pain can frequently be encountered in runners (runners' knee). Most commonly, however, meniscal lesions cause knee pain.

Overuse injuries around the hip and the groin include adductor longus tendinitis and strains, trochanteric bursitis and stress fractures.

Lower back pain can cause problems in runners. Running tends to tighten the posterior low back muscles and fascias. The resulting tendency to low back sway or lordosis increases the risk for a number of low back conditions, including ruptured disc facet syndromes and spondylolysis (Micheli, 1983).

Throwers and pitchers have overuse problems in the elbow region because of valgus stress overload problems. Tennis players often have lateral epicondylitis. Shoulder overuse injuries like rotator cuff problems are commonly seen in throwers and impingement problems in swimmers.

Overuse injuries in muscles

In a muscle strain the muscle is overstretched. In the repair process there is not only a regeneration of muscle fibres but also a simultaneous production of granulation scar tissue. Inelastic scar tissue localized in the muscle will thus develop. The healed muscle consequently includes areas of varying elasticity which later might cause overuse problems. Frequent stretching exercises are needed for prevention of injury.

Muscle pain and soreness Muscle pain is a common symptom but one which is difficult and time-consuming to investigate. Pain in the muscles, which becomes worse after exercise, can be related to muscle damage. If the pain is worse during concentric contractions there is often a metabolic origin, but if it is worse during eccentric contractions a mechanical origin cannot be excluded (Newham, 1982). As a strategy for management it has been found to be important to use the non-capacity of a muscle to adapt favourably to exercise training as a means of convincing the patient that though the pain or fatigue may be extremely troublesome it is not serious.

Exercise-induced soreness is characterized by stiffness, tenderness and pain during active movement and weakness of the affected musculature for a few days after unusually heavy exercise (Fridén et al., 1983). A special relationship exists between muscle soreness and eccentric contractions. The results indicate that the Z disc constitutes the weak link in the myofibrillar contractile chain at high muscle tension. The myofibrillar lesions may be a direct result of mechanical tearing, which may cause the formation of protein components and consequential release of protein-bound ions that result in oedema and soreness via osmosis.

Compartment syndromes

Exercise-induced pain in the lower leg is common in sports. Several names for pain in the medial part of the tibia exist, e.g. medial tibial syndrome, shin splints, tibia periostitis, shin soreness, medial tibial stress syndrome and posterior tibial syndrome. Athletes often experience pain in this region after they have been running for some time in connection with changing running surface, changing shoe type, etc. The cause of this pain is still unknown.

Excessive pronation has been associated with pain in the medial part of the tibia. This syndrome has been considered to be a posterior tibial syndrome secondary to excessive pronation (James et al., 1978). Some consider this pain to be part of a chronic compartment syndrome. This syndrome may exist when exercise raises the intracompartmental pressure sufficiently to produce small vessel collapse which results in ischaemic pain and occasionally neurological deficits (Mubarak, 1982). These symptoms disappear when activity is curtailed and reappear during the next period of exercise. Factors of importance for the increasing compartment pressure may be muscle hypertrophy, which occurs with repeated exercise, or an increase in the intramuscular pressure during strong isometric and isotonic contractions. Whatever the cause, the accumulation of fluid within the interstitial spaces results in either chronic and/or acute compartment syndrome after excursions. In athletes with medial tibial syndrome, however, no increase in the muscular pressure in the deep posterior compartment during or after exercise has been found. Fasciotomy of the deep posterior compartment may, however, be effective in relieving the pain of the medial tibial syndrome. The initial treatment should, however, be modification of the training and shoes, and should include stretching exercises. Anti-inflammatory drugs and sometimes diuretics may be of value.

Pain in the anteriolateral part of the lower leg has been given different names, for example chronic anterior compartment syndrome. A significant increase in intramuscular pressure within the anterior tibial compartment during and after exercise has been found. Fasciotomy of this compartment is probably in many cases the only way to achieve permanent improvement. Reduced physical activity and diuretic treatment can make athletes temporarily symptom-free.

Other causes of pain in the lower leg are stress fractures or stress reactions of the fascia, periosteum and bone.

The basic treatment of lower leg pain and compartment syndromes is limitation of running and alteration of exercise programmes. Shoe modifications and orthotics may sometimes be of value. Obviously, a correct diagnosis forms the basis for identifying a successful treatment programme.

Overuse injuries in tendons

Tendons transmit forces from muscle to bone. In its resting state the tendon has a wavy configuration which will disappear if the tendon is stretched by 2%. At 4–8% strain the collagen fibres slide past one another as the cross-links start to break. As more and more cross-links are broken the weakest fibres rupture and the tendon loses its composite structure at the molecular level (Curwin & Stanish, 1984). Continued application of force results in further fibre failure and ultimately rupture of the tendon.

Injuries to the Achilles, patellar, adductor longus, supraspinatus and biceps brachii tendons are common in sports. Achilles tendon injuries will be used as an example in order to present the principles of treatment of overuse injuries in tendons.

Tendon problems can be divided into: tendinitis, peritendinitis, tendinosus, partial ruptures and total ruptures.

Types of injuries
Tendinitis

These overuse injuries are characterized by a gradual onset of pain. Acute tendinitis involves acute inflammatory symptoms, such as redness, swelling, impaired motion and heat reaction. These acute injuries do not usually constitute a diagnostic problem.

The chronic overuse injuries often involve the so-called pain cycle (Fig. 10.4.3). In the pain cycle the pain disappears during warm-up, allowing

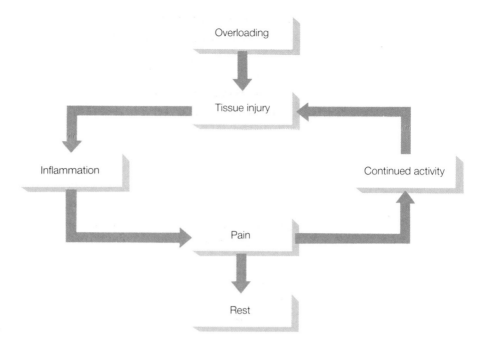

Fig. 10.4.3 The pain cycle.

the athletes to go on with their activities. The athlete develops pain again after the activity but not enough to prevent performance the following day. When the pain no longer disappears with the warm-up, the injury is more or less chronic. Pain indicates an injury and the pain cycle should be interrupted by rest and the injury diagnosed and treated.

During the clinical examination it is usually possible to see a diffuse tenderness and swelling over a rather long area of the tendon; this is also seen in peritendinitis. In injuries concerning the Achilles tendon, these changes are often located 2–6 cm proximal to the insertion of the tendon into the calcaneus in the area of decreased vascularity. Motion is impaired by pain.

Partial ruptures   A partial tendon rupture may heal with chronic inflammatory tissue and give symptoms like chronic tendinitis. These injuries include, however, a history of sudden onset of pain. A partial rupture is characterized clinically by a distinct palpable tenderness which in most cases is combined with a localized swelling. A distinct tenderness and history of trauma differentiate an old partial tendon rupture from tendinitis.

Tendinosus   Tendinosus is a symptomatic tendon degeneration due to ageing, accumulated microtrauma or both; it can be subclassified into interstitial microscopial failures, central necrosis and partial rupture (Clancy, 1982).

Tenoperiostitis   Injuries in the area where the tendon inserts into, or originates from, bone can be called tenoperiostitis, e.g. adductor longus tenoperiostitis. Typical symptoms are pain during active motion. Clinical examination will show a point tenderness over the insertion site and pain against resistance during active motion.

Injury to the Achilles tendon insertion can be recognized as calcaneal apophysitis and to the patellar tendon insertion as Osgood–Schlatter disease. These injuries are characterized by point tenderness in the tendinous insertion into the periosteum and bone. Often there is a bone prominence, which is tender.

In adolescents, injury to the Achilles tendon insertion can be recognized as calcaneal apophysitis or Sever–Haglund disease. It is characterized by point tenderness in the tendinous insertion into the periosteum and bone of the calcaneus.

Bursitis   A bursitis is an inflammation in a bursa. This condition may be caused by friction between, for example, the retrocalcaneal bursa and the Achilles tendon. This tendon inserts in the posterior distal aspect of the tuberosity of the calcaneus. Between the tendon and the posterior part of the tuberosity there is a bursa whose anterior aspect consists of a thin layer of cartilage covering this part of the tuberosity. Chronic Achilles bursitis is associated with tenderness in the anterior aspect of the tendon, often in combination with some fluctuation.

Another commonly affected location is the subacromial bursa in the shoulder, which may impinge between the acromion and the supraspinatus tendon. Degeneration of this tendon may contribute to calcium deposition in the bursa. A 'calcification shoulder' with severe pain may be the result.

Haemobursa   Superficially located bursae, e.g. the prepatellar, the trochanteric and the olecranon bursae may be subject to direct trauma. A haemobursa may form with resultant adhesions, fibrous bodies and calcifications leading to bursitis.

Diagnostic tools   There are some valuable diagnostic tools available, which can be used in conjunction with a thorough manual examination.

Soft tissue X-ray examinations can be helpful. Localized oedema and thickening of the tendon strongly indicate a partial rupture. There may also be oedema extending into Kager's triangle which is limited by the tendon, adipose tissue and calcaneus. The diagnosis of distal partial rupture and chronic bursitis in Achilles tendon injuries can be supported by *ultrasonography*, which reveals decreased echogenesity in the area of the partial rupture, and by *electromyography* (EMG) which shows increased activity on the injured side (Persson & Ljungqvist, 1971). *Bursography* of the retrocalcaneal bursa constitutes a valuable diagnostic method (Allenmark *et al.*, 1982). The presence of a contrast leakage between the tendon fibres indicates a partial tendon rupture in this region. *Arthrography* or arthroscopy can be carried out in bursae in different locations, e.g. the subacromial bursa. *Magnetic resonance imaging* (MRI) is very useful in diagnosing different soft tissue injuries. Experience is, however, limited and examinations expensive.

Often, the manual examination, using the mind, hands and eyes, is the best diagnostic tool.

Principles of treatment

When discussing principles of treatment of these injuries it should be remembered that overuse or chronic injuries in the tendons are persistent and difficult to treat. They have forced many athletes to change their training methods or even to leave sports activities. A treatment programme has to be based on a correct diagnosis.

Some basic principles of importance are:

1 When treating overuse injuries consideration must be given to the healing process (Fig. 10.4.4). Soft tissue injuries, including tendons, heal in stages. At the time of the injury there is damage to the tendon microvasculature resulting in bleeding and increased permeability of the remaining intact vessels. Fluid will accumulate in the injured area. There will be an inflammatory response which will last about 48 hours. This inflammatory response is involved in the healing process, drawing blood cells to the area. Elimination of the inflammatory response by drug administration can delay or interrupt the healing. This inflammatory response should not last longer than 1 to 2 days. If persistent it may result in hypoxia caused by stasis and increased proteolytic activity.

Connective tissue healing is divided into proliferative and formative stages. During the proliferative stage, which lasts for 2 weeks, new collagen and connective tissue are formed. After 12–14 days a full quantity of collagen is formed. This new tissue is remodelled in response

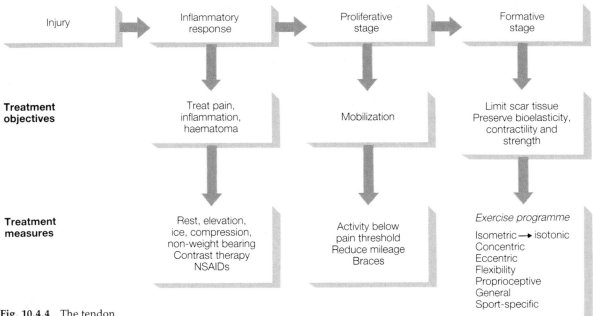

Fig. 10.4.4 The tendon healing process, treatment objectives and measures for overuse injuries. From Renström & Johnson (1985).

to tension during the formative stage. The collagen fibres re-orientate themselves in line with the tensile force applied to the tissue, but the amount of tension that is necessary for optimal orientation is unclear. The aim is to make the collagen as elastic as possible. The rate of collagen fibre formation is directly related to the functional state of the affected area (Curwin & Stanish, 1984). Knowledge about the different stages of healing determines the different models of treatment (Fig. 10.4.4).

2   After acute local treatment of the injury site it is important to make an exact diagnosis before specific treatment is started. Initiation of an exercise programme depends largely on the diagnosis. Ruptures should, for example, not be initially treated with stretching.

3   The athletes respond to their injuries and associated problems differently. Thus, the treatment should be individualized. Patient compliance is the single largest factor determining the success or failure of the treatment. In most cases an exercise programme is prescribed and then consistency with daily exercises must be maintained.

4   The treatment and rehabilitation of an athlete should involve a team including the patient, the doctor, the physiotherapist, the trainer, the coach and the family as rehabilitation programmes can take time and create related psychological problems.

5   Treatment should be started as early as possible in order to prevent acute injuries from becoming chronic.

Basic treatment programme

The aim of acute treatment is to reveal pain, minimize haematoma formation and soft tissue damage and limit inflammation. Acute treatment involves rest, avoidance of weight bearing, elevation, ice and compression bandaging. During the initial inflammatory response, rest and unloading of the area by non-weight bearing is the treatment of choice. Crutches are often recommended.

Rest or activity? Treatment of tendon and other soft tissue injuries can be divided into periods of rest and activity. The initial rest period should be continued usually for 1 to 2 days until the inflammatory response has diminished and until the diagnosis is made. Thereafter the choice is rest or activity.

Prolonged joint immobilization may result in a loss of ground substances found in collagenous connective tissue (Åkeson et al., 1967), which will result in a tissue deficient in elastin. Removal of tension of the newly formed collagen means that the orientation of the collagen fibres will be poor. This will diminish the tensile strength of the healing tissue, which depends on the number, size and orientation of the fibres (Curwin & Stanish, 1984). Joint immobilization will furthermore result in muscle wasting and weakness, joint stiffness and diminished proprioception. Immobilization should be kept to a minimum. This means that immobilization of tendons and other soft tissue injuries basically should be avoided.

Mobilization should start as early as the healing of the injury permits. Mobilization has beneficial effects not only on tendons and other soft tissues but also on the bones and joints. Active or limited exercise means that the injured area should be used, but protected from significant stress which may cause further damage. The remaining parts of the body should, however, be as fully active as possible including conditioning, strength and flexibility training. A runner with an injured tendon can sometimes be very active with cycling or swimming, for example.

Ice or cold treatment Ice or cold should be used in acute injuries in combination with compression bandaging, rest and elevation to reduce the swelling, pain and inflammation. The effectiveness of ice on the circulation deep in the muscles, however, is not yet clear. Its greatest effect is pain relief, because of decreased sensory nerve conduction for 0.5–2 hours after application. This may result in such significant pain improvement, that the athlete may underestimate the severity of the injury. If the athlete then resumes athletic activity his/her injury might be aggravated.

Ice or cold decreases or delays inflammation by reducing the metabolism and enzymatic function; this is achieved after brief periods of ice application of 5–15 min. This should decrease the swelling in the area. Ice should be applied for a limited time, i.e. not more than 15–20 min and repeated every 1 to 2 h in acute cases. In chronic cases ice should be applied after activities which cause discomfort and can then be applied for 30–50 min.

Drugs

Non-steroidal anti-inflammatory drugs

NSAIDs may be useful in the treatment of overuse injuries. The initial physiological inflammatory response in promoting healing is usually limited to 1 or 2 days, indicating that these drugs may be used a couple of days after the injury. These drugs can be used for shorter periods of time, for example 1 week at a time, and the treatment period can then be repeated. These drugs are often effective against pain and stiffness. The athletes should, however, be aware that this medication may mask the symptoms.

Corticosteroids

Injections with corticosteroids should be given with great care. Steroids are very potent anti-inflammatory drugs. They are occasionally indicated in a few chronic overuse syndromes. Sometimes injections can be made into the insertion of a tendon into bone or between the tendon sheath and the tendon or in a bursa. Injections should, however, never be given into the tendon. Nor should they be given to athletes who aim to quickly resume their physical activity, because there is an increased risk of rupture. Steroid injections into a tendon will result in decreased tensile strength, decreased production of collagen and ground substances, and circulatory stasis may be the result. A steroid injection should be combined with rest and reduced physical activity for a couple of weeks.

Anaesthetics

Injections of local anaesthetics can sometimes be of value as a diagnostic aid, when the diagnosis is unclear. Following an injection the injured area can often be more satisfactorily examined. Intravenous injections of heparin for 3–5 days have been shown to be of value in the treatment of acute severe peritendinitis and tendinitis of the ankle and wrist (Rais, 1961).

Exercise and rehabilitation

Exercise is the key in a successful rehabilitation programme if it is properly applied. The aim of the therapy should be to limit the amount of scar tissue formed and to preserve bioelasticity, contractility and strength of the individual components (Ciullo & Zarins, 1983). Repeated exercises will increase the mechanical and structural properties (Woo *et al.*, 1975).

Activity strengthens tendons and other soft tissues, inactivity weakens them.

Strength training   A strength training programme should start very carefully with a gradual increase of the load below the threshold of pain. Initially, *isometric exercises* are recommended and should be carried out without a load. A gradual increase in loads can then be applied. At this early stage it is often sufficient to use the athlete's injured limb as the load. When isometric exercises can be carried out without pain, active motion exercises involving the injured area and gradual increases in load can start.

Dynamic exercises   include both eccentric and concentric contractions. During *concentric exercise*, the muscles contract and shorten their length simultaneously so that their attachments are drawn closer together, for example when flexing an elbow with a weight in the hand. These exercises may start as soon as they can be performed without pain, and may begin relatively early in the rehabilitation programme.

Eccentric exercise   implies that the muscles contract and increase their length simultaneously so that their attachments are drawn apart, e.g. when lowering the arm with a weight in the hand.

There are many different models for dynamic muscle training, e.g. weight training without control of velocity, isokinetic, training with variable resistance, etc.

The musculotendinous unit is subjected to larger loads during eccentric contractions than in concentric ones. Eccentric contraction maximizes the force production and minimizes time delays and energy expenditure.

Eccentric exercises can be used in the rehabilitation phase of chronic overuse injuries (Fig. 10.4.5). It is, however, important to realize that eccentric contractions are involved in the production of chronic tendon problems as part of deceleration. The larger loads developed by eccentric contractions will potentially increase the risk for re-injury, especially in athletes above the age of 40 years. Training with eccentric contractions should therefore initially be carried out without pain or discomfort. After 1–2 weeks of rehabilitation of a chronic injury, the intensity of the exercise could be such that pain or discomfort is experienced towards the end of the training session. The pain indicates that slight overloading of the tendon is occurring, which will increase its strength (Curwin & Stanish, 1984). No pain indicates insufficient loading in which case no improvement in symptoms occurs. However, pain, particularly if it occurs throughout the whole training session, is a sign that too much

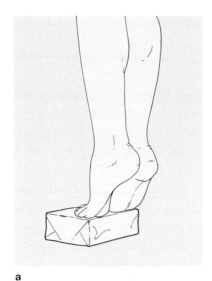 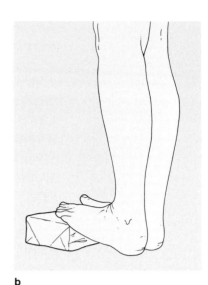

Fig. 10.4.5 Examples of strength exercises in Achilles tendon or gastrocnemius muscle injuries. Concentric contractions (a) and eccentric contractions (b). From Peterson & Renström (1986).

a   b

force is being applied, which in fact may worsen the injury. As the strength of the connective tissue increases, the pain will decrease. As time passes the number of repetitions and the load may slowly increase.

Curwin and Stanish (1984) have designed an eccentric exercise training programme with the following three functional areas:

1   Length. By increasing the resting length of the musculotendinous unit with stretching, it is possible to lessen the strain taking place during the same range of joint motion.

2   Load. Increasing the load will subject the musculotendinous unit to greater stress and the principle of progressive overloading forms the basis of the training programme.

3   Speed of contraction. The force of the musculotendinous unit is related to the speed of muscle contraction and increasing the speed would increase the load on the unit.

Strength training should always be combined with flexibility training (see below), and continuing supervision should be maintained.

Flexibility training   Strength training alone has a negative effect on joint flexibility (Möller, 1984). This can be counteracted by flexibility training and it is therefore important to combine the two types of training. The flexibility of a particular joint is primarily limited by the tightness of the connective tissue, i.e. flexibility is elasticity. The shape and configuration of the bone and joints are also important. Flexibility is basically, however, a musculotendinous condition as there are elastic components in both the tendon and the muscle that will stretch. Flexibility decreases with age, i.e. more emphasis on flexibility training should be done with older age groups. On average, the most flexible person is a girl aged 12 years. When the muscle mass starts to increase at 14–16 years of age, flexibility training should be included in all training programmes.

Flexibility is specific, which means that most of the muscles and tendons involved in the actual sport should be trained. There are different methods of flexibility training including:

1 Ballistic stretching (or dynamic, spring, bound or rebound stretching) involves bouncing of the musculotendinous unit. This method is not often used. Some warn against ballistic stretching because the antagonistic muscle will react with a contraction if it is stretched into the extreme position rapidly and forcefully. This type of stretching is not effective, but it is not as dangerous as some proclaim.

2 Slow static stretching (or static stretch, prolonged plain and hold stretch) involves slowly stretching the muscle as far as possible and then holding that position for 20–60 s.

3 Contract–relax–stretch, which is a modification of the PNF technique. This stretching is a slow stretch to the limit of motion at which a maximum isometric contraction of the muscle is performed for 4–6 s with the aim of encouraging reciprocal inhibition and relaxing of the antagonist muscle. This is then followed by a relaxation for 2–3 s and then a passive stretch to the extreme position and maintenance of that position for 20–60 s.

4 3S system (scientific stretching for sport) means that a muscle is passively stretched and then exposed to an isometric contraction (Holt *et al.*, 1970). This method requires the assistance of another person to hold and stretch the leg.

Practically, stretching should be preceded by a 3–4 min warm-up session. A stretching programme in itself can last 5–10 min. It should, however, be repeated as flexibility is lost rapidly. Stretching should mainly be carried out after training or competition events.

Proprioceptive training   This involves retraining of the interaction between the nervous system and muscle tendons, joints and ligaments. Following, for example, an ankle joint injury during which the nerves in the joint capsule are injured, proprioceptive training can be performed on a tilt board and should be carried out periodically for 6–8 months.

Sport specific training   This involves training of the muscles and tendons involved in a specific sport and it should be carried out before a return to the sport in question.

Conditioning and general exercises of the non-injured areas should be carried out as early as practical following injury.

Physical modalities

Heat thermotherapy

Heat treatment will relieve pain and muscle spasm, increase the local temperature and metabolism, dilate the vessels with increasing blood flow, increase the elasticity of collagen and reduce the stiffness in connective tissues. Heat can potentially increase swelling immediately after an injury. Heat should therefore not be applied until 2–3 days after an acute injury.

Superficial heat modalities include whirlpool contrast bath, paraffin bath, infrared heat, etc. These modalities can increase the heat effect to a depth of 1 cm. They relieve some symptoms of inflammation but there is little scientific evidence that they will shorten the healing time. Local heat can be applied with chemical heat bags.

Heat retainers generate and preserve heat at least at skin level (Myrhage *et al.*, 1981). Through heat conservation they can improve blood circulation. These heat retainers are valuable tools in both prevention and rehabilitation of joint and musculotendinous overuse injuries as they can also be applied and used during physical activity.

Ultrasound waves can make the tissue susceptible to subsequent re-modelling by adjusted tensile forces, which means that this type of treatment should be followed by exercises (Curwin & Stanish, 1984). Ultrasound can also have a heating effect. The use of ultrasound is widely spread, but scientifically little is known.

High-voltage galvanic stimulation is an effective modality in the production of heat within the tissues and may be effective in treating tendinitis and sprains.

TNS (transcutaneous nerve stimulation) or TENS is used for pain relief by skin stimulation and thereby affects the symptoms of overuse syndromes.

Massage

Massage should be avoided in the first couple of days after an injury since it can produce microtrauma and thereby have a negative effect on the healing and coagulation processes. Deep friction massage is used to breakdown scar tissue and is advocated by physiotherapists to be effective. The psychological effect of massage should not be underestimated.

Braces, tape and orthotics

Treatment methods which eliminate the causes of injuries also need to be applied. An injured area should be protected from overloading and weight bearing during the healing phase although some tensile loading may be beneficial. Protection may be given by braces of different kinds. These braces may be divided into stabilizing and other types. The stabilizing braces include preventive, rehabilitative and functional braces (Drez, 1985). Braces may be helpful by providing proprioceptive feedback to the athlete with different instabilities. The real mechanisms and effects of braces are not yet clear.

Taping can be helpful in the prevention and rehabilitation of injuries, especially those involving the ankle and wrist joints.

Foot orthotics are helpful in treating some malalignment conditions, e.g. excessive pronation. The foot orthotics should, however, only control excessive amounts of pronation otherwise the foot becomes rigid and absorbs shock poorly. There are basically three types of orthotics: soft, semiflexible and rigid. Athletes use semiflexible orthotics most commonly.

Surgery Surgery should be avoided and not used until conservative treatment has failed. The aim of surgery is usually to remove the scar tissue, which accompanies repeated trauma, and to encourage revascularization. The scar tissue is formed as a result of increased collagen synthesis in response to repetitive injury, but it is immature and disorganized and it therefore adds little to the strength of the injured area (Curwin & Stanish, 1984). Excision of scar and degenerative tissue can often give good results in, for example, lateral epicondylitis, partial rupture and chronic inflammation of the Achilles tendon, and adductor longus tendon injuries. The rehabilitation period following this type of surgery can, however, be rather long.

Injuries to insertion or origin of muscles and tendons

The insertion of the muscle tendon unit into bone involves a gradual transition from tendon to cartilage, from mineralized cartilage to cortical bone. Very few blood vessels exist in bone-tendon junctions because of fibrocartilage, which creates a barrier (Viidik, 1973). A poor vascularization may be one of the reasons why these injuries often become chronic. Injuries to the bone–tendon junction are often caused by malalignment, repeated exercises with faulty technique, or alteration of the angle between the bone and the muscle belly. Examples of these types of injuries are tenoperiostitis of the adductur longus, lateral epicondylitis in adults and apophysitis of the Achilles tendon insertion in adolescents.

Adolescents and growing individuals sustain different types of overuse injuries than do adults. The adolescents' tendons and ligaments are relatively stronger than their bones. This means that an injury, which in an adult would result in a ligament strain or tendon tear will in an adolescent result in an avulsion fracture or in a traction tenoperiostitis, e.g. Osgood–Schlatter disease or Sever's disease. These types of overuse injuries usually heal when the apophyseal cartilages close up, i.e. when the athlete has grown up.

The diagnosis includes a thorough clinical examination, and an X-ray examination in adolescents. The principles of management of these injuries include acute treatment of the soft tissues with rest, elevation, compression bandaging and ice. The principles for chronic overuse syndromes are the same as mentioned for tendons. In the early treatment phase isometric exercises without load should be carried out below the threshold of pain. Dynamic exercises should start as soon as the pain allows. Careful stretching and eccentric exercises can be carried out within, and sometimes above, the pain threshold. It is important, however, to be particularly careful in adolescents. Non-steroidal anti-inflammatory medication may sometimes be of benefit. If the pain interferes with the training programme a local injection of cortisone may be given in adults but not in adolescents. In resistant cases surgery may become necessary. Tenotomy at the insertion of the bone can sometimes give good results in, for example, adductor longus tenoperistitis and plantar fasciitis.

Overuse injuries in other soft tissues

Friction syndromes

Friction syndromes may result from irritation between the iliotibial band and, for example, the lateral femoral epicondyle or greater trochanteric region.

Runner's knee

Runner's knee is a pain syndrome on the lateral side of the knee. There is a point of tenderness where the iliotibial band slides over the lateral epicondyle. Pain can be reproduced over the lateral femoral epicondyle by fully extending and flexing the knee while placing various stresses on it. Treatment consists of stretching exercises of the iliotibial band. Sometimes orthotics can be used to balance the foot if there is an excessive pronation. Sometimes steroid injections can be used in combination with rest. If these conservative methods have no effect, surgery may be performed to release the area.

Friction bursitis Friction bursitis over the greater trochanter region, the Achilles tendon or the supraspinatus tendon are quite common. Basically the treatment involves local decompression and sometimes aspiration of fluid.

Nerve entrapment syndromes These may develop from overuse as a result of swelling in the surrounding tissues. These injuries are not common. Compression by an os trigonum can cause tarsal tunnel syndrome of the medial plantar nerve, compression of the deep peroneal nerve on the superior part of the talus medial, plantar heel pain, etc. Involved nerves in, for example, the groin region are the genitofemoralis, ilioinguinalis and cutaneous femoris lateralis.

The diagnosis is made based on a history including a sharp severe pain, which can be electric in nature with radiation along the nerve. Clinical examination may show some tenderness over the entrapment area. An injection with local anaesthesia may give pain relief. Conservative treatment includes rest and anti-inflammatory medication, orthotics, etc. Sometimes surgical compression may be necessary.

Overuse syndromes in bones

Stress syndromes of the bone are common in athletes in spite of the fact that the thickness, strength and mineral content of athletes' bones are greater than those of non-athletes. Stress fractures of the lower extremities are more common in athletes than in the general population (Orava, 1980). A stress fracture may be defined as a partial or complete fracture of bone due to its inability to withstand non-violent stress that is applied in a rhythmical, repeated substress hold manner (McBryde, 1982).

Stress fractures can occur in normal bone during normal situations but usually they are sustained by repetitive or slightly increased loading during running. Stress fractures in running can be associated with toe–heel gait, hard-surface running, trunk and lower extremity malalignment, poor conditioning and many other factors, which are described in Chapter 10.1.

The diagnostic key to stress fractures is often a very localized pain and point tenderness. X-rays taken early in the course of the injury may not reveal any abnormality. In doubtful cases a bone scan can, after a day or two, pinpoint the fracture before it becomes radiographical apparent.

Treatment is basically conservative with non-weight bearing or weight bearing within intolerance of pain and avoidance of training. When dealing with a visible fracture line or in a specific location, such as the middle third of the tibia or the femoral neck, more aggressive conservative treatment including casting or surgery should be considered.

Overuse injuries in joints

Patellofemoral pain syndrome

There are some common overuse syndromes located in the knee joint, e.g. patellofemoral pain syndrome. This syndrome can occur at any age but is most frequently seen in teenagers and young adults, and its onset is often insidious. The cause of pain is not clear but appears to arise from the nerve receptors in the subchondral bone (Cox, 1985). Pain results from increased load factors on normal cartilage due to prolonged stress, increased load factors on abnormal cartilage due to less stress, or from increased pressure due to patellar malalignment.

The diagnosis is made from the history, including pain when walking downstairs, pain when driving a car or sitting in a chair (often referred to as 'the movie sign or theatre sign'). The pain is located behind the knee cap. Other symptoms are retropatellar crepitus, and sometimes swelling of the knee joint and a feeling of instability.

Clinical examination will reveal subpatellar tenderness and pain on compression of the patella. Sometimes there is an abnormal mobility of the patella, quadriceps muscle atrophy, crepitous and tenderness over the medial retinaculum. A sign indicating this syndrome is discomfort when the patella is displaced to the lateral side. X-rays may reveal some malalignment; the patellofemoral joint should be shown in the axial view. The quadriceps angle (Q-angle) may be increased and may be caused by lateral displacement of the tibial tubercle, increased femoral anteversion, genu valgum or external tibial torsion, which predisposes the patella to a lateral displacement particularly when a vigorous quadriceps contraction occurs. The increase in the quadriceps angle leads to the excess lateral pressure syndrome. Patella alta may predispose to subluxation of the patella. Vastus medialis insufficiency is common in teenage girls and decreases the ability of the muscle to maintain patellar balance and to prevent subluxation.

The treatment is basically non-operative including correction of the malalignment with orthotics, changes in training, quadriceps exercises, iliotibial band stretching, patellar stabilizing devices, etc. Sometimes operative treatment is indicated. Personal care, careful information and a planned conservative treatment programme will help most patients with patellofemoral pain problems.

Knee synovitis   Knee synovitis is often developed by runners with no apparent intra-articular pathology and no history of injury. A history of increased mileage or vigorous work are often associated. Conservative therapy with anti-inflammatory medication and ice is usually indicated. If this problem seems to be long lasting, arthroscopy should be carried out.

Other joint problems   *Degenerative arthritis* in the hip and knee joints is common in elderly persons. There is no certain increased incidence in athletes and overuse is probably not an important aetiological factor. Normal physical activity is of value as prevention.

Valgus extension stress syndromes in the elbow joints are not uncommon in pitchers. Osteophytes, ligament and capsule calcifications and osteochondritic changes are signs of overuse of the joints.

Intervertebral joint changes in the lumbar spine may be developed in gymnasts. Wrestlers often demonstrate late cervical spine changes.

In the talocrural joints of soccer and football players marginal osteophytes are not uncommon in so-called footballer's ankle.

Conclusion

Overuse injuries are becoming more common in sports, with a greater number of people in training, and higher requirements and higher intensity at all levels of competition. The demands and requirements of both training and competition make it difficult to be competitive even with minor injuries. For top level athletes these injuries constitute a great problem, for they usually also prevent them from training effectively, and can become chronic if the training is continued. When overuse injuries become chronic they are even more difficult to treat and have forced many athletes to retire early. When a correct diagnosis is made, and sensible principles of treatment are applied, most of these injuries can heal with conservative regimens. It is important that the overstress problems of athletes are recognized and not ignored. Even though most of these injuries do not cause problems in everyday life, physicians must understand the importance of physical activity to athletes and the population in general.

These injuries constitute a great diagnostic and therapeutic problem, for the symptoms are often diffuse and uncharacteristic. Our scientific knowledge about these injuries is limited and the treatment is based on practical experience. More research is, therefore, needed to study their aetiology, diagnosis and treatment. Overuse injuries are unnecessary and can usually be prevented.

References

Åkeson, W. H., Amiel, D. & Violette, D. (1967) The connective tissue response to immobility: a study of chondroitin-4 and 6-sulfate and dermatan sulfate changes in periarticular connective tissue of control and immobilized knees of dogs. *Clin. Orthop.* **51**, 183.

Ciullo, J. V. & Zarins, B. (1983) Biomechanics of the musculotendinous unit. Relation to athletic performance and injury. *Clin. Sports Med.* **2**, 71.

Clancy, W. G. (1982) Tendinitis and plantar fasciitis in runners. In R. D'Ambrosia & D. Drez jr (eds) *Prevention and Treatment of Running Injuries*, p. 77. Charles Slack, Thorofare.

Cox, J. S. (1985) Patellofemoral problems in runners. *Clin. Sports Med.* **4**, 699.

Curwin, S. & Stanish, W. D. (1984) *Tendinitis: Its Etiology and Treatment.* The Collamore Press, Lexington.

Drez, D. (1985) *Knee braces* (Seminar report). American Academy of Orthopedic Surgeons, Chicago.

Fridén, J., Sjöström, M. & Ekblom, B. (1983) Myofibrillar damage following intense eccentric exercise in man. *Int. J. Sports Med.* **4**, 170.

Holt, L., Travis, T. & Ohita, T. (1970) Comparative study of three stretching techniques. *Percep. Mot. Skills* **31**, 611.

James, S. L., Bates, B. T. & Ostering, L. R. (1978) Injuries to runners. *Am. J. Sports Med.* **6**, 40.

McBryde, A. M. (1982) Stress fractures in runners. In R. D'Ambrosia & D. Drez jr (eds) *Prevention and Treatment of Running Injuries*, pp. 21–42. Charles Slack, Thorofare.

Mann, R. A. (1982) Biomechanics of running. In Mack (ed) *Symposium on the Foot and Leg in Running Sports*, pp. 1–29. C. V. Mosby, St Louis.

Micheli, L. J. (1983) Overuse injuries in children sports: the growth factor. *Orthop. Clin. North Am.* **14(2)**, 337.

Möller, M. (1984) *Athletic training and flexibility. A study on range of motion in the lower extremity.* Linköping University Medical Dissertations No. 182.

Mubarak, S. J. (1982) Exertional compartment syndromes. In R. D'Ambrosia & D. Drez jr (eds) *Prevention and Treatment of Running Injuries*, pp. 89–107. Charles Slack, Thorofare.

Myrhage, R., Peterson, L. & Renström, P. (1981) Effect på hudtemperatur av linement och värmeskydd under träning (Effect on skin temperature by skin lotion and heat retainer during physical activity). *Swedish Med. Res. Soc.* **Dec**, 195.

Orava, S. (1980) *Exertion injuries due to sports and physical exercise. A clinical and statistical study of nontraumatic overuse injuries of the musculoskeletal system of athletes and keep-fit athletes.* Thesis, University of Oulu, Finland.

Persson, A. & Ljungqvist, R. (1971) Electrophysiological observations in cases of partial and total ruptures of the Achilles tendon. *Electroencephalog. Clin. Neurophysiol.* **31**, 239.

Peterson, L. & Renström, P. (1986) *Sports Injuries: Their Prevention and Treatment.* Martin Dunitz, London.

Rais, O. (1961) Heparin: treatment of peritenomyosis (peritendinitis crepitans acuta). A clinical and experimental study including the morphological changes in peritenon plus muscle. *Acta Chir. Scand.* (Suppl.) **268**, 11.

Renström, P. & Johnson, R. J. (1985) Overuse injuries. *Sports Med.* **2**, 316.

Subotnick, S. I. (1975) Orthotic foot control and the overuse syndrome. *Arch. Ped. Med. Foot Surg.* **2**, 207.

Viidik, A. (1973) Functional properties of collagenous tissues. *Int. Rev. Connect. Tissue Res.* **6**, 127.

Woo, S. L., Matthews, J. V., Akeson, W. H. *et al.* (1975) Connective tissue response to immobility. A correlative study of biochemical and biomechanical measurements of normal and immobilized rabbit knees. *Arthritis Rheum.* **18**, 257.

Further reading

Allenmark, C, Renström, P., Peterson, L. & Irstam, L. (1982) Persistent pain in the distal region of the Achilles tendon. FIMS World Congress, Vienna.

Fridén, J., Sjöström, M. & Ekblom, B. (1981) A morphological study of delayed muscle soreness. *Experientia* **37**, 506.

Orava, S. (1978) Iliotibial tract frictions syndrome in athletes—an uncommon exertion syndrome on the lateral side of the knee. *Br. J. Sports Med.* **12**, 69.

Orava, S. & Puranen, J. (1978) Exertion injuries in adolescent athletes. *Br. J. Sports Med.* **12**, 4.

Stanish, W. D. (1982) Neurophysiology of stretching. In R. D'Ambrosia & D. Drez jr (eds) *Prevention and Treatment of Running Injuries*, pp. 135–45. Charles Slack, Thorofare.

Subotnick, S. I. (1983) Foot orthoses: an update. *Physician Sportsmed.* **11**, 103.

10.5 Clinical implications of youth participation in sports

P. RENSTRÖM & C. ROUX

Introduction

Regular training of children and young adults is becoming more common in sports. Competitive sports are carried out with increasing intensity and at lower ages. In some sports, such as figure skating, swimming and gymnastics, children start regular training from 4–5 years of age. In some sports, training from 2–4 h, 5–6 days a week is not unusual.

The risks of allowing children and adolescents to train and compete regularly can be looked at from different angles—physiological, psychological and orthopaedic.

Physiological and psychological aspects

From morphological, biological and psychological standpoints, it is possible to divide a growing child's life into three major periods. Each has different requirements and possibilities.

5–11 years

This age group lasts from start of school to prepuberty. This age group is characterized by:

1 Weak muscles.
2 Good flexibility.
3 A low level of concentration ability, especially over a longer period of time.
4 The typical movements, gestures and attitudes of a child.

This is the period when the child is initiated into the world of sports. The child should be allowed to participate in team sports, but the emphasis should be on play. The child should not exceed his or her capacity and should participate without pressure; participation in sports should be fun for children. Particularly suitable sports are gymnastics, swimming, football, etc.

11–15 years

This is the prepuberty period, characterized by the acceleration of somatic growth. During this period careful organized participation in competitions increases and is even recommended. It should, however, be remembered that there can be a difference of biological maturity of more than 5 years between adolescents of the same age. This means that during this period young athletes do not always compete against athletes with the same biological development level, although they are of the same age. To win or lose should not be of great importance at this age. Sports are important as adolescents will discover:

1   The feeling of working towards a defined goal.
2   The existence of rules in sports similar to social rules.
3   The importance of sharing experiences and effort with the members of a team.
4   The importance of respecting other competitors.

There are statistics that show that adolescents who practise sports show better academic results than those that do not. This could, however, be an effect of the fact that sports-orientated youngsters are often also more study-orientated.

More than 15 years This is the period when adolescence ends and adult life starts. During this period growth is completed. Muscular development continues up to the age of 17–18 years, and harder training of the muscles, including flexibility training, can start more regularly. Specialization is recommended to start during this period.

Orthopaedic aspects The effects of sports from an orthopaedic point of view can be divided into three groups:

1   Effects on the development of the musculoskeletal system.
2   Injuries due to trauma.
3   Injuries due to overuse.

Injuries because of trauma are well known, but effects on growth development and overuse injuries are new complications in sports for children.

Effects on development of musculoskeletal system

Boys and girls physically develop in the same way up to the age of 10 and the size of their bones and muscles are the same. Between the ages of 10 and 13 years the girls are entering into adolescence during which hormonal changes will start. The growth spurt, i.e. the rapid growth rate in length, usually ends at the age of 14 years (Fig. 10.5.1). Seventy five

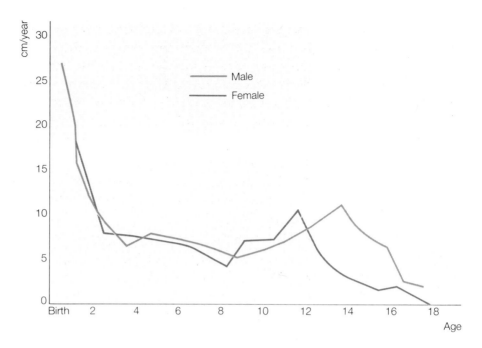

Fig. 10.5.1 Growth in height (cm/year) in young males and females.

percent of the boys will start their growth spurt between the ages of 12 and 15 years. As this growth spurt slows down there is an increase in the muscle mass and the adolescent will dramatically increase in weight and strength. During this period there is a risk of an increase in muscle and tendon tightness about the joints resulting in a reduction of range of motion and the risk of injuries will increase.

The development of the musculoskeletal system in adolescents is governed by its ability to adapt in response to a changed or recurrent load. Adaptation as a result of prolonged one-sided training can cause permanent asymmetric changes. An example of this is the tennis player who, at an early age, begins one-sided and asymmetrical training and loading of his or her racket arm (Fig. 10.5.2). This can result in the development of so-called tennis shoulder, with an increase in the size of the humeral bones and muscles and increased laxity in the joint capsule, ligaments and tendons around the shoulder of the racket arm. The end result is a dropping of the shoulder and a relative lengthening of the arm. In extreme cases a scoliosis can develop.

Another example of the effects of training can be seen in gymnasts. Training over a long period of time increases the range of motion in the vertebral column, bringing about permanent changes in the vertebral bodies and increased mobility in the pelvis.

It is not yet clear what significance these changes will have in the long

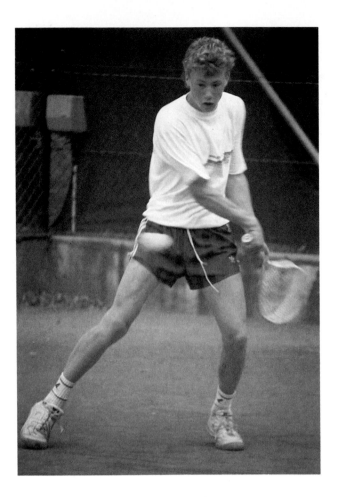

Fig. 10.5.2 Young tennis players often train one-sided, resulting in asymmetrical changes.

run. It is therefore essential that regular hard training in children and adolescents is carried out under medical supervision. One-sided and repetitive training should be avoided in adolescents.

Traumatic injuries

About 40% of all sports injuries happen to children and young adults (Pappas, 1981). In the USA, nearly 4 million individuals under 15 years of age are injured each year while engaged in sports. There is, however, no clear evidence that organized sports are safer or more dangerous than free play (Jackson *et al.*, 1981; Micheli, 1983).

An investigation in Göteborg showed that 6.4% of those coming to emergency clinics at the hospitals were injured because of sports. Fifteen percent of these were under the age of 15 years (Axelsson *et al.*, 1980). The most common causes were soccer, ice hockey, European handball, skating and skiing. In the USA, bicycling, US football, baseball, basketball, roller skating and playground equipment recreation accounted for 75% of all sports injuries to children (Pappas, 1981).

Traumatic injuries to children can be severe (e.g. epiphyseal or avulsion fractures). They are, however, often less severe than those of adults because of two reasons:

1   Children and young adults are physically smaller than adults which means that less forces are involved during the trauma.
2   Children's bones are more resilient and flexible, the ligaments and muscles are more elastic and the joint surfaces are capable of being repaired.

Fractures in children differ from those seen in adults because of the presence of the growth cartilage. Fracture complications can be severe, with angulation and rotation deformities, damage to the growth plate, etc. It is important to make a correct diagnosis and an adequate description of the fracture. This description should include:

1   The anatomical location of the injury.
2   The type of fracture.
3   Tissue changes associated with the injury.

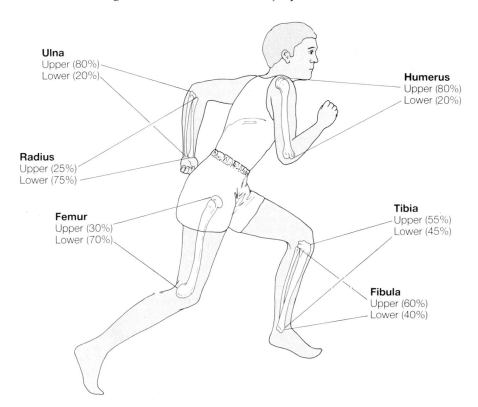

Fig. 10.5.3 Epyphyseal growth zones and contribution to long bone growth.

Injuries to growth centres

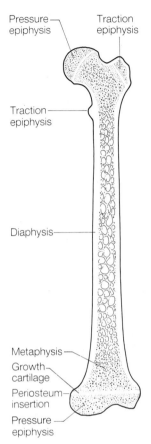

Fig. 10.5.4 Types of epiphyses in long bones.

Growth in the length of the skeleton takes place in the growth zones or epiphyseal cartilages. In the femur, 70% of the growth occurs in the lower growth zone and 30% in the upper growth zone. Corresponding figures for the lower leg are 55 and 45%, respectively (Fig. 10.5.3).

From a macroscopic point of view, growth cartilage is a clear line located between the metaphysis and the epiphysis of the long bones (Fig. 10.5.4). From a microscopic point of view, there are three major lines from the epiphyseal zone to the metaphyseal zone, plus the epiphysis with epiphyseal artery and ossification centre, growth cartilage with growth, maturation, transformation and remodelling functions (Fig. 10.5.5), and the metaphyseal loop.

Normally the weak point of a sliding fracture of the growth cartilage is the peripheral ring (perichondral). A direct trauma against the side of the knee joint would, in a child, most commonly result in an epiphyseal injury, while a similar injury in an adult would result in a tear of the medial collateal ligament and/or the anterior cruciate ligament.

Growth cartilage is located in three places in the child: the epiphyseal plate, the joint surface and the apophyseal insertions of major muscle tendon units. The growth plates are softer than fully formed bones and are therefore more likely to be injured than bone. Any injury to growth centres or cartilage is serious and may result in permanent joint deformity.

An injury may result in a fracture of the joint surface cartilage and the maturing bone beneath the joint surface, and so-called *intra-articular*

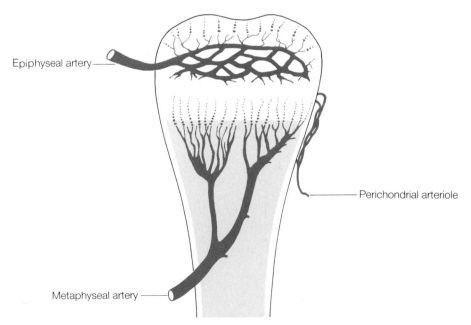

Fig. 10.5.5 Microscopic view of the growth cartilage.

fracture (which is identified by X-ray examination), or in a fracture involving the growth cartilage.

In 10–20% of injuries to the growth plate the normal growth in length may be disturbed.

Fractures of the growth cartilage   These can be divided according to the Salter and Harris classification (Fig. 10.5.6), into horizontal fractures, i.e. types 1 and 2, and vertical fractures, i.e. types 3, 4 and 5.

Horizontal fractures of the growth cartilage

Type 1   These injuries are often caused by a violent trauma. There is a simple detachment and the fracture is benign.

Type 2   These injuries are also often caused by a direct violent trauma. There is an impure epiphyseal detachment and a metaphyseal fragment. The fracture is benign.

These fractures can be treated by reduction under general anaesthesia. The reduction should be perfect, otherwise surgery is indicated. The fractures may be complicated by shortening with 3–4 cm at the end of the growth period. Another, rare, complication is maturation and acceleration of the growth cartilage, which may have to be treated by premature epiphysiodesis.

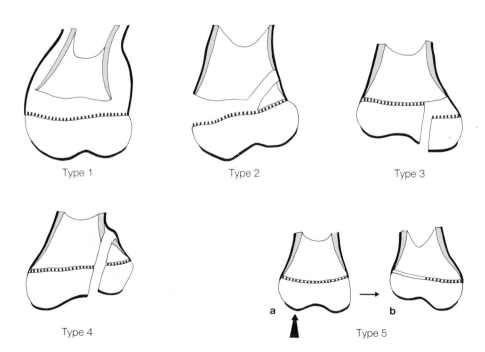

Fig. 10.5.6 Salter–Harris classification of fractures to growth cartilage. Types 1 to 5 are explained in the text.

Type 1   Type 2   Type 3   Type 4   Type 5

Vertical fractures of the growth cartilage   Type 3, 4 and 5 fractures are more rare and potentially dangerous; they may be difficult to detect (especially type 5).

Type 3   This fracture is vertical and detached.

Type 4   This is a vertical fracture passing through the growth cartilage.

Type 5   This is an injury with an accumulation of cartilage growth and longitudinal fissuration. This injury is usually not seen until the growth disturbance starts.

These injuries must be treated *urgently*. They are treated surgically if there is malalignment. Complications are residual valgus or varus malalignment. The surgery should be atraumatic and the epiphyseal cartilage not touched. Information should be given early about the risks for growth problems.

Epiphysiolysis   Growth zones can slip in relation to the bone, and this is called epiphysiolysis or a slipped epiphysis. The most common site is a slipped capital femoral epiphysis where the ball of the joint becomes displaced. This may happen gradually or suddenly. Epiphysiolysis should be treated by surgery. It should be remembered that there is a 25% chance of the same thing happening to the other hip and therefore careful observation is important (Pappas, 1981).

Maturation of the growth plate   The evaluation of the closing of the growth plate can be made by checking the maturation of the round bones of the left wrist. There are four centres in the left wrist and seven in the right. The four carpal centres in the left wrist agree with the chronological age of the body and with the maturation of the tubular bones in both hands. Two tests are commonly used:

1   Risser's test: the normal secondary epiphyseal centre in the crest of the ileum is ranked from zero to five crosses (0 to +++++).

2   Listel's test for secondary ossification centres: superior articular, transverse, spinous and inferior articular processes are examined. These all appear at approximately 16 years of age and fuse with their respective processes at approximately 25 years of age.

Using the Green-Andersson growth rate graphs for the femur and tibia it is possible to analyse any longitudinal discrepancies.

The growth plates are closed in girls usually at the age of 16–17 years and in boys at the age of 17–18. After this they are considered as adults.

Avulsion fractures   In adolescents the strength of the tendons and ligaments is greater than that of the bones, while this situation is reversed in adults. This means that children and young adults usually suffer skeletal injuries as a result of trauma or overuse. The bony attachment of the ligament or muscle may be torn away from its origin instead of the muscle or ligament itself tearing. Such avulsion fractures are often located in the growth centres of the flat bones, and are most common in the front of the pelvis and also in the ischium where the posterior hamstring muscles have their origins. Avulsion fractures often occur suddenly during hard, rapid loading of the muscles. These fractures are true fractures and should be examined by X-ray. If the bony attachments have been torn away and displaced to such an extent that proper healing is doubtful, surgery should be considered. The indications for X-ray examination, computed tomography, MRI, etc. must be wider for children and adolescents than for adults as the diagnosis found may have greater consequences.

Diaphyseal fractures   Bone tissue is softer in adolescents than in adults, and the younger the person the less likely it is to break with malalignment. Fractures in growing individuals show different characteristics. The skeleton also has a better blood supply in children than in adults which reduces the time needed for fractures to heal. The principles of treatment are different from those used in treating adults because:

1   The fractures will heal faster. If a cast is needed it will be worn over a shorter period of time.
2   The fractures will show fewer visible signs remaining in children and young adults.
3   Young adults will sustain different types of fractures.

Bones which have not ceased growing are resilient. They have a higher compliance but perhaps not increased strength per unit area. They can therefore be bent quite vigorously before breaking. An example of this is the so-called greenstick fracture (Fig. 10.5.7).

Diaphyseal fractures in the femur are usually treated by traction for some weeks. Fractures in other locations are treated with a cast. Surgery is sometimes indicated in open fractures and after infections in adolescents.

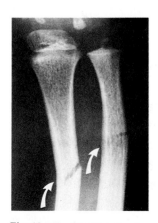

Fig. 10.5.7   An example of a greenstick fracture.

In summary most fractures in children are treated conservatively. Indications for surgery include: acute epiphysiolysis at the proximal femur, displaced fractures of the femoral neck, non-reducible dislocations of the hip, avulsion fractures with a diastasis of more than 5–10 mm, greatly displaced fractures, nerve and vessel complicating fractures, open fractures, etc. Fractures in children should be treated with great care and consideration as they can otherwise lead to lasting and severe complications.

Other traumatic injuries Total ruptures of, for example, Achilles tendon and the anterior cruciate ligaments are commonly seen in adults. As the strength of the tendons and ligaments is greater than that of the bones in adolescents and children it is quite rare to find these injuries in this age group. The young adult, with the same type of trauma, will instead sustain an avulsion fracture.

Soft tissue injuries that are common in spite of this, are injuries to the lateral ligaments of the ankle joint. They heal, however, quickly and usually cause few future problems.

Overuse injuries

Overuse injuries are recognized as being a great problem for older athletes because of degeneration of tendons and other soft tissues. Overuse injuries have, however, also become common in children and young adults resulting from repetitive microtrauma. Overuse injuries constitute a great diagnostic and therapeutic problem because the symptoms are often diffuse and uncharacteristic. Our knowledge about these injuries is limited, and there are many potential causes for these injuries.

Risk factors for overuse injuries can be divided into: (a) intrinsic factors, i.e. malalignment, leg length discrepancy, muscular imbalance, quadriceps and hamstring insufficiency; and (b) extrinsic, i.e. training errors, surfaces, environmental conditions, footwear and equipment (Renström & Johnson, 1985).

Intrinsic factors

Anatomic malalignment Anatomic malalignment is common in adults as a risk factor. Malalignment is commonly present in children but does not usually cause problems. When problems can be correlated to some anatomic malalignment, correction and compensation should be offered.

Flat and pronated feet are often the cause of overuse injuries and can be treated with compensatory orthotics in the shoe (Subotnick, 1975). In the young athlete semirigid orthotics may sometimes be valuable when symptomatic flat feet are present, but it should not be routine. One should, however, rule out associated growth-related musculotendinous imbalances such as tight heel cords.

Leg length discrepancy   Another malalignment which is much discussed is that of leg length discrepancy. These discrepancies are rarely associated with significant problems in young athletes, although an élite adult runner may be affected by a discrepancy of more than 6 mm. For a discrepancy of 10 mm or greater a built-up shoe or inset-type of orthotics may be used (Micheli, 1983).

Excessive lumbar lordosis   Excessive lumbar lordosis or hyperextension of the knees can be corrected by careful directed exercise programmes (Walaszek, 1982). Excessive femoral anteversion may be compensated for by excessive external tibial rotation and foot pronation, which causes knee pain. These malalignments could prevent a young dancer from continuing his or her career.

Musculotendinous imbalance   Musculotendinous imbalance can be a problem of balance between strength and flexibility. From studies of running it is known that a characteristic pattern of a tight, strong quadriceps, a tight, strong gastrocnemius and soleus, and tight, weak hamstrings results from running training alone (Brubaker & James, 1974). This problem has now been seen in children and a specific stretching programme must be used to reverse this tendency.

Extrinsic factors
Training errors   Training errors are the most common cause of injuries in both adults and growing children. Children can play for hours in their backyard without being injured, but with the tendency for an increase in organized sports training, camps, etc. with more intensive and specialized training, the incidence of overuse injuries has increased dramatically. Overuse injuries are often associated with endurance training. Common training errors are running too far, but also changes in intensity, heel work, running technique and fatigue.

Footwear and surfaces   Footwear and surfaces can be of importance, especially as children often use poor and less expensive shoes. Running shoes for children should have a high and hard heel counter, good shock absorbing characteristics and good flexibility in the forefoot.

The playing surface can also be of importance, which is seen, for example, in tennis. On surfaces with high friction, children often sustain more overuse injuries such as medial tibial stress syndromes and Achilles tendinitis. These problems are rarely seen on clay courts. Furthermore there are few tennis shoes made today to suit children playing tennis on high-friction courts. A tennis shoe in a competitive young player does not usually last for more than 6 weeks.

Other factors   Associated diseases or pre-existent injuries can occasionally be factors of importance, e.g. in children who have had Perthe's disease. Hips in children who have had this disease have a loss of rotation and may therefore secondarily develop knee pain.

The growth factor appears to be a risk factor in two aspects (Micheli, 1981). First, the growth cartilage and especially the growing articular cartilage, is less resistant to repetitive microtrauma and more susceptible to shear than adult cartilage. This might, therefore, be a risk factor for injuries (Bright *et al.*, 1974). Second, as mentioned earlier, there is an increase in musculotendinous tightness around the joints and thereby a reduction of the range of motion during the growth spurt. This may certainly increase the risk for injury.

Types of injury

Apophyseal injuries   In a muscle and tendon unit there are certain high-risk areas, such as the attachment of muscles and tendons to bone (the apophyses), the muscle and tendon itself, and also the point at which the muscle and tendon merge (the muscle–tendon junction). In adults, a trauma may cause injury to the muscle and tendon tissue itself; while the corresponding trauma in young adults will cause injuries to the attachment of the muscles or tendon to bone in the apophyseal insertions or the traction apophyses.

Osgood–Schlatter   The site at which injury to the apophyses is most common is the attach-
disease   ment of the patellar ligament to the tibia, Osgood–Schlatter disease. This problem used to be found mostly in boys during their growth spurt but nowadays is also seen in girls aged 10–12 years. The aetiology of these injuries was thought to be an avascular necrosis, i.e. a non-infectious interruption of the blood supply which results in injured tissue. There are, however, indications that these injuries are the result of minor avulsion fractures, secondary to tensioned and laterally deviated quadriceps muscles and the body's healing processes (Micheli, 1983). These conditions are mostly seen in sports like figure skating and gymnastics but also in football and European handball, which include a great deal of jumping and knee bending thus exposing the apophyses to great tensile stress.

Overloading of the apophysis causes inflammation in the attachment of the tendon which manifests itself as pain, tenderness and swelling. An X-ray shows fragmentation of the bone under the attachment of the tendon. These conditions are often associated with tight musculo-tendinous units (Ogden & Southwick, 1976). Actions causing pain should be avoided.

Os calcis apophysitis

Os calcis apophysitis (Sever's disease) occurs in the attachment of the Achilles tendon to the calcaneus and is common in football. The aetiology is often training errors, usually monotonous repetitive training. Mal-alignment and a tight Achilles tendon during the growth spurt are also fairly common factors. The treatment of these injuries consists of rest at an early stage and the use of an orthotic with a heel wedge to decrease the load of the area. It is important to avoid movements that trigger pain.

Tendinitis

Tendinitis of the shoulder, elbow, Achilles tendon, etc. may also be seen in young adults. When the tendon is the site for microtears the body reacts with an inflammation which is the body's normal initial healing response. The treatment consists of rest of the injured area, but other activities can be carried out; ice, compression and non-weight bearing may be of value. One should be careful with medication in children. Sometimes buffered aspirin is of value. Corticosteroid injections should not be used in young athletes. In the rehabilitation phase it is important to perform early muscle exercises, initially including isometric and then dynamic exercises; the dynamic exercises can be divided into eccentric and concentric exercises. Curwin and Stanish (1984) have shown that dynamic eccentric training can safely be done during the early healing phase of tendinitis and they even suggest that this may promote healing. Care is, however, recommended especially in growing individuals as eccentric exercises initiate high force production which if not used carefully can aggravate the injury.

Cartilage injuries

The collagen tissue of the articular cartilage is better supplied with blood vessels but has poorer strength in adolescents than in adults. The growing articular surface of the child can be injured more easily than in adults as a result of sprains and direct blows, especially at the elbow, knee and ankle.

Osteochondritis dissecans

Repetitive trauma could be the cause of many cases of osteochondritis dissecans, especially in the elbow of a child pitcher or in the knee of a football player. In this injury, a part of the articular cartilage that has been damaged may break away and become free, moving inside the joint, which may cause problems. The diagnosis is made with the help of arthroscopy and X-ray. The treatment of choice is rest, sometimes in a splint or cast. In young adults the cartilage is still growing and will usually cover the pivot. Osteochondritis dissecans in young children is mainly a problem of diagnosis not treatment (Pappas, 1981). If the patient still experiences pain after 6 months and the X-ray is unchanged, surgery should be considered.

Patellofemoral pain syndrome   Patellofemoral pain syndrome or chondromalacia patellae is a very common problem in growing children. In the knee, laterally there is a strong fascia lata and medially a relatively lighter tissue which may result not only in longitudinal traction but also in lateral deviation of the patella. If this tendency towards proximal and lateral deviation of the quadriceps mechanism is excessive there might be recurrent lateral subluxation or injuries of the cartilage, like softening fibrillation and erosion. There are also other possible mechanisms. Pain may arise from the medial surface of the patella or around the patella and this is often triggered by running uphill or downhill and by squatting. Prolonged sitting in one place, e.g. in the cinema, might also cause pain. The cause of the problem must always be analysed. If malalignment is present, orthotics, inserts or a brace may be of value.

This pain condition will respond to anti-inflammatory therapy combined with an attempt to strengthen the medial structures of the quadriceps and adductor muscles and to stretch the lateral structures and the hamstrings. If, after 6–12 months of exercise, pain is still felt, arthroscopy and minor surgery may be performed.

Stress fractures   The frequency of stress fractures in young adults is increasing. The injury can be caused by frequently repeated movements under normal load, e.g. long-distance running, or by movements of a lower frequency but with a higher load, e.g. weight lifting. The most dangerous combination is one of high load and high frequency. It is most often associated with maltraining.

Stress fractures can occur in any bone of the body but are most common in the weight bearing long bones of the lower leg, tibia and fibula. They are also seen in the metatarsal bones, in the calcaneus in the tarsal navicular, in the femur, hip, and pelvic bones and vertebral bodies.

Stress fractures should be suspected in athletes who complain of pain during physical activity. Usually there is no pain or discomfort during rest. Distinct local tenderness and sometimes swelling over the painful area are found and a clinical examination should give the diagnosis. To certify the diagnosis, an X-ray examination, sometimes including tomography or a bone scan, is helpful. The treatment is rest until healing.

Spine injuries Back injuries associated with children's sports are increasing and are becoming a problem, especially in gymnastics.

Lordosis of lumbar spine During the growth spurt there appears to be a tendency to develop lordosis of the lumbar spine (Micheli, 1983) which is due to the enhanced growth anteriorly in the vertebral bodies and the secondary tethering of the spine posteriorly by the heavy lumbodorsal fascia. Micheli (1983) has observed a growth-related pattern of posture developing at this time with a tight lumbar lordosis, and a relative flexion contracture at the hips with associated tight hamstrings. Because normal forward excursion of the lumbar spine is limited there is a tendency to develop forward bending at the thoracolumbar junction or the thoracic spine itself. Kraus (1976) has suggested that increased lumbar lordosis increases the tendency of both posterior element failure at the pars interarticularis (see below) and disc failure. This theoretical explanation supports the clinical observations of back problems seen in young athletes; these generally fall into one of three categories:

1 Stress fracture of the pars interarticularis (see below) called spondylolysis.
2 Hyperlordotic mechanical low back pain.
3 Disc herniation.

All these changes will cause pain mainly in the lumbar spine and are accelerated during sport.

Almost 50% of all young athletes with lumbar pain for more than 3 months are found to have spondylolysis (Jackson *et al.*, 1981).

Spondylolysis Spondylolysis is a break in the narrow bony neck (the pars interarticularis) between the articular processes of the vertebra. It is often caused by repeated hyperextension of the lumbar spine carried out, for example, in gymnastics. Young female gymnasts performing front and back walk-overs, vaults, flips and dismounts have a high incidence of the condition. Defects in the pars interarticularis occur in 2.3% of the normal white female population compared to 11% in female gymnasts (Jackson *et al.*, 1981). The symptoms are aching pain in the lower back which is often unilateral. The pain is worsened by twisting and hyperextension. The diagnosis is made from clinical findings, X-ray examinations and bone scans. The treatment is restricting vigorous physical activity in the acute phase, sometimes with bed rest, early bracing, and an antilordotic exercise programme and hamstring stretching.

Spondylolisthesis   Further damage might cause spondylolisthesis which is a slippage of one vertebrae on another. It is more commonly seen in young people between 9 and 14 years of age and it is usually L5 that slips forward on S1. If there is a large slippage of up to 50%, the athlete's sacrum becomes vertical. Flexibility will then lessen and the hamstrings become tight making the athlete incapable of top level gymnastic performance (Kulund, 1982). The treatment is the same as for spondylolysis.

Scheuermann's disease   Scheuermann's disease mostly affects young men between 10 and 25 years of age. In this disease, X-ray examination shows irregularities in the superoanterior part of the epiphysis that result in vertebral wedging. These young adults often complain of pain during sitting and after sports but the pain often decreases during sports activities.

Thoracolumbar back pain   Back pain can develop at the thoracolumbar junction, frequently associated with repetitive sports activity. The cause for this pain may be repetitive microtrauma or compression fractures of the vertebral bodies anteriorly (Hensinger, 1982). These conditions are treated with a low back and hamstring flexibility programme and early bracing.

Other injuries   There are many other special injuries that might occur in children and young adults such as the *little leaguer's elbow* which is an overuse injury sustained by young throwers in baseball. The mechanism is repetitive valgus stress applied to the elbow with throwing, resulting in compression laterally and traction medially. The result might be loose bodies in the joint, osteochondritis dissecans of the capitellum, deformation or premature closure of the proximal radial epiphysis, overgrowth of the radial head and, on the medial side, irritation of the medial epicondyle. These injuries are always preventable and if observed early they can be treated with no long-term sequelae.

Shoulder problems, e.g. *impingement syndrome*, may be caused by activities involving repetitive use of the arm above the horizontal level, e.g. in swimming and tennis. This syndrome is secondary to increased volume of the structures located between the rotator cuff muscles and the coracoacromial ligament and the anterior edge of the acromion itself. In throwing and breast-stroke in swimming an internal rotation contracture of the shoulder may develop because of a tight posterior and loose anterior capsule (Micheli, 1983). This imbalance may lead to impingement. The symptoms are pain after activity and after some time also during activity. There is a point tenderness and painful abduction arc of motion. The treatment is modified activity, stretching and surgery.

Training of young individuals

Principles of treatment

The treatment of overuse injuries are controversial and the principles described in Chapter 10.4. It must be emphasized that the treatment of injuries in young athletes should be individualized. The aim of acute treatment is to relieve pain, minimize haematoma formation and soft tissue damage and limit inflammation.

The question after the acute phase is whether to prescribe rest or activity. Joint immobilization will result in muscle wasting and weakness, joint stiffness and diminished proprioception and should be avoided if possible. Repeated exercises increase the mechanical and structural properties of the tendon (Woo *et al.*, 1975). Therefore, mobilization should be started as early as the healing of the injury permits.

The exercise programme should start very carefully with a gradual increase of the load within the limits of pain. Initial careful isometric exercises can be carried out without load. Dynamic exercises may include both eccentric and concentric contractions and they can be carried out as soon as they can be performed without pain. Eccentric contractions of the muscles can maximize force production and minimize time delays and energy expenditure. Some care is, however, advisable as the larger loads of eccentric contractions will potentially increase the risk for re-injury. Strength training after injury should, in principle, initially be carried out without loads. The frequency should be increased before load and the training should be all encompassing. Strength exercises should always be combined with flexibility exercises.

Strength training

Children and young adults can respond dramatically to muscular strength training because there is relatively more effect on the muscles than on the skeleton. In strength training with a high load level, muscular strength develops faster than the strength of the skeleton, which can lead to avulsion fractures, i.e. where the tendon or attachment of a muscle to the bone is torn away because of the muscular force generated.

Strength training can involve isometric, isokinetic, eccentric, etc. training. The strength gained via isometric training is very specific to the joint angle at which the training is performed and it is therefore of limited value in sports. Young individuals should be cautious with loaded isometric work as this means that the muscles are working without appreciably changing their length. After an injury, however, some isometric exercises can be of value.

Light dynamic exercise, such as running and walking, is in most cases efficient. Training with heavy weights should be avoided by individuals who are still growing. The load on the vertebral column during weight training can be so great that the vertebrae are affected. Only the weight of the body should be used as a load in strength training in young individuals. Not until the skeleton has stopped growing, which in girls happens at about the age of 16 years and in boys 17–18 years, should systematic strength training with heavy weights start.

Flexibility training   Strength training alone has a negative effect on joint flexibility (Möller, 1984). Children are in themselves very flexible but after the growth spurt when the muscles start to grow they tend to rapidly become inflexible. This should therefore be counteracted by flexibility training. There are several different methods of flexibility training including ballistic stretching, slow static stretching and contract–relax stretching. The most widely used is slow static stretching. The most efficient method is, however, contract–relax stretching with a maintenance of the stretched position for more than 30–45 s.

Endurance training   There is a widespread opinion that endurance training has a better effect the earlier in life it starts. Scientific evidence has not been able to verify this and recent findings indicate that for children there is no loss in effect by delaying systematical physical fitness training until they are in their teens.

Heat treatment

Heat increases the extensibility of collagen in connective tissue, decreases joint stiffness, relieves muscle spasm and gives pain relief. Local heat can be applied with chemical heat bags or electrical pads. Heat retainers preserve heat, at least at the skin level. These heat retainers are valuable tools in both prevention and rehabilitation of joint muscle and tendon injuries as they can be applied during activity.

Conclusion

Most of the injuries in young athletes can be prevented. Knowledge of the special characteristics of the musculoskeletal system is of great importance. The trainer, the coach and the parents must be aware of the risks that exist for children in the long, as well as in the short, term with different types of training. Sports must remain being play for children and a means of maintaining physical health for adulthood.

Young individuals have some characteristics which distinguish them from adults. In the playing of sports, specific age groups are often formed. This creates a classification which is purely chronical and thereby ignores the complete physiological picture of a growing youngster. There can be a difference of biological maturity of more than 5 years between young people in the same age group. Thus a group of 13-year-old girls or boys can include youngsters whose biological maturity is on the same level as that of 15–16-year-old or 10–11-year-old boys or girls.

Anyone involved in training with growing young people should have a sound knowledge of the physical development of these athletes. The training and competition programme must be individualized, considering the growth level and the biological and physiological maturity.

Considering injuries in growing children, it is important to realize that there are many special risk factors involved as children are not small adults. Injuries in children require extra care and examination because deleterious diseases can be disguised and because the end result can be a disaster if maltreated. Increased awareness and knowledge about these problems is essential. Let us all help our children participate in sports safely by considering these facts.

References

Axelsson, R., Renström, P. & Svensson, H. O. (1980) Akuta idrottsskador på ett centrallasarett. *Läkartidningen* **77**, 41.

Bright, R. W., Burnstein, A. H. & Elmore, S. M. (1974) Epiphyseal plate cartilage—a biomechanical and histological analysis of failure modes. *J. Bone Joint Surg. (Am)* **56**, 668.

Brubaker, G. E. & James, S. L. (1974) Injuries to runners. *J. Sports Med.* **2**, 189.

Curwin, S. & Stanish, W. D. (1984) *Tendinitis, Its Etiology and Treatment.* The Collamore Press, D.C. Heath & Co., Lexington.

Hensinger, R. N. (1982) Back pain and vertebral changes simulating Scheuermann's disease. *Orthop. Trans.* **6**, 1.

Jackson, D. W., Wiltse, L. L., Dingeman, R. & Hayes, M. (1981) Stress reactions involving the pars interarticularis in young athletes. *Am. J. Sports Med.* **9(5)**, 304.

Kraus, H. (1976) Effect of lordosis on the stress in the lumbar spine. *Clin. Orthop.* **117**, 56.

Kulund, D. (1982) *The Injured Athlete.* Lippincott Co., Philadelphia.

Micheli, L. J. (1981) Young runners. *Pediatr. Alert* **6**.

Micheli, L. J. (1983) Overuse injuries in children sports: the growth factor. *Orthop. Clin. North Am.* **14(2)**, 337.

Möller, M. (1984) *Athletic training and flexibility. A study on range of motion in the lower extremity.* Linköping University Medical Dissertations No. 182.

Ogden, J. A. & Southwick, W. D. (1976) Osgood Schlatter's disease and tibial tubercle development. *Clin. Orthop.* **116**, 180.

Pappas, A. (1981) In W. Southmayd & M. Hoffman *Sports Health.* Quick Fox, New York.

Subotnick, S. L. (1975) Orthotic foot control and the overuse syndrome. *Arch. Pediatr. Med. Foot Surg.* **2**, 207.

Walaszek, A. (1982) Physical therapy rehabilitation of dance injuries. In W. J. Gillespie (ed) *Sports Medicine, Sports Science: Bridging the Gap.* The Collamore Press, Lexington.

Woo, S. L., Matthews, J. V., Akeson, W. H. et al. (1975) Connective tissue response to immobility: a correlative study of biochemical and biomechanical measurements of normal and immobilized rabbit knees. *Arthritis Rheum.* **18**, 257.

Further reading

DeHaven, K. E. (1978) Athletic injuries in adolescents. *Pediatr. Ann.* **7**, 95.

Jackson, D. W. (1982) Spine problems in the runner. In R. D'Ambrosia & D. Drez jr (eds) *Prevention and Treatment of Running Injuries*, pp. 43–54. Charles Slack, Thorofare.

Renström, P. & Johnson, R. J. (1985) Overuse injuries in sports. A review. *Sports Med.* **2**, 316.

Stanish, W. D. (1981) *Treatment of chronic tendinitis with eccentric exercise training.* Presented at the American Academy of Orthopedic Surgery Meeting, Las Vegas, Nevada, 24 February 1981.

10.6 Principles of rehabilitation after injuries

G. GRIMBY & R. THOMEÉ

Introduction

This chapter discusses the following points:

1 General consequences of muscle structure and function in different phases after sport injury.
2 A summary of different treatment principles used in the different phases.
3 Examples of training procedures for specific post-traumatic conditions.

Changes in muscle structure and function

The structural and functional consequences for muscle of an injury of the locomotor system can generally be divided into three phases.

Phase one The first phase is characterized by the immediate effects of immobilization and inhibition of muscle activation. Various patterns can be seen depending on the type of immobilization. In an immobilization with a fixed joint angle, the muscle atrophy pattern seems to depend on the relative length of the muscle and, therefore, the type and amount of impulses from the stretch receptors. Thus, it has been observed, that with a muscle in a slack condition, such as at immobilization with a straight knee or a plantar flexed foot, there is a dominance of atrophy of the slow twitch (type I) fibres. These, therefore, seem to be most dependent on the impulses from the stretch receptors. With no joint immobilization but a general disuse, the atrophy of fast twitch (type II) fibres will dominate. One would expect that such a patient does not make contractions strong enough to recruit the high-threshold motor units innervating the fast twitch fibres. Various mixtures of atrophy between these two extreme situations may occur and a combined atrophy of both muscle fibre types are not uncommon. In the literature different patterns of fibre-type atrophy associated with joint damage and/or immobilization has therefore been described (Young & Stokes,

1986). Different non-invasive methods have been suggested to follow specific type of muscle fibre atrophy such as the use of the force–velocity relationship, but without much proven usefulness in clinical situations. As further discussed in connection with different training regimens it would be of some practical use to have an idea of specific type of muscle atrophy, for the choice of training programmes. This is, however, still an area of uncertainty. There has also been a discussion whether conversion of slow twitch (type I) to fast twitch (type II) muscle fibres may occur. There is some evidence that this might be the case during an immobilization period, but these changes may not have any major clinical relevance. For major changes in fibre composition much more dramatic alterations must occur in the recruitment pattern, such as after a prolonged electrical stimulation.

Pain in a joint results in voluntary inhibition of activity in muscle acting across that joint. However, it is not necessary to experience pain to get inhibition. The activity in other receptors from the joint and adjacent structure may give similar effects as seen in animal experiments and human studies (e.g. Stokes & Young, 1984). It was thus demonstrated, that a very small amount of joint effusion may give a reflex inhibition of the musculature. There might be selective inhibitions of motor units, which could explain part of the dominant atrophy for a specific fibre type, such as with slow twitch fibre (STF) atrophy seen after joint damage.

There is a vicious circle causing muscle weakness (Fig. 10.6.1) (Stokes & Young, 1984). It shows the relationship between joint damage, immobilization, reflex inhibition and muscle wasting. The reflex inhibition

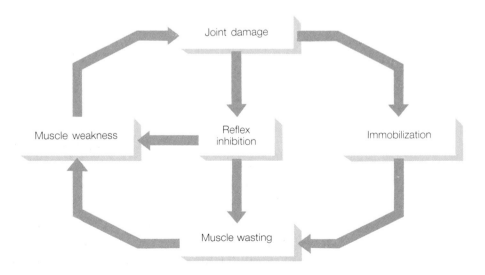

Fig. 10.6.1 Schematic presentation of different mechanisms leading to muscle wasting and muscle weakness. Redrawn from Stokes & Young (1984).

can, therefore, result in an immediate reduction of voluntary muscle activation causing a muscle weakness as in the early postoperative period after knee surgery, and also, in the longer perspective, a muscle atrophy which further augments the muscle weakness. Reduction in inhibitory influence, such as blocking with epidural or local anaesthesia, can immediately increase the voluntary muscle activation, as demonstrated by electromyography. As already pointed out, there is not a direct relationship between the degree of pain and the amount of muscle inhibition. In a later postoperative phase, inhibition might be as severe as at the first postoperative day, but with now a virtually pain-free patient (Shakespeare *et al.*, 1985).

Phase two   In the second phase, when the patient can be mobilized, the effect of inhibition and disuse may still have an effect on muscle structure and function. There are individual variations due to the type of injury and therefore due to the type of disuse and inhibition. In patients with remaining pain, a longstanding atrophy of type I fibres has been noted (Edström, 1970). The phase is characterized by the results of the muscle wasting occurring during the previous period; it is not unusual to have up to 30–50% quadriceps atrophy after knee injury. The quadriceps atrophy usually dominates over the atrophy of the hamstrings muscle (e.g. Arvidsson *et al.*, 1981; Thomeé *et al.*, 1987).

The degree of muscle wasting cannot be accurately diagnosed by measurements of circumference as measured with a tape measure and can in fact be grossly underestimated. The reason for this is that the fat and bone structure are constant. With a reduction of the circumference of the muscle tissue, there will be an increase in the width of the subcutaneous fat layer masking part of the effect of muscle wasting on the total circumference. In the thigh there are also differences in the degree of muscle wasting between different muscles with a predominance of quadriceps compared to hamstrings atrophy. The muscle mass can be regained through activity and training, although this cannot be accurately followed by circumference measurement. Measurement with computerized tomography is not easily available and the clinician has to depend on palpation and indirect conclusions based on functional measurements concerning the amount of muscle wasting.

It is important that inhibitory factors are eliminated during this phase, otherwise an optimal recruitment of motor units cannot be achieved. Otherwise proper stimulus for the synthesis of muscle proteins, which should be one of the main issues during the rehabilitation in this period, may not be given.

Phase three The third phase can arbitrarily be defined to start when the muscle has regained sufficient volume, strength and endurance to approach a minimal level needed for various functional activities. Different individuals have different functional needs, and the limitations will therefore vary. A common feature, however, is the need for further improvement in muscle structure and activation, as well as improved motor control and coordination.

It has been demonstrated that there might remain quite marked differences in muscle strength between the two sides of the body, which are subjectively unnoticed. Thus, a 20% reduction, or even more, of quadriceps muscle strength has been recorded in the previously injured side compared with the uninjured side in people who have returned to full normal activity and considered themselves as completely recovered. Even in athletes, such differences between sides can be seen. There are reasons to assume that side differences and imbalance between the muscle strength of agonists and antagonists may increase the risk for new injuries (Fleck & Falkel, 1986). The ratio of hamstrings of quadriceps muscle strength of 0.56–0.80 has been identified as normal, and it has been suggested that athletes with a lower than normal ratio should be placed on a training programme to improve the weak area and in that way hopefully prevent subsequent injuries. In other muscle groups similar ratios may be found and interpreted within the training regimen. The knowledge concerning muscle imbalance, however, is still poor.

In some types of injuries, such as ankle injuries, one of the major issues is the reduction of proprioceptive control. In such situations training of motor control and coordination should be given higher priority than training of muscle strength. There is a definite need for objective measurements of muscle function before full athletic activity is allowed, and the physicians should look for an adequate checklist with respect to the particular type of sport. It has clearly been demonstrated that subjective assessment of functions are not sufficient.

The degree of lack of function is relative and dependent on the aim for muscle performance of the individual. A person involved in recreational activities such as golf, jogging or swimming has other needs than a highly trained athlete. Athletes involved in sports needing high motor performance or intensity such as ice hockey or downhill skiing, or where very precise motor skills are needed such as in throwing, jumping or gymnastics, require a more intense and specific rehabilitation programme.

Principal aspects of treatment

It must be emphasized that the different phases are not distinctly separated and that there may be a more or less obvious overlap of different treatment approaches between the different phases.

Phase one In the first phase, emphasis should be placed on the reduction or elimination of any reflex inhibition (see Arvidsson *et al.*, 1986). Factors such as pain, joint effusion and inflammation can be reduced by proper clinical management. Training should be done in a pain-free range of motion. Local anaesthesia, analgesics or the use of TNS (transcutaneous nerve stimulation) or TENS will reduce pain-released inhibition. However, as already mentioned, factors not related to perception of pain may cause inhibition and blocking of afferented impulses may have a functional positive effect here as well.

To achieve a more than voluntary activated muscle force, electrical muscle stimulation can be used during the immobilization phase. The electrical stimulation should be combined with simultaneous voluntary muscle activation to achieve an optimal muscle effect. It can be assumed that at the same time afferent impulses from the electrical stimulation have a TNS effect with reduction of inhibition. The electrical stimulation may further enhance voluntary muscle activation and have a psychological effect in some people who hesitate to produce a maximal muscle contraction voluntarily. Present clinical experience is that a combination of electrical stimulation of the quadriceps muscle and simultaneous voluntary contraction during immobilization in a cast after anterior cruciate ligament surgery will result in significantly less reduction in quadriceps muscle strength than in a control group with only voluntary contractions, and also that there is less muscle wasting as measured with computerized tomography (Wigerstad-Lossing *et al.*, 1988). This type of electrical stimulation can also limit the reduction in relative area of type I fibres and the muscle enzymatic activity during the immobilization period. When using electrical stimulation it is important to use proper techniques, e.g. a frequency of about 30 Hz, stimulation periods not causing fatigue, and sufficiently high stimulation intensity. The use of stimulators with very high frequencies (2500 Hz) does not seem to be of any benefit. It is also suggested that stimulators with constant current output should be used to give a reproducible response.

With immobilization in a cast only isometric contractions are possible. If these are timed with short pauses (of a few seconds) between each contraction, the total metabolic load can be kept high over several minutes. In this way endurance training effects can also be achieved, which can be demonstrated in the mitochondrial function (see above concerning electrical stimulation and Grimby et al., 1973). This may to some degree counteract the reduction in STF size and numbers.

If there is a mobilization which allows dynamic activity, such as with a mobile cast, dynamic exercises can be used to prevent reduction in strength as well as in endurance. Besides maintenance of joint mobility it is also easier to use training programmes aimed at maintaining motor recruitment pattern. When the recruitment pattern deteriorates, different facilitation techniques can be used to get a better recruitment of motor units, e.g. proprioceptive neuromuscular facilitation (PNF) techniques. These can, however, be better utilized when full mobility is allowed. Emphasis must be placed on achieving a better neural activation of the musculature; the training effects are specific for the type of sport. It is therefore important to give training through the full range of allowed motion, specifically emphasizing weak areas of function.

Phase two　In the second phase, the treatment should at first be concentrated on the recovery of muscle mass. Before this can be efficiently achieved it is necessary to assure that there are no major inhibitory influences and that there is an adequate motor recruitment so that the major part of the muscle is activated at a maximal voluntary effort. It must be assumed that the stimuli for an increased protein synthesis leading to an increasing muscle mass is the tension developed in the musculature. With that background it can be assumed that training can be rather unspecific and different training equipment can be used.

Isokinetic devices have received much attention in recent years. The basic principle is that the degree of resistance is determined by the person undergoing training. The angular velocity can be varied from slow to high velocities. As soon as the preset velocities are reached further effort will only result in larger resistance. Thus, training can be performed submaximally or maximally and overloading is avoided. The return can be loaded or unloaded and when a concentric model is used the risk for overload during the return with eccentric work, as in weight training, is avoided. With increasing velocity, the force developed will be reduced and less compression force on the joint surfaces and less tension in tendons and ligaments will occur. Training with high velocities may be advantageous in certain conditions and will also allow a specific training of fast motor units. It has been demonstrated that the effects of fast training velocities seem to be an increase in strength at slow angular velocities as well, whereas training at slow speeds have less effect on performance at high velocities. The specificity of the training programme will probably vary in different phases of rehabilitation, but the comments above have some general implications. The main rule is that different training speeds should be used and, especially if fast twitch fibre (FTF) atrophy is expected, high velocities may be beneficial.

Another benefit of the isokinetic system is that maximal resistance can be achieved through the full range of motion and therefore the total work produced will be larger than during weight training. Different studies have also demonstrated a superior training effect of an isokinetic programme compared to a weight training programme. With intense isokinetic training over a 6–8 week period an increase of about 25% in strength can be achieved on the injured side for knee extension as well as for knee flexion (Grimby et al., 1980; Thomeé et al., 1987). Several factors can explain such an increase — improved neuronal activation which may be partly due to reduced inhibitory influence and to muscle fibre hypertrophy.

However, by using biomechanical principles the weight training model can also be improved. By adaptation of the angle between the weight bearing arm and the resistance arm of up to 90°, the torque angle curve produced of calf weight can be approximated to that produced by the knee extension muscles for a considerable part of the joint movement. For other examples of using biomechanical principles in arranging a training procedure, the reader is referred to, for example, Harms-Ringdahl et al. (1985).

It should, however, be noted that isokinetic training will only give maximal resistance during movement and isometric training must be added. Eccentric training has aroused considerable interest in recent years with the construction of special equipment for particular types of training. The force produced during eccentric contractions is larger than in concentric contractions and it has therefore been suggested that this could be a still better stimuli for protein synthesis and the recovery of muscle mass. Besides, in certain conditions such as retropatellar pain, inhibition may dominate for part of the eccentric movement and it seems that training could change such a specific weakness. Further studies are necessary to get sufficient knowledge on the clinical implications of eccentric training. It must also be remembered that overload during eccentric work can easily cause muscle damage with dearrangement of the Z-line and pain a few days after the exercise (Fridén et al., 1983 and others). The use of eccentric exercise must therefore be carefully controlled and used with caution in untrained situations, although there is less risk of negative effects in trained patients.

Different emphasis can be placed on different types of training regimens depending on the type of muscle fibre atrophy. If the aim is to achieve a training effect, particularly in the high-threshold motor units, very high intensities must be used in order to recruit these motor units and in short bursts in order to avoid fatigue. On the other hand, for training with the emphasis on low-threshold motor units repetitive exercises at submaximal levels should be used to achieve an improvement in the metabolic adaptation in the oxidative slow twitch fibres. For full muscle recovery different types of training programmes are needed.

There may also be negative effects of a specific training programme. For example, too strong an emphasis on high-intensity strength training may limit the recovery of the capillarization and oxidative enzymatic capacity necessary for high-endurance performance. Such a training programme may increase the size of the muscle fibres, but not the capillarization, thus increasing the diffusion distances.

In certain conditions, for example after ankle joint injury, where loss of proprioceptor reflexes are the major problem, coordination training has a dominant role. The balancing board has been demonstrated to be a useful tool here (Tropp, 1985).

It is also of utmost importance to regain a full range of motion using stretching exercises as emphasized by Möller (1984) and others. Contract–relax stretching related to PNF techniques seems to give the best results; slow stretching is useful to increase range of motion. Stretching ought to be preceded by a general warm-up. It seems to be of particular importance to use stretching when heavy strength training is included as the latter may otherwise reduce the range of motion.

Phase three   In the third phase, basic training programmes to achieve and maintain gross motor functions must continue, but more and more emphasis should be placed on specific training for certain activities. The training programme should use specific exercises directed to the needs of the specific sports activity. Training of coordination precision should be included.

Conclusion   Looking at the general aims of the training programme in the different phases, emphasis in the first phase is placed on achieving the best neural activation of the musculature as possible, which means that part of the training is rather specific. In the second phase, training is rather unspecific and the emphasis is on the recovery of muscle mass, whereas in the third phase the neurogenic factors are emphasized again with more specific training for certain motor performances.

Examples of training programmes after different sports injuries

Knee ligament surgery

The long rehabilitation period of up to 1 year or more after anterior cruciate ligament surgery is a condition that has well-defined phases, as described earlier.

Phase one

Surgery is followed by some sort of immobilization. This is usually in a rigid cast or some type of brace that allows movement in a limited range of motion.

Rigid cast   If a rigid cast is used the training programme can be as follows:

1   Quadriceps isometric contractions.
2   Hamstrings isometric contractions.
3   Straight leg raises.
4   Toe exercises if a full leg cast is used.
5   Toe and ankle exercises if a leg cast is used.
6   Hip exercises in some type of pulley machine.
7   Abdominal and lower back strengthening exercises.
8   Balance exercises if weight bearing is permitted.

Training should be done in short periods (5–15 min) several (four to six) times per day to avoid overuse. The aim is to stimulate neural activity, and to try to limit hypotrophy, joint effusion and pain.

If possible use electrical stimulation. A hole is made in the cast over the vastus medialis and rectus femoris. Stimulate with a surge current with a frequency of 30–50 Hz. The stimulation period should be 5–10 s and the patient should make a simultaneous voluntary contraction followed by a 5–10 s rest for a total of 5–10 min. This session should be repeated several times per day if possible.

Mobile brace   If a mobile brace is used the training programme can be as follows:

1   Same exercises as above.
2   Dynamic strengthening exercises for knee extension.
3   Dynamic strengthening exercises for knee flexion.
4   Isometric contractions in different knee angles.

Be careful not to overload the operated knee which can result in general synovitis and increased joint effusion. It is also not uncommon that the patient experiences patellofemoral discomfort or pain. The training programme must take into consideration both the aim of the training and how the patient's knee reacts to the different exercises. Gradually the load and intensity of training is increased and the exercises are made more and more demanding.

Phase two   When the cast is removed and the full range of motion is allowed, the second phase of training starts. Usually this is 4 to 6 weeks after surgery. The primary goal of training is to regain the full range of motion and to try to stop the muscle wasting process and to start the muscle building process instead. As range of motion increases the intensity of strength training can also increase; between 3 and 6 months after surgery more intense strength training can take place with increasing loads. A general strength and conditioning programme for the rest of the body should be constructed in order to maintain or improve general body endurance. If possible use pool exercises and a cycle ergometer.

Phase three   In the third phase more and more emphasis is placed on functional activities where movement pattern, muscle synchronization, coordination and balance become very important.

The programme can now consist of:

1   Continued strength training from the second phase.
2   Different strengthening exercises done with bodyweight as resistance.
3   Various running activities — circles, figures of 8, zig-zag, starts and stops, turns in all directions, different types of terrain, etc.
4   Various jumping activities — mini-trampoline, rope jumping, vertical jumps, plyometrics, etc.
5   Sports technique — exercises that facilitate motor control but with less load or intensity.

Shoulder muscle–   A supraspinatus partial rupture or acute overuse injury usually results in
tendon injury   a long period of inability to participate in sports involving throwing, team handball, basketball, volleyball, raquet sports, swimming, etc.

Phase one   In conservative treatment the first phase is dominated by a marked inhibition, and there is impingement pain due to tenderness and local swelling. Training in a pain-free range of motion is essential to limit the muscle-wasting process. Submaximal repetitive exercises give a local increase in blood flow resulting in less friction and a reduction in stiffness and local swelling. Methods to reduce the inhibition such as analgesics and TNS may help.

Immobilization and disuse lead quickly to muscle wasting and thereby a muscle imbalance. If the muscle imbalance is not corrected before return to sports the risk for re-injury is very high.

Exercises in the first phase could be as follows:

1 Internal and external rotation of the shoulder (Fig. 10.6.2a). The elbow should be kept tight into the body and flexed to 90°. Use a light rubber band to give resistance. Alternate between internal and external rotation with no rest in between for 15–20 repetitions and three to four sets in each direction.

2 When possible add straight arm pulls with the rubber band as resistance in flexion, extension and adduction. Do 15–20 repetitions and two to three sets for each direction. Use a very light resistance to get an increase in local blood flow.

The programme should be done three to five times per day.

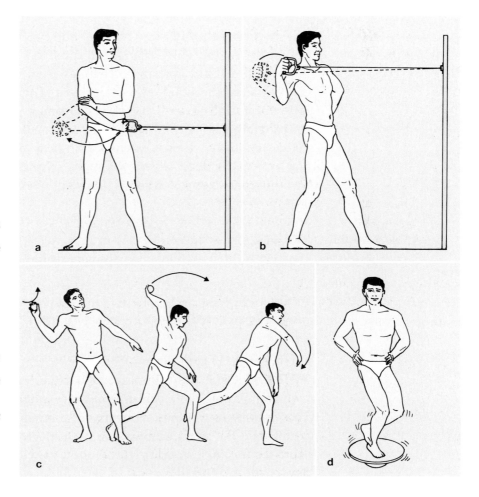

Fig. 10.6.2 (a) External rotation of the shoulder. Keep the elbow tight to the waist and flexed to 90° through the whole movement. (b) External rotation of the shoulder with the arm abducted to 90°. In the beginning the arm can be horizontally adducted 30–60°, and then gradually horizontally abducted. (c) Throwing movement. Note that in the first part the arm externally rotates eccentrically (prestretch) followed by a concentrical internal rotation at the same time as the arm is moving forward in extension. At the end of the movement the internal rotation is quickly slowed down by an eccentric contraction by the external rotators (= supraspinatus among others). (d) Balance exercises while standing on a platform.

Phase two   The second phase concentrates on strength training with a large variety of exercises in order to increase strength through the full range of motion for all the shoulder muscles in general and for the rotator cuff muscles specifically.

The programme can now consist of:

1   Isometrics.
2   Strength training of surrounding muscles.
3   Internal and external rotation as described in the first phase. The elbow can gradually be adducted to 30, 45, 60 and 90° of adduction (Fig. 10.6.2b) in order to put greater and greater demand on the rotatory muscles.
4   Include adduction to the straight arm pulls. Gradually increase to a full range of motion.
5   Horizontal abduction and adduction exercises.
6   Barbell exercises.

Phase three   The third phase emphasizes coordination training with increased speed of movement and quick changes in direction. The purpose is to try to improve the ability to handle changes from eccentric contractions to concentric in technique-related exercises. Therefore ball exercises with different bouncing and throwing movements should be included in the programme (Fig. 10.6.2c). Exercises should stimulate all movements in the shoulder — flexion, extension, abduction, adduction, and internal and external rotation — with different starting and stopping positions and different sizes and weights of balls.

Ankle distortion injuries   This injury is often very poorly treated. A marked loss of proprioceptive function is often seen in ankle ligament distortion injuries.

Phase one   In the first phase the joint effusion is often pronounced. The training programme should, therefore, concentrate on reduction of the effusion and regaining full range of motion. Ankle and toe exercises with many submaximal repetitions (20–50 for each movement) should be done several times per day.

Phases two and three   The training programme through the second and third phases is dominated by proprioceptive training (Fig. 10.6.2d). Strengthening exercises for ankle evertors (pronators) as well as for the ankle dorsi-flexors and plantar flexors could be added.

The exercise programme can now consist of:

1 Warm-up exercises with three sets of 15 repetitions of each of the following exercises: (a) toe flexion–extension; (b) ankle plantar and dorsiflexion; and (c) ankle/foot supination–pronation.

2 Strengthening exercises for the dorsiflexors, ankle/foot supinators and pronators using a rubber band as resistance.

3 Toe raises standing and sitting for the gastrocnemius and soleus muscles.

4 Toe flexion and extension exercises using a towel that is pulled in under the ball of the foot.

5 Balance and coordination exercises standing on one leg: (a) with arms free; (b) with arms crossed; (c) with closed eyes; and (d) writing the alphabet in the air with the other leg.

6 Standing on one or both feet on a balance platform or on a mini-trampoline.

7 Bouncing and jumping exercises on a mini-trampoline.

8 Various walking exercises, e.g. walking on the toes or heels.

9 Various jogging and running exercises as described in the knee-rehabilitation programme.

10 Various jumping exercises.

11 Various sports activities.

For all rehabilitation programmes of sports injuries, general and specific tests of strength, endurance, flexibility and function are extremely important to assure that the injury is completely healed. The best long-term insurance is a thorough and complete rehabilitation. A return too soon to sports after injury is very hazardous and the risk for re-injury is high.

References

Arvidsson, I., Eriksson, E., Häggmark, T. & Johnson, R. J. (1981) Isokinetic thigh muscle strength after ligament reconstruction in the knee joint: results from a 5–10 year follow-up after reconstructions of the anterior cruciate ligament in the knee joint. *J. Sports Med.* **2**, 7.

Arvidsson, I., Eriksson, E., Knutsson, E. & Arnér, S. (1986) Reduction of pain inhibition on voluntary muscle activation by epidural analgesia. *Orthopedics* **9**, 1415.

Edström, L. (1970) Selective atrophy of red muscle fiber in the quadriceps in long-standing knee-joint dysfunction injuries to the anterior cruciate ligament. *J. Neurol. Sci.* **11**, 551.

Fleck, S. J. & Falkel, J. E. (1986) Value of resistance training for the reduction of sports injuries. *Sports Med.* **3**, 61.

Fridén, J., Sjöström, M. & Ekblom, B. (1983) Myofibrillar damage following intense eccentric exercise in man. *Int. J. Sports Med.* **4**, 170.

Grimby, G., Björntorp, P., Fahlén, M., Hoskins, T. A., Höök, O., Oxhöj, H. & Saltin, B. (1973) Metabolic effects of isometric training. *Scand. J. Clin. Lab. Invest.* **31**, 301.

Grimby, G., Gustafsson, E., Peterson, E. L. & Renström, P. (1980) Quadriceps function and training after knee ligament injury. *Med. Sci. Sports Exerc.* **12**, 70.

Harms-Ringdahl, K. (1985) Shoulder externally rotating exercises with pulley apparatus. *Scand. J. Rehab. Med.* **17**, 129.

Möller, M. (1984) *Athletic training and flexibility.* Thesis, Linköping University. Medical Dissertation No. 182.

Shakespeare, D. T., Stokes, M., Sherman, K. P. & Young, A. (1985) Reflex inhibition of the quadriceps after meniscectomy. Lack of association with pain. *Clin. Physiol.* **5**, 137.

Stokes, M. & Young, A. (1984) The contribution of reflex inhibition to arthrogenous muscle weakness. *Clin. Sci.* **67**, 7.

Thomeé, R., Renström, P., Grimby, G. & Peterson, L. (1987) Slow or fast isokinetic training after knee ligament surgery. *J. Orthoped. Sports Phys. Ther.* **8**, 475.

Tropp, H. (1985) *Functional instability of the ankle joint.* Thesis, Linköping University. Medical Dissertation No. 202.

Wigerstad-Lossing, I., Grimby, G., Jonsson, T., Morelli, B., Peterson, L. & Renström, P. (1988) Effects of electrical muscle stimulation combined with voluntary contractions after knee ligament surgery. *Med. Sci. Sports Exerc.* (accepted for publication).

Young, A. & Stokes, M. (1986) Reflex inhibition of muscle activity and morphological consequences of inactivity. In B. Saltin (ed) *International Series of Sport Sciences, Vol. 10. Biochemistry of Exercise VI.* Human Kinetics, Champaign.

PART 11

EXERCISE IN THE PREVENTION AND MANAGEMENT OF INTERNAL DISEASE

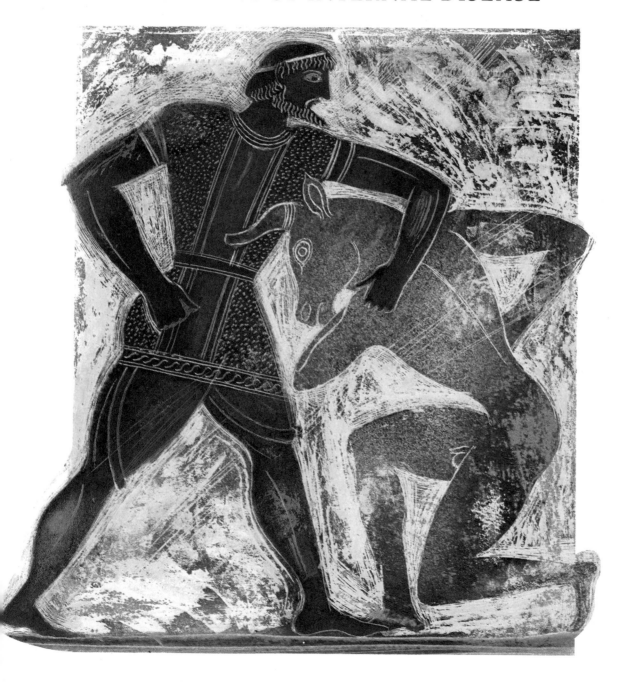

11.1 Cardiovascular disease

A. VENERANDO, P. ZEPPILLI & G. CASELLI

Introduction

Sports practice results in many physiological and psychological benefits: an increase in physical performance capacity and muscular strength, the percentage of body fat is kept under control, the skeletal and joint systems are kept more flexible, favourable biochemical and neural hormonal adjustments take place and, finally, the psychological condition of the person improves. However, sports activity requires effort and chronic conditioning, which is aimed at improving individual tolerance to effort, but actually represents an extra load on the cardiovascular system. Nevertheless, sports activities are not absolutely contraindicated in patients suffering from cardiovascular diseases, as they can be useful in improving the quality of life as long as indications and prescriptions are correctly adopted.

Before examining the different exercise possibilities that cardiac patients have, it is useful to emphasize some general concepts and rules:

1 Sport in cardiac patients, when possible and not contraindicated, must be carried out at a level compatible with the disease and able to stimulate physiological effects in the muscles, the cardiovascular system and elsewhere in the respiratory system. To do this in a simple way, sports activity should be carefully correlated with simple biological indexes such as heart rate and blood pressure, which must not be so high as to elicit symptoms in the patient. Patients must therefore learn how to count their pulse, and to evaluate and recognize their own fatigue threshold and the phase that precedes the occurrence of symptoms so that they can interrupt physical work.

2 Sports activity should start at a low level and gradually be increased in line with progressive conditioning.

3 Patients should be instructed on emergency measures and there should be open communication between the physician and the patient undergoing sports treatment.

4 Depending on personality, the majority of subjects find it preferable and more pleasurable for sports activities to be done in a group rather

than alone. There is also the advantage that a companion is available in the event of injury or cardiac emergency. On the other hand, metabolic cost and cardiac load of team games are more difficult to assess in a precise way.

5 It is important that prescription of sports activity takes into consideration the diet and habits of the subject and the drugs that he or she might have to take.

6 Dynamic-type or isotonic/aerobic sports are usually preferred. Isometric or strength sports have not yet been well defined and should be avoided in patients with ischaemic heart disease, hypertension or other cardiovascular pathologies.

7 Sports activities must be adapted according to general rules for broad groups of cardiovascular pathology, and must also be tailored to the individual, taking into account the type of professional activity, the degree of physical fitness, age, sex, etc. It is important to bear in mind that sport must maintain in the healthy subject a healthy status, while in the cardiac patient it must allow the maintenance of the best possible physical and psychological conditions compatible with the disease.

Safety measures that must be taken when prescribing a sports programme to a cardiac patient are the same as with a healthy subject. They consist of a clinical and instrumental examination of the patient's condition, as well as an evaluation of the likelihood of possible contraindications such as acute disease or chronic uncontrolled illness, extracardiac anatomic and functional abnormalities, some drugs, psychological disturbances, etc. However, not all these conditions are definitive contraindications for a sports activity programme. For instance, a situation like decompensated diabetes or a recurrence of bronchitis, may be only temporary contraindications to sports activity.

Prevention measures and exercise prescriptions applicable to the main groups of cardiovascular pathology, e.g. congential, rheumatic and ischaemic heart disease, hypertension and arrhythmias, will be schematically illustrated.

Congenital heart disease

When dealing with congenital heart disease and sports activities it is necessary to emphasize some general characteristics of the patient with an inborn malformation of the heart. The first is that in the large majority of these patients the myocardium is normal, and is able to compensate for this specific defect so that many patients can reach adult age without symptoms. This can explain why some patients with mild defects, for instance mild pulmonary stenosis or atrial septal defects, can tolerate exercise and sports activities. The second is that since the myocardium is normal and has an adequate coronary blood supply (with the exception of aortic stenosis), exercise electrocardiograms are generally normal and the direct determination of the cardiovascular performance capacity (maximal aerobic capacity or $\dot{V}_{O2\ max}$) is not only easy and safe to perform but also is the only means to assess the functional limitations of the patient. Indirect methods, such as the determination of physical working capacity at a heart rate of 170 beats/min (PWC_{170}) may also be utilized but these methods are obviously less reliable.

Since there are many different congenital lesions of the heart it is very difficult and impractical to define indications and prescriptions for patients with each of these defects. For the purpose of this chapter, only the most common situations will be considered.

Right ventricular outflow obstruction

The site of obstruction to the right ventricle outflow may be valvular (congenital deformed pulmonic valve) or subvalvular (muscular hypertrophy), or associated. Most young adults, like some children, with mild to moderate pulmonic stenosis are asymptomatic at rest and maintain a good tolerance to effort for long periods.

Concerning the indications for sports activities, the right ventricle pressure and transvalvular gradient should first be ascertained. If during exercise the transvalvular gradient is about, or less than, 50 mmHg and the flow increase at least four to five times the basal value, sports activity is possible. The methods of evaluation are:

1 Electrocardiogram (ECG): no signs of right ventricular hypertrophy.
2 Echocardiogram (ECHO): normal dimensions of right ventricular cavity and absence of significant wall hypertrophy.
3 Maximal exercise stress test (ex-ECG): normal $\dot{V}_{O2\ max}$; normal blood pressure increase; work quantity well correlated to age and body size; no arrhythmias.
4 Holter monitoring: no significant arrhythmias.

Indications: Skill activities, team games and aerobics.
Contraindications: Anaerobic and strength activities.
Prescriptions: Skill activities and team games, which can also be done competitively; aerobic activities, but only at submaximal rates (<70% of maximal aerobic capacity) three times a week.

In operated patients with or without residual insufficiency, adequate relief of symptoms indicates that sport is proposable. If the transvalvular gradient is equal to, or less than, 50 mmHg during exercise, the right ventricular function can be evaluated according to the preceding protocol and the indications, contraindications and prescriptions remain the same as for unoperated pulmonary stenosis.

Left ventricular outflow obstruction

Aortic stenosis

Sports activity is contraindicated in patients with aortic stenosis (Fig. 11.1.1) with the exception of those with minimal disease (manifest by a gradient of less than 20 mmHg at rest), because of: (a) the risk of arrhythmias and sudden death; and (b) unfavourable effects on the evolution of the cardiopathy.

After surgical treatment, contraindications may persist owing to: (a) the impossibility of adequate output increase during exercise through the prosthesis; (b) the risk of haemolysis and/or haemorrhage with a mechanic prosthesis and anticoagulants; and (c) the risk of sudden death.

However, the possibility of undertaking skill activities and sports in patients who have had successful operations should be tailored to individual cases, particularly when the ex-ECG shows no signs of ischaemia, no arrhythmias on effort and an adequate blood pressure increase at peak exercise.

Bicuspid aortic valve

This congenital malformation is characterized by the presence of an aortic valve with two, usually deformed, leaflets (Fig. 11.1.2). A bicuspid aortic valve is not a significant obstacle to the outflow until sclerosis and calcification occur, usually in later years. Sports activities can be permitted if the obstruction has not developed and there is no valvular insufficiency. The methods of evaluation are:

1   Clinical examination: exclusion of physical signs of stenosis (grade II and over murmur) or insufficiency (diastolic murmur) and associated defects (aortic coarctation).
2   ECG: normal.
3   ECHO: normal morphology of left ventricle; no wall hypertrophy; no associated defects.
4   ex-ECG: normal $\dot{V}O_{2\ max}$ and blood pressure increase; good correlation of work quantity with age and body size; no arrhythmias.
5   Holter monitoring: no arrhythmias.

Indications: All sports activities are possible.

Prescriptions: All activities can be competitive. To evaluate the stability of haemodynamic-pattern patients with bicuspid aortic valves, they should be re-examined every 12 months.

Aortic coarctation

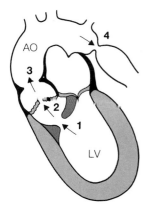

Fig. 11.1.1 Schematic representation of the congenital defects causing left ventricular outflow obstruction. 1, Subvalvular aortic stenosis (fibromuscular type); 2, valvular aortic stenosis; 3, supravalvular stenosis (diaphragm-like); 4, coarctation of the aorta. AO = aorta; LV = left ventricle.

The site of aortic coarctation is generally near the origin of the left subclavian artery (juxtaductal area) so that there is a higher arterial pressure in the upper limbs and lower pressure and pulses in the lower limbs. The stenosis is responsible for the trans-stenotic pressure gradient and the degree of pressure overload of the left ventricle and aortic arch, which influence the incidence and severity of complications (cerebro-vascular accidents, rupture of aorta with trauma, and long-term effects on target organs of hypertension). If surgical treatment is not indicated (gradient <30 mmHg), the possibility of sports activity can be evaluated:

1 ECG: normal.

2 ECHO: no left ventricular hypertrophy; normal contractility; no aortic root dilatation.

3 ex-ECG: blood pressure within the normal limits; normal $\dot{V}_{O_2\ max}$; good correlation of work quantity with age and body size; no arrhythmias.

Indications: Skill activities and aerobic.

Contraindications: Strength (e.g. weight lifting) and anaerobic activities. Participation in sports with a danger of chest trauma should be avoided.

Prescriptions: Skill and aerobic activities can be done at competition level in patients with mild coarctation. However, every 12 months re-evaluation of patients should be performed to exclude complications. In all patients, if there is an abnormal increase of blood pressure during exercise, one can prescribe non-competitive submaximal sport activity (≤60% of aerobic capacity) three times a week.

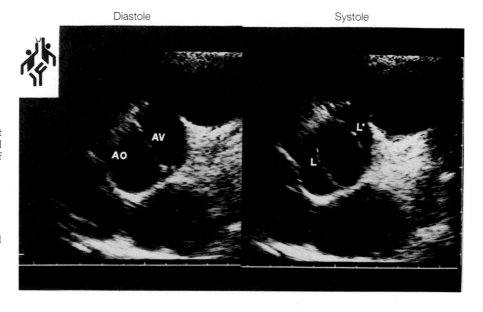

Fig. 11.1.2 Two-dimensional echocardiogram of a 15-year-old boy. At the age of 13 he had surgical correction of a coarctation of the aorta. Two years later, while playing football, he complained of palpitations and dyspnoea. Physical examination and ECHO revealed a bicuspid aortic valve with mild stenosis and moderate insufficiency. AO = aortic root; AV = aortic valve; L and L' = the two cuspids.

Congenital heart disease with left-to-right shunt
(Fig. 11.1.3)

Atrial septal defect (ASD)

The severity of the left-to-right atrium shunt depends on the width of the septal defect and on the resistance of the pulmonary circulation. The volume overload at low pressure induces dilatation of the right ventricle and, if severe and prolonged, pulmonary hypertension. In the ostium secundum defect the shunt occurs at the mid-atrial septum. In the ostium primum defect the shunt occurs at the base of the septum and it may be associated with a reflux from the left ventricle to the left atrium across a cleft in the anterior leaflet of the mitral valve. Ostium primum is the most frequent form of the endocardial cushion defects syndrome, which includes more severe forms such as the complete atrioventricular canal.

Ventricular septal defect (VSD)

The severity of the shunt depends on the diameter of the defect: an area ≤ 0.5 cm/m^2 gives an elevated resistance in the mesotelesystole, a mild shunt and a characteristic harsh, holosystolic murmur with a normal second heart sound. A defect with a larger area gives a greater shunt, a volume overload of both ventricles and later pulmonary hypertension. In this case evaluation of sports activity should be made only after surgical correction.

Patent ductus arteriosus (PDA)

The severity of the shunt depends on the diameter and length of the ductus. Patients with a small PDA are asymptomatic with normal heart size and ECG. With increasing size of the PDA, the pulmonary blood flow and pressure increase and pulmonary hypertension develops in some cases. In this case, indications for sport can be evaluated only after surgical correction.

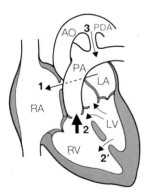

Fig. 11.1.3 Schematic representation of the most common congenital defects causing left-to-right shunt. 1, ASD; 2 and 2′, VSD; 3, PDA. The most important haemodynamic consequence of the shunt is the increase of pulmonary blood flow (large arrow) which may lead to pulmonary hypertension. AO = aortic root; LA = left atrium; LV = left ventricle; PA = pulmonary artery; RA = right atrium; RV = right ventricle.

If no significant pulmonary hypertension existed prior to surgery, morphological and functional evaluation of the ventricle involved will be sufficient to document the regression of pre-existing volume overload. The methods of evaluation are:

1 Physical examination: (a) ASD—return to variable second heart sound with reduced intensity of pulmonary component; (b) VSD—same as in ASD with third heart sound disappeared; and (c) PDA—same as in VSD with disappearance of the continuous murmur.
2 ECG: no significant anomalies of conduction. Surgery on atrial and ventricular septum may lead to lesions of the conduction system with atrioventricular block or fascicular damage. Patients with ASD who have undergone surgery may develop sinus node dysfunction (leading to symptomatic bradycardia or bradycardia–tachycardia syndrome).
3 ECHO: normal ventricular morphology and contractility.
4 ex-ECG: normal arterial blood pressure increase; normal $\dot{V}_{O_2\ max}$; quantity of work done adequate for age and body size; no arrhythmias.

5 Holter monitoring: no significant arrhythmias (Lown grade 0, 1 or 2) (Lown *et al.*, 1975).

Indications: All sports activities, at competitive level if wanted, can be performed by patients with minimal defects or in successfully operated patients with complete regression of haemodynamic load and without residual defects.

Contraindications: Power and contact sports should be contraindicated for at least 6–12 months after surgery (sternotomy).

Prescriptions: Aerobic activity at a submaximal level (60% of maximum aerobic capacity) and skill activities can be done by patients with moderate defects or well-selected patients with large defects.

Congenital heart disease with right-to-left shunt

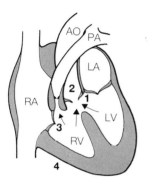

Fig. 11.1.4 Schematic representation of the anatomic defects in the tetralogy of Fallot. 1, Ventricular septal defect; 2, dextroposition of the aorta; 3, infundibular pulmonary stenosis; 4, right ventricular hypertrophy. Abbreviations as in Fig. 11.1.3.

Right-to-left shunt leads unavoidably to cyanosis and reduced exercise tolerance, which may be severe in many cases. Sports participation is not usually possible for these patients, unless it is of very low intensity. The most common form of cyanotic congenital heart disease is tetralogy of Fallot. This malformation is characterized by a ventricular shunt of varying degree, according to the dextroposition of the aorta and the severity of pulmonary stenosis (Fig. 11.1.4). There is a tendency to perform a total corrective operation in early childhood, and survival without symptoms has become more common, so that more and more patients are able to participate in sports.

Indications: In successfully operated patients, aerobic and skill sports can be played but only at the amateur level. Participation in school sports programmes can be allowed too.

Contraindications: All competitive sports should be contraindicated. Operated patients frequently have a residual right ventricle to pulmonary artery gradient, fibrosis of the right myocardium, ventricular conduction disturbances and a documented risk of sudden death. Therefore, only low-intensity competitive sports should be considered, in carefully selected and well-studied cases.

Prescriptions: The above mentioned activities should be done at an intensity not greater than 60% of the maximum aerobic capacity, three times a week.

Marfan's syndrome

The complete form of the disease consists of aneurysmal dilatation of the aortic root, dislocation of the crystalline lens and skeletal anomalies. The incomplete form, in which the skeletal and ocular anomalies are less evident, is more common in young people; it can be recognized by the presence of cardiac lesions, the floppy valve syndrome, and initial aortic root enlargement.

Contraindications: All forms of sports activities, with the exception of very low-intensity aerobic or skill activities at amateur level, because of the possible adverse effects of an increased output and blood pressure on the natural evolution of this cardiopathy.

Mitral prolapse and the floppy valve syndrome

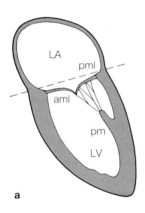

a

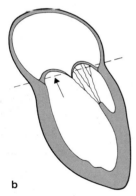

b

Fig. 11.1.5 Schematic representation of the mitral valve anatomy in the normal situation (a) and in primary mitral valve prolapse (b). In mitral prolapse one (or both) mitral leaflet protrudes above the atrioventricular plane (dotted line) into the left atrium during the systole. aml = anterior mitral leaflet; LA = left atrium; LV = left ventricle; pm = papillary muscle; pml = posterior mitral leaflet.

Mitral prolapse consists of a protrusion of one or both leaflets (Fig. 11.1.5) of the valve into the left atrium during systole and, in the large majority of cases, of a mesotelesystolic click and/or murmur on auscultation. This anatomical entity may be accompanied by symptoms such as chest pain, palpitation and dyspnoea, but most patients are asymptomatic. Mitral prolapse may be secondary to Marfan's syndrome, ischaemic cardiopathy or hypertrophic cardiomyopathy but usually it appears as isolated (primary mitral prolapse).

Primary mitral valve prolapse (Fig. 11.1.6) may present with different clinical manifestations, varying from completely silent forms to those with disabling symptoms and complications (rare), e.g. mitral insufficiency, life-threatening arrhythmias, infective endocarditis and sudden death.

The floppy valve syndrome is characterized by a plurivalvular prolapse, usually of the mitral and tricuspid valve or of the mitral and aortic valve, and represents a more diffuse form of the myxomatous degeneration of the cardiac structures. It may present as the only cardiac alteration in Marfan's syndrome or as an isolated pathology.

In both primary mitral prolapse and the floppy valve syndrome the following methods of examination are used:

1 Physical examination: isolated click and/or endsystolic murmur.
2 ECG: normal.
3 ECHO: absence of any aortic root pathology; normal dimensions of atrial and ventricular cavities; normal ventricular function.
4 ex-ECG: normal increase of systolic blood pressure, heart rate and $\dot{V}_{O_2\ max}$. Work quantity in proportion to age and body size; no ischaemic alterations; no arrhythmias.
5 Holter monitoring: no significant arrhythmias (Lown grade 0, 1 or 2) (Lown *et al.*, 1975).

Indications: All sports, even at competitive level, are permitted in uncomplicated primary mitral prolapse. A yearly examination of the subject is recommended to assess the stability of the valvular alteration or the appearance of arrhythmias. In the floppy valve syndrome, competitive skill activities and aerobic sports at amateur level can be considered. In cases with haemodynamically significant mitral regurgitation, indications are the same as for mitral insufficiency (see below).

Contraindications: All sports are proscribed in secondary mitral prolapse or in the floppy valve syndrome where it is a clinical manifestation of Marfan's syndrome.

Prescriptions: The limits for aerobic activities are 70% of the maximum aerobic capacity with a frequency of three times a week.

Acquired valvular heart disease

There are many different kinds of acquired valvular heart disease leading to different types and degrees of haemodynamic loading of the cardiovascular system. Diagnosis of the type of valvular disease may be easy on the basis of cardiac auscultation alone, which reveals the characteristic murmur of the disease. Estimation of the severity of the disease, however, may be difficult, particularly in asymptomatic patients; the combined use of clinical history, physical examination, ECG and ex-ECG, chest radiograph and ECHO with Doppler techniques at rest, should provide sufficient information to assess the clinical status and functional capacity of the patient.

Patients classified in grade 3 or 4 (New York Heart Association scale) on the basis of this examination should be excluded from any sports activity. In patients belonging to other classes, sports activity may be considered; it probably exerts a preventive action against further deterioration of physical condition. In all cases, however, competitive sports

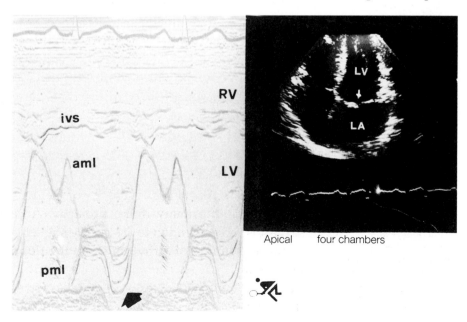

Fig. 11.1.6 One- (left) and two- (right) dimensional echocardiogram of a 26-year-old tennis player with a history of chest pain and palpitations. The ECHO shows an anatomically severe prolapse of both mitral leaflets (arrows). aml = anterior mitral leaflet; ivs = interventricular septum; LA = left atrium; LV = left ventricle; pml = posterior mitral leaflet; RV = right ventricle.

Apical   four chambers

activities, with the exception of low-intensity aerobic and skill activities, must be avoided. We have very little information on the influence of strenuous exercise on the progression of the severity of valvular lesions and of ventricular dysfunction. Patients who have been operated on for valvular disease should be assessed in a similar manner.

Mitral stenosis

Aetiology of mitral stenosis is almost always rheumatic. There is a decreasing incidence of mitral stenosis and the problem of indicating sports activity is therefore a rare one. For practical purposes, since patients with significant mitral stenosis can rarely tolerate prolonged or excessive effort, only amateur sports activities such as callisthenics, gentle swimming and walking should be permitted regardless of other investigative results. Some selected patients with mitral stenosis in class 1 or 2 (NYHA scale) can be allowed to practise competitive sports with low energetic demands (e.g. bowling, cricket, golf, riflery, etc.).

In asymptomatic patients with sinus rhythm, functional evaluation by ex-ECG may be useful to assess functional capacity. Additional information on the severity and complications of the valvular lesion will be provided by ECHO, with Holter monitoring for the detection of arrhythmias. A periodic re-evaluation of the asymptomatic patient to ascertain the progression of the disease is mandatory.

Mitral insufficiency

Mitral insufficiency is usually better tolerated than mitral stenosis. It can have different aetiologies, myxomatous valve degeneration (see mitral prolapse), rheumatic heart disease, infective endocarditis, etc. When it is long lasting, with mild to moderate haemodynamic changes, then the possibility of amateur and competitive sports activities can be considered.

The severity of mitral insufficiency is related to the magnitude of the regurgitant fraction which conditions the severity of the volume overload of the left ventricle and left atrium. During dynamic exercise there is no significant change, or else a mild decrease, in the regurgitant fraction because the forward and retrograde flow increase to the same extent. Static exercise, by increasing the arterial pressure, probably worsens the regurgitation.

Methods of evaluation include:

1 Clinical examination: absence of symptoms; grade of murmur inferior to 3/6.
2 ECG: sinus rhythm; absence of signs or left ventricular and atrial overload.
3 ECHO: normal or slightly enlarged left ventricular and atrial cavities; minimal to moderate reflux with Doppler echo.

4 ex-ECG: adequate increase of blood pressure, heart rate and normal $\dot{V}O_{2\ max}$; work quantity adequate to age and body size; no arrhythmias.
5 Holter monitoring: no arrhythmias.

Indications: Asymptomatic patients with normal investigative results can participate in all competitive sports, usually with the exception of strenuous sports activities such as competitive distance running, professional cycling, cross-country skiing, etc. Patients with moderate mitral insufficiency can participate in competitive skill activities and team games.

Contraindications: Strength or static-isometric sports should be avoided.

Prescriptions: Low-intensity amateur activities, e.g. callisthenics, golf, swimming and walking, can be made by patients with moderate to severe mitral insufficiency. Periodic re-evaluation is mandatory.

Aortic insufficiency Aortic insufficiency, like mitral insufficiency, has different aetiologies, e.g. a congenital bicuspid aortic valve (see 'Congenital heart disease' above), rheumatic disease, myxomatous valve degeneration, infective endocarditis and Marfan's syndrome. Aortic regurgitation increases diastolic volume of the left ventricle with chronic volume overload, which ultimately may lead to left ventricular failure. During dynamic exercise, the decrease in diastolic filling period together with the fall in peripheral vascular resistance increases forward flow and decreases the regurgitant volume. Severe aortic regurgitation may lead to inadequate coronary blood supply during exercise, leading to angina, syncope and life-threatening ventricular arrhythmias.

If either clinical or instrumental investigative methods demonstrate a good tolerance to effort with no ECG, ECHO or roentgenographic signs of hypertrophy or increased volume of the heart, the same indications adopted for mitral insufficiency can be followed. Methods of evaluation, contraindications and prescriptions are also the same.

Aortic stenosis The criteria reported for congenital forms are also valid for acquired (rheumatic or sclerotic) aortic stenosis.

Patients with valvular prostheses Since the tendency is toward early surgery for valvular heart disease, more and more young patients are operated on who wish to participate in sports. We must remember, however, that the use of anticoagulants may represent a haemorrhagic risk in the practice of sports. Digitalis and its derivatives may cause arrhythmias of various types and degrees and, in addition, patients with mechanic prostheses may run the risk of haemolysis. Moreover, aortic and mitral prostheses may limit maximal cardiac output during effort.

Therefore, patients with prosthetic or bioprosthetic mitral and aortic valves should only perform amateur sports with low to moderate energetic demands, such as swimming, cycling and running at a level not higher than 60–70% of maximal aerobic capacity. These patients should not engage in sports where there is a danger of body collision.

Ischaemic heart disease

One of the most important components of physical readaption (rehabilitation) in ischaemic heart disease is physical activity. This activity must be included with all other therapeutic measures, such as drug therapy, body fat control through diet, smoking cessation, etc. In this context we can consider possible utilization of sports activities.

Myocardial infarction

Before permitting and prescribing sport in a patient after well-healed myocardial infarction (MI), one must establish selection criteria and the kind of sport that each patient can be allowed to play. Even if it is true that all patients may theoretically undergo a programme of individually selected physical activities, criteria for choice of activity, indications, contraindications and prescriptions must be more firmly established.

Patients with healed MI deserve careful screening in order to assess the risks and potential benefits of sport. Under careful supervision, patients may eventually attain levels of functional capacity that permit participation in such vigorous activities as distance running. In general, people who have suffered from MI and wish to take up a sport have previously participated in sports and have a positive attitude towards it. In these patients, the psychological benefits of resuming their previous sports activity can be very strong; patients may even disregard symptoms or avoid preventive medical screening in order to do so.

In order to assess the risks and benefits of prescribing sports activities to patients with MI, an evaluation of clinical history and physical/laboratory examinations has to be made:

1 Clinical history will ascertain the eventual presence of residual angina, its duration since MI, symptomatic arrhythmias, medication and exertional hypotension or syncope. Sometimes it can be difficult to ascertain and identify unstable angina, which contraindicates sport. Standard questioning may not always reveal forms of changing anginal pain. The physician screening must appreciate the symptoms and try to differentiate them. Signs of reduced ventricular function, as exertional dyspnoea, and of impaired myocardial reserves or the occurrence of rest and exercise arrhythmias must be identified.

2 Physical examination: careful examination of the cardiovascular system may identify patients at risk by cardiac auscultation, blood pressure measures, etc.

3 Laboratory investigations: such as ECG, ECHO, ex-ECG and Holter monitoring, may reveal findings of reduced left ventricular function, exertional ischaemia and complex arrhythmias, which indicate undue sports risks.

Indications: Sport can be indicated in patients who are well healed and rehabilitated from an acute episode, asymptomatic, in good muscular form, and in a stable condition using clinical and instrumental indices.

Contraindications: Sport is contraindicated when symptoms or signs of clinical and instrumental instability or abnormal results of laboratory investigations are found. Ventricular aneurysm or diffuse alterations of contractility also contraindicate sport.

Prescriptions: Before prescribing sports activities it is useful to give advice and to encourage some training activity (weekly sessions) which will help the patient achieve a good level of physical fitness. Once that is obtained, and after an ex-ECG examination of physical working capacity and respiratory parameters, sport can be prescribed. Sports activities of choice are aerobic and, eventually, team games. Isometric or strength exercises or activities including prolonged bursts of isometric contractions must be avoided.

It should be remembered that sports activities can be useful in maintaining the physical condition acquired during previous periods of rehabilitation and also useful in improving psychological conditions. It is important to emphasize that if patients want to obtain long-lasting beneficial effects from sport, it is necessary to persevere, with physical activity and sport being included in daily life. Perseverance is, of course, dependent upon educational and social factors which are often beyond the possibility of medical intervention. Walking, cycling, swimming and cross-country skiing, may be done according to individual preference, aptitude and resources. Sports activities must be under surveillance and competitive activity should be excluded because of the psychological motivation which such activity entails. Some patients tolerate well sports such as tennis and downhill skiing, but it does not seem wise to advise this kind of sport on a large scale, particularly for 'type A' personalities.

A clinical examination, ECHO and ex-ECG must be periodically performed (at least every year).

Patients after coronary bypass surgery

The prescription of sports activities is similar to that in infarction cases, both for duration and aims. This will allow the patient to maintain a good level of fitness. Patients who do not have residual angina can undertake sports activities, that are more intense and less controlled, with marked advantages. For these patients, after the coronary reserve has been carefully evaluated with ex-ECG and, eventually, myocardial perfusion scintigrams, a gradual and progressive increase in length and intensity of training can be undertaken.

In patients with mild residual angina, prescription of sports activities can only be done after an ex-ECG which will assess the effort limitation. Particular attention must be paid to the maximal heart rate that is attained as well as to the changes in arterial pressure, ECG abnormalities and possible arrhythmias. The maximal working capacity should be expressed in terms of maximal oxygen uptake or in terms of the work rate sustained in the steady state. All non-invasive investigations like Holter monitoring and ECHO must be done before starting sports activities.

With regard to the indications and prescriptions, activities should not attain more than 80–90% of maximal aerobic capacity, and maximal heart rate should not exceed 90% of the maximum heart rate attained during ex-ECG. A control test must be carried out periodically. Patients must be made aware of certain drawbacks of isometric or static efforts.

Cardiomyopathies

Present classification of cardiomyopathies include primary or idiopathic cardiomyopathies and cardiomyopathies secondary to agents known as toxic (alcohol, some drugs, etc.), infective causes, etc.

Primary or idiopathic cardiomyopathies are presently distinguished into three pathological forms:

1 Hypertrophic cardiomyopathy (Fig. 11.1.7).
2 Dilated (congestive).
3 Restrictive.

Hypertrophic cardiomyopathy, above all, may be encountered in the juvenile population and it represents one of the most frequent causes of sudden unexpected death from sport in young people.

Contraindications: Sports activity is excluded in all forms of cardiomyopathies, for haemodynamic reasons as well as for the frequent association of serious rhythm disturbances and the documented risk of sudden death.

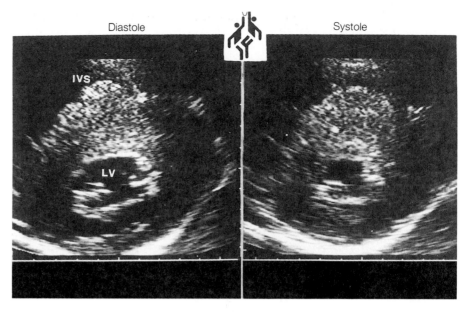

Fig. 11.1.7 Two-dimensional echocardiogram of a 17-year-old asymptomatic amateur basketball player. The short-axis view of the left ventricle (LV) shows severe hypertropic cardiomyopathy. The anterior interventricular septum (IVS) had a diastolic thickness of 38 mm (normal range for this age, 7–11 mm).

Acute myocarditis and pericarditis

Sports activity can be proposed only when the myocardial and/or pericardial inflammation has resolved. Once clinical recovery has been ascertained, and before permitting the initiation or resumption of sports activity, it is necessary to evaluate *ex novo* the eventual effects of the disease on ventricular morphology and function. It is important to emphasize that some acute myocarditis may ultimately lead to dilated cardiomyopathy.

Methods of evaluation are:

1 Physical examination: normal.
2 ECG: normal, with no ST–T wave changes.
3 ECHO: normal ventricular function.
4 ex-ECG: normal systolic blood pressure increase; normal heart rate and $\dot{V}_{O_2\ max}$; work done in proportion to age and body size; no ECG alterations or exercise arrhythmias.
5 Holter monitoring: no arrhythmias (Lown's class 0, 1 or 2) (Lown *et al.*, 1975).

Indications: If the protocol results are normal, the patient may participate in all competitive sports. Periodic re-evaluation is necessary.

Arrhythmias

In order to evaluate the possibility of a patient having arrhythmias to participate in sports activities it is necessary to take into consideration different aspects:

1 The type and severity of the cardiopathy, if present.
2 The characteristics of the arrhythmia—their origin, supraventricular or ventricular, heart rate reached, duration of the episodes, accompanying symptoms, frequency of relapses, etc.
3 The possibility of provoking and/or documenting the arrhythmic episode.
4 The responsiveness of the arrhythmia to drugs.
5 The type and intensity of cardiocirculatory demand required by the sports activity.

Above all, the major difficulties lie in the impressions gathered from a patient's history, the ability to obtain a correct and sufficient recording of the arrhythmia and sometimes to document the existence and type of eventual associated organic heart disease.

In studying arrhythmias, the fundamental diagnostic tool is the ECG. Its discriminatory capabilities can be improved using simple provocative tests, such as sympathetic and vagal stimulation and inhibition. Other methods of investigation include ex-ECG, Holter monitoring and intra-cavitary ECG. ECHO is the most simple and reliable non-invasive method for excluding the existence of an organic substrate for arrhythmias. The most valuable method of investigation is Holter monitoring, especially when utilized during the course of a patient's specific daily activities and training programme.

Premature beats and tachyarrhythmias

Premature atrial (PAB) and ventricular (PVB) beats

The significance of PAB and PVB is in their relationship to the general cardiac and clinical situation of the patient. PAB and PVB can trigger other types of arrhythmias; this is especially valid for PVB which can unleash major ventricular tachyarrhythmias leading to sudden death. On the other hand, PAB and PVB may frequently present in patients without any sign of cardiopathy, as an expression of extracardiac causes or functional cardiovascular derangement.

Indications: Any type of sports activity is consented for patients with simple PAB or PVB (Lown's classification classes 0, 1 and 2, evaluated by 24-hour Holter monitoring). Lown's class 3 PVB should be further evaluated to exclude minimal arrhythmogenic substrates. Recently, it has been shown that some patients with Lown's class 3 and 4 PVB who

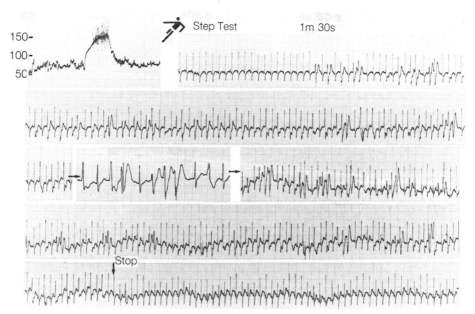

150-
100-
50

Step Test   1m 30s

Stop

Fig. 11.1.8 Exercise electro-cardiogram (Harward step test) of a 26-year-old soccer player with mitral valve prolapse (lead V5, paper speed 10 mm/sec, and the heart rate trend in the top left). Ventricular ectopy occurred after 1 min exercise with increasing complexity, bigeminy, couplets and triplets (see between arrows, paper speed 25 mm/sec).

were thought to have a normal heart, have revealed at catheterization occult coronary artery disease, initial dilated cardiomyopathy or arrhythmogenic right ventricular dysplasia. Therefore, indications for these patients should be made only after an accurate evaluation.

Contraindications: All competitive sports are contraindicated in cases of classes 3, 4 and 5 of Lown's classification especially when PVB are frequent and precipitated or worsened by effort (Fig. 11.1.8).

Prescriptions: Sports activities can be practised even at competitive level in cases of minor grade PAB and PVB. In the other cases, amateur and submaximal (<70% of the maximum aerobic capacity) activities are possible, under medical treatment if necessary.

Atrial fibrillation

Atrial fibrillation may occur in patients without signs of organic cardiopathy or in patients with predisposing electric conditions, such as the Wolff–Parkinson–White syndrome (see below), even though it is usually a consequence of valvular, ischaemic or sclerotic-degenerative cardiopathies. Aside from the basal cardiac situation, the possibility of playing sports also depends on the haemodynamic consequences of a potentially rapid ventricular rate.

Recurrent paroxystic atrial fibrillation indicates the use of electro-physiological studies to exclude the presence of accessory pathways which could facilitate rapid ventricular rates.

Indications: Aerobic and skill sports, provided that the ventricular rate is slow and/or well controlled by therapy and that physical activity does not induce an excessive increase in heart rate. The same is also true for isolated episodes of paroxysmal atrial fibrillation as long as it is haemodynamically well tolerated.

Contraindications: Competitive sports should be avoided in stable atrial fibrillation, particularly when due to organic heart disease. Anaerobic and power sports are also contraindicated.

Prescriptions: Skill sports may be practised even at competitive level, as long as they do not take place in a risky environment. Aerobic sports are allowed only at an amateur and submaximal level (60% of maximum aerobic capacity), three times a week.

Atrial flutter   In general, this is a tachycardia which is poorly tolerated haemodynamically because of the rapid atrial rate and the difficulty in controlling the ventricular rate. In particular situations, the passage of all atrial impulses to the ventricle, with a very rapid ventricular rate, can be verified. Prescription of physical activity in such situations is therefore not proposable. However, physical activity and sport may be consented to in cases of isolated episodes of atrial flutter if it is haemodynamically well tolerated, has little tendency to recur and the patient shows no clinical signs of cardiopathy or the Wolff–Parkinson–White syndrome.

Indications, contraindications and *prescriptions* are usually the same as for atrial fibrillation.

Focal and re-entrant   Besides the general cardiac and clinical situation of the patient, the
paroxysmal   clinical significance of such arrhythmias depends on the ventricular rate
supraventricular   and the number and duration of the episodes. Ventricular rate, duration
tachycardia   of the episode and the basal cardiac situation condition the haemodynamic tolerance. So, low-rate tachycardia may be poorly tolerated by patients with valvular or myocardial disease while high-rate tachycardia can be well tolerated by children and young adults without organic heart disease.

In some cases, particularly of re-entrant supraventricular tachycardia, an intracavitary electrophysiological study may be indicated to identify the location and type of circuit and the eventual presence of accessory pathways.

Indications: Skill and aerobic sports, provided that paroxysms of tachycardia are not frequent, do not last more than 30 s (the longer the episode the more frequent the haemodynamic repercussion), do not cause a rapid ventricular rate (>110% of the maximum predicted heart rate for age or maximum heart rate achieved in a symptoms-limited exercise stress test), are not specifically caused by exertion, and benefit from pharmacological treatment.

Contraindications: Anaerobic and power sports.

Prescriptions: Aerobic sports should be practised at a submaximal level (60% of the maximum aerobic capacity). To judge the possibility of practising competitive sports it is advisable to carry out an intracavitary electrophysiological study to exclude additional arrhythmogenic substrates as occult accessory pathways. If no such pathways are evident, competitive sports activity can be consented to, provided that it is conducted in a non-risky environment.

Cardiac pre-excitation (Wolff–Parkinson–White syndrome) This deserves a separate discussion. In these cases, amateur sports activity can be consented to only in asymptomatic patients without organic heart disease regardless of the type of pre-excitation (short P–R interval, Wolff–Parkinson–White syndrome, etc.). Symptomatic patients and asymptomatic subjects desiring to participate in competitive sports should undergo a complete electrophysiological study to evaluate:

1 The anterograde refractory period of the accessory pathway.

2 The presence of a multiple bypass.

3 The entity of atrial irritability, i.e. the facility of provoking sustained atrial tachyarrhythmias with programmed atrial stimulation.

4 The average ventricular rate and the minimum R–R interval between two pre-excited beats during spontaneous or induced atrial fibrillation.

Actually, the evaluation of atrial irritability and the ventricular response during atrial fibrillation are considered to be the best indications of risk in these patients. More recently, transoesophageal electrical stimulation of the heart has provided a semi-invasive means of assessing these characteristics, not only at rest but also during exercise stress tests.

Since patients and subjects with Wolff–Parkinson–White syndrome may have cardiac arrest or sudden death as the first manifestation of the anomaly, electrophysiological data are very important in determining their fitness for sports activity.

Ventricular tachycardia Ventricular tachycardia may present with different forms of varying prognostic values. Common ventricular tachycardia (VT) has the worst prognosis because of the usually high ventricular rate and significant haemodynamic consequences. It is usually associated with organic heart disease, such as ischaemic cardiopathy or cardiomyopathies, and therefore sports activity is excluded.

A special form of VT, *torsaide de pointe*, can herald ventricular fibrillation, and has the same or even worse clinical significance as common VT.

Slow VT can be found, instead, in young subjects with no signs of cardiopathy, and is associated with a reduction in sinus node automaticity due to an increased vagal tone. Such VT is considered benign. It is usually overdriven by the heart rate increase which occurs with exercise and it does not constitute any contraindication to sports activities, even at competitive level.

Iterative VT is a haemodynamically well tolerated form of VT. It is generally intermittent, does not achieve rates higher than 130–150 beats/min, does not tend to worsen, disappears on exertion, and above all is not necessarily associated with a cardiopathy. In such cases, under eventual anti-arrhythmic treatment, sports activities with minimal to moderate cardiocirculatory demands (submaximal aerobic sports at 60% of maximum aerobic capacity, and skill sports) may be considered in subjects without signs of organic heart disease.

Naturally, the problem of practising sports is not considered for patients who have had documented ventricular fibrillation or resuscitated cardiac arrest (aborted sudden death).

Bradyarrhythmias and atrioventricular conduction disturbances

Bradycardia and sinoatrial blocks

Bradycardia is a situation frequently encountered in clinical practice. Mild, moderate and even marked bradycardia, with rates of less than 40 beats/min, is also frequently found in athletic subjects and very rarely poses problems. But the occurrence of marked bradycardia in young or elderly people who practise no sports and who sometimes have poorly defined symptoms of malaise, dyspnoea, etc., or even episodes of fainting or syncope, is quite different. In these cases it is necessary to exclude intrinsic or extrinsic (excessive vagal tone) sinoatrial node disease (sick sinus syndrome) using both pharmacological and ergometrical tests. Holter monitoring has, above all, proven to be the most important ambulatory diagnostic tool for these arrhythmias. The occurrence of characteristic symptoms of the sick sinus syndrome—marked sinus bradycardia, sinoatrial blocks or sinus arrests—and the bradycardia–tachycardia syndrome (i.e. the alternance of paroxysmal supraventricular tachyarrhythmias and bradyarrhythmias), must discourage the practice of all sports activities. Symptomatic patients may also be studied electrophysiologically for indications of eventual pacing treatment.

Atrioventricular blocks

Atrioventricular blocks (AVB) are usually divided into first degree, second degree (Mobitz 1, Mobitz 2, 2 : 1 and advanced block), and third degree or complete AVB. According to the anatomophysiological location, AVB can be divided into: pre-His, intra-His and sub-His bundles. Periodic first degree AVB and second degree pre-His AVB are a relatively frequent finding in highly-trained endurance athletes, and may also be encountered in asymptomatic, apparently healthy children and young adults during the preparticipation screening for sports. Methods of evaluation are:

1   Clinical history: no syncopal or presyncopal attacks; no familial history of bradyarrhythmias, AVB or intraventricular conduction disturbances.

2   ECG: with non-invasive provocative (sympathetic stimulation) and pharmacological tests (atropine). Complete disappearance of AVB after sympathetic stimulation or vagal inhibition (atropine) are considered favourable responses. Vagal stimulation manoeuvres may worsen the degree of blockage but this should be considered as an aspecific response unless very prolonged ventricular pauses are induced (these manoeuvres must be avoided in elderly patients, and should be made under strict medical surveillance).

3   ex-ECG: disappearance of AVB; adequate heart rate increase.

4   Holter monitoring: no periods of advanced or complete AVB, marked bradycardia or sinus arrest.

Indications: All sports activities, even at competitive level, can be consented to in subjects with first and second degree Mobitz 1 AVB of functional origin and with normal investigative results. In organic AVB, skill and aerobic activities at an amateur level can be permitted provided that exertion does not affect the degree of the block. In cases of complete

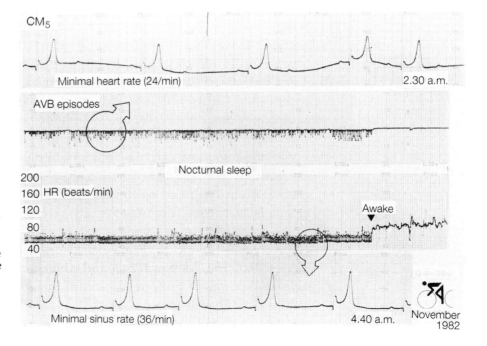

Fig. 11.1.9 Nocturnal Holter monitoring of a 35-year-old amateur cyclist with a high-degree atrio-ventricular block. Tracings were taken in 1982 when he was symptomless. Very recently, in spite of electro-cardiographic findings quite indistinguishable from those of 1982, he has had two episodes of presyncopes with a witnessed 'very low pulse rate' requiring the cessation of training.

congenital AVB, where the substituting pacemaker can guarantee an adequate heart rate and cardiac output increase, skill and aerobic activities at an amateur level can also be considered. The same indications can only be valid for patients with pacemakers when there is a good clinical and haemodynamic situation.

Contraindications: Anaerobic and power sports, especially when there is a danger of body collision, must be avoided in patients with organic AVB or with pacemakers.

Prescriptions: All sports activities can be allowed in asymptomatic patients with functional AVB. However, since some subjects thought to have functional AVB may have syncopal attacks and a worsening of the block with an increase in the training intensity, periodic re-evaluation must be done (Fig. 11.1.9). In patients with organic AVB, skill sports can be practised even at competitive level, while aerobic activities should be performed only at an amateur and submaximal level (50–60% of the maximum aerobic capacity) three times a week.

Intraventricular conduction disturbances

For intraventricular conduction disturbances, the prognostic orientation for prescription of sports activities is one of caution. This is particularly true for patients with left bundle branch block (LBBB) or right bundle branch block (RBBB) with an associated left posterior hemiblock (LPH). These disturbances are frequently an expression of organic heart disease and present an uncertain natural history. In such cases, competitive sports must be discouraged. Skill and aerobic sports, conducted at an amateur and submaximal level, limited to young, asymptomatic patients without any apparent organic cardiopathy or with a haemodynamically well compensated organic heart disease, may be permitted.

An RBBB associated with a left anterior hemiblock (LAH), in absence of any evident cardiac pathology is considered to have a prognosis of minor gravity. An intracavitary electrophysiological study is, however, necessary to verify the residual functionality of the conduction system and to judge the patient's fitness for sports.

Prominent problems are not usually presented by isolated RBBB, LAH or LPH. In these cases, naturally, the favourable prognosis and judgement for sports activities must be confirmed by the normal results of non-invasive investigations, e.g. ECHO, exercise test and Holter monitoring, demonstrating the absence of any myocardial disease and associated

arrhythmias. Since such conduction disturbances may be the first manifestation of a progressive degenerative disease of the conduction system,
periodic re-evaluation must be done.

Arterial hypertension

Arterial hypertension is one of the most common cardiovascular diseases
in Western countries. Ninety percent or more of hypertensive patients
have essential hypertension and the remaining ones have secondary
forms, usually of renal origin.

The haemodynamic picture of the first stage of essential hypertension
is characterized by an increased cardiac output with an unchanged
peripheral vascular resistance. This stage is frequently found in young
patients and it usually presents with isolated, often labile, systolic
hypertension and, very often, with a hyperkinetic heart.

In the second stage, an increased peripheral resistance is established
which maintains a stable, elevated arterial pressure. This stage is characterized by chronic systolic and diastolic hypertension and progressive
target organ (kidney, eye, etc.) damage.

In prescribing sports activities, the level of arterial pressure is not the
sole criterion. Possible organ complications produced by hypertension
must be evaluated; this is particularly important for: (a) the kidney, since
damage here can accentuate the relative renal ischaemia that occurs
during exercise; and (b) the heart, since, for instance, heart hypertrophy
can be aggravated by chronic exercise and because hypertension by itself
is a risk factor for cardiovascular disease.

Investigative methods include:

1 Physical examination: this is necessary to exclude some forms of
secondary hypertension (e.g. absent femoral pulses with coarctation of
the aorta or palpable kidneys in polycystic renal disease). Accurate
assessment of blood pressure values at rest must be made, on at
least three separate occasions. Patients having diastolic blood pressure
values between 90 and 104 mmHg have mild hypertension, from 105 to
114 moderate hypertension, and >115 mmHg severe hypertension.
Patients with systolic values >160 mmHg have isolated systolic hypertension.

2 Blood chemistry: for serum creatinine, uric acid, potassium and
cholesterol; complete urinalysis with normal results.

3 Eye examination: normal.

4 ECG: no left ventricular hypertrophy or strain (high QRS voltage and/ or ST depression); no atrial abnormalities.

5 ECHO: ventricular hypertrophy absent or of modest degree; left ventricular function normal; atrial cavity and aortic root normal.

6 ex-ECG: evaluation of blood pressure. Tolerated upper limits of peak blood pressure may be 250/115. With higher values, patients should be more carefully evaluated for sports activities regardless of the presence or absence of organ damage; no ECG signs of ischaemia; no arrhythmias.

Indications: Aerobic and skill sports.

Contraindications: Anaerobic and power sports should be contra-indicated as they, unlike dynamic exercises, may cause a considerable increase of blood pressure during activity and benefits for the hyper-tensive patient are very doubtful.

Prescriptions: Competitive practice of the indicated sports above is consented for patients without organ complications (first stage). For patients with organ complications or secondary hypertension only amateur aerobic activity (at 60% of the maximum aerobic capacity) three times a week is permitted, in addition to skill sports, eventually with pharmacological protection.

Appendix 1:   General contraindications to sport in internal diseases

1 *Acute diseases*: myocardial infarction, respiratory infections, fever, phlebitis, embolism, etc.

2 *Chronic uncontrolled diseases* (whether associated or not with cardio-vascular involvement): renal insufficiency, hepatic insufficiency, diabetes, rheumatic diseases, gout, severe anaemia, etc.

The following conditions must be considered as *temporary contra-indications* only:

1 Excessive anxiety, severe sunstroke and drunkenness, neurological troubles and vertigo, oedemas of unknown origin, dehydration, etc.

2 Unresolved orthopaedic problems.

3 Adverse environmental conditions, e.g. hot and humid, too cold, fog and smog, rain.

4 Large meals and excessive intake of xanthines (coffee, tea, Coca-Cola).

5 The use of certain medicaments, e.g. bronchodilators, atropine, anorexia drugs.

Appendix 2:   Practical instructions for sports activity in cardiac patients

1 Maintenance of reasonable fitness is the aim, rather than achievement, of an athletic standard.

2 Unaccustomed sports exercise either prolonged, or sudden and short-lived, may be harmful. Heavy exertion may be dangerous especially if it does not involve movement (isometric or static exertion).

3 With any new exercise, its duration should be gradually increased to start with and only later the intensity.

4 During restful vacations it is unwise to discontinue training altogether, while during busy holidays the temptation to be overactive should be resisted.

5 The patient should not start sports activities if he/she feels even slightly unwell and unusually tired; even minor ailments should be improved before gradually attaining again the accustomed degree of exertion.

6 If angina, undue breathlessness or palpitations should ensue during sports activities, it is wise to reduce intensity and if slowing down is ineffective, one should stop and rest. Dizziness, light headache, 'rubber-legs', significant palpitations, new chest discomfort or other symptoms developed during or following exercise, should be promptly reported to the patient's physician. However, it should be remembered that standing still immediately after exercise can cause such symptoms. For that reason, strenuous exercise should not be interrupted suddenly but should be tapered gradually.

7 Musculoskeletal complaints are usually the result of excessive exertion. Reducing the intensity helps to distinguish a temporary mild disorder from a potential injury.

8 For those at work, the best times for sports activities are in the morning before work and after work before the evening meal. If the patient takes a bath or shower after exercise, the water must be warm, as extremes of temperature may cause excessive cardiocirculatory reactions and arrhythmias.

References

Conference proceedings (1985) Cardiovascular abnormalities in the athlete: recommendations regarding eligibility for competition (16th Bethesda Conference). *J. Am. Coll. Cardiol.* **6(6)**, 1189.

Eichner, E. R. (1983) Exercise and heart disease. Epidemiology of the 'exercise hypothesis'. *Am. J. Med.* **75**, 1008.

Fagard, R. H. & Bekaert, I. E. (1986) *Sports Cardiology. Exercise in Health and Cardiovascular Disease.* Martinus Nijoff Publishers, Dordrecht.

Haskell, W. L. (1984) Cardiovascular benefits and risk of exercise: the scientific evidence. In R. H. Strauss (ed) *Sports Medicine.* W. B. Saunders, Philadelphia.

Lown, B., Calvert, F., Armington, R. & Ryan, M. (1975) Monitoring for serious arrhythmias and high risk of sudden death. *Circulation* (Suppl.) **51–2**, 111.

Rulli, V. & Vajola, S. F. (eds) (1986) *Sport Activity and Cardiovascular Diseases.* L. Pozzi, Rome.

Strauzenberg, S. E. (1984) Recommendations for physical activity and sports in children with heart disease. A statement by the Scientific Commission of the International Federation of Sports Medicine (FIMS) approved by the executive Committee of the FIMS. *Int. J. Sports Cardiol.* **1**, 1.

11.2 Respiratory disease

K. D. FITCH & A. R. MORTON

The effect of exercise on respiratory disease must be viewed from two angles. While exercise has an important role in the management of some pulmonary disorders, it may at times provoke unfavourable consequences of lung function. Three chronic lung conditions will be examined—asthma, chronic obstructive lung disease and cystic fibrosis.

Asthma

Asthma, one of the most common respiratory disorders, is a major cause of morbidity in childhood and adolescence and has a significant mortality throughout life. Asthma has been defined by the American Thoracic Society (1962) as 'a disease characterised by an increased responsiveness of the trachea and bronchi to various stimuli and manifested by a widespread narrowing of the airways that changes in severity either spontaneously or as a result of therapy'.

The airways may be narrowed by one or more of the following: contraction of the bronchial smooth muscle, swelling of the mucous membrane and an increased mucus secretion. The result is an increased resistance in the airways, which may necessitate recruitment of accessory respiratory muscles in order to maintain a now noisy bronchial airflow or wheeze. The bronchoconstriction and mucosal oedema serve to increase the unfavourable transmural pressure gradient of the intrathoracic airways such that closure of small airways may occur. This results in 'air trapping' which increases the residual volume and decreases the vital capacity of the lungs.

Infection, irritating dusts, air pollutants, exposure to allergens (such as pollens, house dust, animal danders and specific foods) and nervous tension can all induce episodes of asthma in some people. Not all asthmatics respond to the same allergens. In fact some people, called intrinsic asthmatics, do not respond to any.

Vigorous physical activity can often lead to acute exacerbation of asthmatic symptoms, the degree of bronchoconstriction correlating well with the severity of the person's asthma. In rare cases, exercise is apparently the only stimulus that provokes asthma. Historically, asthma sufferers have avoided or have been excluded from exercise, but recent studies of the pulmonary effects of various exercise regimens, the long-term benefits of physical training and the protective effect of certain drugs against exertional asthma suggest that avoiding exercise is unwarranted and even detrimental to asthmatic people.

Exercise in provoking asthma

In many, and perhaps all, asthmatics, bronchoconstriction can be provoked by exercise. However, individuals vary greatly in this response. A few patients develop asthma only on rare occasions. On the other hand, some people, in the absence of pharmacological protection, become symptomatic almost every time they exercise.

There is a characteristic pattern of change in lung function which occurs during and after exercise in most asthmatics (Jones *et al.*, 1962). The forced expiratory volume in the first second (FEV_1) or peak expiratory flow rate (PEFR) is increased immediately after 6–8 min of submaximal exercise, followed by a reduction which reaches its maximum within 5 to 10 min of cessation of activity. The FEV_1 or PEFR then gradually returns towards the pre-exercise level in approximately 60 min (Fig. 11.2.1).

The immediate post-exercise increase in FEV_1 or PEFR may be due to

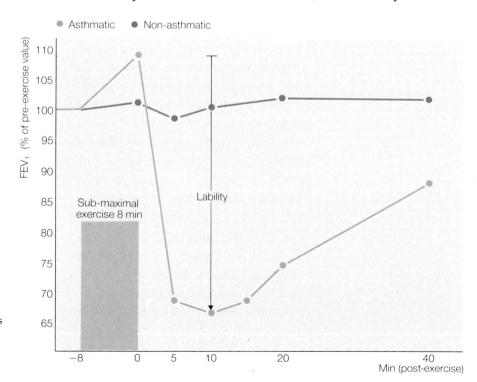

Fig. 11.2.1 Typical changes in FEV_1 following 8 min of submaximal exercise in an asthmatic and a non-asthmatic subject.

the bronchodilatory effect of increased circulating catecholamines (Jones *et al.*, 1963). Airway obstruction may develop during exercise but more commonly occurs afterwards. This is termed exercise-induced asthma (EIA) or exercise-induced bronchoconstriction (EIB). A 15% or greater fall of FEV_1 or PEFR from the pre-exercise volume is necessary to be termed EIA or EIB (Burr *et al.*, 1974).

Although non-asthmatics may show a slight increase in FEV_1 or PEFR immediately after exercise, followed by a slight reduction, these changes are seldom significant (Fig. 11.2.1). Despite 25 years of intensive research the mechanisms of EIA remain unclear. Recently, a great deal of emphasis has been placed on the temperature and humidity of inspired air as a major influence on airway response to exercise. Inhalation of cold air (Strauss *et al.*, 1977) and dry air (Bar-Or *et al.*, 1977) during exercise have both been shown to enhance the severity of post-exercise airways constriction. However, recent research has indicated that when the water content of inspired air was held constant, varying the temperature by as much as 25°C had no significant effect on EIA, while breathing hot humid air significantly inhibited EIA. Thus, water loss—not simply cooling of the airways due to heat loss—appears more important in EIA and the mechanism may be related to changes in osmolarity of the fluid lining the respiratory tract (Hahn *et al.*, 1984).

In addition to people with asthma or a known tendency to EIA, others may experience EIA when exercising in unfavourable exercise conditions (see Table 11.2.1). Such individuals include those with a history of childhood asthma or wheezy bronchitis, those with atopic disorders such as eczema or hay fever (allergic rhinitis) and those whose immediate family have asthma or atopy. The risk of such people developing EIA are summarized in Table 11.2.1.

Table 11.2.1 Risk of developing exercise-induced asthma.

Increased risk	Reduced risk
Continuous exercise	Intermittent exercise
Running	Swimming
Higher exercise intensity	Lower exercise intensity
Inferior physical fitness	Enhanced aerobic fitness
Cold, dry air	Warm, moist air
Air pollutants	Recent (within 3–4 hours) EIA (refractoriness)
Pollens, grasses	
Recent respiratory infection	
Taking β-blocking drugs	

Pharmacotherapy for exercise-induced asthma

To minimize or abolish EIA, it is imperative that a good control of asthma be achieved. This may necessitate a variety of measures, physical, immunological and pharmacological. The classes of drugs used in the management of asthma and their routes of administration are listed in Table 11.2.2.

Glucocorticoids, both oral (e.g. prednisone) and aerosol (e.g. beclomethasone dipropionate), are excellent drugs to stabilize asthma but have little effect if administered before exercise to prevent EIA. The H_1 antagonists have no significant role in the management of asthma, but are often prescribed to control symptoms associated with other manifestations of atopy, e.g. nasal, dermatological. Aerosol ipratroprium bromide is a belladonna alkaloid which is a useful bronchodilator for patients who cannot tolerate or do not respond to β-2 adrenoceptor stimulants, but is considered to be more effective in patients with chronic bronchitis.

The cornerstone of drug prevention of EIA consists of the β-2 adrenergic stimulants or β-2 agonists. There is little to choose between any of these agents, although it should be noted that fenoterol is not permitted for use when anti-doping controls are likely because of its metabolism to parahydroxyamphetamine (C. Clausnitzer, personal communication). β-2 agonists should be administered by inhalation immediately prior to exercise. However, in young children who cannot manipulate hand-held aerosols, oral administration of salbutamol, terbutaline or fenoterol can be recommended. Nevertheless, the aerosol is preferred to the oral route because of more rapid onset of action, superior efficacy, greatly reduced dosage and reduction of side effects such as tremor (Fig. 11.2.2).

β-2 agonists may be combined with either sodium cromoglycate (aerosol) and/or theophylline. The latter is administered orally and should achieve serum levels of 10–20 μg/ml to ensure a therapeutic effect.

Table 11.2.2 Classes of drugs used in the management of asthma and exercise-induced asthma.

Drug	Route of administration
Sodium cromoglycate*	Aerosol
Glucocorticoids	Oral, i.v. and aerosol
Methyl xanthines*	Oral and i.v.
Belladonna alkaloids	Aerosol
H_1 antagonists	Oral
Sympathomimetic amines*	Oral, i.m., i.v. and aerosol

* Of value in the prevention of EIA.

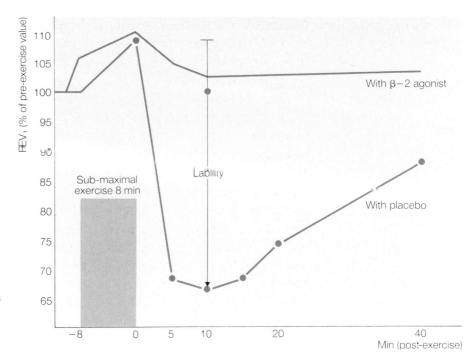

Fig. 11.2.2 Typical changes in FEV$_1$ following 8 min of submaximal exercise after inhalation of a β-2 agonist and a placebo.

These two drugs are approximately equal in their protection against EIA but inferior to β-agonists.

Until recently the asthmatic athlete had been subject to changing restrictions and prior notification of pre-exercise drug use. A review of anti-asthmatic drugs and their lack of any ergogenic effect on sports performance has been recently published (Fitch, 1986). In 1986, the Medical Commission of the International Olympics Committee rescinded the need to notify the use of β-2 agents given to asthmatics prior to competition, but restricted the administration of these agents to aerosol administration. Table 11.2.3 summarizes the current status of drugs available to the asthmatic athlete who is subject to anti-doping procedures.

Sport and exercise in the management of asthma

While exercise has been demonstrated to induce asthma, sports and regular physical activity are accepted components in the total management of asthma. A number of studies evaluating the effect of exercise training have been undertaken and these have recently been reviewed (Bar-Or, 1985).

To achieve physical conditioning in asthmatics, a variety of exercise programmes have been shown to be effective. Because of its reduced asthmagenicity, swimming is the optimal exercise, especially in the more

Table 11.2.3 Drugs to treat asthma and exercise-induced asthma.

Drug	Route of administration
Permitted*	
Cromyglycate (cromolyn)	Aerosol
Theophylline	Oral
Beclomethasone dipropionate	Aerosol
β-2 agonists	Aerosol
Salbutamol	
Terbutaline	
Orciprenaline (metaproterenol)	
Rimiterol	
Biltolterol	
Banned	
Fenoterol	
Isoprenaline (isoproterenol)	
Adrenaline	
Ephedrine	

* Permitted by the IOC Medical Commission.

severe asthmatic (Fitch & Morton, 1971). Aerobic activities with an exercise intensity requiring 65–75% of maximal oxygen uptake (approximately 75–85% of predicted maximal heart rate) are recommended (Silverman & Anderson, 1972). Warm-up should precede the principal activity, which should be intermittent or be interval in nature, due to the reduced risks of EIA (Morton *et al.*, 1982). Exercising when the ambient air is drier or colder than normal is likely to result in increased EIA (Hahn *et al.*, 1984). Exercise sessions should be conducted three to five times per week for 30–60 min and conclude with a warm-down session. Pre-exercise medication to reduce or prevent EIA is essential, especially in the more severe asthmatic prone to EIA.

Regular and frequent aerobic exercise at a moderate to heavy intensity produces the same physiological benefits for the asthmatic as for the non-asthmatic. Enhanced aerobic fitness increases the tolerance and threshold levels of asthmatics so that a higher level of provocation is required to produce EIA. Bronchial hyper-responsiveness appears to be unaltered. Medication requirements decline and psychological and sociological benefits, with resulting improvement in self-image and greater recognition and acceptance by both peer groups and parents, have been observed (Fitch *et al.*, 1976).

The availability of efficient pre-exercise medication with β-2 agonists and/or cromoglycate to abolish or minimize EIA has been a major factor in permitting asthmatics to achieve excellence in sport. Of the last three Australian Olympic teams (1976–84), a mean of 8.4% of athletes (range

7.2–9.5%) have had asthma. Between 1956 and 1984 there has been an unbroken run of success by asthmatics in winning Olympic medals, mostly but not all in the swimming pool (Fitch, 1984).

Conclusion The response of asthmatics to exercise varies from person to person and, to some extent, even in the same person at different times. However, asthmatics should participate in regular exercise and sports programmes with a minimum of restrictions. To maximize the level of participation they should use suitable pre-exercise medication in the form of aerosol β-2 agonists and/or cromoglycate, and should EIA occur, it may be reversed by an aerosol β-2 agonist. The success of asthmatics at the highest levels of sport is testimony to the benefits of exercise in overcoming their disability and a stimulus for others to commence including physical activity and sports in their daily lives.

Chronic obstructive lung disease

Breathlessness and wheezing are the most important symptoms which indicate the presence of chronic airflow obstruction (CAO), commonly termed chronic obstructive lung disease (COLD). Other terms such as chronic obstructive airways disease, chronic obstructive pulmonary disease and chronic non-specific lung disease are synonymous with COLD.

Chronic obstruction to airflow may be the result of narrowing of the conducting airways or destruction of the lung parenchyma (emphysema). Chronic cough and sputum due to hypersecretion of mucus in the bronchial airways indicate chronic bronchitis which frequently, but not always, accompanies CAO. Cigarette smoking is by far the most common cause of both CAO and chronic bronchitis. The current theory is that smoking cigarettes damages lung cells releasing proteolytic enzymes, which in turn degrade the extracellular matrix of the lung, resulting in emphysema. Asthma (or variable airflow obstruction) may also cause CAO, especially if poorly managed. Other causes of COLD include environmental pollutants, especially those in industry and cystic fibrosis (Musk, 1987).

Measurement of lung function is fundamental to the diagnosis and assessment of COLD. Spirometry will detect the presence and severity of airflow obstruction. To evaluate the presence of any reversible component of CAO, spirometry is initially performed before and after the aerosol administration of a β-2 agonist such as salbutamol. Irreversibility of

CAO cannot be established until at least a 10-day course of oral gluco-corticoids has been administered in adequate dosage (e.g. 40 mg prednisone daily) and spirometry repeated.

In the management of COLD, the cessation of smoking is the most essential feature. The aim is to achieve optimal lung function, and spirometry is a valuable aid in long-term management. Even small increases in lung volume after the use of aerosol bronchodilators may be accompanied by an acceptable reduction of breathlessness. The aerosol administration of beclomethasone dipropionate will reduce the side effects of systemic glucocorticoids in patients who benefit from oral corticosteroids. Theophylline is useful in some patients and may provide the additional benefit of reducing respiratory muscle fatigue (Aubier *et al.*, 1981).

Because exertion increases breathlessness, patients with COLD tend to become less and less active. Inevitably this results in a progressive decline of cardiovascular and musculoskeletal fitness and breathlessness becomes steadily greater with reducing levels of exertion until the patient is dyspnoeic at rest. This vicious cycle can be halted by a supervised exercise programme. COLD patients should be encouraged to undertake regular exercise within the limitations of their disease (Belman, 1986).

Several pathophysiological factors restrict exercise in patients with COLD. Damage to the tissues responsible for the elastic recoil of the lungs limits respiratory flow rates and contributes to air trapping (as indicated by an elevated residual volume) during the hyperventilation of exercise. Inefficient ventilation is also caused by mismatching of ventilation and perfusion (some regions of the lung being hypoventilated and others hyperventilated) and by an increase in the physiologic dead space. Hyperinflated lungs flatten the diaphragm which is then a less efficient respiratory muscle. Finally, the oxygen cost of breathing may be as much as three times greater in COLD than in normal individuals at rest and during exercise. These and other factors demonstrate the major difficulties that confront COLD patients during exercise (Shayevitz & Shayevitz, 1986).

A distance test involving a 12 min walk allowing the person to stop and rest as required, provides valuable baseline data from which to write the exercise programme and to compare the post-training results (McGavin *et al.*, 1976). During the test, various parameters may be monitored, such as heart rate, ear oximetry and the more complicated $\dot{V}_{O_2 \, max}$. Other investigators have preferred a 3 or 6 min walk test for more severely affected patients, with supplemental oxygen administered if required.

Exercise prescription should be individually tailored following the 12-min walk test and the training target is 70–85% of predicted maximum heart rate for age. Warm-up, flexibility exercises and cool-down are integrated with the predominate exercise, usually walking. COLD patients have been evaluated during cycling on a cycle ergometer (Brundin, 1974), walking on a treadmill (Chester *et al.*, 1977), a 5BX-type programme (Mungall & Hainsworth, 1980), free range walking (Shayevitz & Shayevitz, 1986), and prone immersion exercise (tethered swimming) (Jankowski *et al.*, 1976). The potential benefits which may occur from exercise reconditioning have been reviewed by Hughes and Davison (1983). Accepted gains include increased physical endurance and a greater distance walked in 12 min. Higher oxygen uptake and superior skill in motor performance result in the ability to undertake the same tasks at lower levels of ventilation, oxygen cost and heart rate. Additional consequences are enhanced mobility and reduction of anxiety, depression and social isolation. Thus, both physical and emotional gains combine to improve the quality of the lives of many COLD patients.

Little or no benefit from exercise training has been observed in ventilatory capacity and pulmonary hypertension, and effects on survival have yet to be evaluated. The hazards of exercise in COLD include exercise-related cardiac arrhythmias, systemic hypotension and increased P_{CO_2}. A potential danger is progressive muscle fatigue of a disadvantaged diaphragm, potentially leading to respiratory failure. Nevertheless, such dangers have been outweighed by the benefits of regular supervised exercise training in COLD to the extent that it is becoming an accepted component of the total management of these patients.

Cystic fibrosis

Cystic fibrosis (CF) is a lethal genetic disorder presenting in early childhood and principally affecting the exocrine glands. In the lungs, it is associated with viscous secretions which tend to produce airways obstruction. Recurrent life-threatening chest infections and subsequent parenchymal damage are common. Much of the disability and mortality of CF are consequences of the pulmonary disorder. Modern treatment with diet, antibiotics, mucolytics, inhalation therapy, physiotherapy and pancreatic enzyme supplementation has greatly improved life expectancy. Children, adolescents and even young adults with CF have recently been exposed to exercise training in an attempt to improve the quality of their lives.

A number of studies have demonstrated that CF patients have tolerated well, and benefited significantly from, exercise programmes involving jog-walking (Orenstein *et al.*, 1981), swimming (Zach *et al.*, 1981; Edlund *et al.*, 1986), tethered swimming (Clement *et al.*, 1979), and swimming and canoeing (Keens *et al.*, 1977). Increased exercise tolerance, maximum oxygen uptake, pulmonary gas exchange and ventilatory muscle endurance have been evident with concomitant improvement in lung volumes observed by some, but not all, authors. A preliminary study (Zach *et al.*, 1982) has suggested that regular exercise, notably swimming, may prevent a reduction of the labour-intensive and tedious physiotherapy in CF patients. This has been confirmed recently with a 12-month home exercise programme that was individually prescribed for a number of patients (Blomquist *et al.*, 1986). A universal finding in these studies has been an increased sense of well-being and independence of the participating CF patients and often by their relatives. The need for pre-exercise bronchodilators is infrequent; some patients do require aerosol β-2 agonists but many do not (Canny & Levison, 1987). In theory, unfavourable consequences of exercise training in CF would include arterial oxygen desaturation in the more severely affected and poor heat adaptation due to excessive sodium and chloride content in sweat. The former demands that exercise prescription must be tailored to the physical capabilities and restrictions of the individual CF patient. The latter necessitates adequate fluid and electrolyte replacement during and after exercise, especially in hot environments (Bar-Or, 1985). While it is premature to suggest that suitable regular exercise may increase life expectancy in CF, it has been established that CF patients tolerate exercise-training programmes well and with few unfavourable consequences, and thus the quality of their lives does appear to be enhanced.

References

American Thoracic Society (1962) Definitions and classification of chronic bronchitis, asthma and pulmonary emphysema. *Am. Rev. Respir. Dis.* **85**, 763.

Aubier, M., De Troyer, A., Sampson, M., Macklem, P. T. & Roussos, C. (1981) Aminophyllin improves diaphragmatic contractability. *New Engl. J. Med.* **305**, 249.

Bar-Or, O. (1985) Physical conditioning in children with cardiorespiratory disease. *Exerc. Sport Sci. Rev.* **13**, 305.

Bar-Or, O., Neuman, I. & Dotan, R. (1977) Effects of dry and humid climates on exercise-induced asthma in children and pre-adolescents. *J. Allergy Clin. Immunol.* **60**, 163.

Belman, M. J. (1986) Exercise in chronic obstructive pulmonary disease. *Clin. Chest Med.* **7**, 585.

Blomquist, M., Freyschuss, U., Wiman, L–G. & Strandvik, B. (1986) Physical activity and self treatment in cystic fibrosis. *Arch. Dis. Child.* **61**, 362.

Brundin, A. (1974) Physical training in severe chronic obstructive lung disease. *Scand. J. Respir. Dis.* **55**, 25.

Burr, M. L., Eldrige, B. A. & Borysiewicz, L. K. (1974) Peak expiratory flow rates before and after exercise in school children. *Arch. Dis. Child.* **49**, 923.

Canny, G. J. & Levinson, H. (1987) Exercise response and rehabilitation in cystic fibrosis. *Sports Med.* **4**, 143.

Chester, E. H., Belman, M. J., Bahler, R. C., Baum, G. L., Schey, G. & Buch, P. (1977) The effect of physical training on cardiopulmonary performance in patients with chronic obstructive pulmonary disease. *Chest* **72**, 695.

Clement, M., Jankowski, L. W. & Beaudry, P. H. (1979) Prone immersion physical exercise therapy in three children with cystic fibrosis. *Nurs. Res.* **28**, 325.

Edlund, L. D., French, R. W., Herbst, J. S., Ruttenberg, H. D., Ruhling, R. O. & Adams, T. D. (1986) Effects of a swimming programme on children with cystic fibrosis. *Am. J. Dis. Child.* **140**, 80.

Fitch, K. D. (1984) Management of allergic olympic athletes. *J. Allergy Clin. Immunol.* (Suppl.) **73**, 722.

Fitch, K. D. (1986) The use of anti-asthmatic drugs: do they affect sports performance? *Sports Med.* **3**, 136.

Fitch, K. D. & Morton, A. R. (1971) Specificity of exercise in exercise-induced asthma. *Br. Med. J.* **4**, 577.

Fitch, K. D., Morton, A. R. & Blanksby, B. A. (1976) Effects of swimming training on children with asthma. *Arch. Dis. Child.* **51**, 190.

Hahn, A., Anderson, S. D., Morton, A. R., Black, J. L. & Fitch, K. D. (1984) A reinterpretation of the effect of temperature and water content of inspired air in exercise-induced asthma. *Am. Rev. Respir. Dis.* **130**, 575.

Hughes, R. L. & Davison, R. (1983) Limitation of exercise reconditioning in COLD. *Chest* **83**, 241.

Jankowski, L. W., Roy, L. E., Vallee, J. & Boucher, R. (1976) Effect of prone immersion physical exercise (PIPE) therapy in patients with chronic obstructive pulmonary disease (COPD). *Scand. J. Rehab. Med.* **8**, 135.

Jones, R. S., Buston, M. H. & Wharton, M. J. (1962) The effect of exercise on ventilatory function in the child with asthma. *Br. J. Dis. Chest* **56**, 78.

Jones, R. S., Wharton, M. J. & Buston, M. H. (1963) The place of physical exercise and bronchodilator drugs in the assessment of the asthmatic child. *Arch. Dis. Child.* **38**, 539.

Keens, T. G., Krastins, I. R. B., Wannamaker, E. M., Levinson, H., Crozier, D. N. & Bryan, A. C. (1977) Ventilatory muscle endurance training in normal subjects and patients with cystic fibrosis. *Am. Rev. Respir. Dis.* **116**, 853.

McGavin, C. R., Gupta, S. P. & McHardy, G. J. R. (1976) Twelve minute walking test for assessing disability in chronic bronchitis. *Br. Med. J.* **1**, 822.

Morton, A. R., Hahn, A. G. & Fitch, K. D. (1982) Continuous and intermittent running in the provocation of asthma. *Ann. Allergy* **48**, 123.

Mungall, I. P. F. & Hainsworth, R. (1980) An objective assessment of the value of exercise training in patients with chronic obstructive airways disease. *Q. J. Med.* **49**, 77.

Musk, A. W. (1987) Chronic obstructive lung disease. *Aust. Fam. Physician* **16**, 589.

Orenstein, D. M., Franklin, B. A., Doershuk, C. F., Hellerstein, H. F., Germann, K. J., Horowitz, J. G. & Stern, R. C. (1981) Exercise conditioning and cardiopulmonary fitness in cystic fibrosis. *Chest* **80**, 392.

Shayevitz, M. B. & Shayevitz, B. R. (1986) Athletic training in chronic obstructive pulmonary disease. *Clin. Sports Med.* **5**, 471.

Silverman, M. & Anderson, S. D. (1972) Standardisation of exercise tests in asthmatic children. *Arch. Dis. Child.* **47**, 882.

Strauss, R. H., McFadden jr, E. R., Ingram jr, R. H. & Jaeger, J. J. (1977) Enhancement of exercise-induced asthma by cold air. *New Engl. J. Med.* **297**, 743.

Zach, M. S., Oberwaldner, B. & Hausler, F. (1982) Cystic fibrosis: physical exercise versus chest physiotherapy. *Arch. Dis. Child.* **57**, 587.

Zach, M. S., Purrer, B. & Oberwaldner, B. (1981) Effect of swimming on forced expiration and sputum clearance in cystic fibrosis. *Lancet* **ii**, 1201.

11.3 Metabolic disease

A. VENERANDO, G. CALDARONE & A. PELLICCIA

Physical activity in the therapy and prevention of obesity

There are many different aetiopathological mechanisms involved in excessive increase in bodyweight but the main cause seems to be a decreased energy output together with an excessive energy input. This is only true, however, for obesities not caused by dysfunctions of the endocrine system.

A marked reduction of physical activity can in some cases be the only cause for being overweight; in fact in some cases even under a well-controlled diet it is very difficult to lose weight (Bloom & Eidew, 1967). The increase in appetite is not only the result of incorrect eating habits, but is also a direct effect of an alteration of the appetite centre situated in the hypothalamus, which seems to be induced by prolonged inactivity. Sedentarism in this case is the only cause for being overweight. Therefore, dieting is not sufficient for an obese person to reach his or her ideal bodyweight, so a specific training programme has to be associated with the diet (Bjorntorp et al., 1973; Oscai, 1973; Lewis et al., 1976; Leon et al., 1979; Bronwell & Stunkard, 1980; Thompson et al., 1982; Stunkard, 1983).

In order to come up with an adequate training programme for an obese person it is of fundamental importance to evaluate how healthy the subject is and his/her residual physical capacity. This clinical and instrumental check-up will allow the physician to see if there are any contra-indications that could limit the training programme, and also to evaluate the actual conditions of the cardiovascular, respiratory and musculo-skeletal systems of the subject. In this way a very specific and person-alized training routine can be planned (Table 11.3.1). The motivation and

Table 11.3.1 Prescription of physical activity.

Evaluation of the subject's physical fitness (clinical and instrumental)

Evaluation of the initial tolerance to physical activity and the residual capacity (instrumental)

Personalized training programme

general psychological state of the obese patient must also be taken into consideration in order to reduce the frequent phenomenon of 'quitting', which is very often at the basis of many failures (Gibson *et al.*, 1983; Hage, 1983).

Physical reconditioning of the obese must be programmed in such a way that there is:

1 An improvement of the body fat mass to lean tissue mass ratio.

2 A reactivation of the muscles that have become hypotonic and hypotrophic due to inactivity.

3 A restoration of the physiological mobility of the major joints, especially the cervical, lumbosacral, shoulder girdle and knees.

4 A reconditioning of the cardiovascular and respiratory systems and the adaptations that will follow (i.e. resting bradycardia, low blood pressure, improved venous return, ability to withstand even strenuous exercise, tendency to normalize altered metabolic indexes) (Venerando, 1980).

These major points are easily achieved by subjects that are only slightly or moderately overweight, whilst it is harder for subjects with severe obesity to take part in any type of training programme.

Training programme The training programme for the physical reconditioning of the obese can be divided into three major parts (Table 11.3.2) (Caldarone & Giampietro, 1985).

Part 1 The first part of the programme must only consist of exercises that are directed to restoring the mobility of the upper and lower limbs and the vertebral column. These exercises should be performed through callisthenics, rhythmically but at a low frequency and intensity so as to reduce the pain which always arises whenever physical activity is started after a long period of sedentarism. Once a good mobility of the limbs is achieved the callisthenics exercises can be alternated with a lightweight

Table 11.3.2 Training programme.

Part 1	Restoration of the joints and muscular stimulus	Isometric and isotonic exercises
Part 2	Improvement of the cardiorespiratory and musculoskeletal systems	Mainly dynamic exercises
Part 3	Permanent and long-lasting efficiency of the major systems	Regular practice of an aerobic or an alternated type of physical activity

programme, which will induce muscular reconditioning through an antigravitational stimulus. One can use small dumbells, medicine balls and any other type of equipment that is easy to use.

This initial part of the training programme will have a duration which is directly proportional to the degree of obesity. However the main characteristics of the training programme are the progressive increase of the workloads and the continuity. Not following one of these two points will result in a rapid loss of any of the beneficial effects obtained previously.

The series of exercises should have a duration of 2–3 min and must be alternated by a resting period of approximately 30–60 s. Every exercise should be repeated three to five times. During the course of the training programme the patient will be able to reach 5–6 min series of continuous exercises, always alternated with 30–60 s resting periods (Table 11.3.3). The patient starts in a standing position with legs straight and spread apart, the arms held straight in front. The exercise is performed in the following way: pronation and supranation of the hands, flexion of the forearms on the arms, and rotation of the arms around the shoulders and of the head around the neck. One can then proceed with the flexion of the torso on the legs, both foward and then laterally. At this point it is better that the subject lies down and begins the exercises of rotation of the feet around the ankles, flexion and extension of the legs on the thighs, and of the thighs on the pelvis and then of the torso on the legs. With the subject in a supine position, he or she can unite and extend the lower limbs and then alternately move one leg at a time without bending the knees, then by extending the arms and flexing the torso try to touch his/her toes with the fingers.

After a period of callisthenics only, which varies according to the degree of obesity and inactivity, from 2 weeks to a maximum of 4 weeks (with a daily frequency), one can then introduce some workouts with weights. It is better to start by using easy-to-use equipment, which in the

Table 11.3.3 Motor training programme part 1. Duration: 4–8 weeks; frequency: daily.

Stretching exercises	8–10 min
Callisthenic exercises	2–6 min series, repeated 3–5 times, alternated with 30–60 resting periods; every day for 2–4 weeks
Exercises with small weights, e.g. dumbells, medicine balls, etc.	2–6 min series repeated 3–5 times with weights from 1 kg to 5 kg alternated with 1 min resting periods; every day for 2–4 weeks

beginning should not weigh more than 1 kg. First the patient will start by exercising the upper and lower limbs (e.g. placing wrist and ankle weights) rhythmically and alternatingly. Going on with the programme the weights can be increased to reach 4–5 kg. The restoration of an adequate muscular tone and trophism is mainly taken care of by anti-gravitational exercises with progressive increments of the workloads; this represents the most suitable stimulus to recondition the muscles.

Besides using weights it is also important to remember all those exercises where a person's own bodyweight is used as stimulus; these exercises can only be used once one has reached a good degree of physical fitness. Also part of this first section of the training programme are the stretching exercises which should be performed at the beginning of each training session in order to improve the mobility of the joints and the extension of the musculotendinous structures (8–10 min exercises).

Part 2 The second part of the motor-training programme is aimed at increasing the efficiency and capacity of the cardiovascular, respiratory and musculo-skeletal systems. From mainly isotonic exercises, such as those prescribed in the first part of the training programme in which the muscular contractions were followed by changes of only some segments and not of all the body, the patient now goes on to exercises that are more demanding and complete and which are mainly based on 'movement'. It is particularly difficult to perform these exercises initially because even for low-intensity workloads there is a rapid onset of muscular fatigue together with disproportionate tachycardia and tachypnoea. Therefore, the training programme must start with stimuli that are well below submaximal, but on the other hand, they have to be able to induce an increase of the heart rate to at least 60% of the theoretical maximum heart rate. This means that even if the workout is of low intensity it has to be a 'training stimulus' and the degree of training is given by the increase of cardiac and respiratory workload (Table 11.3.4).

The energy required for rhythmical and prolonged exercises is provided

Table 11.3.4 Training programme part 2. Duration: 6–12 months; frequency: 3–6 days a week.

Stretching and callisthenic exercises	8–10 min
Aerobic-type activities	From 15 to 60 min a session, with increments of 5 min a week and at an intensity of 50–70% of the maximum theoretical heart rate ($HR_{max} = 220 - $ age)
Cooling down exercises	5–10 min

by carbohydrates and by the NEFA (non-esterified fatty acids) that produce ATP in the constant presence of oxygen, i.e. in an aerobic metabolism. Haematosis and, therefore, the transportation and utilization of oxygen are directly correlated to the capacity of the cardiovascular and respiratory systems. A higher need for oxygen leads to an increment of the capacity and efficiency of these systems and to a utilization of both carbohydrates and fats.

The most suitable type of physical activity for the obese person who wants to achieve these results is walking at a fast pace and low-intensity jogging (Moody *et al.*, 1969; Boileau *et al.*, 1971; Gwinupp, 1975; Foss *et al.*, 1976; Kukkonen *et al.*, 1983). These two physical activities can be performed freely and are able, if performed continuously and at an adequate rhythm and intensity, to reach these goals (Anderson, 1984). They both have a lot of favourable characteristics, such as the prescription of progressively increasing workloads with the possibility to adapt these workloads to the subjects' capabilities. The running course can be more or less difficult according to the distance that one has to cover, the difficulties that can arise (i.e. running on a flat surface, an undulating course or uphill), the velocity and the rhythm; the exercise can be slowed down or even stopped in order to allow the subject to recover and eventually restart the exercise. Jogging is an exercise that can take place anywhere, on any type of surface, adapting the clothes to the different climatic conditions, with no need of particular structures or equipment and not restricted to particular hours.

At the beginning of the programme it is a good habit to run or walk for not more than 15 min at a slow pace and rhythm. Before starting to run it is advisable to warm-up for at least 8 min; stretching and callisthenics are recommended. After following this programme for a week (8–10 min warm-up and 15 min of running or walking) one can increase the duration of the exercise by 5 min and so forth so as to reach an end result of 50–60 min.

These results can only be achieved with complete participation of the obese subject. The weight loss, together with the feeling of having recuperated one's body's capacities, should gratify the patient to such a point that the training programme will be considered fun and the diet restrictions will be tolerated without excessive sacrifices.

Exercises with these characteristics (i.e. duration, intensity and rhythm) must be performed at least three times a week, to a maximum of six times (always taking into account the degree of physical fitness of the subject). For those who are willing to take part in more than three training sessions a week it is a good habit to allow a day of complete rest so that the patient can recuperate from the fatigue and therefore have a more efficient resumption of physical activity (supercompensation phenomenon).

It is important to mention that in subjects with severe obesity, instead of running or walking it is better for them, especially in the initial phases, to do some swimming or cycling. In fact these types of physical activities allow for even prolonged training sessions without putting the articulations of the vertebral column and of the lower limbs under further strain, other than that already present due to being overweight.

Part 3 The third part of the programme is probably the most gratifying and pleasant one for the patient. The first two phases, if correctly performed, will allow for a series of modifications of the various organs and systems which will allow the subject to engage even in difficult exercises without the rapid onset of pain and fatigue (Table 11.3.5). The major modifications, or adaptations, are seen in the cardiovascular, musculoskeletal and respiratory systems; they were started in the second part of the training programme. The metabolism, diet and correct training programme will improve or even normalize the haematological indexes which are frequently altered in the obese subject.

The improvement of all these parameters will allow the subject to eventually choose the physical activities that he/she prefers without having to follow the exercises prescribed in the first two parts of the training programme. However, the subject should always try to take part in 'endurance' sports activities. These sports activities have the characteristic of increasing the quality of resistance, which means the subject is able to exercise for a long period of time without being limited by the rapid onset of fatigue.

The physiological requirements are: a good alveolar haematosis, a rapid transport of oxygen through the cardiovascular system and a good utilization of oxygen by the muscles. These are the adaptations that one requires to be able to obtain a good cardiac efficiency (resting bradycardia,

Table 11.3.5 Training programme part 3. Duration: unlimited; rate: three to six times a week.

Callisthenics and stretching	10–15 min
Endurance exercises (running, swimming, cycling, etc.)	20–30 min
Specific sport activities (team sports, tennis, golf, etc.)	30–60 min

gradual and proportionate increase of the heart rate in response to muscular work), a normalization of the blood pressure values (due to a reduction of the peripheral resistances), a good venous return (provided by the pump effect induced by muscular contractions), increased and improved ventilatory dynamics, an adequate utilization of blood oxygen in the periphery (due to the increased oxidative capacities of the mitochondrion induced by training).

The sport activities that induce these types of adaptations are: walking, running, swimming, cycling, rowing, roller skating and cross-country skiing (Wilmore, 1980; Schuster, 1983). Other sports that should also be considered are those that are not only 100% endurance exercises, but that alternate mainly aerobic exercises with mainly anaerobic ones. These are 'mixed sports', such as the majority of team sports (football, basketball, volleyball, etc.) and tennis. In these sports activities there is always a part of the training programme that is directed towards improving endurance. In choosing suitable sports it is important to take into account the training programme, which can tend to concentrate on endurance training.

The frequency of the training sessions must be from three to six times a week. Each training session should start with warm-up exercises (stretching and callisthenics), which should last about 10–15 min, followed by a series of exercises aimed at improving one's endurance (low-intensity running) which last 20–30 min. The last phase of the training session consists of a specific sport (team sports, tennis, golf) which should last at least 20 min. For the mainly aerobic sports activities, after the warm-up session, the specific training should have a duration of 30–60 min.

Conclusion   Obesity can be cured by adopting a controlled diet and by many other methods all the way down to surgery. However, physical activity especially aimed to obtain an increased energy output is one of the best and most efficient strategic therapies. This strategy should also be utilized in the prevention of obesity. If well programmed and personalized, the training programme will be able to physically recondition the overweight subject, improving his/her articulations, cardiovascular system and, if present, any metabolic disorders (Oja, 1983; Pelliccia et al., 1983). The results obtained, together with the sensation of a more efficient body, will also improve the subject's psychological condition. This can be particularly important as obese people are usually dissatisfied with their bodies and image.

The training programme must be prescribed just as any other type of therapy, it must not be generalized, but has to be specific for each subject and has to be performed under the supervision of qualified experts. It also has to be performed regularly and with a rhythm and intensity such that it will induce the right modifications and adaptations (American College of Sports Medicine, 1980).

Physical activity in the therapy and prevention of hyperlipoproteinaemias

Hyperlipoproteinaemias are both a qualitative and quantitative alteration of plasma lipids. They can be caused by an altered metabolism of the lipoproteins (primary hyperlipoproteinaemias) or by a disorder of various organs and systems that, as a collateral effect, can produce an alteration of the plasma lipids (secondary hyperlipoproteinaemias). Primary hyperlipoproteinaemias can be caused by genetical and hereditary alterations, they can be multifactorial, or as seen in the majority of the cases they are the result of both genetical alterations and incorrect life-styles and eating habits. Secondary hyperlipoproteinaemias can be caused by disorders of the thyroid gland, kidney diseases and liver diseases. They can also be associated with diabetes and alcoholism.

For the classification of the hyperlipoproteinaemias, this chapter will refer to that proposed by Fredrickson and colleagues (1967), which is still a valid diagnostical and therapeutical classification of these metabolic alterations (Table 11.3.6). High-density lipoproteins (HDL), which were

Table 11.3.6 Hyperlipoproteins classification according to Fredrickson *et al.* (1967).

			Pathogenesis
Type I	Chylomicrons ↑ ↑	Triglycerides ↑ ↑	Lack of lipoproteinlipase
Type IIa	LDL ↑ ↑	Cholesterol ↑ ↑	Increased production of LDL
Type IIb	VLDL ↑ LDL ↑ ↑	Triglycerides ↑ Cholesterol ↑ ↑	Increased production of LDL, increased synthesis of triglycerides
Type III	LDL ↑	Cholesterol ↑ Triglycerides ↑	Synthesis of intermediate lipo-proteins between VLDL and LDL
Type IV	VLDL ↑ ↑	Cholesterol ↑ Triglycerides ↑ ↑	Increased synthesis of triglycerides
Type V	VLDL ↑ ↑ Chylomicrons ↑ ↑	Triglycerides ↑ ↑	Increased synthesis of VLDL and triglycerides

VLDL = very low-density lipoproteins; LDL = low-density lipoproteins.

not taken into account in Fredrickson's classification, are added. Hyperlipoproteinaemias types I, III and V are relatively rare, whilst types IIa, IIb and IV are more common. Particular attention must be directed towards these last three types of hyperlipoproteinaemias since they are frequently associated with coronary and peripheral atherosclerosis (especially types IIa and IIb) and also with obesity, diabetes and hyperuricaemia (especially type IV).

Exercise has a preventive and therapeutic effect on hyperlipoproteinaemia caused by incorrect eating habits and sedentarism. In fact it has been shown that well trained subjects have low plasma levels of triglycerides and total cholesterol, which is mainly LDL cholesterol (this is the lipoprotein fraction that is frequently correlated with atherosclerosis and coronary heart diseases). Moderate physical activity, however, that does not represent an adequate training stimulus, does not produce any significant alteration in the plasma lipids.

Diabetes, obesity and smoking can be a limitation to the practice of intensive physical activity in hyperlipoproteinaemic subjects. Other limiting factors can be the various complications that can arise from this disease, such as coronary heart disease and atherosclerosis (peripheral and cerebral). Therefore it is important before the subject undertakes any type of training programme that he or she is carefully evaluated. This evaluation should consist of the following steps:

1   A detailed personal and family history (i.e. myocardial infarction, stroke, etc.).
2   A stress ECG.
3   An evaluation of any arrhythmias if present.
4   A urine analysis and if necessary also a creatinuria analysis.

Once the presence of coronary or vascular disease has been ruled out the subject should undergo an orthopaedical examination in order to prevent any musculotendinous pathologies arising from functional overload.

Prescription of sports activities   The criteria used to choose the type of physical activity which is most suitable for the subject must take into consideration the preferred type of physical activity and also his or her experience, if any, in sports. Studies have shown that if the subject is motivated and attracted by the sport then he/she will practise it regularly. The only restriction is that the sports activity must be an aerobic one, such as jogging, running, cycling, swimming and cross-country skiing, when possible. To these sports one can also add, depending on each case, sports such as football, basketball, volleyball, tennis, circuit and weight training. This will make the training programme more personalized and interesting (Lampman *et al.*, 1977, 1978, 1980; Huttunen *et al.*, 1979; Hartung *et al.*, 1981).

It must also be added that sports activities with a low metabolic demand, such as golf, target firing and bowls, are useless in correcting hyperlipoproteinaemias.

Intensity, duration and frequency of sports activities

When a subject starts a training programme after a long period of sedentarism it is very important that it is started gradually so as to avoid any complications, especially those arising from the musculotendinous system. Therefore, it is important that there is a reconditioning period that lasts at least 2–3 weeks, consisting of stretching exercises and callisthenics, before engaging in any type of sports activity. The intensity should be regulated on the basis of the subject's heart rate, which can be recorded during exercise or in the 10 s immediately following exercise. The recommended heart rate should be approximately 70% of the theoretical maximum heart rate. The intensity of the exercise can then be adapted to each individual on the basis of the cardiovascular response.

The duration of the exercise must also be correlated to the subject's physical fitness. We recommend that the exercise lasts at least 20 min at a continuous pace. This does not include the 5–10 min warm-up and cool-down exercises. The training sessions should be at least three times a week, and each should correspond to an approximate energy expenditure of 4200 kJ so as to reach a weekly expenditure of around 19000 kJ. This expenditure should be sufficient to increase the levels of HDL cholesterol. These modifications should occur 4–8 weeks after the beginning of the aerobic training programme.

In cases in which the subject starts a training programme for rehabilitation or with no competitive goal then the training programme can be directly controlled by the subject without the continuous supervision of a trainer (Lampman *et al.*, 1978). If, instead, the subject takes part in competitive sports activities (i.e. there are no major cardiovascular problems) then the athlete can follow a specific schedule which has previously been planned out together with a trainer. Provided that the amount of aerobic exercises in the training programme is elevated then the physical activity will contribute to normalizing the altered lipoproteic pattern. If the programme does not take into consideration aerobic activities then they should be included, always taking into consideration the above mentioned recommendations.

Effects of sports activities on plasma lipoproteins

It is important to periodically control the plasma lipoproteins in order to evaluate the effects of physical activity, and to then modify the duration, intensity and frequency of the training programme accordingly. The end result obtained from an aerobic sports activity and an adequate diet should be the normalization or partial correction of the altered lipoproteins (Oscai *et al.*, 1972; Lampman *et al.*, 1977, 1980; Garman, 1978; Huttunen *et al.*, 1979; Wood & Haskell, 1979; Lopez *et al.*, 1974; Hartung *et al.*, 1981; Wood *et al.*, 1983; Hartung, 1984).

The following effects can be expected:

1 VLDL (very low-density lipoproteins): Medium-intensity aerobic training even if only performed for a few weeks is capable of reducing the plasma concentrations of VLDL and of the triglycerides. These effects have been seen both in subjects with normal levels of plasma lipoproteins and in subjects with type IV hyperlipoproteinaemia. The effects of exercise seem to be the activation of the enzyme lipoproteinlipase, which is present in type I muscular fibres and in the myocardium. This enzyme is responsible for the hydrolysis of the triglycerides. It also seems that exercise increases the storage of this enzyme in the muscle fibres. There is also a drop in the hepatic production of VLDL due to a reduction of the precursors in the plasma.

2 LDL: Exercise results in a reduction of LDL and cholesterol which occurs both in normolipaemic subjects and also in hyperlipoproteinaemic subjects (type IIa). To achieve this effect it is necessary to follow a medium- or high-intensity training programme for at least 2 months. LDL derives from the hydrolysis of VLDL and therefore reduction can depend on a lower conversion of VLDL or on an increased catabolism of LDL.

3 HDL: Exercise results in an increased plasma concentration of HDL and cholesterol (transported by the HDL). This is seen in normal subjects and also in hyperlipoproteinaemic subjects (types II and IV).

Table 11.3.7   Effects of training on plasma lipoproteins and lipids (Hartung, 1984).

	Cross-sectional studies		Longitudinal studies	
	Men	Women	Men	Women
Total cholesterol	↓ /≈	↓ /≈	↓ /≈	↓ /≈
Triglycerides	↓	↓	↓	↓
LDL	↓	↓	↓	↓
HDL	↑	↑	↑	↑ /≈

↓ = decrease; ↑ = increase; ≈ = approx. constant.

The effects seem to be positively correlated to the variations in aerobic power ($\dot{V}O_{2\ max}$) and also with the intensity and duration of the training programme and seem to be inversely proportioned to the initial levels of HDL. Data on the subfractions of HDL (HDL_2 and HDL_3) are still limited but they indicate that aerobic exercise increases HDL_2 (which is inversely correlated to atherosclerosis) and reduces HDL_3.

Conclusion A summary of the effects of exercise on plasma lipoproteins is presented in Table 11.3.7. The modifications of the plasma lipoproteins mentioned above seem to depend directly on the type of sports activity rather than on a reduction of body fat, bodyweight or a reduced caloric intake. Therefore, physical activity is strongly recommended in the treatment of hyperlipoproteinaemias in association with pharmacological and dietological treatment (Lampman *et al.*, 1977, 1980; Hartung, 1984).

In type IIa, IIb and IV hyperlipoproteinaemias, engaging in an aerobic training programme is probably the best method of treatment and prevention. In these types of hyperlipoproteinaemias exercise has been shown to normalize (in moderate cases) the anomalous lipoproteic profile.

By adding a suitable diet the results can be improved even further (Table 11.3.8). The major points that should be taken into account when prescribing a diet (Connor & Connor, 1977; Hartung, 1984) are:

1　A reduced intake of lipids (less than 30% of total calories).
2　Cholesterol intake lower than 300 mg/day.
3　Partial substitution of saturated fats with polyunsaturated ones, so that the polyunsaturated : saturated ratio is lower than 0.80, or better still 1.

Alcohol in small amounts will raise the level of HDL, just as physical activity will, but this method is not suggested because of the side effects that can arise. The association of physical activity and a hypolipidic diet is important since it maintains a high level of HDL which would otherwise tend to be low.

Table 11.3.8 Effects of diet on plasma lipoproteins and lipids.

	Increase in fat	Decrease in cholesterol	Decrease in P/S	Alcohol
Total cholesterol	↑	↓ /≈	↓ /≈	≈
Triglycerides	↓ /≈	≈	↓	↑
HDL	↓ /≈	↓ /≈	≈	↑
LDL	↓	↓	↓	↓

P/S = polyunsaturated/saturated (fatty acid ratio); ↓ = decrease; ↑ = increase; ≈ = approx. constant.

Physical activity in the therapy and prevention of diabetes mellitus

Diabetes mellitus is characterized by an altered utilization of glucose by the body tissues, due to an insufficient activity of the hormone insulin. This can be brought about by low levels of this hormone (non-insulin-dependent diabetes mellitus, NIDDM) or by its complete absence (insulin-dependent diabetes mellitus, IDDM). Since it is a metabolic disease, the alterations caused by diabetes can involve any organ or tissue. These alterations can be directly related to various causes, such as hyper-glycaemia and to alterations due to metabolites produced as a result of the insulin deficiency, as well as other disorders.

The therapy for diabetes mellitus is aimed at the normalization of some of the altered haematochemical parameters, such as the blood glucose level that has a very restricted range from 50 to 170 mg% (the lowest values are recorded during fasting, whilst the highest values are recorded after a meal). The therapy is based on three major points:

1   Diet.
2   Antidiabetic drugs (oral drugs and insulin).
3   Physical activity.

Physical activity is probably the most important factor in the therapy of IDDM and in the prevention of NIDDM. In the first case, physical activity is very important since diabetes often starts in young subjects, especially prepubertal children and adolescents, where physical activity plays a dominant role (Caldarone, 1984).

Insulin mainly affects the liver, adipose tissue and muscular tissue. In the liver, insulin activates many enzymes which take part in the meta-bolism of sugars. In the muscle cells and adipose tissue, insulin mediates the entrance of glucose into the cells. It also stimulates the enzyme phosphofructokinase in the muscle cells, which encourages glycolysis, and glycogen-synthase, which is an enzyme necessary in the formation of glycogen (Holloszy, 1977; Benzi, 1985). An active muscular tissue requires more sugars to produce energy. Sugars are present in excess in the diabetic patient because of the fact that insulin helps in transporting glucose into these cells.

Therefore, physical activity enhances the glycidic metabolism that in the diabetic patient is low and insufficient. It also reduces the blood glucose level, whereas sedentarism has the opposite effect since it increases the need for insulin (Leon et al., 1979). From a metabolic point of view, exercise increases the hepatic production of glucose but it also increases the captation of glucose by the muscle cell. Studies have shown that physical activity increases by more than 30% the sensibility of the muscle cells to insulin, due to an increased number of insulin receptors on the cell membrane (Archer *et al.*, 1973; Bar, 1976; Soman *et al.*, 1978; Koivisto *et al.*, 1980). Exercise also has a preventive effect on vascular complications of diabetes.

In the past it was thought that the metabolic damage caused by insular pancreatic insufficiency was incompatible with any type of physical activity. More recently, however, it has been found that not only can the diabetic subject tolerate intense muscular workloads but that he/she can also, through a well planned and continuous training programme, obtain a more stable and efficient metabolic equilibrium. IDDM can result in different metabolic responses, which vary from subject to subject, and therefore the diet regimen for each patient has to be personalized and continuously modified; the same must apply to the training programme.

In short-lived and intense muscular activity the energy required is produced by high-energy substrates which are already present in the muscular cell. If physical activity is prolonged, regardless of intensity and rhythm, then the energy substrates must reach the muscle cell via the bloodstream. In this case the glucose present in the bloodstream, produced by hepatic glycogenolysis, and the NEFA deriving from lipolysis, represent the energy substrates. Therefore prolonged muscular activity, even if at a submaximal level, is able to metabolize glucose and fatty acids which derive from storage tissues.

NIDDM is commonly seen in sedentary subjects, who are very often overweight and with a constitutional tendency towards hyperglycaemia. Of all the various aetiologies in the onset of NIDDM, probably the most common is the lack of exercise. This can lower the tolerance to the elevated carbohydrate load; it can also indirectly lead to NIDDM since it enhances the onset of other metabolic disorders such as obesity and altered lipid metabolism (Venerando, 1980). So moderate, continuous and prolonged exercise is a sure prevention in the eventual onset of hyperglycaemic syndromes in adult and senile subjects.

However the general statement that the diabetic patient derives beneficial effects from the practice of some type of physical activity is not sufficient to establish who are the subjects that need to take part in a training programme and also those who can take part in it. It also does not indicate the rate, rhythm, intensity and type of physical activity that has to be prescribed. In diabetes, as in other diseases, physical activity must be prescribed just as any other type of therapy (Gibson, 1983; Hage, 1983; Caldarone & Giampietro, 1985). For this, it is necessary to establish the quantity and type of physical activity which is suitable, taking into account the type of diabetic patient (i.e. IDDM patients, metabolically compensated or uncompensated, or NIDDM patients). Physical activity should only be prescribed in metabolically-compensated diabetics, those who are not in this situation should be compensated, via a diet and/or associated drugs. IDDM and NIDDM patients, provided that they are well compensated, should take part in some type of physical activity once they have undergone a thorough medical and instrumental check-up. This check-up is necessary to evaluate the pathological condition of the subject and also his/her residual physical capacities. From these results it is possible to prescribe a personalized training programme.

Young diabetics can start a training programme having first undergone a general reconditioning programme, i.e. callisthenics and short running routines. After that the patient should carry out circuit training at low or medium intensity, at a continuous rate, with short resting periods and with a continuous change of the exercises. This develops both the musculoskeletal and cardiovascular systems. At this point the subject can choose the sports activity that he/she prefers and that suits his/her anthropometric characteristics the best (Chiumello, 1978; Caldarone, 1984).

Sports activities that require a massive and rapid muscular demand are proscribed (e.g. any type of sprinting activity—running, swimming, roller skating, etc.). Even skill sports activities that require a considerable muscular demand must be proscribed (e.g. gymnastics, ice skating, fencing, tennis and Alpine skiing). Other skill activities that have to be proscribed, even if the muscular component is not very demanding, are motor and car racing, sailing and windsurfing; one can prescribe horse riding, golf, target shooting and archery. Even in this last group of exercises the same principle applies; that the patient must at the same time take part in some type of aerobic activity (i.e. jogging, walking, cycling, etc.). Young diabetics can perform, with absolute safety, sports activities demanding continuous muscular activity, even if prolonged, as long as the exercise is submaximal. These are the characteristics of endurance sports such as running, marching, cycling, roller skating, swimming and cross-country skiing. Of the various physical activities that are not classified as sports activities but that are very popular we suggest jogging and aerobics. Team sports are also popular, and have alternating aerobic and anaerobic metabolism. If the actual training programme of some of these team sports is carefully considered, then some of these can be practised by young diabetics (e.g. football, basketball and handball).

Adult diabetics, once they have undergone a thorough medical and instrumental check-up, can also take part in various types of sports activities but only after a long reconditioning period. A prolonged sedentary life-style will have produced a number of problems and functional limitations which are characteristic of 'non-use' (Bloom & Eidew, 1967; Milvy *et al.*, 1977). Particular care must be taken in exercises that involve the upper and lower limbs and the vertebral column. These exercises must initially be callisthenic and eventually be done with equipment that can help the articulations (e.g. small dumbells). These will then have to be alternated with exercises that utilize moderate workloads so that the antigravitational effects can induce adequate muscular adaptations.

Even in this phase one has to respect the two fundamental characteristics of muscular work in the diabetic subject; these are a rhythmical progression of the workloads and continuity. At this point one can prescribe a sports activity which will, necessarily, have to be limited. The sports activities that older diabetics can take part in are those known as endurance ones. Long-distance running is probably the number one choice, since it can be easily programmed for duration, intensity and rhythm, it can be performed without the need of particular structures, at any time, in any climatic conditions and on any surface. Road cycling, long-distance swimming and cross-country skiing are valid alternatives.

References

American College of Sports Medicine (1980) *Guidelines of Graded Exercise Testing and Exercise Prescription*, 2nd edn. Lea & Febiger, Philadelphia.

Anderson, B. (1984) *Stretching*. Shelter Publications, Bolinas, CA.

Archer, J. A., Gorden, P. & Gavin, I. R. (1973) Insulin receptor in human circulating lymphocytes: application to the study of insulin resistance in man. *J. Clin. Endocrinol. Metab.* **36**, 627.

Bar, R. S. (1976) Fluctuations in affinity and concentration of insulin receptors on circulating monocytes of obese patients. *J. Clin. Invest.* **58**, 1123.

Benzi, G. (1985) *Mitochondrial enzyme adaptation to endurance*. Center for study and research, F.I.D.A.L., Rome.

Bjorntorp, P., De Jounge, K., Krottieswski, M., Sullivan, L., Sjöstrom, L. & Stenberg, J. (1973) Physical training in human obesity. III. Effects of long term physical training on body composition. *Metabolism* **22**, 1467.

Bjorntorp, P., Sjöstrom, L. & Sullivan, L. (1978) The role of physical exercise in the management of obesity. In J. F. Munro (ed) *The Treatment of Obesity*. M.T.P. Presslim.

Bloom, W. L. & Eidew, M. F. (1967) Inactivity as a major factor in adult obesity. *Metabolism* **16**, 679.

Boileau, R. A., Buskirk, E. R., Horstman, D. H., Mendez, J. & Nicholas, W. C. (1971) Body composition changes in obese and lean men during physical conditioning. *Med. Sci. Sports* **3**, 183.

Bronwell, K. & Stunkard, A. (1980) Physical activity in the development and control of obesity. In A. Stunkard (ed) *Obesity*, p. 300. W. B. Saunders, Philadelphia.

Caldarone, G. (1984) L'attività fisica. *Il Diabete Eubiotica* **38**, pp. 41–43. Eubiotica Publ., Torino.

Caldarone, G. & Giampietro, M. (1985) L'attività fisica nel trattamento dell'obesità. *Med. Sport* **38**, 365.

Chiumello, G. (1978) L'attività fisico-sportiva nella prevenzione e terapia dell'obesità a del diabete in fantile. *Med. Sport* **31**, 151.

Connor, W. E. & Connor, S. L. (1977) Dietary treatment of hyperlipidemia. In B. M. Rifkind & R. I.

Levy (eds) *Hyperlipidemia: Diagnosis and Therapy*. Grune & Stratton, New York.

Foss, L. M., Lampman, R. M. & Schteingart, D. (1976) Physical training program for rehabilitating extremely obese patients. *Arch. Phys. Med. Rehabil.* **57**, 425.

Fredrickson, D. L., Levy, R. I. & Lees, R. S. (1967). Fat transport in lipoproteins: an integrated approach to mechanism and disorders. *New Engl. J. Med.*, **276**, 32.

Garman, J. F. (1978) Coronary risk factor intervention—a review of physical activity and serum lipids. *Am. Correct. Ther. J.* **32**, 183.

Gibson, S. B., Gerberich, S. G. & Leon, A. S. (1983) Writing the exercise prescription: an individualized approach. *Phys. Sports Med.* **11**, 87.

Gwinupp, G. M. D. (1975) Effect of exercise alone on the weight of obese woman. *Arch. Intern. Med.* **135**, 667.

Hage, P. (1983) Prescribing exercise: more than just a running program. *Phys. Sports Med.* **11**, 123.

Hartung, G. H., Squires, W. G., Gotto jr, A. M. (1981) Effect of exercise training on plasma high-density lipoprotein cholesterol in coronary disease patients. *Am. Heart J.* **101**, 181.

Hartung, G. H. (1984) Diet and exercise in the regulation of plasma lipids and lipoproteins in patients at risk of coronary disease. *Sports Med.* **1**, 413.

Holloszy, J. O. (1977) Biochemical adaptation in muscle. Effects of exercise in mitochondrial oxygen uptake and respiratory enzyme activity in skeletal muscle. *J. Biol. Chem.* **242**, 2278.

Huttunen, J. K., Länsimies, E., Voutilainen, E., Ehnholm, C., Hietanen, E., Penttilä, I., Siitonen, O. & Rauramaa, R. (1979) Effect of moderate physical exercise on serum lipoproteins: a controlled clinical trial with special reference to serum high density lipoproteins. *Circulation* **60**, 1220.

Koivisto, V. A., Soman, V. R. & Felig, P. (1980) Effects of acute exercise on insulin binding to monocytes in obesity. *Metabolism* **29**, 168.

Kukkonen, K., Rauramaa, R., Siitonen, O. & Hanninen, O. (1982) Physical training of obese middle-aged persons. *Ann. Clin. Res.* **14**, 80.

Lampman, R. M., Santinga, J. T., Bassett, D. R., Mercer, N., Flora, J. D., Foss jr, M. L. & Thorald, N. G. (1978) Effectiveness of unsupervised and supervised high intensity physical training in normalizing serum lipids in men with type IV hyperlipoproteinemia. *Circulation* **57**, 172.

Lampman, R. M., Santinga, J. T., Bassett, D. R., Mercer, N., Flora, J. D., Foss jr, M. L. & Thorald,

N. G. (1980) Type IV hyperlipoproteinemia: effects of a caloric restricted type IV diet versus physical training plus isocaloric type IV diet. *Am. J. Clin. Nutr.* **33**, 1233.

Lampman, R. M., Santinga, J. T., Hodge, M. F., Block, W. D., Flora, J. D. & Bassett, D. R. (1977). Comparative effects of physical training and diet in normalizing serum lipids in men with type IV hyperlipoproteinemia. *Circulation* **55**, 652.

Leon, A. S., Conrad, J., Hunninghake, D. B. & Serfass, R. (1979) Effect of vigorous walking program on body composition and carbohydrate and lipid metabolism of obese young men. *Am. J. Clin. Nutr.* **32**, 1766.

Lewis, S., Haskill, W. L., Wood, P. D., Manoogian, N., Bailey, J. E. & Pereira, M. (1976) Effects of physical activity on weight reduction in obese middle-aged women. *Amer. J. Clin. Nutr.* **29**, 151.

Lopez, S. A., Vial, R., Balart, L. & Azzoyave, G. (1974) Effects of exercise and physical fitness on serum lipids and lipoproteins. *Atherosclerosis* **20**, 1.

Milvy, P., Forbes, W. F. & Brown, K. S. (1977) A critical review of epidemiological studies of physical activity. *Ann. NY Acad. Sci.* **301**, 519.

Moody, D. L., Kollias, J. & Buskirk, E. R. (1969) Evaluation of aerobic capacity in lean and obese women with four test procedures. *J. Sports Med. Phys. Fitness* **9**, 1.

Oja, P. (1983) Comparison of the physiological effects of different forms of physical activity. *Finnish Sport Exerc. Med.* **2**, 62.

Oscai, L. B. (1973) Role of exercise in weight control. In J. H. Wilmore (ed) *Exercise and Sport in Science Reviews*, Vol. 1, p. 103. Academic Press, New York.

Oscai, L. B., Patterson, J. A., Bogard, D. L., Beck, R. J. & Rothermel, B. L. (1972) Normalization of serum triglycerides and lipoprotein electrophoretic patterns by exercise. *Am. J. Cardiol.* **30**, 775.

Pelliccia, A., Daniele, G., Giampietro, M. & Caffarini, G. (1983) Effetti medico-preventivi dell'esercizio fisico e sportivo di tipo prevalentements aerobico. *Med. Sport* **36**, 127.

Schuster, K. (1983) Aerobic dance, a step to fitness. *Phys. Sports Med.* **7**, 98.

Soman, V. R., Koivisto, V. A. & Grantham, P. (1978) Increased insulin binding to monocytes after exercise in normal man. *J. Clin. Endocrinol. Metab.* **47**, 216.

Stunkard, A. J. (1983) Physical activity and obesity. *Finnish Sports Exerc. Med.* **2**, 99.

Thompson, J. K., Jarvie, G. & Laney, B. (1982) Exercise and obesity: etiology, physiology and intervention. *Psychol. Bull.* **91**, 55.

Venerando, A. (1980) L'attività fisica nel trattamento dell'obesità. In *Obesità*, p. 357. S.E.U. Publ., Rome.

Wilmore, J. H., Davis, J. A., O'Brien, R. S. & Vodak, P. A. (1980) Physiological alterations consequent to 20 week conditioning programs of bicycling, tennis and jogging. *Med. Sci. Sports Exerc.* **12**, 1.

Wood, P. D. & Haskell, W. L. (1979) The effect of exercise on plasma high density lipoproteins. *Lipids* **14**, 417.

Wood, P. D., Haskell, W. L. & Blair, S. N. (1983) Increased exercise level and plasma lipoprotein concentration: a one year, randomized, controlled study in sedentary, middle-aged men. *Metabolism* **32**, 31.

PART 12

MEDICAL CARE OF SPORTS TEAMS

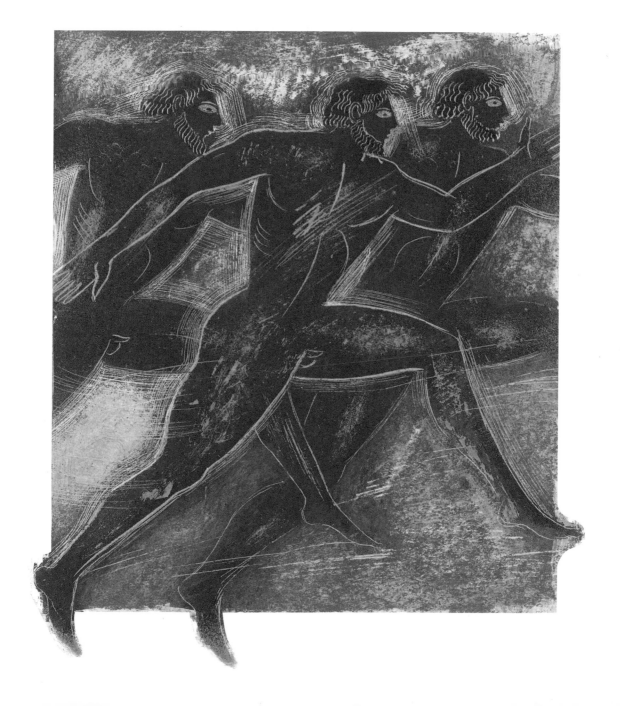

12.1 Relationships between athlete, physician, trainer and coach

D. HANNEMANN

Introduction

For all sportspeople under regular training and competition, basic sports fitness and medical assessments and preventive check-ups two to three times a year are an important precondition of sporting activities. Besides checking the general state of health (complete clinical status), the functioning of the following should also be checked:

1 Cardiovascular and respiratory systems.
2 Renal and urinary systems.
3 Metabolic system.
4 Locomotor system.
5 Central nervous system.

These are assessed by means of medical parameters, including prophylactic inoculations if required (e.g. tetanus) and special examinations (X-ray, etc.). In the course of this regular medical care the sports physician simultaneously has an influence on the way of life, on food habits and on suitable clothing. He or she advises athletes and coaches on medical aspects of training which should be observed. This clinico-medical activity is largely of a prophylactic character (i.e. healthy people receiving medical care) and includes the following three fields:

1 The determination of physical powers and maximum stress. This concerns both the human organism as a whole and the individual organic and functional systems. As a clinical task, it is prevailingly a diagnosis of the condition of the athlete and part of the subjective responsibility of the physician. The collection and evaluation of function–physiological, biophysical, biochemical and other parameters, the inclusion of pathophysiological or pathomorphological findings and the problems of the general environment and of the way of life make up the main pillars of this complex medical assessment. Analogously to clinical practice, the sports medical check-up and assessment of maximum stress requires a necessary range of clinical and paraclinical, if possible

non-invasive, methods of examination which enable the physician not only to differentiate between healthy and ill, but to define qualitative performance properties of single functional systems.

2 The effect achieved by the physician is decisively determined by how far it is possible to include the medical findings into the training process. Therefore it is necessary that the physician observes the training programme and exchanges results with the coach and the physiotherapist. For important competitions, the attending physician should apply and implement rules of general hygiene to cope with the stress and living regimen. At the same time, together with the masseur and physiotherapist, he or she ensures that preparation for the competition and recovery after the competition are carried out properly.

3 Medical care for possibly occurring injuries and diseases. This requires a close cooperation between various special branches (traumatology, internal medicine, surgery, radiology, etc.) in order to combine the latest knowledge of clinical practice with the existing sports-specific practices for the rapid curing and recovery of the athlete.

Cooperation between athlete, physician and coach

In the course of training the coach has the most intensive contact with the athlete. Besides the training activities, he or she observes and takes note of the physical and mental condition of the athlete. Important knowledge of the reaction and behaviour of the athlete in regular and special situations is thus gained. During longer periods of training, in training camps and at important contests the presence of the sports physician/ team physician is desirable. It is important to pay attention to the state of health of the athlete, to fatigue and overstrain symptoms, as well as to hygiene behaviour and a proper diet. Together with the coach the sports physician influences the proper ratio of strain and recovery.

Medical check-ups before competitions

According to the competition rules of different sports federations and organizations of the IOC, basic medical examinations and check-ups are necessary for athletes under regular training and involved in competitions; these have to be entered in the starting booklets or in the membership cards. In some kinds of sport (e.g. boxing, wrestling) medical check-ups immediately before the competition are compulsory. The coach has to take care that all the athletes undergo these compulsory medical examinations. Special aspects of the check-ups are usually fixed in the competition rules of the particular sports federation.

Cooperation in the training process

As mentioned above, regular basic and preventive check-ups make up the cornerstones of the medical observations of the athlete. The results of the examinations will be explained to the athlete and evaluated with the coach. Possible consequences for the organization of the training programme will be worked out. Of special importance are the careful therapy and rehabilitation of infectious diseases, in particular influenzal infections. In these cases check-ups at short intervals (two to three times a week) and observation of strain including control of the cardiovascular response and a continuous evaluation should be carried out in conjunction with the coach. A similar thorough and concerted approach is required by both the physician and coach in, for example, juvenile osteochondrosis which is fairly frequently found in young athletes. Under strict observance of the functional consequences of the training by the coach and with reliable medical supervision, the further sporting career of the affected young athlete may often be maintained; however the first consideration is to ensure the functioning of the axial organ.

Using regular check-ups, considered as longitudinal studies in connection with knowledge of the specific structure of the movements, the sports physician will obtain a very detailed picture of the physically strong and weak points of the individual athlete. In the last 10 years, increasing cooperation has been seen between coach, trainer, physician and masseur prior to planning the long-term training of top athletes, in order to preserve the health of the athlete and reach best training results as a single unit. The results of the sports medical examinations are directly connected with the methodical knowledge and experience of the trainer in the organization of a training aimed at preserving and promoting health and at developing highest performance capacities. If this cooperation takes place where the training is carried out, the sports physician can simultaneously use his or her skills to exert influence on a physiologically reasonable preparation for training (warming up, stretching, contraction), and on proper behaviour by the athlete between training elements and on consequent training follow-up.

12.2 Safety and hygiene in sport

P. N. SPERRYN

Safety in sport

The player Players and spectators need protection. Selection and proper training, correct clothing and equipment and attention to event safety protect the competitor and are reinforced by fair but strict application of the rules. Spectators should expect protection from dangerous equipment and behaviour.

Selection Fair sport depends on fair matching of opponents. Athletes should ideally be selected into suitable events and out of inappropriate ones. The physiques best suited to the different disciplines are well established and the young hopeful can be encouraged to pursue sports which give the best chance of good achievement and thereby also minimize the risk of event-related injury. Many sports injuries are caused by unsuitable activity for an individual, e.g. gymnastics for a heavily built or stiff-limbed child, or heavy weight lifting by a weak or slender boy.

Age and size groups in each sport should be kept under review to avoid unfair and potentially dangerous mismatching, especially in contact sport where forceful impact between mature and immature bodies increases injury risk.

Screening, medication and doping Medical screening should detect ill-health and injuries which undermine the athlete's health and safety in training and competition. Implementation of screening programmes depends on local resources, but chronic neglected injuries are common in all athletes and conditions such as anaemia are frequently overlooked as causes of poor performance, especially in females.

Medical examinations may lead to treatment. Care should be taken to ensure that any medication prescribed does not infringe current doping regulations. The physician should be familiar with any side effects of medicines which may impair or even endanger the athlete's performance. Screening is an appropriate time for educating the athlete and his or her coach on the dangers of doping, and random or routine dope tests can be undertaken.

Equipment **1** *Clothing* should be chosen for comfort and efficiency, considering climate as well as any protective functions. Cotton's sweat absorbency is superior to synthetic fibres in hot or humid conditions. Well-ventilated outfits help to prevent heat-stroke, especially where requirements of protection conflict with the need for heat loss, e.g. fencing, American football. White uniforms help to reflect heat in a bright hot climate.

2 *Protective padding* can add a considerable burden to the hot athlete's sweat mechanisms and should always be designed with light weight and ventilation in mind.

3 *Safety helmets* increased the risks of neck injury until sports doctors recognized this and redesigned new models. Helmets must not only be worn in risk sports, but must be firmly attached to the head—the high incidence of head and neck injury in horse riding is an example of neglecting these precautions. Doctors should consider their moral obligation to draw the attention of legislators to such public safety measures.

4 *Footwear* has been the subject of much development and even more promotion in the decade since mass running emerged as a population-wide sport. Education is greatly needed—of makers no less than athletes—to prevent the high incidence of foot injury due to poorly fitting shoes and such dangerous design features as the high firm heel-tabs formerly described as 'Achilles protecting' but in reality frequently the cause of friction lesions of the Achilles tendon. Simple excision of this tab prevents further friction. Shoes are the vital interface between the athlete and the environment and different surfaces call for different soles, studs or spikes as well as different materials in order to prevent the athlete slipping or falling during the event.

5 *Sports surfaces* are important in injury prevention, especially in their resilience, traction and stability. The design and construction of landing pits and mattresses is crucial to safety in gymnastics and jumping events. The maintenance and supervision of trampolines, with provision of 'catchers', is essential in prevention of spinal injury.

Each type of surface presents a different challenge to the athlete and, in addition to footwear changes to compensate for ground variations, the athlete has to make slight event technique alterations to accommodate to changing foot–surface interaction. Injury easily follows misjudgements and enough time should be given to allow full adjustment to a new surface.

Wound infection can occur on grass pitches and the danger of tetanus means that all athletes (and indeed all citizens) should be routinely inoculated with tetanus toxoid. This can be incorporated into the screening and continuing medical care of athletes. Synthetic turf causes troublesome friction burns and appropriate clothing gives some protection. Less appreciated is the fact that the low-level microclimate in synthetic turf arenas may be extremely hot—to the point of endangering the player through hyperthermia. Playing uniforms should be chosen to match this environmental stress.

6 *Implements,* such as javelins, discoi, hammers and cricket balls still kill athletes; even shoe spikes (cleats) can cause severe injury. This can be avoided through the rigid application of event discipline in each sport, together with the provision and correct maintenance of throwing cages and similar protective devices in the arena.

The severity of contact injury is reduced by protective clothing and padding appropriate for each sport. Young players should be made to become completely accustomed to wearing such items and any bravado in playing without proper protection should be strongly discouraged. Public education may be necessary to encourage the wearing of specific items such as, for example, eye-goggles in squash, where there is an ever-present danger of the flexible small rubber ball entering the orbit to destroy the globe. Helmets and goggles are required in, for example, cricket and ice hockey and in the latter, the spectators must be protected by screens of adequate height to avoid the chance of the puck flying out of play into the crowd.

7 *Vehicles* can kill spectators and participants in motor sports. Anti-roll bars and safety harnesses in the vehicle must be effective and crash

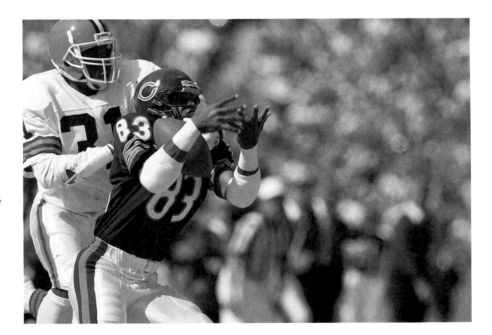

Fig. 12.2.1 Injuries can be curtailed and even prevented in many contact sports but complete safety cannot be guaranteed in a collision sport such as American football despite wearing the correct protective clothing. Courtesy of Ace Photo Agency.

barriers provided at the track. Spectators must be be kept away from the track in rally events. Motor cycles are frequently instruments of death, but racing dangers can be minimized by safety barriers, crowd control, helmets and padding, and especially cancellation of events in dangerous track conditions such as ice, rain, and surface mud or oil.

8 *Horses* can kill by kicking or throwing. Helmets (*vide supra*) and adequate fencing are essential safety measures.

Event safety   In addition to adequate protective cages and fencing, event discipline should limit the number of people in the arena at any time. Officials and competitors should be allowed onto the field or track only for their actual competition. Overcrowded tracks, swarming with casual observers and inattentive bystanders make it difficult to control safety in throwing events (and obstruct vision). Adequate barriers between crowds and participants are sometimes essential, whether in games like soccer or at boxing contests, where spectators may hurl missiles (e.g. bottles and cans) at the competitors.

Climatic conditions   Unduly, hot, cold or humid weather can endanger the competitor. The physiological aspects are dealt with elsewhere (Parts 2–5), but the organizational aspects of competition are often unsympathetic to athletes, a tendency which seems to be worsening with increasing commercial pressures imposed by the media at major events. For instance, severe endurance events like marathons should be held at the safest time of day to protect the runners, regardless of television convenience. It is highly debatable whether some such events should be held at all at some venues, e.g. at altitude, in view of the grave physiological disadvantage (not fully mitigable by acclimatization) imposed on many individuals.

Rules and enforcement   Foul play increases the rate and severity of sports injuries. The rules are designed to ensure fair and safe competition. Referees and judges must be trained to be impartial and implement firmly the rules in all circumstances. Proper punishment must be enforced if players are to respect and observe the rules and this applies to suspension for foul play as much as to life suspension for cheating by doping.

Incidentally, it should be recognized that many referees are themselves at risk in sport because of their poor personal health. Medical care and screening is appropriate in their selection too!

The spectator   Stadium collapse and major fires have occurred and public safety dictates that all spectators must be able to rapidly vacate any public arena. The necessary design features are best incorporated into public building legislation.

Stadia may lack easy direct access for rescue vehicles and attendants to reach sick or injured persons or to transport them rapidly to safety. Organizers of public events should check their legal liability in such cases and seek to mitigate danger by well-drilled rehearsals or emergency procedures. The provision of trained first aid attendants is also essential for both player and spectator safety.

Crowd control and discipline has become a major problem throughout the world and poses political and public order problems outside the scope of this work. However, such features as the design and placing of barriers and strong partitions within crowd spaces, entry control and alcohol restrictions all have an important part to play in keeping sport safe.

Hygiene in sport

Infections Bacterial infections are common in the young and in sport. Crowded conditions encourage the spread of staphylococcal and streptococcal infections, enteritis and 'traveller's diarrhoea'. These call for the provision of adequate clean space for living and changing accommodation. Control of cooking and serving conditions and provision of clean drinking water are minimum requirements. Travelling athletes should be taught to avoid uncooked foods, unclean or unbottled drinks, ice cream, salads and unpeeled fruits, the common causes of diarrhoea. Cholera vaccine is indicated in certain areas and team managers must check inoculation requirements before team departure. The use of prophylactic medication against diarrhoea is at least highly controversial and discouraged by the majority of medical authorities. Antibiotics themselves often cause diarrhoea as well as allergic reactions and should be reserved for actual illness.

Venereal infections are common in the young and sexually active population and athletes should be educated accordingly as well as being treated promptly and effectively.

Fungal infections are also common, notably the epidermophytoses causing athletes' foot or inguinocrural infection (tinea pedis, tinea cruris). Early diagnosis is simple and effective and a prime aim of medical screening. Cross infection through clothing, towels and floors has to be prevented by cleansing floors, baths and showers with suitable disinfectants (e.g. hypochlorite), using shoes and slippers in public facilities rather than bare feet, and treatment with antifungal creams (e.g. benzoic acid compound ointment, salicylic and benzoic acids in wax—Whitfield's ointment) or powders (e.g. chlorphenesin or zinc undecenoate), using the latter also for preventive dusting of feet and footwear.

Viral infections range from influenza, through warts and verrucae to hepatitis and now AIDS. Planned immunization against common infections is a universal public health aim, but it is worth remembering that susceptibility to common infections varies greatly around the world. Some travelling athletes may be unexpectedly vulnerable to infections considered minor in distant populations, hence the importance of planned immunization as a part of the long-term medical care of athletes.

Warts and verrucae need medical treatment as well as public health control by cleansing of public living, washing and swimming facilities. Walking in bare feet helps to spread these infections and those infected should use coverings approved by their doctors or by temporary withdrawal from public facilities.

AIDS has become the cause of much ill-informed panic. It is scientifically established that swimming pools, showers and changing rooms do not, *per se*, spread AIDS. The AIDS virus is fragile, does not long survive outside the body and is also highly vulnerable to any standard pool disinfectant such as ozone or chlorine.

Inoculations These are essential (*vide supra*). Tetanus immunization should be mandatory. Local public health legislation varies and should be checked in advance of any planned travel so that athletes have time to recover from the often unsettling discomforts of inoculations.

12.3 Medical examination of athletes

R. LEACH

Routine physical examinations of athletes are time consuming and may be costly. Therefore, if such physical examinations are to be performed there must be very good reasons for so doing, and examinations should be done in the most efficient and fruitful manner possible.

The reasons for doing physical examinations of athletes are straightforward. It must be determined if there is any physical defect or condition which would jeopardize an athlete playing a particular sport. There is a great deal of self-selection in athletics in the sense that most athletes who play a particular sport are healthy and have the physical attributes that allow them to play that sport, particularly at the higher levels. At the lower levels this is not necessarily true. People who are chronically ill are less likely to participate in sports. People who have physical defects which would adversely affect their performance or their pleasure are also less likely to participate in sports.

Medical problems   There are, however, a number of medical conditions which individuals may unknowingly have and which might surface under certain athletic or stressful situations. There are other medical conditions which could be well known to the athlete and which for reasons of their own, the athlete might either ignore or even hide from coaches, team mates and physicians. Exercise-induced bronchitis is an example of a condition which may cause symptoms under the stress of athletic performance but would not greatly interfere with normal living. A person with this condition might not recognize the fact that it exists or that it is a particular problem until the time of athletic performance at which point the health of that person and the performance of the sport would be adversely affected. Another condition which may exist without that individual being aware of it is Marfan's syndrome. Many people with Marfan's syndrome, because of their particular body build, are likely candidates for sports such as basketball, volleyball, etc., which benefit from a person being tall. These sports may put stress on the cardiovascular system of a person with Marfan's syndrome which could have severe adverse effects on that person's health. Some young athletes, particularly those who are beginning sports may have conditions that are well known to them, such as allergies, diabetes or even a gastrointestinal ulcer and may be dealing with it well in their normal life, but athletic performance may cause a problem. In other instances the athlete may, for their own peculiar reasons, not want people to be aware of these conditions. A routine physical examination and the all-important history should pick up such physical problems.

New conditions may arise during the course of an athletic career which need treatment. Serious illnesses such as Hodgkin's disease and diabetes mellitus can be picked up as the result of a routine physical examination of an athlete prior to a major competition. Athletes having a physical or mental condition which is well controlled in normal life, may have a problem during the stress of a long or particularly competitive athletic season, particularly before a major athletic event such as the Olympic Games. Certain conditions are sometimes seen in particular athletic populations. Weight control is a major problem for sports such as wrestling, gymnastics and figure skating. The conditions of anorexia nervosa and bulimia are seen in athletes who perform in those sports. A properly performed interval history should elicit enough information to lead to the proper diagnosis, and physical examinations also performed at appropriate intervals will allow abnormal weight changes to be picked up.

Confidence between athlete and physician

One other excellent reason for doing a physical examination is to allow the physician and the athlete to become acquainted, even if it is only on a relatively limited time basis. In this fast-paced world and in the world of athletics, injuries happen all too often and very quickly. For an athlete, it is particularly frightening to have an injury because of the fear of being so severely hurt that their career is threatened. It is a source of some solace to an athlete or a team to have a physician who is personally known. The physical examination allows an opportunity for the physician to talk with an athlete and, in some instances, to discuss a problem which the athlete has been worried about. There can be a build-up of confidence which can be very valuable over the course of a competition or a season. The further away from home the athlete is, the more likely he or she is to want to have a doctor with whom they are acquainted. Virtually all sports teams have new competitors coming to them each year, and the routine physical examination gives the first opportunity for these athletes to meet the physician and trainers who will be responsible for their medical care.

Frequency of examination

Which athletes should have physical examinations, and whose responsibility is it to perform such an examination? Millions of children and adults throughout the world play sports on an unorganized basis and their health is the responsibility of their parents or of themselves. However, when a child or an adult participates in organized sporting activities under the leadership or auspices of a team, federation, university, etc., some of the responsibility for that athlete's health is taken by the organization. It would seem reasonable that all athletes upon entry into a particular sporting group should have a physical examination by a physician responsible to that organization or by the athlete's own physician with a report of that examination going to the organization.

The American Medical Association has in recent years acknowledged that a complete physical examination each year for healthy people is not an efficient use of time and effort for either the patient or the physician. People who are playing sports are generally in a healthy state and thus one would not normally expect to pick up many illnesses in such a group. Most physicians who are associated with a team will not have the time nor the facilities to do as complete a physical examination as an internal medicine specialist might do, or as complete a medical analysis as would be seen in a major clinic. Circumstances will vary tremendously with the team and facilities. A professional basketball team in the USA with only 12 players to look after and with access to a great deal of medical care would be more likely to have a complete physical examination. On the other hand, a small high school in the same country with a large number of young athletes coming out for a variety of sports in the autumn will not have the personnel or facilities available to do a complete examination. A potential way of solving this problem is to have the entry-level athlete have a physical examination prior to competition, done by his or her own physician. This would include a comprehensive past and present history, and the athlete would bring a copy of the examination report and history on entry to a new athletic team.

Forms

The history form may well prove to the most important aspect of the physical examination. It should be filled out by the athlete and/or the parents or guardian. This form will alert the team physician to any major physical problems which have already arisen or are likely to arise on the basis of past or family history.

This raises another aspect of the physical examination—record keeping. Physical examinations and histories are not of value if adequate records are not kept. These records must be updated yearly and filed appropriately so that they can be checked in the case of an injury or an illness and during the annual physical check-ups. A past history of illness or injury and certainly of any operations is invaluable in treating an athlete with an injury or illness. The records must be made as simple as possible so that the task of filling them out does not become too complicated either for the athlete or for the physician. Somebody must be made responsible for the care of these records and their updating. This applies whether it is on a yearly basis or on a short-term basis, such as for an international meet or Olympic Games, etc.

Which athletes?

In a country such as the USA, the author feels that any athlete who is to play athletics on an organized level in a high school, college, national or professional team, should have a physical examination and complete history upon first entry to that particular team. The National Collegiate Athletic Association, the ruling body of intercollegiate athletics in the USA, has ruled that a physical examination must be done the first year a player enters a sport. The following yearly examinations do not have to be as complete, but do require a check for any new illnesses or injuries. There is a major problem for schools as there are thousands of participants in high school and college athletics for each year, and the man hours required to do complete physical examinations and histories on each of these players could be prohibitive.

The team physician must be prepared to do the initial physical examination which would include a brief consideration of the athlete's general health and a more specific look at those areas which are particularly liable to injury. It would seem reasonable to always measure the height, weight and blood pressure of the incoming athlete. After that, any obvious abnormalities in the ear, nose and throat region should be looked for and a routine check of the heart and lungs undertaken. Male athletes should be checked for the possibility of an inguinal hernia and a routine examination of the extremities and joints is indicated. In some instances, a much more detailed examination of the musculoskeletal system can be done which would be helpful in predicting the possibility of an injury pattern. However, this will not be possible for all teams and physicians. Much of what is done on the physical examination is determined by the personnel and time available and the circumstances. It is quite different for physicians working with university teams who have adequate help and a period of time set aside to do the physical examinations, as compared to checking athletes for a major competition.

Competition examinations

For major international competitions such as the Olympic Games, World University Games and the Asian Games, it seems unlikely that any athlete who was successful enough to enter these games would be severely ill or have major problems. However, there should be a relatively short history and physical examination form filled out by the athlete which should be looked at by the team physician. The athlete should be interviewed at the time by a team physician and a quick physical check of any areas of previous injury or areas causing worry should be done at that time. Particular attention should be paid to recent injuries or illnesses as opposed to doing an overall physical examination. An injury, even a minor one, may need immediate or continued therapy to allow participation in the games. Again, the time spent during the examination allows the athlete to meet the medical team with whom he or she will be working during the time of a major competition.

Timing of physical examinations

There are several factors to consider in the timing of physical examinations of athletes. The first is that one wants to choose the optimum moment to find any problems that the athlete may have in regard to training and to competing in a particular athletic season. The second factor is that one must be aware of the time, effort and cost that routine physical examinations can engender; the benefit for the athletes should be maximized while being aware of the output of time and energy by medical personnel.

Traditionally, athletes are examined at the time of their entry into a particular school or team activity. In other words, if a young athlete is playing sport at a high school or college, the athlete should be examined at the beginning of the training period for that sport during the first year of entry. This would allow any chronic injuries or significant past history to be immediately evaluated and any needed treatment could be instituted. One would not usually expect to pick up many acute injuries at this point, although as many athletic seasons now seem to be 12 months a year, it is certainly possible that people could be training throughout the year and acute injuries observed. This same type of entry-level physical examination should be done on athletes coming in to new teams, such as a national team. In this instance one would expect the athlete to have been receiving good medical care; in order to have achieved such athletic prominence, the athlete must have been playing with an organized team—which would have such medical care.

In each of these instances, the physical examination achieves the objective of allowing the athlete and the medical staff to make contact. An athlete who has a chance to talk to the physician and other medical and training personnel, is much more likely to feel comfortable and to seek out medical attention, particularly if the problem seems small or possibly even embarrassing to the athlete. Sometimes it is difficult for a new person in a system to establish contact, and chronic injuries, minor illnesses or particular worries may slip by without receiving appropriate attention.

The question as to the proper timing for examinations of athletes who are entering into major competitions, e.g. national or international championships or major games such as the Olympic Games, World University Games or Asian Games, is a more difficult one. It seems likely that a person going to a major championship is going to be in sound physical shape for that competition. A major, full physical examination routinely carried out prior to such a competition is not an efficient use of resources. It is, however, a time when the treatment of chronic injuries has to be continued, although with a realization that there is little that can be achieved. Acute injuries probably result in an inability to perform. For some athletes the major problems are those connected with anxiety and mental problems from being under intense stress.

For these reasons, a short physical examination may be of great help to these athletes. The medical team should have a concise and simple form which the athletes fill out prior to arrival in which they detail any acute and chronic injuries, putting down anything for which they are continuing to receive care and any medications which they are on or are likely to need. There should be a brief past history giving information likely to be of value during this relatively short period of time. This history would be handed in to a member of the medical unit attached to this team. This would allow two things. It would allow contact between the athlete and a member of the medical team. It would also allow the athlete to know where the medical facilities are and the times they are readily available. At all games, there is always a medical facility set up by the host nation or city and the place and hours of availability should be made known to all athletes.

After the physician looks at the medical history, a brief physical examination should be performed. If the athlete has a more major problem or wants to discuss some medical matters of a personal nature, then the athlete can do it at this time or can come back already knowing the medical personnel and the availability of such personnel.

The time prior to major games is always busy and sometimes emotionally difficult. It is a time when the athletes are jealous of their own time for training and for relaxation. It is therefore important to make maximal use of both the athlete's and the medical personnel's time.

Appendix A: Physical examination form.

Courtesy of the University of Iowa.

Date: _____ Sport: _____

Name: _____ S.S.no.: _____

Sex: _____ Height: _____ Weight: _____ Pulse: _____ B/P: _____ Birth date: _____

Visual acuity: R _____ L _____ Near vision: R _____ L _____

	Regions	Normal	Abnormal	Explanation
Eyes:	Conjunctiva			
	Pupils			
	E.O. muscles			
Ears:	Hearing			
	Canals			
	Drums			
Nose & throat:	Gums			
	Pharynx			
	Nares			
Teeth & jaw:				
Skull, scalp, face:				
Neck:	Thyroid			
	Lymph nodes			
Chest:	Pulmonary			
	Breasts			
	Axillary nodes			
Heart:	Apical impulse			
	Rhythm			
	Thrills			
	Murmurs			
Abdomen:	Scars			
	Masses			
	Liver			
	Spleen			
Groin:	Hernia			
	External			
	Lymph nodes			
Anal:	Hemorrhoid			
	Pilonidal cyst			
	Other:			
Musculoskeletal:	Neck			
	Back			
	Shoulder			
	Elbow			
	Wrist/Hand			
	Knee			
	Ankle/Foot			
Skin:	General			
	Inguinal			
	Feet			
	Acne			
Nervous:	Knee jerk			
Pelvic (females):	Bus			
	Introitus			
	Vagina			
	Cervix			
	Uterus			
	Adnexa			
	RV			

Laboratory: Hemoglobin _____ **Urinalysis:** Albumin _____ **Pulmonary functions:** FVC _____
Hematocrit _____ Sugar _____ FEV_1 _____
White blood count _____ Microscopic _____
Sickledex _____

Other: Please comment on those Medical History Questionnaire answers you consider significant.

Participation in intercollegiate athletics at the University of Iowa is an extremely strenuous activity. This candidate's condition is _____ is not _____ suitable for such participation. **Other comments:**

Date: _____ Examining physician: _____ Signature: _____

Appendix B: Interim health questionnaire for athletes.

Courtesy of the University of Iowa.

Name: _____   Sport: _____

Local/campus address: _____   Phone: _____

Student I.D. No: _____

In case of emergency:

Name: _____   Relationship: _____

Address: _____   Phone: _____

_____

_____

	Circle One*	
1. Have you been hospitalized in the past year?	Yes	No
2. In the past year have you had any injury or illness?	Yes	No
3. Are you currently under the care of a physician or taking any kind of medicine on a daily or regular basis?	Yes	No
4. Do you, your parents or physician at home believe that there should be any limitation to full participation in sports?	Yes	No
5. Do you have any allergies to medicine?	Yes	No
6. Do you wear glasses or contact lenses?	Yes	No
(a) contact lenses	Yes	No
(b) glasses	Yes	No
7. Have you had any change in your vision in the past year?	Yes	No
8. Have you been knocked unconscious at any time this past year?	Yes	No
9. Do you wish to talk with a physician?	Yes	No
10. Women athletes: Do you have any menstrual problems?	Yes	No

*Please explain all 'yes' answers:

_____

_____

_____

_____

_____

Student's signature: _____   Date: _____

Reviewed: _____   Date: _____

Physician

Appendix C: Report of medical history form.

Courtesy of the University of Iowa.

SIDE ONE

Sex: M ☐   F ☐

| Last name (Print) | First name | Middle | Social security number |

| Home address (number and street) | City or town | State | Zip code | Date of birth |

| Name, relationship, and address of next of kin | Home telephone number |

| Next of kin's business address | Business telephone |

| What health insurance do you have? | Name of insurance company | No of policy |

Are you a veteran?

Family history

	Age	State of health	Occupation	Age at death	Cause of death
Father					
Mother					
Brothers					
Sisters					

Have any of your relatives ever had any of the following?

	Yes	No	Relationship
Cancer			
High blood pressure			
Sickle cell trait			
Tuberculosis			
Diabetes			
Kidney disease			
Heart disease			
Arthritis			
Stomach disease			
Asthma			
Hay fever			
Convulsive disorder			
Emotional disorder			

Personal Medical History: ANSWER ALL QUESTIONS. **Comment on all positive answers on reverse side of sheet**

HAVE YOU HAD?	Yes	No		Yes	No		Yes	No		Yes	No
Mumps			Head injury with unconsciousness			Rheumatic fever			Rupture, hernia		
Chicken pox						Heart murmur			Weakness, paralysis		
Eye trouble			Hay fever			Disease or injury of joints			Venereal disease		
Ear, nose, throat trouble			Asthma						Albumin/sugar in urine		
			Tuberculosis			Back problems					
Surgery—type			Allergy			Tumor, cancer			Urinary infection		
Genetic disorder			Drug			Jaundice or hepatitis			Kidney stones		
Handicaps			Other			Stomach or intestinal trouble			Convulsive disorder		
			(Specify)						FEMALES ONLY		
			High blood pressure			Recurrent diarrhea			Menstrual irregularity		
						Gallbladder trouble or gallstones			Contraceptive medication or device used.		
									Type:		

Comment on all positive answers on reverse side of sheet	Yes	No
A. Has your physical activity been restricted during the past five years? (Give reasons and durations)		
B. Are you now receiving or have you ever received treatment or counseling for mental health reasons?		
C. Have you had any serious illness or injury or been hospitalized other than already noted? (Give details)		
D. Have you consulted or been treated by clinics, physicians, healers, or other practitioners within the past five years? (Other than routine checkups?)		
E. Do you have any question in regard to your health, family history, or other matters, such as pre-marital counseling, which you would like to discuss with a member of the staff of the Health Service?		
F. Are you taking any medications regularly?		

Remarks or Additional Information
(Use back of this sheet)

I AM ALLERGIC TO THE FOLLOWING MEDICATIONS

I HAVE THIS 'MED-ALERT' CONDITION

Student's signature   Date

Appendix C continued.   SIDE TWO

Required immunization information

IMMUNITY TO MEASLES AND RUBELLA IS A REQUIREMENT FOR REGISTRATION UNLESS BIRTHDATE IS PRIOR TO 1957. DATES FOR IMMUNIZATIONS MUST BE RECORDED.

1. Did you have active disease of measles?   Yes _____   No _____

   If yes, date: _____

2. Measles immunization (1969 or later) Date: _____
   (Only valid if date of immunization is 1969 or later.)

3. Rubella immunization (1969 or later) Date: _____
   (Only valid if date of immunization is 1969 or later.)

4. Rubella immune titre: Yes _____   No _____
   If yes, send lab report or copy of report with this form.

5. Tetanus _____ (date) (valid only if within 10 years.)

6. Diphtheria _____ (valid only if within 10 years.)

7. Polio _____ (date)

8. Mumps _____ (date)

9. Tuberculin skin test _____ (date) Results: negative (   ) positive (   )
   (Valid only if within 1 year.) If positive, send copy of chest x-ray report. If positive, and have had or are on INH treatment, send copy of report of treatment.

   Sickle cell anaemia is an inherited disease in black people and can be detected by a 'sickeldex' screening test. Sickeldex   negative ☐   positive ☐

_____   Photocopy of immunization record also acceptable.
    Signature of physician or authorized immunizing official

Comment on all positive answers from the front side of this sheet

_____

_____

_____

_____

_____

_____

_____

_____

_____

_____

_____

_____

_____

_____

_____

12.4 Infectious diseases in tropical climates

I. DIOP MAR

From the point of view of parasitic and other infectious diseases, there is no pathology specific to the athlete, but it must nevertheless be borne in mind that the practice of certain sports can mean that the athlete is more exposed to the risk of infection than is the non-athlete. Moreover, travel facilities in the modern world and constant human interaction mean that the northern hemisphere is no longer safe from diseases formerly specific to tropical countries.

In the context of supervision of athletes and preventive treatment—through clinical measures, medicaments and vaccines—this chapter is divided into the roles played by water, ground, animal and insect vectors and intercontinental travel.

Water

Water is a major source of infection, whether it is used for drinking or bathing purposes. Bottled water is a safeguard, particularly when travelling; all drinks not meeting hygiene standards should be rejected. The consumption of uncontrolled water and bathing in outside swimming pools and the sea can give rise to various diseases:

1   Bacterial: leptospiroses, salmonelloses, shigelloses, cholera, etc.
2   Viral: poliomyelitis and other enteroviral infections (Cocksackie, echo) and adenoviral follicular conjunctivitises.
3   Parasitic: amibiasis, bilharziosis (schistosomiasis), etc.

Table 12.4.1 covers the main water-transmitted diseases.

Ground

Infection originating in the ground is usually due to microbic agents of the Pectridium group, as is the case with gangrene or tetanus, which may follow even the slightest of injuries. The risks of contamination for athletes vary, depending on whether they are performing on consolidated

Table 12.4.1 Main infectious and parasitic diseases transmitted by water.

Morbid condition	Pathogenic agent	Mode of transmission	Dominant symptoms	Treatment	Prevention
Leptospiroses	*Leptospira icterohaemorraghicae, L. grippotyphosa,* etc.	Bathing in fresh water contaminated by rat urine; penetration of the organism by leptospira through skin or mucous membranes	Fever, algias, jaundice, lymphocytic meningitis, haemorrhaging	Antibiotics: penicillins, tetracylines	Prohibition of bathing in rivers suspected of being contaminated
Salmonelloses	*Salmonella typhi* or *S. paratyphi A, B, C*	Absorption of water or food contaminated by germs of faecal origin	Fever, gastroenteritis, encephalopathy to a greater or lesser degree	Chloramphenicol, ampicillin, cotrimoxazole, etc.	Hygiene, TAB vaccination
Shigelloses	*Shigella dysentriae, Sh. flexneri, Sh. boydii, Sh. sonnei*	Absorption of water or food contaminated by germs of faecal origin	Dysentery with stools containing blood and mucus	Chloramphenicol, ampicillin, cotrimoxazole, etc.	Food hygiene
Cholera	*Vibrio cholerae, V. El Tor*	Absorption of water or food contaminated by germs of faecal origin	Diarrhoea, ricewater stools, dehydration, collapse	Tetracycline, chloramphenicol, co-trimoxazole	Hygiene, chemoprophylaxis; vaccination not very effective
Acute anterior poliomyelitis	Poliovirus I, II, III	Direct contamination from person to person or indirect contamination through polluted food and water	Asymetric paralysis	Symptomatic; no specific treatment	Food hygiene, avoidance of bathing in rivers, vaccination
Amibiasis	*Entamoeba histolytica*	Drinking water and food eaten raw	Dysentery with stools containing blood and mucus	Dehydroemetine, metronidazole, tinidazole, secnidazole, ornidazole	Food hygiene
Bilharziasis	*Schistosoma haematobium, S. mansoni, S. japonicum*	Repeated contacts with fresh water: contracted through the skin	Haematuria, dysentery	Niridazole, oxamniquine, praziquentel	Avoidance of freshwater bathing in zones where it is endemic; vaccine being studied

surfaces or ground consisting of hard-packed earth, which is considered more dangerous, polluted by human or animal excrement.

Gas gangrene arises as a result of penetration of the organism through a wound by microbic germs, which are strictly anaerobic and cause deep lysis and necrosis of the tissues. Precautions must be taken in the form of proper disinfection of all wounds, avoidance of premature sutures in anfractuous wounds and application of preventive penicillin therapy.

Tetanus can arise following even a minimal wound, graze or pinprick. The toxin secreted by *Pectridium tetani* spreads through the organism, provoking the contractures and paroxystic crises characteristic of the disease. It may be prevented by meticulous care of all injuries, and the injection of antitetanus serum or a booster injection of tetanus toxoid if the patient has already been vaccinated.

Animals and insects

There are a large number of animal diseases which can be transmitted directly or indirectly to human beings. The practice of certain sports such as hunting, riding and caving, for example, creates favourable conditions for human contamination.

Hunting Horses, dogs and game are all sources of contamination. Because of the existence of rabies vulpina sylvatica in certain areas, albeit limited, a rabid fox can attack hunter, dog and horse; the man should be immediately vaccinated and the dog put down, even if it has already been vaccinated.

Certain zoonoses are found in the hare and wild rabbit, for instance: (a) tularaemia, contracted by clumsy handling of game and easily treated with antibiotics; and (b) boutonneuse fever caused by rickettsia, transmitted by the sting of a tic which can be carried by the wild rabbit, which, when hunted, seeks refuge in gardens and poultry yards in the countryside.

Mention should also be made of certain staphylococcal suppurations contracted from rabbits, which can be hard to get rid of and may lead to a septicopyaemia in certain predisposed patients.

Riding Riding and outings on horseback in small clubs are becoming increasingly popular; it is important, however, to point out a number of risks related to contact with horses. The biggest risk is tetanus. The horse harbours in its intestine the tetanus spore which, eliminated with the excrement, contaminates the ground of hippodromes and various routes also used by walkers and runners. It is therefore important to prescribe an anti-tetanus injection for members of riding clubs and all those practising open-air sports in places also frequented by horses.

The horse may also be affected by arboviroses transmissible to human beings. These are of varying gravity, ranging from Venezuelan encephalitis, a disease very widespread in central America and with a high mortality rate, which sometimes leaves survivors with lasting after effects, to the much more benign West Nile arbovirus, found in the Mediterranean region and transmitted by a mosquito, the symptoms of which are a so-called 3-day fever, followed by a long convalescence marked by severe asthenia.

The fight against mosquitos is one necessary preventive measure. It is also important, in order to limit the spread of the disease, to ensure that horses travelling from one country to another for international competitions such as the Olympic Games are in good health.

Horses may also be affected with scabies or contagious tineas (ringworm). It is necessary to be able to detect and treat these in order to avoid infection of the rider.

Intercontinental travel

As a result of fast means of transport, modern times are characterized by long journeys outside people's habitual areas of residence. Consequently, what used to be known as exotic pathology is no longer restricted to the inhabitants of tropical countries, but also affects those living in countries with a temperate climate.

An athlete taking part in intercontinental international competitions is not safe from such threats. Disorientation, jet lag, changes in climate (season, temperature, humidity, wind) upset the functioning of the body and make it more vulnerable to microbic aggression. It is advisable to inform the athlete about these problems and to encourage him or her to take a number of precautions in order to maintain a good physiological equilibrium, indispensable to the practice of sport. Before leaving on a journey, an athlete should acquire elementary but absolutely necessary notions of hygiene, be vaccinated and, during the stay abroad, protect him/herself by means of chemoprophylaxis.

Personal hygiene precautions

These primarily concern diet: salads, sea food and ice cream should be avoided. Game, especially warthogs killed on safari, should be well cooked to avoid trichiniasis. Outside urban centres where water is controlled, bottled or canned mineral water should be drunk where possible, or, failing that, water which has been boiled or treated with bleach (2 drops/litre) or hydrochlonazone (1 tablet/litre). Water treated in this way may also be used for careful washing of raw vegetables. These precautions serve as protection against shigelloses, salmonelloses, cholera, amibiasis, certain intestinal flagelloses, ascariasis, taeniases (tapeworm) and Medina filariasis contracted by the consumption of infested crustaceans.

Advice should be given to refrain from bathing in fresh water, walking barefoot in mud or crossing streams and brooks, in order to avoid urinary or intestinal bilharziosis (schistosomiasis). Athletes should be encouraged to protect themselves against the stings of certain disease-carrying arthropods by the use of mosquito nets, insect repellants and insecticides.

Finally, athletes should be advised to protect themselves from sexually transmitted diseases, particularly by the use of sheaths.

Vaccinations

Some vaccinations are compulsory and others recommended.

Compulsory vaccinations

The Rockefeller Institute 17D vaccine is the only one used against yellow fever at the present time; its period of validity is 10 years beginning 10 days after vaccination. The anticholera vaccination is valid from the sixth day after the last injection until the sixth month. Many countries have ceased to demand this vaccination.

The antismallpox injection used to belong to this group, but it is no longer demanded since the eradication of the disease.

Recommended vaccinations

These concern acute anterior poliomyelitis, tetanus and typhoid fevers, to which may be added hepatitis B and, in exceptional cases, exanthematous typhus and the plague, although this no longer really constitutes a threat.

Chemoprophylaxis

Antimalaria chemoprophylaxis is indispensable for anyone entering an area where malaria is endemic. It consists of taking an amino-4-quinoline such as chloroquine at a dosage of one 100 mg tablet/day for 6 days out of seven. This preventive treatment should begin on the day of departure and be continued for 6 to 8 weeks after the traveller's return to the place of residence (Europe, North America, etc.).

To a lesser degree, prophylactic treatment can provide protection against amibiasis, filariasis and sleeping sickness:

1 Against amibiasis: Recommended by some doctors who suggest the taking of 2 bromooxine capsules/day during the stay. It could also have an effect on what is known as travellers' diarrhoea.

2 Against filariasis: In zones where filariasis is hyperendemic, diethyl-carbamazine may be prescribed (one 100 mg tablet/week).

3 Against sleeping sickness: A single pentamidine injection (4 mg/kg bodyweight) gives protection against trypanosomiasis caused by *Trypanosoma gambiense* for a period of 6 months. It is less effective against *T. rhodesiense*.

Conclusion

To sum up, there is a need for awareness of the risks incurred by athletes in relation to transmissible diseases, but it is important to see them in perspective and take precautions, which, for the most part, consist of vaccination and elementary rules of hygiene.

12.5 Infectious diseases in temperate climates

R. H. STRAUSS

The purpose of this chapter is to describe the diagnosis, treatment and prevention of a small number of infectious diseases that are commonly found among sports participants. Many of these diseases will impair performance if not recognized and treated at the start, and some are made worse by overuse.

Microorganisms can infect the body and cause disease. Viruses cause the common cold, herpes and many other illnesses. They are the simplest microorganisms, reproduce only within the cells that they attack, and are unaffected by most antimicrobial drugs. Bacteria exist in various shapes and clusters and can reproduce outside other cells. They cause common skin, throat and other infections that often can be treated effectively with antibiotics. Fungi cause skin infections such as athlete's foot. They grow outside cells, more slowly than bacteria. Antifungal drugs are helpful in fighting these microorganisms.

Skin

Bacterial infections   Occasionally a bacterial infection will get started where there has been a small break in the skin, such as a scrape or abrasion.

Prevention   The best way to prevent infection is to wash the wound well with ordinary soap and water soon after the injury, either immediately or when showering after practice. There is no evidence to show that iodine or other antiseptic solutions are helpful. Putting hydrogen peroxide on the wound looks impressive, but is not as effective as washing the wound with ordinary soap and water. Alcohol should not be used on an open wound because it kills healthy tissue.

For the first few hours, a small amount of blood and clear yellow serum may leak from the wound. During this time the wound can be covered with a clean dressing. A topical antibiotic ointment can be applied but is probably unnecessary. After the leakage has stopped, usually within 24 hours, the wound should be left uncovered as much as possible in order to air dry. The continued use of bandages tends to promote the growth of bacteria through retention of moisture, heat and debris. However, during the time the athlete is actually participating in his or her sport, it is often wise to keep the wound covered with a bandage for its protection. Showering after practice or competition allows the wound to be gently cleaned each day.

With normal healing, the wound will be a little red and sore. If infection sets in, the wound, after a day or so, will not dry up with scab formation; instead, pus may form and leak from the wound. Also, the surrounding skin may become increasingly red. More intense medical attention is then necessary, as described below.

Cellulitis   An enlarging area of redness surrounding the wound indicates that an infection is spreading in the skin, and this is often called cellulitis. The infection may spread even further by involving the lymph channels and lymph nodes. For example, red streaks may be seen running up the skin of the arm or leg, and the lymph nodes under the arm or in the groin may become enlarged or tender. These are danger signs that require immediate treatment. Fever may follow, and if the patient is not treated, death may occur from widespread infection.

Treatment   The infection can usually be halted before it is widespread by a combination of local cleansing and oral antibiotic therapy. Culture of the exudate should be considered. The wound should be soaked in clean warm water, to which a small amount of soap can be added, for approximately 15 min four times daily. At this time, the wound should be gently cleansed.

An antibiotic should be administered, either orally or by injection. This type of infection is frequently caused by staphylococci. Penicillin is sometimes effective against these bacteria, but, unfortunately, some staphylococci are resistant to penicillin. Therefore, it is best to use an antibiotic that is effective against such resistant bacteria. For example, dicloxicillin 250 mg orally every 6 hours is an effective drug for moderate infection. More severe infection may require twice this dose or may even require hospitalization and intravenous antibiotic therapy. Tetanus immunization should be current.

The affected part should be rested, and the athlete may be out of action for several days.

Impetigo   Impetigo is a superficial skin infection caused by streptococcal or staphylococcal bacteria. It usually appears on the face or upper body as sores with honey-coloured crusts. It is highly contagious and is transmitted among athletes by direct contact or by infected towels or other material.

Prevention   The infected individual should not have contact with others until the crusts are gone (healed) because they are infectious. The use of common towels to wipe off sweat should be avoided.

Treatment   The infected area is cleaned as described above. In addition, an appropriate antibiotic should be used—for example, erythromycin 250 mg four times daily (approximately every 6 hours) for 10 days.

Folliculitis   Hair follicles, particularly on the legs, sometimes become infected by bacteria. When these infections are small and localized they frequently are treated effectively simply by keeping the area clean and dry. Treatment with an antibiotic can be added if necessary.

Furunculosis (boils)   A boil is a localized infection, usually caused by staphylococci, that can range from a tender red papule to a large fluctuant abscess. Treatment consists of frequent warm compresses and, often, an oral antibiotic such as dicloxicillin or cephalexin 250 mg four times daily. If the abscess 'points' (comes to a head) it can be incised and the pus drained. The athlete should be allowed to rest the involved part and should not have direct contact with other athletes until the infection is under control.

Acne   Changes in hormonal balance during maturation result in some people in an overproduction of oils and fatty acids by the skin. These accumulate to form black heads (comedones) and promote infection (pimples), especially on the face and shoulders. Sports can make the situation worse because of the sweating and increased oil production associated with exercise, especially in warm environments.

Treatment   The treatment consists of keeping the skin clean and removing excess oil. First, the affected skin should be washed with soap each morning, after practice, and at bedtime. In addition, a drying agent such as benzoyl peroxide 5% or 10% can be used once a day. An oral antibiotic taken for several weeks or months can be helpful. Tetracyline 250 mg or 500 mg orally twice daily can be used.

Athlete's foot (tinea pedis)   This extremely common problem is caused by several types of fungus that exist almost everywhere but need a warm, moist environment in which to grow. Some people seem to have a natural immunity, while others get the infection repeatedly.

Treatment   Itching and peeling skin between the toes is usually the first sign. Each day the feet should be washed and dried well between the toes and an antifungal solution or cream such as miconazol (Micatin) or tolnaftate (Tinactin) should be applied. Medicated powders do not penetrate the skin well enough to treat the infection effectively. Application of a drying agent, such as benzoyl peroxide, once a day will often help to speed recovery. The infection will usually start to get better after a few days, but it is necessary to continue the antifungal treatment for approximately 1 month in order to eliminate the fungus from the skin.

Cracking of the skin may allow the feet to become superinfected with bacteria. This may lead to pain, swelling and redness which must be treated as described previously for bacterial infections. Once the bacterial infection is under control, longer term treatment for the fungus can continue.

Prevention   The feet should be washed and dried well at least once daily. Clean socks should be worn. People with a tendency to get this infection can dust an antifungal powder between the toes after drying.

Jock itch (tinea cruris)   This common fungal infection of the groin is caused by microorganisms similar to those that cause athlete's foot and is treated in the same way. It appears as an itching, red rash, particularly on the skin adjacent to the scrotum.

Herpes simplex (cold sores, fever blisters)   This viral infection commonly occurs as a vesicle or blister at the margin of the lips. However, its distribution can be much wider, particularly among wrestlers, in whom it appears as 1–2 mm wide vesicles on a red, inflamed base. The first time that an individual is infected, he or she may experience fever, tiredness and swollen lymph nodes. These generalized signs are usually much milder or non-existent when the lesion recurs at a later time. (See below under 'Sexually transmitted diseases'.)

Treatment   The patient usually recognizes that a lesion is about to recur because the skin feels irritated several hours before vesicles appear in the location in which they have been experienced previously. As soon as the warning signs are recognized, the patient should begin to take acyclovir (Zovirax) 200 mg orally five times daily for 5 days. This treatment significantly shortens the course of the recurrence or initial infection but does not cure the disease. That is, the virus continues to be harboured within the body and may be activated by sunburn, fever, irritation or stress. When blisters are present, they can be dried more quickly by the application of a drying agent such as benzoyl peroxide twice daily. Untreated, an episode of the disease lasts about 2 weeks; with treatment, it tends to last half as long.

Prevention   Avoid skin-to-skin contact with people who have an active herpes lesion. Drinking from the same cup should also be avoided.

Canker sore   A canker sore is a small, painful ulcer within the mouth that can appear following a small cut or abrasion or for no apparent reason. The cause is unknown.

Treatment   The canker sore heals by itself in 1 to 2 weeks, and treatment seems to help very little. A paste containing a topical anaesthetic or hydrocortisone can be dabbed onto the ulcer and may ease the discomfort. Certain foods such as citrus fruits make the ulcer feel worse and should be avoided.

Common warts   Common warts are caused by a virus and are mildly contagious. They can appear almost anywhere on the body and sometimes disappear for no apparent reason.

Treatment   Warts are treated by destroying them. The important point is to destroy the wart but not the surrounding skin. Many home remedies, such as the application of salicylic acid, attempt to do this. Probably the most effective method is to freeze the wart with liquid nitrogen. Several applications, separated by a few weeks, are often necessary.

Plantar warts are those that are located on the bottom of the foot. They are painful for the same reason that a stone in the shoe is painful. It is best to remove them when they are small, but not usually during the competitive season of an athlete because removal often makes walking or running difficult for several days. During the season, the plantar wart can be pared down periodically to keep walking comfortable.

Molluscum contagiosum   Molluscum contagiosum is also caused by a virus and occasionally is transmitted among athletes by skin-to-skin contact. The lesions are small (2–5 mm in diameter), pearly, raised papules with an indentation at the centre.

Treatment   These lesions are readily cured without scarring by removing the waxy contents. This is easily done with the tip of a blade or by another method of unroofing the lesion and expressing the core.

Ears

Otitis externa
(swimmer's ear,
infected canal)

When people swim a great deal, or in warm weather, the ear canal tends to remain damp. This allows infection to occur, usually from bacteria. The result is an itching or painful ear canal that feels worse if the outer cartilage of the ear (the pinna) is tugged on. The canal itself appears inflamed and an exudate may be present.

Treatment   Debris should be removed from the canal by irrigation with warm water. The infected canal generally can be treated effectively by instilling otic drops three or four times daily. For example, a suspension of polymyxin B-neomycin-hydrocortisone (Cortisporin) can be used. Although it is considered best to keep water out of the ear during healing, most competitive swimmers can continue to practise if they simply instill the antibiotic drops in the ear following each practice.

Prevention   People who tend to get this infection can generally prevent it by using ear drops that dry the canal following swimming. A cheap and effective solution is rubbing alcohol (70% isopropyl or ethyl alcohol). Using a dropper, the ear canal is filled with alcohol and then immediately emptied in order to remove water. Alternatively, ear plugs can be used to keep water out of the canal during swimming.

Otitis media (middle
ear infection)

Infection of the middle ear is probably no more frequent among athletes than among the general population. The patient usually complains of ear pain and a sensation of fullness or decreased hearing. Examination usually reveals that the canal is not red or tender but the tympanic membrane (ear drum) is red. Fever may be present.

Treatment   Treatment with an oral antibiotic is usually curative. For example, pencillin or ampicillin 250 mg four times daily for 10 days can be used. An antihistamine–decongestant combination is sometimes used at the same time in an attempt to help clear any middle ear effusion. However, if the athlete is going to participate in a competition at which drug testing is carried out, the physician should not prescribe a decongestant because this may disqualify the athlete. Also, the antihistamine may make the athlete drowsy and decrease performance.

Eyes

Conjunctivitis (pink eye)   Inflammation of the conjunctiva can be caused by allergies, viral infections, or bacterial infections. When the infection is bacterial, pus appears at the corner of the eye. When the patient wakes up in the morning the eye is often crusted and difficult to open.

Treatment   One drop of an antibiotic solution such as sulfacetamide in the eye four times daily is generally effective. Alternatively, a solution of polymyxin B-neomycin-gramiciden (Neosporin) can be used. Improvement should be observed within approximately 1 day after the treatment is started. Antibiotic drops are preferred to ointments, particularly in students and athletes, because the ointment causes blurred vision for several hours whereas the drops do not. Treatment should continue until symptoms have been absent for 2 days.

Stye (hordeolum)   A stye is a common infection of the hair follicle at the base of an eyelash.

Treatment   Warm compresses should be applied several times daily and antibiotic drops should be used as described above.

Respiratory system

Common cold (upper respiratory infection)   In this annoying disease a virus infects the lining of the respiratory tract where it causes swelling and secretion of fluid. As everyone has experienced, this may cause a runny nose, sneezing, stopped-up ears, sore throat, hoarseness and cough. Victims often feel weak but have little fever.

Prevention   The disease is transmitted from person to person by infected secretions in the form of droplets in the air, which are then inhaled; by the sharing of items such as drinking glasses; or by direct personal contact. Avoiding communal water cups and towels can help to decrease transmission. An individual becomes temporarily immune to the particular virus that infected him or her, but because there are several hundred different viruses that cause the common cold, he or she is not immune to colds in general.

Treatment   There is no cure for the common cold. Antibiotics, such as penicillin, do not work because they do not affect the virus. Colds tend to last about 1 week and the symptoms can be treated, although not always effectively. Some age-old advice may be the best treatment: get plenty of rest, especially if you feel tired; drink fluids to ensure normal hydration; and take aspirin or acetaminophen every 4 hours for headache, sore throat or fever.

Some individuals seem to be helped by an oral combination of antihistamine and decongestant. A nasal spray such as phenylephrine may help nasal congestion temporarily. Such sprays should be used for only 2 or 3 days because their effectiveness decreases with use. When the drug is overused, a 'rebound' effect may cause worse congestion. Throat lozenges or sprays which are surface anaesthetics help to alleviate the sore throat.

The cough may be alleviated by placing a vaporizer in the patient's room. Cough syrups can help to liquify secretions so that they can be coughed up more easily. Such remedies are, at best, moderately effective. A mild cough suppressant can be taken, particularly at night in order to allow sleep. Symptoms that last more than a week or so, such as a cough, sometimes represent superinfection by bacteria and may be treated with an antibiotic.

Sports participation   Many people ignore a mild cold and continue to work or exercise. An athlete should not participate when he or she has a fever or significant cough or feels tired or achy. Because antihistamines, such as those in cold remedies, often cause drowsiness, they may decrease athletic performance. Decongestant pills and sprays are stimulants related to epinephrine and, when drug testing is done, may disqualify the participant as will narcotics such as those in certain cough-suppressant medications.

Streptococcal pharyngitis (strep throat)   One of the many causes of a sore throat is infection of the pharynx and tonsils by the streptococcus bacterium. Infection by group A β-haemolytic streptococcus is potentially dangerous because it can lead to rheumatic fever and heart disease at a later time. These complications may be prevented if the infection is treated early with an antibiotic. The patient usually has a sore throat, especially when swallowing, exudate (pus) on the tonsils, swollen lymph nodes in the neck, fever, headache and weakness. Sometimes a bright red rash covers parts of the skin, in which case the term scarlet fever is used. It is still, basically, a streptococcal infection of the throat. Other diseases such as colds and mononucleosis can begin with a sore throat. A throat culture or other test for the streptococcal infection is necessary in order to establish the diagnosis.

Treatment   The usual treatment is oral penicillin V 250 mg four times daily for 10 days. Alternatively, an injection of long-acting (benzathine) penicillin may be used. When the patient feels ill, he or she should rest, take fluids and take aspirin or acetaminophen for fever. Gargling with warm salt water (½ teaspoon salt in a cup of water) eases throat pain. Erythromycin can be used in patients who are allergic to penicillin.

Prevention   Transmission is by droplets in the air or on infected materials, or by direct contact. Such contact with infected persons should be avoided.

Gastrointestinal system

Viral gastroenteritis   Several viruses tend to disturb the normal function of the stomach and intestines. Symptoms of this common disease include loss of appetite, nausea, vomiting, diarrhoea, cramps, abdominal pain, and a generally achy feeling. It usually lasts only a few days and, as with all viruses, has no cure.

Treatment   The most important treatment is simple. The patient should rest and, at first, drink only clear liquids, mainly water with sugar and electrolytes. Clear liquids include soft drinks which contain sugar, jello and clear soups. Milk products should be avoided. When symptoms are severe, antispasmotics such as diphenoxylate (Lomotil) or loperamide (Imodium) may be added. However, these drugs should be used with caution because they may prolong certain gastrointestinal infections.

Food poisoning (staphylococcal)   A common type of food poisoning is caused by contamination of food by the staphylococcus bacterium, especially in warm weather. Dairy products such as cream fillings or meats may become contaminated from the infected skin or respiratory tract of a food handler. If the food is not kept refrigerated, the bacteria can multiply over several hours and produce a toxin that causes vomiting and diarrhoea an hour or so after being eaten. These unpleasant effects usually last only a few hours. The staphylococcal bacteria do not multiply inside the digestive tract, so the body simply gets rid of the poison.

Treatment   Medicines used to reduce the vomiting and diarrhoea are not usually given because they may prolong the illness. Occasionally, treatment of severe dehydration may require administration of fluids by vein.

The disease is prevented by proper food handling. It can strike large groups eating the same food, as at picnics.

Traveller's diarrhoea   People who live in temperate climates and who travel to warmer latitudes sometimes get diarrhoea a few days after arriving. This is thought to be from infection by a strain of the bacterium *Escherichia coli* that is new to the traveller or by other bacteria or viruses. *E. coli* normally lives in the human intestine but the new strain causes diarrhoea for a few days before the disease cures itself.

Prevention   This disease is difficult to prevent, but chances of avoiding it are improved by eating in establishments that are known to prepare food hygienically and by avoiding water and ice cubes of unknown quality. When in doubt, avoid fresh salads, eat only those fruits that you have peeled yourself, eat foods that are served hot, and drink bottled beverages.

Treatment   Drinking liquids, such as soft drinks containing sugar, and soups helps to replace lost water and salt and prevent dehydration. Diarrhoea, in the absence of fever or blood in the stool, can be relieved by short-term use of diphenoxylate (Lomotil), loperamide (Imodium) or bismuth subsalicylate (Pepto-Bismol). An effective treatment appears to be the oral antibiotic fixed combination trimethoprim 160 mg and sulpha-methoxazole 800 mg (Bactrim DS) taken twice daily. This same drug combination can be taken once daily as a preventive measure prior to and during a brief period when the traveller is passing through an area in which he or she may be exposed to this disease.

Infectious mononucleosis

Infectious mononucleosis occurs occasionally among young adults. It is caused by the Epstein–Barr virus and is transmitted to individuals through the mouth or respiratory tract by close personal contact or inhalation of viral particles. Fortunately, it is not very contagious, so other family members or room-mates generally do not catch the disease. The incubation period is several weeks.

Symptoms of the disease generally last from 2 to 4 weeks. The syndrome often begins with a feeling of tiredness followed by sore throat, fever and enlarged, tender lymph nodes usually noted first in the neck. Lymph nodes under the arms and in the groin also frequently become enlarged and tender. The sore throat that accompanies this syndrome may cause confusion with other diseases.

A blood test usually reveals a level of atypical lymphocytes greater than 5–10% and an increase in the number of normal lymphocytes. A rapid slide test (Monospot), when positive, confirms the diagnosis. By the second week of illness an enlarged spleen is palpable in some patients. The liver occasionally is mildly enlarged and tender and liver function tests may be mildly abnormal.

Treatment   There is no specific treatment for mononucleosis. The sore throat can be alleviated with analgesics and gargles. Corticosteroid therapy generally is not helpful but has been used by some physicians when the tonsils are so swollen that swallowing is difficult. Bedrest is appropriate when the victim feels tired or has a fever. Otherwise, moderate activity such as walking is permissible.

Return to sports   When the patient is symptomatic, sports participation and strenuous exercise should be avoided. The main problem as to when to allow a return to sports centres on enlargement of the spleen. Rupture of the spleen is a rare, but potentially fatal, complication of infectious mononucleosis. Rupture of the spleen has rarely occurred later than 3 or 4 weeks following the onset of illness. Therefore, reasonable guidelines for return to activity would seem to be as follows: If the spleen was palpable to the clinician during the acute phase of the disease, the spleen should have regressed so that it is no longer palpable. If serious question remains about splenic size, ultrasound or another diagnostic test can be done. The patient should be asymptomatic and significant fatigue and malaise should be absent. The patient should gradually increase physical exertion over a number of days as tolerated by personal feeling of well-being. On average, most athletes do not return to participation for 3 or 4 weeks after the onset of the disease.

Sexually transmitted diseases

The incidence of sexually transmitted diseases among athletes appears to be the same as in others of the same age and socioeconomic group. The use of condoms can help to prevent the transmission of gonorrhoea, non-gonococcal urethritis, herpes simplex and venereal warts.

Gonorrhoea   In males, gonorrhoea usually appears as a discharge of yellow–white pus from the penis accompanied by urethral burning on urination. Females may have no symptoms or may overlook a moderate urethral or vaginal discharge caused by gonorrhoea. Gonorrhoeal infections of the throat and rectum also occur.

Treatment   In the male, the diagnosis should be established by microscopic smear of the discharge which reveals Gram-negative intracellular diplococci. A culture on appropriate medium will confirm the diagnosis. In the female, a culture is necessary to establish the diagnosis. A treatment that is usually effective is the administration of oral probenecid 1 g, followed by the injection of 4.8 million units of procaine penicillin. Alternative therapy is necessary if the causative organism is resistant to penicillin. Because of the frequent coexistence of a second infecting organism such as chlamydia, tetracycline 500 mg orally four times daily for 7 days is often recommended in addition to the penicillin.

Non-gonococcal urethritis (NGU)   This is a relatively common problem among males. It generally is caused by chlamydia. Usual symptoms are a small amount of mucoid discharge from the urethra and mild urethral burning with urination.

Treatment   The presence of gonorrhoea should be ruled out by the smear and culture described above. A culture or immunofluorescence test can be performed for the causative organism. However, once gonorrhoea is ruled out by smear, treatment is usually started immediately. A common treatment is tetracyline 500 mg orally four times daily for 7 days.

Genital herpes   This disease is caused by the herpes simplex virus. Generally, type 1 is observed above the waist and type 2 below the waist, although this distinction is becoming less clearcut. The lesion consists of one or more small blisters on an erythematous base. These blisters frequently occur on the penis or on the labia but can be contracted almost anywhere on the body. The diagnosis can be confirmed by a viral culture or Tzanck test.

Treatment   The treatment is the same as described for herpes simplex earlier in this chapter.

Venereal warts   These lesions are caused by a virus that results in warts most often on the penis and labia.

Treatment A solution of podophyllin 20% in tincture of benzoin is applied to the warts and washed off after approximately 4 hours. This is repeated at weekly intervals and usually results in a cure within a few weeks. In resistant cases, the small residual warts can be frozen with liquid nitrogen.

Pediculosis pubis (crab lice) The crab louse is transmitted mainly by intimate contact, although it can be transmitted by clothing, towels or other vectors. This louse is usually limited to the pubic and perineal region of the body but can also affect other hairy areas. The louse clings to the skin and sucks blood. It results in itching and can be observed with a magnifying glass. Sometimes the victim observes the louse and may describe it as a 'moving freckle'.

Treatment The patient should apply lindane 1% (Kwell) shampoo from the neck down and leave it in place for 5 min, then rinse thoroughly. Clothes and bedding must be washed well with hot soapy water so that the individual does not become re-infected. A single treatment is generally effective.

Scabies Scabies is caused by a mite that burrows under the skin and causes severe itching. Tortuous red burrows may appear on the hands, waist, pubic area or other areas of contact. If untreated, this disease may last for years, and may be complicated by infection.

Treatment Lindane 1% (Kwell) lotion is applied from the neck down and left in place overnight. Signs and symptoms may require more than a week to clear because of the body's reaction to the mites within the skin. A topical corticosteroid can help to decrease itching during this period.

Return to sport

The return to sport following specific infections was discussed above.

Preventive measures Are athletes more or less susceptible to illness than non-athletes? There is probably little difference, although few studies have addressed this question. However, athletes in the same team are in close contact with each other every day. Therefore, contagious diseases tend to spread more rapidly among team members than among the general population. Contagion can be minimized by encouraging athletes not to drink from the same cups and not to share personal items such as towels. In addition, diseases that are spread by skin-to-skin contact pass more readily among athletes in whom physical contact is frequent. The skin condition of such athletes should be monitored by medical personnel. Team-mates who are ill should not return until their disease is no longer contagious.

Many people simply ignore the symptoms of a mild viral upper respiratory infection (cold) and continue their daily activities. Athletes do this as well, and there appear to be few ill effects. However, if the viral infection is accompanied by fever, fatigue or malaise, exercise should be curtailed.

Individualizing return to sport

Athletes usually are anxious to return to their sport as soon as possible following an illness. There is general agreement that an athlete should resume exercise only after the symptoms of the disease have disappeared. After fever has subsided, it is probably best to wait an additional 24 h before returning to exercise.

Mild fatigue may be present following illness due to the deconditioning effect of inactivity as well as to the disease itself. The athlete should gradually increase the level of exercise over several days, depending on how well he or she feels each day.

Acknowledgement

This paper was adapted in part from the author's chapter 'Nontraumatic medical problems' in R. H. Strauss (ed) *Sports Medicine and Physiology*. W. B. Saunders, Philadelphia, 1979.

Further reading

Eichner, E. R. (1987) Infectious mononucleosis: recognition and management in athletes. *Physician Sportsmed*. **15(12)**, 61.

Simon, H. B. (1987) Exercise and infection. *Physician Sportsmed*. **15(10)**, 134.

Strauss, R. H. (ed) (1984) *Sports Medicine*. W. B. Saunders, Philadelphia.

12.6 Nutrition and dietetics*

D. L. COSTILL

The foods we eat contain the chemically-bonded energy needed to sustain life and permit bodily movement. These molecular bonds, however, are relatively weak and provide only a low-energy source, that cannot be used directly for muscular contraction. Rather, the energy that bonds these food molecules together must be chemically released and stored in the form of a high-energy phosphate, adenosine triphosphate (ATP). Assembling and disassembling these energy compounds is facilitated by special proteins termed enzymes. When acted on by the enzyme ATPase, the ATP molecule releases a great deal more energy (32 kJ/mol or 7.6 kcal/mol of ATP) than was originally contained in the low-energy foods.

Energy systems

Another high-energy phosphate molecule, phosphocreatine (PCr), is also used to store energy within the cells. Unlike the energy derived from the breakdown of ATP, PCr does not appear to be used directly to accomplish work within the cells. Instead, it is used to rebuild the ATP molecule, thereby maintaining a relatively constant supply of this high-energy compound. Thus, when energy is released from ATP by the splitting of a phosphate group, the ATP molecule can be reconstructed by reducing PCr to creatine and inorganic phosphate (Pi), thereby providing energy for ATP production. During the first few seconds of a maximal sprint, ATP is maintained at a relatively normal level, whereas PCr declines steadily throughout the activity. However, at exhaustion both ATP and PCr are quite low, unable to provide the energy for further contractions and relaxations.

Since the stores of ATP and PCr can only sustain the energy needs of the muscle for a few seconds during an all-out sprint, the muscles must rely on other processes for ATP formation. Aside from the ATP–PCr system, there are two other sources for ATP production: (a) glycolysis, ATP production from sugar stored in muscle (i.e. glycogen) without the

* Certain material contained in this chapter has previously appeared in Wilmore, J. & Costill, D. (1987) *Training for Sport and Activity*, Vol. 3, Allyn & Bacon Inc., Boston; and Costill, D. L. Dietetics and nutrition for sports performance, *Int. J. Sports Med.* (in press).

use of oxygen; and (b) oxidation, the formation of ATP from carbohydrate, fat and protein molecules with the aid of oxygen.

During the early minutes of exercise and when the intensity of the muscular effort is high, the body is unable to provide sufficient oxygen to regenerate the needed ATP. To compensate, both the ATP–PCr and glycolytic energy systems generate ATP without the aid of oxygen, a process termed anaerobic metabolism. In this system, muscle glycogen, sugar stored within the fibres, is broken down through the action of special glycolytic enzymes, resulting in the production and accumulation of lactic acid. Unfortunately, this system of energy production is relatively inefficient, providing only 3 mol of ATP from the anaerobic breakdown of 1 mol (180 g) of glycogen. On the other hand, in the presence of oxygen, aerobic metabolism can generate 39 mol of ATP from 1 mol of glycogen.

In addition to being inefficient glycolysis results in the incomplete breakdown of glycogen, producing lactic acid. In all-out sprint events that last 1 or 2 min the demands on the glycolytic system are high, causing muscle lactic acid levels to rise from a resting value of 1 mmol/kg of muscle to over 25 mmol/kg. The high acid content of the muscle fibres inhibits further breakdown of glycogen and may interfere with the muscle's contractile process.

As mentioned earlier, the energy bound into the ATP molecule is derived from the breakdown of the foods we eat: carbohydrates, fats and protein. When this process of disassembling fuels is conducted in the presence of oxygen, it is said to be oxidative or aerobic. As we have seen, the anaerobic production of ATP, without oxygen, is quite inefficient and inadequate for exercise lasting more than a minute. Consequently, aerobic metabolism is the primary method of energy production during endurance events, placing heavy demands on the athlete's ability to deliver oxygen to the exercising muscles.

Within each muscle fibre, there are special 'power-house' like structures called mitochondria, which use carbohydrates (CHO), fats and proteins in combination with oxygen to produce large amounts of ATP. In this process the energy bonding the carbon, oxygen and hydrogen (H^+) atoms together is liberated by the action of the oxidative enzymes, resulting in the formation of ATP. If left unattended, the hydrogen component of these fuels would be free to disrupt the function of the cells. In the presence of oxygen, however, two hydrogen molecules bond with oxygen to form water, thereby allowing the energy system to flow uninterrupted. Carbon dioxide, formed from the carbon and oxygen within the fuels, is another by-product of oxidative metabolism. When dissolved in the water of the body it forms carbonic acid that upsets the normal cellular homeostasis. Fortunately, carbon dioxide diffuses easily out of the cells and is transported by the venous blood back to the lungs, where it can leave the body in the expired air.

Energy demands of sports

Training for competitive sports may increase one's daily energy expenditure by 25–50%. Long-distance runners, for example, commonly run 15–40 km/day at an average expenditure of 230 270 kJ/km (55–65 kcal/km) (Jung et al., 1987). Distance runners may, therefore, expend 3780–10 080 kJ/day (900–2400 kcal/day) during training. The energy expenditure in other exercise modes, such as cycling, differs from that seen in runners. The energy cost of cycling 160 km at 40 km/h is approximately 120 kJ/km (28.6 kcal/km), or about 4900 kJ/h (1170 kcal/h), a total energy cost of 19 650 kJ (4680 kcal). This suggests that during training cyclists may average more than 25 200 kJ/day (6000 kcal/day) (Sjøgaard et al., 1986). The upper extremes of energy expenditure for skilled competitive cyclists, who have cycled 540 km in 19.3 h is estimated at 39 900 to 58 200 kJ (9500–13 850 kcal) (Kardel & Costill, 1981).

Competitive swimmers in training have been reported to swim 5 to 15 km/day. It has been estimated that these athletes expend roughly 5250 to 15 750 kJ (1250–3750 kcal) during each training session, or about 72 to 210 kJ/kg bodyweight (17–50 kcal/kg bodyweight) per session. In combination with the energy expended for normal living (~125 to 150 kJ/kg bodyweight/day), it can be estimated that the total energy expenditure for swimmers, and perhaps other athletes in heavy training, may range

Table 12.6.1 Estimated energy and carbohydrate (CHO) expenditure during running, swimming and cycling for a 70 kg individual.

Activities	Estimated energy		
	kJ/min (kcal/min)	Total kJ (total kcal)	CHO (g)
Running			
2 mile (3.2 km)	84 (20)	903 (215)	50–55
10 km	735 (17.5)	2940 (700)	150–170
Marathon	63 (15)	11 760 (2800)	500–550
Swimming (front crawl)			
200 m	105 (25)	210 (50)	12 15
1500 m	84 (20)	1680 (400)	90–100
Cycling			
1 hour	71.5 (17)	4285 (1020)	230–250

from 197 to 357 kJ/kg bodyweight/day (47–85 kcal/kg bodyweight/day) (Dengel *et al.*, 1987). A 65 kg athlete would, therefore, have a daily energy expenditure of 12830 to 23200 kJ (3055–5525 kcal).

A large fraction of the energy for training and competition is derived from endogenous CHO, principally muscle and liver glycogen. In activities lasting 60 min or longer, the energy derived from CHO may vary from 50 to 90% of the total energy burned. Thus, a 65 kg athlete who expends 8400 kJ in training might burn 4200 to 7560 kJ of CHO, or 250 to 450 g of CHO. In combination with one's normal daily requirements for CHO (e.g. 300 to 350 g/day), such an athlete would use 550 to 800 g/day, or 8.5 to 12.3 g/kg bodyweight. This is in contrast to a normal intake of only 4.5 g of CHO/kg bodyweight/day. Table 12.6.1 provides examples of the energy and CHO demands for running, swimming and cycling.

Carbohydrates

The production of adenosine triphosphate (ATP) during intense muscular effort depends on the availability of muscle glycogen and blood glucose. Although it is possible to perform light exercise with low levels of these carbohydrates, depletion of these fuels makes it impossible for the muscles to meet their ATP requirements and to sustain the contractile tension needed for work performance (Costill *et al.*, 1973; Hultman, 1979). Fats and proteins contribute to the energy pool used during muscular activity, but these fuels alone cannot support the demands of acute exercise; carbohydrate is the primary fuel for exercise. Even in the presence of adequate muscle glycogen only minor demands are placed on the body's protein and fat reserves. It has been calculated that even in a marathon race less than 1% of the body's total fat and protein stores might be oxidized, whereas total glycogen depletion may occur during the activity (Costill & Miller, 1980).

At the onset of exercise, muscle glycogen is the primary source of carbohydrate used for energy. This point is illustrated by the data in Fig. 12.6.1, which show the rapid decline in muscle glycogen during the early stage of a 3 h treadmill run. Although the test was run at a steady pace, the rate of glycogen used from the gastrocnemius muscle was greatest during the first 90 min of activity. Thereafter, the use of glycogen slowed as stores became depleted. The subject felt only moderate distress during the early part of the run, when the rate of muscle glycogen use was most rapid. Only when muscle glycogen was nearly depleted was severe fatigue experienced.

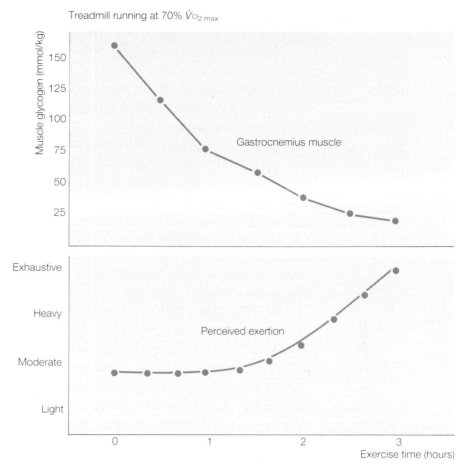

Treadmill running at 70% $\dot{V}_{O_2\,max}$

Fig. 12.6.1 Muscle glycogen content and the subject's rating of effort during a 3-h treadmill run. Note that during the first half of the run, glycogen was used at a higher rate than during the final 90 min of the exercise.

The rate of muscle glycogen depletion depends on a number of factors, including exercise intensity, physical conditioning, exercise mode, environmental temperature, and the pre-exercise diet (Christensen & Hansen, 1939). When the flow of oxygen to the working muscle does not adequately meet the demands for oxidative metabolism, there is greater reliance on CHO for energy. An exponential relationship has been shown between the rate of muscle glycogen utilization and exercise intensty (%$\dot{V}_{O_2\,max}$). Little muscle glycogen is oxidized (0.3 mmol/kg/min) when walking at 20 to 30%$\dot{V}_{O_2\,max}$, whereas repeated maximal contractions can elevate the rate of glycogen use to more than 40 mmol/kg/min.

Many factors effect the rate of glycogen depletion during prolonged exercise. Two hours of cycling at 30%$\dot{V}_{O_2\,max}$, for example, will only reduce muscle glycogen by about 20%, whereas performing at 75% $\dot{V}_{O_2\,max}$ results in almost total depletion (Hermansen *et al.*, 1967). These results further emphasize that there is a marked increase in muscle glycogen use when the work intensity approaches maximal and/or supramaximal work levels.

Early studies by Christensen and Hansen (1939) showed that at exercise levels below 95% of the runner's $\dot{V}_{O_2\ max}$, both carbohydrates and fats are used as fuels. Above this intensity, however, carbohydrates appear to be used almost exclusively; thus, a fast pace in the early stage of an exercise bout may lead to glycogen depletion and premature exhaustion. When muscle glycogen levels are very low, the intensity of the exercise must be reduced to lessen the demands on CHO, thereby, allowing the muscles to rely more on fat.

The higher the initial muscle glycogen stores, the longer the subject can continue to exercise at a given load ($>70\%\dot{V}_{O_2\ max}$). With an initial glycogen content of about 100 mmol/kg w/w, Bergstrom $et\ al.$ (1967) observed that subjects could tolerate a $75\%\dot{V}_{O_2\ max}$ workload for 115 min. When muscle glycogen was reduced to 35 mmol/kg by a low carbohydrate diet, a 75% work effort could be sustained for only 60 min. A 3-day carbohydrate-rich diet resulted in a muscle glycogen content of 200 mmol/kg and a subsequent work time to exhaustion of 170 min.

The glycogen content of muscle has an effect on maximal power output in short-term exercise as well as events lasting more than 1 h (Flynn $et\ al.$, 1987); however, decrements in glycogen content appear to have only a minor influence on sprint performance unless the levels fall below 40 mmol/kg. In the final stages of an endurance event, for example, when the athlete may have to sprint to the finish, the levels of muscle glycogen may be the deciding factor between winning or losing.

Exercise in hot weather can also increase the demands on CHO use by the muscles. Fink $et\ al.$ (1975) have shown a 76% increase in muscle glycogen use during 75 min of exercise in the heat (air temperature = 41° C; humidity = 15%) as compared to similar exercise in the cold (air temperature = 9° C; humidity = 55%). This increased reliance on muscle glycogen appears to be caused by a reduction in muscle blood flow and an increase in intramuscular temperature. Thus, it is apparent that environmental factors may also influence the rate of CHO usage during exercise.

In man, the storage of liver and muscle glycogen depends almost exclusively on the dietary consumption of carbohydrates. As noted earlier, during periods of prolonged exercise and fasting the liver must mobilize its reserves in order to maintain blood glucose. As a consequence of strenuous exercise lasting 60 min, liver glycogen was found to decrease 55% from 244 to 111 mmol/kg tissue (Hultman & Nilsson, 1971). Studies have shown that liver glycogen stores will decrease rapidly when a resting individual is deprived of carbohydrates for only 24 h. In combination with a low carbohydrate diet, hard training may empty the liver glycogen stores. Unlike some animals, man is unable to generate a significant amount of muscle or liver glycogen by gluconeogenesis. The rat, for example, can use various precursors (e.g. glycerol, lactate, etc.) to resynthesize liver glycogen even when deprived of food. Humans, however, must rely on the intake of carbohydrate foods to replace these stores. A single CHO meal has been shown to quickly restore liver glycogen to normal.

The amount of muscle glycogen stored is controlled by the individual's level of activity, training status and the dietary content of CHO. Untrained subjects, who are rested and well nourished, have been found to possess muscle glycogen values ranging from 70 to 110 mmol glucosyl units/kg w/w (Blom et al., 1986). Endurance-trained athletes, on the other hand, have muscle glycogen ranging from 140 to over 230 mmol/kg w/w (Hultman et al., 1971). The higher levels of muscle glycogen seen in the trained individuals appear to be due to the combined influence of chronic exercise, glycogen depletion and CHO intake.

The key enzyme in the regulation of glycogen storage in muscle is glycogen synthetase (UDP-glucose: α-1,4-glucan α-4-glucosyltransferase; EC 2.4.1.11). An inverse relationship ($r = -0.88$) between muscle glycogen content and synthetase I activity has been reported in normally active subjects. Consequently, when muscle glycogen is depleted at the end of exercise the synthetase I activity is dramatically elevated. This enzyme is further activated by insulin and/or glucose infusion; thus, it is not surprising that after exercise it stimulates a rapid resynthesis of muscle glycogen when carbohydrates are ingested. The highest rate of muscle glycogen resynthesis (0.4–0.5 mmol glucosyl units/kg/min) occurs in glycogen-depleted muscle during glucose infusion.

Blood-borne glucose also serves as a major contributor to the metabolic energy pool for muscular activity. At rest the uptake of glucose by muscle accounts for less than 10% of the total oxygen consumption by muscle. During moderate to strenuous cycling exercise, however, the net glucose uptake by the leg muscles increases ten to 20-fold above the resting value (Wahren et al., 1971). During the latter stages of prolonged exercise, the fraction of energy derived from blood glucose increases and may account for 75–90% of the muscle's carbohydrate metabolism (Wahren et al., 1971). This large drain of blood glucose necessitates a concomitant increase in hepatic glucose output, delaying the onset of exertional hypoglycaemia. Since the liver is the major contributor of glucose to the blood, the increased demands imposed by muscular activity result in a rapid reduction in liver glycogen and a greater reliance on gluconeogenesis.

It has been demonstrated that during 4 h of moderate exercise, liver glycogen may be depleted by 75% with an increasing production of glucose from such precursors as lactate, pyruvate, glycerol and gluco-genic amino acids (Wahren, 1966). Despite these mechanisms for en-hanced glucose production and release, as exercise continues beyond 40 to 60 min a gradual imbalance between hepatic production and per-ipheral utilization of glucose may occur (Wahren, 1977). Thus, athletes who compete in events lasting 3 h or longer may become hypoglycaemic; with blood glucose values less than 2.5 mmol/l.

Despite the dramatic drop in liver glycogen, hepatic glucose release remains closely matched to glucose utilization by muscle. Consequently, blood glucose levels do not fall until liver glycogen stores decrease to very low levels. This fine control of blood glucose during exercise is achieved as a consequence of a decrease in the release of insulin from the pancreas and an increase in the muscles' sensitivity to circulating insulin. During prolonged exercise, plasma insulin may drop to 50% of the resting level. In addition, acute bouts of exercise increase the muscles' sensitivity to glucose and insulin. The mechanisms responsible for this finer control of blood glucose and the management of carbohydrate feedings during exercise is not fully understood, but is probably linked to the increase in membrane permeability and an increase in the number of receptors for insulin along the muscle cell membrane.

Carbohydrate intake before exercise

The importance of a rich carbohydrate diet in the days that precede an exhaustive endurance event is well established, and will be discussed later (see below under 'Carbohydrate loading'). However, CHO feedings from 15 min to perhaps 1 h before the exercise may have a detrimental effect on performance (Coyle *et al.*, 1985). As shown in Fig. 12.6.2, glucose feedings taken less than 60 min before exercise may result in a dramatic rise in blood glucose and insulin followed by an increase in CHO oxidation and a rapid fall in blood glucose within the first few minutes of exercise (Foster *et al.*, 1979). Coyle *et al.* (1985) have suggested that glucose levels are reduced because of the antilipolytic effects of insulin on the fat cell and the persistent effect of insulin on hepatocytes and muscle.

Recent studies, however, have shown that the consumption of sugar, in the form of a solid confectionary bar, 30 min before exercise will maintain blood glucose (McMurray *et al.*, 1983). Muscle glycogen use

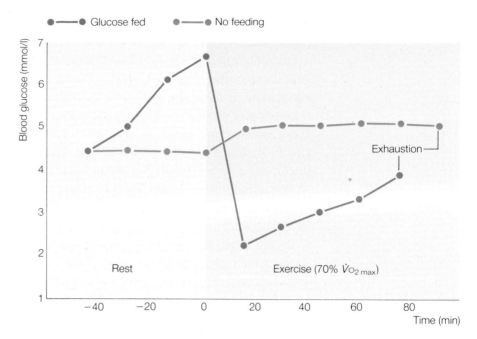

Fig. 12.6.2 Effects of a glucose feeding (70 g) taken 45 min before the start of exercise. Note the rise in blood glucose after the feeding and the rapid fall in glucose during the first 15 min of exercise (Costill & Miller, 1980).

and total CHO oxidation were not affected by the pre-exercise feeding. Similarly, Devlin *et al.* (1986) observed that a snack food (43 g CHO, 9 g fat and 3 g protein) taken 30 min before exercise did not impair endurance performance. Unlike the earlier studies, both of these investigations employed intermittent exercise, which could affect the rate of hepatic glucose release and the uptake of glucose by the contracting muscles.

Ingestion of fructose during the last few minutes before exercise has been shown to produce a less dramatic rise in serum insulin and glucose (Decombaz *et al.*, 1985; Koivisto *et al.*, 1985). Furthermore, fructose does not appear to reduce the levels of circulating free fatty acids to the same extent as glucose. Koivisto *et al.* (1981) observed a high relationship between pre-exercise blood glucose and the subsequent decline in blood glucose during the onset of muscular activity. Since the insulin response to fructose is less pronounced than that observed after glucose or sucrose feedings, it has been suggested that it might serve as a better pre-exercise feeding.

Levine *et al.* (1983) described a sparing of muscle glycogen following the pre-exercise ingestion of a solution containing 75 g fructose when compared to an equal dose of glucose or a placebo water trial (control). Surprisingly, the smaller use of muscle glycogen after the fructose feeding was accompanied by a higher respiratory exchange ratio (RER) than during the control experiment. In addition, these investigators failed to find an exercise hypoglycaemia in either of the sugar-feeding trials (glucose or fructose).

Decombaz et al. (1985) studied the metabolic responses during 60 min of exercise after ingesting glucose and fructose solutions that were labelled with naturally enriched ^{13}C. Blood glucose and hormonal responses (i.e. insulin) to these feedings were similar to previous studies (Hargreaves et al., 1984). In agreement with the study by Hargreaves et al. (1984), sprint performance at the end of 2 h of exercise was not improved as a result of the sugar feedings. Glycogen use during the fructose trial was 67 mmol/kg w/w, compared to 97 mmol/kg w/w in the control trial. This mean difference was not statistically significant ($P > 0.05$). Unfortunately, the pre-exercise glycogen values differed by 33 mmol/kg w/w. Since the rate of glycogen utilization during exercise is dependent on the initial concentration, the differences noted in the study by Decombaz et al. (1985) could differ as a consequence of the pre-exercise level.

The advantage of fructose over glucose as a pre-exercise feeding, therefore, appears doubtful. It should be noted that large fructose feedings (≥ 75 g) may produce an osmotic diarrhoea from incomplete intestinal absorption (Crapo & Kolterman, 1984). In addition, fructose feedings have been shown to elevate blood lactate, which could have some effect on acid–base balance and performance.

Up to this point we have considered only sugar feeding in the 30–60 min period before a bout of exercise. Another topic of interest to those in sport is 'when should the pre-competition meal be taken?' Since an overnight fast will dramatically reduce the liver glycogen supply, pre-exercise meals are essential for endurance performance (Nilsson & Hultman, 1973). Coyle et al. (1985) observed that a high CHO meal (140 g) administered 4 h before 105 min of cycling at 70% $\dot{V}_{O_2\,max}$ resulted in a higher initial level of muscle glycogen (42%) compared to the level after a 16 h fast. Although this feeding was taken 4 h before the exercise, there was still a rapid drop in blood glucose levels and an accelerated rate of CHO oxidation throughout the exercise. Despite the higher initial levels of muscle glycogen (42%) in the CHO feed trial, the glycogen level at the completion of the exercise was similar to that at the end of the fasting trial. Since the subjects appeared to burn glycogen faster when they started with elevated muscle glycogen values, one might expect little performance advantage from this pre-exercise feeding.

On the contrary, Neufer et al. (1987) has shown an improvement in performance when a light CHO meal (200 g CHO) was taken 4 h before exercise and the subjects ate a confectionery bar (45 g CHO) immediately before exercise. Male cyclists performed 45 min of cycling at 77% $\dot{V}_{O_2\,max}$ followed by a 15 min performance ride on an isokinetic cycle ergometer. The total amount of work performed in the final 15 min ride was significantly greater when the light CHO meal was consumed before the exercise (194 735 ± 9448 Nm) than after an overnight fast (159 143 ± 11 407 Nm). Although no differences were found in the amount of glycogen used during the CHO meal and fasting trials (53.9 ± 3.3 and 56.4 ± 3.3 mmol/kg w/w, respectively), the rate of CHO oxidation was significantly greater during exercise in the CHO meal trial (4.45 ± 0.14 g/min) compared to the fasting treatment (2.94 ± 0.28 g/min). Although the precise explanation for the improved performance with the CHO feedings in combination with the meal is not clear, it has been suggested that the feedings aid in maintaining the hepatic energy reserves and the maintenance of blood glucose for muscle metabolism.

The preceding discussion presents a somewhat confusing picture of the effects of pre-exercise CHO feedings on blood glucose concentrations, CHO oxidation and exercise performance. Nevertheless, the findings can be summarized, as in Table 12.6.2. Although some studies have suggested that pre-exercise feedings (0–5 min before exercise) may cause a reduction in muscle glycogen use, this point remains debatable.

Carbohydrate intake during exercise The occurrence of hypoglycaemia during long-distance running and cycling was noted early in this century and has since been considered as one of the factors responsible for fatigue in long-term exercise (Levine *et al.*, 1924). There is general agreement that CHO given during exercise will elevate blood glucose and enhance endurance performance (Fig.

Table 12.6.2 Effects of pre-exercise CHO feedings on blood glucose, muscle glycogen use and exercise performance. All trials are compared to trials without a feeding.

Condition	Blood glucose	Muscle glycogen	Performance
Glucose 30–45 min before exercise	↓	⟷	↓
Fructose 30–45 min before exercise	⟷	⟷	←↑→
Glucose, fructose, or snack CHO 0–5 min before exercise	←↑→	⟷	↑
Glucose or CHO meal 3–4 h before exercise	←↑→	⟷	↑

Arrows denote an increase ↑, decrease ↓, or no change ⟷ compared to fasting conditions.

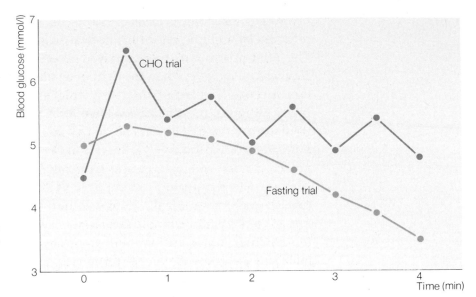

Fig. 12.6.3 Blood glucose during 4 h of cycling at 50% of $\dot{V}_{O_{2max}}$ with and without CHO feedings at hourly intervals. Time of feedings are shown with upright arrows.

12.6.3). Mitchell *et al.* (1987) observed that sprint performance at the end of 2 h of intermittent exercise was equally improved with 33.5, 39.4 and 50.1 g of CHO taken each hour (g CHO/h) compared to a water trial. Likewise, Hargreaves *et al.* (1984) demonstrated that a solid feeding (confectionary bar) of 42.5 g CHO/h improved sprint performance following 4 h of intermittent exercise. Smaller doses of CHO, on the other hand, have failed to improve endurance. Fielding *et al.* (1985) reported that a smaller dose of CHO (21.5 g/h) improved the subjects' sprint time after 4 h of cycling when they were fed every 30 min during the trial (10.75 g/ 30 min). However, when the 21.5 g was given every hour, the improvement in sprint performance failed to reach significance ($P<0.05$). These data suggest that a dose of 21.5 g/h may be the minimal CHO dosage to elicit an improvement in exercise performance. Since most of the other investigations have administered considerably larger doses of CHO, it is not surprising that they have found consistent benefits to endurance with combinations of feedings given immediately before and during the exercise.

The form of CHO ingested during an exercise bout does not appear to be of major concern. Both liquid and solid CHO feedings are equally well tolerated and assimilated during prolonged exercise (1–4 h). Neufer *et al.* (1987), for example, has shown that feeding CHO as either liquid or solid improved endurance performance to a similar degree, though these feedings had no effect on the rate of muscle glycogen use.

The digestive processes and metabolic rates for different sugars have been examined at rest and during prolonged exercise (Wahlqvist *et al.*,

1978; Flynn *et al.*, 1987). Since 1920, glucose was proposed to be absorbed more quickly than starch, a glucose polysaccharide (Allen, 1920). Under resting conditions, subjects appear to experience a sharper rise in blood glucose following the intake of 70 g of glucose than when a similar quantity of starch is administered. Wahlqvist *et al.* (1978), however, has shown that this difference is probably more affected by the dietary form (i.e. liquid vs. solid) than the differences in glucose chain length. Studies of ^{14}C glucose and ^{14}C fructose ingestion at rest and during exercise have shown that they begin to appear in the blood 5 to 7 min after consumption. This suggests that any differences in the rate of gastric emptying and/or absorption for these sugar molecules must be small and have no effect on delivery to the muscles. It should also be noted that despite the CHO form ingested (i.e. glucose, fructose or glucose polymer), glucose remains the primary form of blood sugar (e.g. 99% of total CHO). Attempts to determine the influence of glucose, fructose and glucose polymer solutions on exercise performance have found no differences in performance between the different feedings. Thus, there does not appear to be any major advantage of one CHO form over another in the ability to enhance performance during endurance exercise. Regardless of the type of sugar ingested, all appear to be converted to glucose during the process of intestinal absorption or by the liver with no measurable difference in the rate of appearance in the blood.

Although it is generally agreed that CHO ingestion during prolonged exercise will enhance performance, the mechanism responsible for this improvement is not fully understood. It has been suggested that the CHO feedings may produce a sparing of muscle glycogen, though other investigators support the idea that the CHO is used directly as fuel only after muscle glycogen levels are substantially depleted. An early study by Bagby *et al.* (1978) demonstrated that both liver and muscle glycogen sparing occurred as a result of glucose infusion during exercise in rats. Glucose feedings also improved running time to exhaustion in these animals. Similarly, glucose infusion has also been shown to delay the rate of glycogen depletion during exercise in humans (Bergstrom & Hultman, 1967b). Oral administration of CHO (42.5 g CHO/h) in humans has also been reported to reduce the rate of muscle glycogen use (Hargreaves *et al.*, 1984).

Measurements of leg and/or splanchnic arteriovenous differences do not allow for a determination of the energy contributions of the exogenous CHO feedings. Recent studies using naturally labeled ^{13}C glucose have made this determination possible (Pirnay *et al.*, 1981). These investigations suggest that ingested glucose is readily available for oxidation throughout the exercise bout. Nevertheless, the exact pathways and fates for orally administered CHO are still unclear and must await further study.

Thus, there is general agreement that CHO feedings during exhaustive endurance exercise, lasting for an hour or more, will enhance performance. There is substantial evidence which indicates that the intake of CHO either as a single feeding at the start of the exercise, or as frequent feedings throughout the activity, contribute extensively to CHO oxidation during the activity. Comparisons of glucose, fructose and sucrose feedings during exercise have failed to demonstrate any differences between their rate of oxidation or the contribution of these sugars to endurance performance.

Gastrointestinal absorption during exercise

There are obvious benefits to be gained by ingesting carbohydrate solutions during prolonged exercise, especially during hot weather. These solutions can minimize the degree of dehydration that normally results from heavy sweating, thereby reducing the stress placed on the circulatory system. Since little water and practically no carbohydrate can be absorbed directly from the stomach, the rate of water and sugar delivered to the small intestine is critical. Despite a wealth of research conducted to describe the factors that influence the rate of gastric (stomach) emptying and intestinal absorption, there is considerable confusion and debate concerning the most ideal composition of fluids for use during exercise.

The gastric emptying and intestinal absorption of carbohydrate solutions has been studied extensively at rest and during varied levels of muscular effort (Hunt & Pathak, 1960; Hunt & Knox, 1969). Early studies suggested that moderate to heavy exercise inhibited gastric emptying to a small degree (Costill & Saltin, 1974), whereas intestinal absorption of carbohydrate solutions might be drastically impaired by exercise. In addition, Rowell et al. (1964) showed that splanchnic blood flow was only 30–40% of the resting value at workloads demanding $70\% \dot{V}_{O_2 \, max}$. Williams et al. (1964) showed that the urinary output of orally ingested 3-O-methyl-D-glucose, an actively transported sugar, is reduced during exercise in the heat. Since urinary output of orally ingested D-xylose, a passively absorbed sugar, is not affected by similar exercise, these workers postulated that exercise reduces blood flow to the gut and that this, in turn, reduces active but not passive intestinal absorption.

Recent investigations, however, have failed to confirm these earlier findings and have even suggested that gastrointestinal absorption of sugar solutions may be accelerated during intense physical activity (Mitchell *et al.*, 1987). In light of these contradictions, it seems appropriate that we contrast the early and recent studies of gastric emptying to determine the limitations of exercise and the ingestion of sugar solutions. In 1967 Åstrand (1967a) examined the consumption of a 40 g% lemon-flavoured glucose solution by Swedish cross-country skiers at 5 to 6 km (25 min) intervals throughout a 50 km race. Although the total volume of fluid ingested was in excess of 1 litre, representing ~400 g of sugar in about 4 h of skiing, none of the men experienced any sensations of gastric filling or discomfort. Similarly, Costill *et al.* (1970) observed that marathon runners could empty 83–90% of a glucose-electrolyte solution (2000 ml, 4.4 g% glucose, 20 mmol/l Na^+, 15 mmol/l K^+) that was consumed at 5 min intervals during 2 h of treadmill running (70% $\dot{V}_{O_2 \, max}$). Under resting conditions the rate of gastric (stomach) emptying appears to be affected by the volume, temperature, osmolality, sugar content and energy content of the drink. Studies by Costill and Saltin (1974) indicated that these factors are unaffected during exercise, provided the energy demands are less than 60–70% $\dot{V}_{O_2 \, max}$. Above that work level there is a steady slowing of gastric emptying. It should be noted that these studies were all performed with a nasogastric tube positioned before the exercise and prior to the ingestion of the test solutions. This procedure generally causes some discomfort and may have influenced the rates of gastric emptying. When subjects are allowed to exercise and consume fluids without the discomfort of a nasogastric tube, the rate of gastric emptying seems to be substantially greater.

More recently, Coyle *et al.* (1978) compared the emptying rate of three commercially available solutions with a placebo water drink. They observed that the highest CHO solutions (4.5 g glucose-fructose/100 ml) significantly slowed the rate of gastric emptying. Foster *et al.* (1980) also found that solutions containing the greatest amounts of CHO emptied more slowly than water. However, a 5 g/100 ml (g%) glucose polymer (maltodextrin) solution was found to empty faster than a similar concentration of glucose. It appears that the advantage of the polymer's higher molecular weight and lower osmolality on gastric emptying is only experienced when the solute concentration is 5 g% or less. In either case, the rate of CHO delivery was shown to be inversely related to the concentration of the drink.

In addition to glucose polymers, the response of gastric emptying also seems to be affected by other sugars (Hunt & Knox, 1968). Whereas glucose appears to empty at a linear rate, fructose has been shown to leave the stomach at an exponential rate. Glucose solutions emptied at a constant rate of 0.1 g/min while fructose was observed to empty at a rapid rate during the first 20 min after ingestion, yielding a mean emptying rate of 0.2 g/min.

It has been suggested that a combination of glucose polymer and fructose might provide an optimal replacement of fluids and CHO. Seiple *et al.* (1983) compared two drinks containing 3 g% glucose polymer and 2 g% fructose with a drink containing 5 g% glucose polymer and 2 g% fructose. They observed no significant difference in the rate of gastric emptying of the two solutions. However, Neufer *et al.* (1986) observed that during 15 min of treadmill running a glucose polymer-fructose solution (4.5 g% maltodextrin; 2.6 g% fructose) emptied faster than a solution containing 5.5 g% maltrin and 2 g% glucose. This suggests that glucose may exert a greater inhibitory effect on gastric emptying than a similar concentration of fructose.

Contrary to these findings, Mitchell *et al.* (1987) recently observed no difference between the gastric emptying rates of three different CHO solutions containing 5–7.5% mixtures of maltodextrins, glucose, fructose and sucrose. On average, 94–96% of the ingested drinks were emptied from the stomach during the 2 h intermittent exercise period. In addition, Segal *et al.* (1985) reported that there was no difference in gastrointestinal transit time for a flavoured water placebo and an 18 g% glucose solution taken during intermittent exercise at 74% $\dot{V}_{O_2 \, max}$. Thus, movement of carbohydrate solutions out of the stomach during prolonged exercise

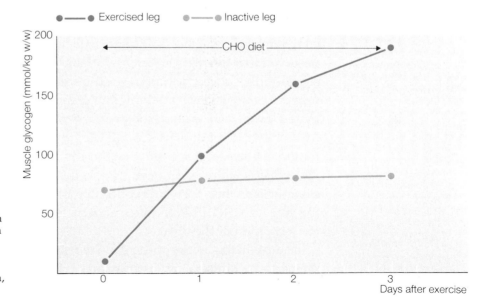

Fig. 12.6.4 Effect of prior exercise and glycogen depletion (exercised leg) on the rate of muscle glycogen resynthesis. Note that the non-exercised leg did not benefit from the rich CHO diet (Bergstrom & Hultman, 1966).

does not appear to be as great a problem as suggested by early studies. Although there are a number of anecdotal reports of gastric distress associated with fluid ingestion during exercise, these problems may be isolated individual complications.

Carbohydrate intake after exercise

The rate of muscle glycogen resynthesis after exhaustive exercise is related to the muscle's glycogen synthase activity and the dietary CHO content. Furthermore, a high CHO diet will not increase muscle glycogen storage above normal (80–120 mmol/kg w/w) unless the diet is preceded by a depletion of muscle glycogen and a concomitant increase in synthase activity. This point was first demonstrated by Bergstrom and Hultman (1966). As shown in Fig. 12.6.4, one-leg cycling lowered the glycogen only in the exercised leg. When the subject ate a CHO-rich diet for 3 days, only the exercised leg showed a supercompensation of muscle glycogen stores.

Early studies of muscle glycogen storage during repeated days of endurance running concluded that only a partial resynthesis of glycogen occurred when the subjects were fed a mixed diet containing 250–350 g of CHO/day (Costill *et al.*, 1971). As shown in Fig. 12.6.5, there was a consistent day-by-day decline in the muscle's (vastus lateralis) glycogen stores despite the CHO intake. During a similar training regimen (cycling), however, we have noted that a diet rich in CHO (550–600 g/day) effectively restored muscle glycogen in the 22 h between exercise sessions.

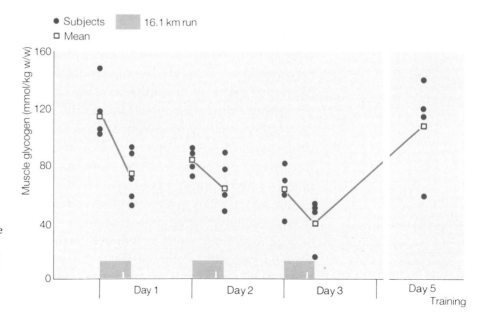

Fig. 12.6.5 Muscle glycogen depletion on three successive days of hard training (16.1 km/day). The subjects consumed a mixed diet containing 55% of energy as CHO (Costill & Miller, 1980).

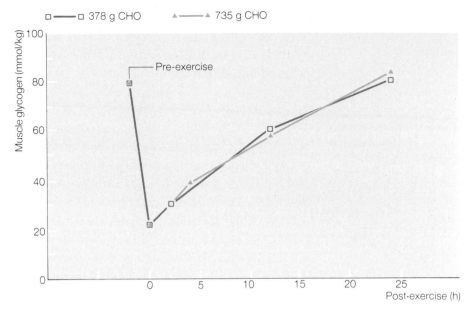

Fig. 12.6.6 Mean muscle glycogen concentrations for two dietary regimens following exhaustive exercise. Note that despite the difference in CHO ingestion there was no difference in the rate of muscle glycogen resynthesis (Costill & Miller, 1980).

MacDougall *et al.* (1977) observed that after exercise which lowered muscle glycogen to 28% of its pre-exercise value, a mixed diet (13 000 kJ/ 24 h) resulted in complete resynthesis within 24 h (Fig. 12.6.6). They noted, however, that within this time period, the rate of resynthesis could not be accelerated by a higher than normal CHO intake.

It should be noted that there are marked differences in the metabolic rates of simple (e.g. glucose) and complex (e.g. starch) CHO. Measurements of serum cholesterol and triglyceride values show an increase when sugars were fed and a decrease when the diet contained the same calories in the form of starch. Absorption of a large dose of glucose, resulting in a temporary hyperglycaemia, may overload the Embden–Meyerhof pathway and impose a heavier load on the hexose-monophosphate shunt. This would favour the production of large quantities of NADPH, tending to enhance the formation of free fatty acids and cholesterol. Complex CHO, such as starch, produce a lesser use of the hexose-monophosphate shunt, since they cause a smaller rise in blood glucose and insulin. It should be noted, however, that these responses to simple and complex CHO were observed in relatively untrained subjects. It is speculative to assume that the responses would be similar in endurance-trained men and women. To the contrary, endurance-trained subjects generally demonstrate a diminished hyperglycaemia and a lower insulin response to a given oral glucose load than do untrained subjects (Lohmann *et al.*, 1978). Thus, endurance athletes demonstrate a greater tolerance to CHO, diverting the majority of such feedings to glycogen storage with little disturbance in their serum lipids.

In light of these differences in simple and complex CHO, one might anticipate a difference in the rate and quantity of glycogen resynthesis following diets rich in glucose or starch. Early studies by Bergstrom and Hultman (1967a) showed that the infusion of glucose and fructose in exercised men resulted in about the same glycogen resynthesis with both sugar forms. More recently, well trained men who were fed either glucose or starch diets (70% of calories) for 2 days after an exhaustive exercise bout, demonstrated little difference in glycogen resynthesis. There was, however, a tendency for the starch diet to produce a greater glycogen storage after 2 days of rest. Additional research is needed to confirm this finding of enhanced glycogen storage with starch.

Comparisons of glycogen resynthesis with glucose, fructose and sucrose feedings have been made by several investigators. Blom et al. (1982) compared glucose, sucrose and fructose feedings (0.7 g/kg body-weight) given every hour for 8 h. Muscle glycogen was measured immediately after, and 8 h after, exhaustive exercise. Glycogen resynthesis was similar after 8 h of glucose and sucrose feedings, but a significantly slower rate of storage was observed following the fructose ingestion. These findings were confirmed by Conlee et al. (1982) who examined the effect of glucose and fructose feedings on muscle glycogen resynthesis in rats after 1 h of exercise. Muscle glycogen recovered at a faster rate for the first 2 h of recovery in the glucose-fed animals. Liver glycogen resynthesis, on the other hand, occurs more rapidly with fructose than with glucose feedings (Nilsson & Hultman, 1973). It is felt that this occurs because fructose is mainly metabolized in the liver. Thus, while glucose appears to promote muscle glycogen resynthesis more rapidly after exhaustive exercise, liver glycogen may be restored faster with fructose feedings.

Carbohydrate loading

Although, studies conducted in the late 1960s demonstrated that exercise–diet manipulation could double the muscle glycogen stores normally observed in inactive subjects, Christensen and Hansen (1939) were the first investigators to use various CHO diets to enhance endurance performance. They observed that men on a high CHO diet for 3 days performed heavy work loads for more than twice as long as men on a high fat diet. Based on studies by Bergstrom et al. (1967a), Åstrand (1967b) proposed that the optimal plan to achieve maximal glycogen storage (glycogen loading) in preparation for endurance competition would be to perform an exhaustive training bout 1 week before competition (i.e. depletion exercise), followed by 3 days on a diet rich in fat and protein. This kept muscle glycogen levels low and elevated glycogen synthetase activity. Thereafter, the athlete consumed a high carbohydrate diet for the final days leading up to the competition. It was proposed that the intensity and volume of training performed during this week-long regimen should be reduced to prevent additional consumption of muscle glycogen and to permit 'maximal' glycogen storage.

This regimen has been shown to effectively elevate muscle glycogen to values above 200 mmol/kg w/w, more than twice the normal levels (i.e. 80–100 mmol/kg w/w) seen in inactive subjects who were fed only a mixed diet. The benefits of this regimen for competitive performance were subsequently demonstrated by Karlsson and Saltin (1971). Using a cross-over design, two groups performed the depletion phase of the loading regimen and then consumed either a high CHO diet (~70% CHO) or a mixed diet for 3 days before a 30 km running race. The best performances were observed following the CHO loading regimen.

Unfortunately, the 3 days of low CHO intake causes the athlete to become irritable, hypoglycaemic and unable to train. In addition, the depletion exercise performed 7 days before the competition may not be

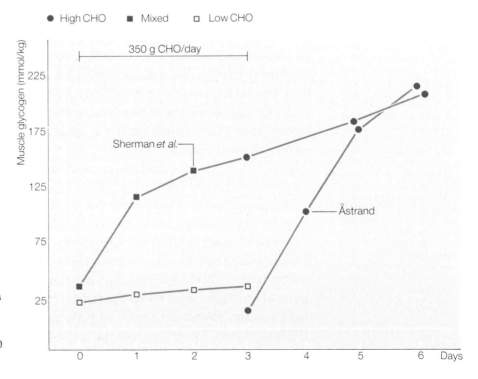

Fig. 12.6.7 A comparison of two dietary regimens designed to maximize muscle glycogen storage. The major difference between these two diets occurs in the first 3 days. In the regimen described by Åstrand (1967a) the subjects were fed a low CHO diet, whereas that proposed by Sherman *et al.* (1981) used a normal mixed diet on days 0 to 3.

in the best interest of the athlete. As noted earlier, the trauma associated with such muscular efforts may interfere with glycogen resynthesis, and might also subject the athlete to any number of overstress injuries. Consequently, Sherman *et al.* (1981) studied a less drastic diet routine. They observed that when a mixed diet was used for 3 days instead of the low CHO phase of the regimen, muscle glycogen achieved the same, high levels as in the routine described by Åstrand (1967b). A comparison of the dietary regimen proposed by Sherman *et al.* (1981) and Åstrand (1967b) is shown in Fig. 12.6.7. Thus, it appears that neither the glycogen depletion exercise nor the 3 days of low CHO diet are necessary for maximal muscle glycogen storage. In our studies we have observed that all endurance-trained athletes are able to achieve muscle glycogen levels above 190 mmol/kg w/w simply by resting for 2 to 3 days, while eating a diet rich in CHO (~8 to 10 g CHO/kg bodyweight).

Since approximately 2.6 g of water is stored with each gram of glycogen, CHO loading often produces a 1–2 kg increase in bodyweight (Costill & Miller, 1980). It has been suggested that acute changes in bodyweight may be a practical method to monitor muscle glycogen storage. Unfortunately, such gross indications of body water content are confused by changes in body fat and extracellular water balance. Nevertheless, early morning weight, taken after emptying the bladder and before breakfast, may provide an indication of the individuals readiness for endurance exercise.

Carbohydrate loading only benefits the athlete in long-term events (> 1 h), where fatigue and exhaustion result from a lack of muscle glycogen. In all-out exercise bouts lasting for less than an hour fatigue may be caused by changes in muscle acid–base balance and/or other disturbances in cellular homeostasis. However, athletes who train for several hours each day must be aware of the large CHO demands imposed by such exercise and the need to replenish their muscle and liver glycogen stores between training sessions (Costill *et al.*, 1971).

Proteins and fats

Proteins are nitrogen-containing compounds formed by amino acids. They constitute the major structural component of the cell, antibodies, enzymes and many hormones. Protein is necessary for growth, but it is also necessary for: the repair and maintenance of body tissues; the production of haemoglobin (iron + protein); the production of enzymes, hormones, mucus, milk and sperm; the maintenance of normal osmotic balance; and protection from disease through antibodies. Proteins are also potential sources of energy, but they are generally spared when fat and carbohydrate are available in ample supply. Over 20 amino acids have been identified, and of these, eight or nine are considered to be essential as a part of the daily food intake. While many of the amino acids can be manufactured or synthesized by the body, these essential or indispensable amino acids either cannot be synthesized by the body or cannot be synthesized at a rate sufficient to meet the body needs, and thus become a necessary part of the diet. If any one of these is absent from the diet, protein cannot be synthesized or body tissue maintained. Protein sources in the diet that contain all of the essential amino acids in the proper ratio and in sufficient quantity are referred to as complete proteins. Meat, fish and poultry are the three primary complete proteins. The proteins in vegetables and grains are referred to as incomplete proteins, as they do not supply all of the essential amino acids in appropriate amounts.

Approximately 5–15% of the total calories consumed per day are in the form of protein. This is considered by many to be two to three times the actual amount of protein necessary for proper body function. The daily recommended allowance published in 1980 by the US National Research Council is 45 and 56 g/day for the teenage and adult male, respectively, and 44–46 g/day for the teenage and adult female. Since the allowance is dependent on the individual's bodyweight, an allowance of 0.8 g/kg bodyweight is considered appropriate for the adult. These recommendations are substantially lower than the 1968 recommendations.

Is it necessary for athletes who are training for strength and muscle bulk to increase their normal dietary intake of protein? Does protein supplementation enhance athletic performance? It is generally agreed that little protein is consumed (<9% of total energy) as fuel for muscular work. If fats or carbohydrates are available, they are selected in preference to proteins as sources of energy. The early studies found little or no difference in performance between diets low, normal and high in protein. Darling *et al.* (1944) studied the effects of a low protein diet (53 g/day) on endurance performance, compared with diets containing normal (95–113 g/day) and high (151–192 g/day) levels of protein. No differences between diets were found for endurance, serum protein, erythrocyte count or haemoglobin content. Pitts *et al.* (1944) reported no reduction in endurance following a diet low in protein compared to diets of normal and high protein content.

In her comprehensive review, Haymes (1983) has concluded that a protein intake of 1.0 g/kg bodyweight/day may be inadequate for the diets of athletes in training. Increased protein intake may be important during the early stages of training to support increases in muscle mass, myoglobin, enzyme content and erythrocyte formation, and the optimal intake during this period may be as low as 1.2 g/kg bodyweight/day. For weight lifters or athletes undergoing intense strength training, optimal intake may be as high as 2.0 g/kg bodyweight/day.

Fats are composed of about 98% triglycerides, with the remainder including traces of mono- and diglycerides, free fatty acids, phospholipids and sterols. Triglycerides are composed of three molecules of fatty acids and one molecule of glycerol. While fat has generally been thought of in negative terms, i.e. a person is too fat, or the blood fats are elevated placing the person at risk of coronary artery disease, fat in fact provides many useful functions in the body. It is an essential component of cell walls and nerve fibres; a primary source, providing up to 70% of the total energy when the body is in the resting state; a support and cushion for vital organs; involved in the absorption and transport of the fat-soluble vitamins; and an insulative layer subcutaneously for the preservation of body heat.

There are two types of fatty acids: saturated and unsaturated. The difference between the two is in the bonding between carbon and hydrogen atoms. Unsaturated fats contain one (monounsaturated) or more (polyunsaturated) double bonds between carbon atoms in a chain of carbon atoms. Each double bond in the chain takes the place of two hydrogen atoms. When the carbon chain is saturated with hydrogen atoms, i.e. two hydrogen atoms for each carbon atom, this is called a saturated fatty acid. In practical terms, a saturated fat is in the form of a solid, i.e. animal fat, and an unsaturated fat is in the form of a liquid, i.e. fish and vegetable oil. Saturated fats are derived primarily from animal sources and unsaturated fats from plant sources. Saturated fats have been associated with an increased risk of coronary artery disease.

Fat supplies approximately 40–45% of the total caloric intake of the American population, and this represents a substantial increase over the percentage of fat consumed in the early 1900s. In addition, fat from animal sources has increased markedly, and that from vegetable sources has decreased. Most nutritionists recommend that approximately 25% of the caloric intake should be in the form of fat, but this should not exceed 30–35%. While many agree that the reduction of fat intake should come from saturated fats, there is presently a great deal of controversy on specific recommendations for the intake of saturated fats, particularly in reference to egg and dairy products.

Minerals and vitamins

Athletes are always looking for an edge, something that will give them an advantage. Since the difference between winning and losing can often be measured in fractions of a second, no athlete wants to feel that he or she did not try everything possible to achieve his or her best performance. Manipulating the diet and taking extra quantities of various vitamins and minerals seem to be relatively harmless methods to make the body work at its best. But do these really help?

As noted earlier, vitamins are essential for normal body function. Unfortunately, athletes have no way to judge their vitamin levels until they become deficient. Only then do the rather unpleasant symptoms appear. The characteristic sores and loss of vision associated with a deficiency in vitamin B_2 (riboflavin), for example, are a rare event in our society and unheard of among athletes. Earlier evidence has shown that, on the average, most athletes consume equal or greater amounts of vitamins than the RDA (recommended daily allowance). Some individuals, however, have been observed to consume diets containing less than the RDA for vitamins B_6, B_{12}, pantothenic acid and folic acid. Some distance runners were found to be taking less than 50% of the recommended amount for these vitamins, based on the number of calories they were eating. One explanation for the low levels may be that some of the athletes studied were vegetarians or ate diets low in such animal products as meats, cheese, milk and eggs, which are the principal sources of vitamin B_6, B_{12} and pantothenic acid.

There have been a number of studies that found increased endurance with megadoses of vitamins C, E and B-complex, but there are far more studies demonstrating that vitamins in excess of the RDA will not improve performance in either strength or endurance activities. Experts generally agree that popping vitamins will not make up for a lack of talent or training or give one an edge over the competition.

As a matter of fact, too much of a good thing can be harmful. Extremely large doses of vitamins A and D may produce some undesirable effects. Overdoses of vitamin A, for example, may cause a loss of appetite, loss of hair, enlargement of the liver and spleen, swelling of the long bones, and general irritability—scarcely ideal conditions for any athlete. These symptoms, however, have never been reported in athletes, even those taking two to three times the RDA for these vitamins.

All in all, it appears that the RDA values for the various vitamins are about optimal for normal body operations, though possibly on the conservative side. Certainly, there is no convincing evidence to prove that vitamin pills taken to supplement a balanced diet will improve athletic performance. Megadoses of vitamins may be of some value, if for some reason you wish to increase the vitamin content of your urine, since that is where most of the excess ends up. Perhaps that is why it is said that athletes produce the most expensive urine in the world.

Minerals are the second most widely used diet supplement by athletes. Since perspiration tastes salty, many athletes fear a large loss of body salts during periods of heavy sweating. Actually, sweat is quite dilute when compared to other body fluids. There is, however, a wide individual variation in the quantity of electrolytes lost in sweat. Although fewer electrolytes are lost in the sweat of highly trained and heat-acclimatized runners than untrained individuals, the mineral content of the diet can have an effect on the electrolyte concentration of sweat. A low salt diet results in a low salt sweat. The body adjusts the electrolyte content of sweat to keep pace with dietary intake. It seems that even without mineral supplements, the body can get all it needs from the natural minerals in food.

Iron is an essential component of haemoglobin, the oxygen-carrying component of blood, and of myoglobin, the oxygen-transporting pigment of muscle. Since iron-deficiency anaemia is known to impair endurance performance, it is important to distinguish between true anaemia and the plasma volume dilution associated with repeated days of training in warm weather. Training tends to increase the volume of plasma more than the number of red blood cells, producing a drop in haemoglobin concentration with no apparent effect on oxygen transport or endurance. Plasma water changes dramatically with both acute and chronic exercise, whereas the number of red cells remains relatively constant. Thus, changes in plasma volume can alter the concentration of red blood cells and haemoglobin, giving the false impression of anaemia or an excess of blood cells.

Several studies have reported that between 36 and 82% of female runners are anaemic or iron deficient. In light of this high frequency of iron deficiency in females, it seems logical to suggest that they include iron-rich foods in their diets. In addition, athletes suspected to be anaemic or iron deficient should be tested for serum ferritin, a measure of the body iron stores and a method to determine the athlete's need for extra dietary iron. Iron supplementation should, however, be directed by a physician, since prolonged administration of iron can cause an iron overload, a potentially serious condition.

Many athletes wish to lose body fat while continuing to train hard. Unfortunately, to lose excess fat the body must be forced to rely more heavily on its fat reserves for energy, while taking in little fuel. This results in an energy deficit and a gradual reduction in the body's fat weight. Though such a diet–exercise regimen accelerates the rate of fat loss, it fails to allow for adequate replacement of muscle and liver glycogen stores. As a result, the athlete may feel heavy and is easily fatigued, able to train only at a relatively slow pace and with a reduced total work output.

During periods of voluntary weight loss the individual must take care to obtain the essential vitamins and minerals while consuming fewer than required calories. Malnutrition among these individuals may occur when they consume foods low in these necessary ingredients. Under these conditions it may be helpful to use vitamin and mineral supplements.

Attempts to lose weight should be scheduled for periods when the athletes are not preparing for competition. During these periods they can afford to perform lower intensity exercise for longer periods, thereby stimulating the burning of calories, mostly fat. Though exercise aids in losing weight, the only way known to ensure the removal of body fat is 'partial-starvation'. Too bad it isn't as easy or as enjoyable to get rid of body fat as it is to put it on!

Fluid balance for optimal performance

The ability to lose body heat during exercise depends, for the most part, on the formation and evaporation of sweat. The amount of sweat lost during exercise, in turn, depends on the exercise intensity, body size and environmental heat stress. Exercising in warm weather may evoke sweat losses in excess of 2 l/h. Despite efforts to drink fluids during an event such as a marathon, sweating and the loss of water in the air breathed may reduce body water content by 13–14%.

Studies have shown that dehydrated individuals are quite intolerant of exercise and heat stress. Distance runners, for example, are forced to slow their pace by 2% for each percent of weight lost as a consequence of dehydration. Both heart rate and body temperature are elevated during exercise when the individual is dehydrated more than 2% of bodyweight.

The impact of dehydration on the cardiovascular system is quite predictable. Plasma volume is lost and the ability to provide adequate blood flow to the skin and muscles is reduced. Under such circumstances, it is common for subjects to collapse, showing the usual symptoms of heat exhaustion. It is difficult to understand how some athletes tolerate several hours of hard running in warm weather. In addition to the body water lost during endurance events, many nutrients are known to escape with sweat. The following discussion will examine the effects of heavy sweating on body water and the mineral composition of body tissues.

Human sweat has been described as a 'filtrate of plasma', since it contains many of the items present in the water portion of blood, including sodium, chloride, potassium, magnesium and calcium. However, even though sweat tastes salty, it actually contains far fewer minerals than do body fluids. Sweat is considered hypotonic, i.e. it is a very dilute version of body fluids.

Sodium and chloride are the ions primarily responsible for maintaining the water content of the blood. The concentrations of sodium and chloride in sweat are roughly one-third those found in plasma and five times those found in muscle. The ionic concentration of sweat may vary

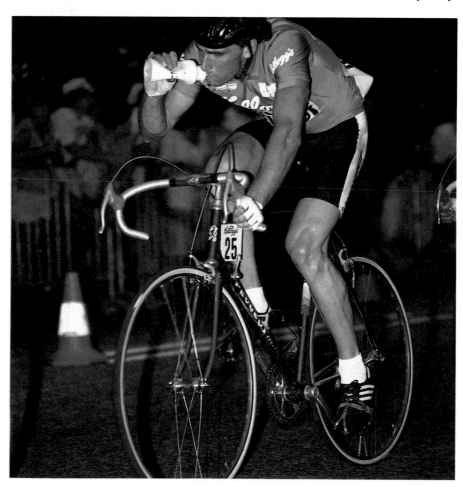

Fig. 12.6.8 Drinks should be readily available during events of extended duration such as road cycling, particularly in warm weather, as it is important for athletes to avoid dehydration. Courtesy of Ace Photo Agency.

markedly between individuals and is strongly influenced by the rate of sweating and the athlete's state of training and heat acclimatization.

At the high rates of sweating reported during endurance events, sweat contains relatively high levels of sodium and chloride, but little potassium, calcium and magnesium. A sweat loss of nearly 4 kg, representing a 5.8% reduction in bodyweight, resulted in sodium, potassium, chloride and magnesium losses of 155, 16, 137 and 13 mmol, respectively. Based on estimates of the athlete's body mineral contents, such losses would only lower the body's sodium and chloride content by roughly 5–7%. At the same time, total body levels of potassium and magnesium, two ions principally confined to the inside of the cells, would decrease by about 1%.

The other major source of mineral loss is routine urine production. In addition to cleaning the blood of cellular waste products, the kidneys also control the body's water and electrolyte content. Under normal conditions, the kidneys excrete about 50 ml of water per hour. During exercise, however, blood flow to the kidneys decreases, and urine production drops to near zero. Consequently, electrolyte losses by this avenue are quite diminished during exercise.

There is another facet of the kidneys' management of electrolytes. If an individual eats 250 mmol of sodium and chloride per day, normally the kidneys will excrete an equal amount of those electrolytes to keep their levels constant. Heavy sweating and dehydration, however, cause the release of aldosterone, a hormone from the adrenal gland that stimulates the kidneys to reabsorb sodium and chloride. Since the body loses more water than electrolytes during heavy sweating, the concentration of these minerals in the body fluids rises. That means that instead of showing a drop in plasma electrolyte concentrations, there is actually an increase. Although this may seem confusing, the point is that during periods of heavy sweating, the need to replace body water is far greater than the need to replace electrolytes.

There are obvious benefits in drinking fluids during prolonged exercise, especially during hot weather. Drinking will minimize dehydration, lessen the rise in internal body temperature, and reduce the stress placed on the circulatory system. Even warm fluids, near body temperature, provide some protection against overheating, but cold fluids seem to enhance body cooling. It takes some of the deep body heat to warm a cold drink to the temperature of the stomach and blood.

A number of sports drinks, containing electrolytes and carbohydrates, are currently on the market and grossing more than US $100 million each year. Unfortunately, many of the claims used to sell these drinks are based on misinterpreted and often inaccurate information. Electrolytes, for example, have long been touted as important ingredients in sports drinks. But, as noted earlier, these claims may be exaggerated, since a single meal can usually replace the electrolytes lost during exercise. The body needs water to bring its concentration of the electrolytes back into balance. While the importance of minerals such as sodium, potassium and magnesium should not be underestimated, blood and muscle biopsy studies have shown that heavy sweating has little or no effect on water and electrolyte concentrations in body fluids during events that last for several hours.

One might wonder if the intake of too much water could overdilute the blood electrolytes, leading to a body deficit? Apparently not. Even marathoners who lose 2.5–4 kg of sweat and drink nearly 2 litre of water, retain normal plasma sodium, chloride and potassium concentrations. Marathoners and ultramarathoners who run 24 to 40 km per day in warm weather and do not season their food, do not develop electrolyte deficiencies.

Some experts have suggested that during an ultramarathon (80 km or more), some individuals may experience unusually low blood sodium levels. A case study of two runners who collapsed after an ultramarathon race in 1983 revealed that they had blood sodium values of 123 and 118 mmol/l, remarkably lower than the normal values of 135–148 mmol/l. One of the runners experienced a grand mal seizure; the other man became disorientated and confused.

Although the cause of these after effects is unclear, the initial diagnosis tends to implicate the lack of body sodium. An examination of the runners' fluid intake (21–24 litre) and estimates of their sodium intake (224–145 mmol) during the run suggested that they diluted their body sodium levels by consuming fluids that contained little sodium. Nevertheless, studies during marathon and exercise bouts lasting up to 6 hours suggest that electrolytes are not an essential ingredient for sports drinks.

So what should the athlete drink during training and competition? Under the extreme stress of hot weather, water is the primary need and the preferred drink. It empties from the stomach with minimal delay, is easy to obtain, and reduces the dehydration associated with heavy sweating. Under cooler conditions, a carbohydrate drink will provide the energy lift needed for peak performance in events lasting an hour or longer. In events lasting less than an hour, there is less need for water ingestion and little benefit from the intake of carbohydrates.

It is important to remember that human thirst is a poor indicator of the body's water and electrolyte balance. No matter how efficiently the kidneys do their job, body fluid balance depends on a strong thirst sensation to stimulate fluid intake. Unfortunately, man's drive to replace body fluids is far less effective than that seen in animals. Burros, for example, will replace a 18 kg body water loss in 5–6 min of continuous drinking, whereas humans who sweat away 2.5–3.5 kg of body mass are satisfied after drinking only 0.5 litre (1 pint) of fluid. If the athlete's thirst is used as the only gauge of water need, it may take 12 to 24 h to replace such a sweat loss. During exercise and heavy sweating, athletes should be encouraged to drink more than their thirst demands.

References

Allen, F. M. (1920) Gross anatomic relations of the pancreas and diabetes. *J. Exp. Med.* **31**, 381.

Åstrand, P. O. (1967a) Diet and athletic performance. *Fed. Proc.* **26**, 1772.

Åstrand, P. O. (1967b) Interrelation between physical activity and metabolism of carbohydrate, fat and protein. In G. Blix (ed) *Nutrition and Physical Activity*. Uppsala.

Bagby, G. J., Green, H. J., Katsuta, S. & Gollnick, P. D. (1978) Glycogen depletion in exercising rats infused with glucose, lactate or pyruvate. *J. Appl. Physiol.* **45**, 425.

Bergstrom, J. & Hultman, E. (1966) Muscle glycogen synthesis after exercise: an enhancing factor localized to the muscle cell in man. *Nature* **210**, 309.

Bergstrom, J. & Hultman, E. (1967a) A study of the glycogen metabolism during exercise in man. *Scand. J. Clin. Lab. Invest* **19**, 218.

Bergstrom, J. & Hultman, E. (1967b) Synthesis of muscle glycogen in man after glucose and fructose infusion. *Acta Med. Scand.* **210**, 1.

Bergstrom, J., Hermansen, L., Hultman, E. & Saltin, B. (1967) Diet, muscle glycogen and physical performance. *Acta Physiol. Scand.* **71**, 140.

Blom, P., Vaage, O., Kardel, K. & Hermansen, L. (1982) Effect of different carbohydrates on rate of muscle glycogen resynthesis after prolonged exercise. *Med. Sci. Sports Exerc.* **14**, 136.

Christensen, E. H. & Hansen, O. (1939) Arbeitsfåhigkeit und Ernåhrung. *Skand. Arch. Physiol.* **81**, 160.

Conlee, R. K., Lawler, R. & Ross, P. (1982) Effect of fructose or glucose ingestion on glycogen repletion in muscle and liver after exercise or fasting. *Med. Sci. Sports Exerc.* **14**, 137.

Costill, D. L., Bowers, R., Branam, G. & Sparks, K. (1971) Muscle glycogen utilization during prolonged exercise on successive days. *J. Appl. Physiol.* **31**, 834.

Costill, D. L., Gollnick, P. D., Jansson, E. C., Saltin, B. & Stein, E. M. (1973) Glycogen depletion patterns in human muscle fibers during distance running. *Acta. Physiol. Scand.* **89**, 374.

Costill, D. L., Kammer, W. F. & Fisher, A. (1970) Fluid ingestion during distance runing. *Arch. Environ. Health* **21**, 520.

Costill, D. L. & Miller, J. M. (1980) Nutrition for endurance sport: carbohydrate and fluid balance. *Int J. Sports Med.* **1**, 2.

Costill, D. L. & Saltin, B. (1974) Factors limiting gastric emptying during rest and exercise. *J. Appl. Physiol.* **37**, 679.

Coyle, E. F., Coggan, A. R., Hemmert, M. K., Lowe, R. C. & Walters, T. J. (1985) Substrate usage during prolonged exercise following a preexercise meal. *J. Appl. Physiol.* **59**, 429.

Coyle, E. F., Costill, D. L., Fink, W. J. & Hoopes, D. G. (1978) Gastric emptying rates for selected athletic drinks. *Res. Quart.* **49**, 119.

Crapo, P. A. & Kolterman, O. G. (1984) The metabolic effects of 2-week fructose feeding in normal subjects. *Amer. J. Clin. Nutr.* **39**, 525.

Darling, R. C., Johnson, R. E., Pits, G. C., Consolazio, F. C. & Robinson, P. F. (1944) Effects of variations in dietary protein on the physical well being of men doing manual work. *J. Nutrition* **28**, 273.

Decombaz, J., Sartori, D., Arnaud, M. J., Thelin, A-L., Schurch, P. & Howald, H. (1985) Oxidation and metabolic effects of fructose or glucose ingested before exercise. *Int. J. Sports Med.* **6**, 282.

Dengel, D. R., Flynn, M. G., Costill, D. L. & Kirwan, J. P. (1988) Determinants of success during triathlon competition. *Res. Quart.*, (in press).

Devlin, J. T., Calles-Escandon, J. & Horton, E. S. (1986) Effects of preexercise snack feeding on endurance cycle exercise. *J. Appl. Physiol.* **60**, 980.

Fielding, R. A., Costill, D. L., Fink, W. J., King, D. S., Hargreaves, M. & Kovaleski, J. E. (1985) Effect of carbohydrate feeding frequencies and dosage on muscle glycogen use during exercise. *Med. Sci. Sports Exerc.* **17**, 472.

Fink, W. J., Costill, D. L. & Van Handel, P. J. (1975) Leg muscle metabolism during exercise in the heat and cold. *Europ. J. Appl. Physiol.* **34**, 183.

Flynn, M. G., Costill, D. L., Hawley, J. A., Fink, W. J., Neufer, P. D., Fielding, R. A. & Sleeper, M. D. (1987) Influence of selected carbohydrate drinks on cycling performance and glycogen use. *Med. Sci. Sports Exerc.* **19**, 37.

Foster, C., Costill, D. L. & Fink, W. J. (1979) Effects of preexercise feedings on endurance performance. *Med. Sci. Sports* **11**, 1.

Foster, C., Costill, D. L. & Fink, W. J. (1980) Gastric emptying characteristics of glucose and glucose polymer solutions. *Res. Quart.* **51**, 299.

Hargreaves, M., Costill, D. L., Coggan, A., Fink, W. J. & Nishibata, I. (1984) Effect of carbohydrate feedings on muscle glycogen utilization and exercise performance. *Med. Sci. Sports Exerc.* **16**, 219.

Haymes, E. M. (1983) Proteins, vitamins, and iron. In M. H. Williams (ed) *Ergogenic Aids in Sport*, pp. 27–55. Human Kinetics, Champaign.

Hermansen, L., Hultman, E. & Saltin, B. (1967) Muscle glycogen during prolonged severe exercise. *Acta Physiol. Scand.* **71**, 129.

Hultman, E. (1979) Muscle fuel for competition. *Phys. Sports Med.* **7**.

Hultman, E., Bergstrom, J. & Roch-Norlund, A. E. (1971) Glycogen storage in human skeletal muscle. In B. Pernow & B. Saltin (eds) *Muscle Metabolism During Exercise*, pp. 273–88. Plenum Press, New York.

Hultman, E. & Nilsson, L. H. (1971) Liver glycogen in man: effect of different diets and muscular exercise. In B. Pernow & B. Saltin (eds) *Muscle Metabolism During Exercise*, pp. 143–51. Plenum Press, New York.

Hunt, J. N. & Knox, M. T. (1968) Regulation of gastric emptying. In C. F. Code (ed) *Handbook of Physiology*, Vol. IV, pp. 1917–35. American Physiological Society, Washington DC.

Hunt, J. N. & Knox, M. T. (1969) The slowing of gastric emptying by nine acids. *J. Physiol.* **201**, 161.

Hunt, J. N. & Pathak, J. D. (1960) The osmotic effects of some simple molecules and ions in gastric emptying. *J. Physiol.* **154**, 254.

Jang, K. T., Flynn, M. G., Costill, D. L., Kirwan, J. P., Houmard, J. A., Mitchell, J. B. & D'Acquisto, L. J.

(1987) Energy balance in competitive swimmers and runners. *J. Swim. Res.* **3**, 19.

Kardel, K. & Costill, D. (1981) Energiforbruk under Styrkeproven. *Pa Hjul.* (Norway) **June**.

Karlsson, J. & Saltin, B. (1971) Diet, muscle glycogen, and endurance performance. *J. Appl. Physiol.* **31**, 203.

Koivisto, V. O., Harkonen, M., Karonen, S., Groop, P. H., Elavainio, R., Ferrannini, E., Sacca, L. & Defronzo, R. A. (1985) Glycogen depletion during prolonged exercise: influence of glucose, fructose or placebo. *J. Appl. Physiol.* **58**, 701.

Koivisto, V. O., Karonen, S. & Nikkila, E. A. (1981) Carbohydrate ingestion before exercise: comparison of glucose, fructose and sweet placebo. *J. Appl. Physiol.* **51**, 783.

Levine, L., Evans, W. J., Cadarette, B. S., Fisher, E. C. & Bullen, B. A. (1983) Fructose and glucose ingestion and muscle glycogen use during submaximal exercise. *J. Appl. Physiol.* **55**, 1767.

Levine, S. A., Gordon, B. & Drick, C. L. (1924) Some changes in the chemical constituents of the blood following a marathon race. *JAMA* **82**, 1778.

Lohmann, D., Liebold, F., Heilmann, W. *et al.* (1978) Diminished insulin response in highly trained athletes. *Metabolism* **27**, 521.

MacDougall, J. D., Ward, G. R., Sale, D. G. & Sutton, J. R. (1977) Muscle glycogen repletion after high-intensity intermittent exercise. *J. Appl. Physiol.* **42**, 129.

McMurray, R. G., Wilson, J. R. & Kitchell, B. S. (1983) The effects of glucose and fructose on high intensity endurance performance. *Res. Quart. Exerc. Sport.* **54**, 156.

Mitchell, J. B., Costill, D. L., Fink, W. J., Houmard, J. A., Flynn, M. G. & Beltz, J. D. (1988) Effect of carbohydrate ingestion on gastric emptying and exercise performance. *Med. Sci. Sports Exerc.*, (in press).

Neufer, P. D., Costill, D. L., Fink, W. J., Kirwan, J. P., Fielding, R. A. & Flynn, M. G. (1986) Effects of exercise and carbohydrate composition on gastric emptying. *Med. Sci. Sports Exerc.* **18**, 658.

Neufer, P. D., Costill, D. L., Flynn, M. G., Kirwan, J. P., Mitchell, J. B. & Houmard, J. (1987) Improvements in exercise performance: effects of carbohydrate feedings and diet. *J. Appl. Physiol.* **62**, 983.

Nilsson, L. H. & Hultman, E. (1973) Liver glycogen in man: the effect of total starvation or a carbohydrate-poor diet followed by carbohydrate refeeding. *Scand. J. Clin. Lab. Invest.* **32**, 325.

Pirnay, F., Krzentowski, G., Crielaard, J. M., Palli-karakis, N., Lacroix, M., Mosora, F., Luyckx, A. S. & Lefebre, P. J. (1981) Oxidation of orally administered naturally labeled ^{13}C-glucose during prolonged muscular exercise. In J. Poortmans & G. Nisset (eds) *Biochemistry of Exercise*, pp. 196–207. University Park Press, Baltimore.

Pitts, G. C., Johnson, R. E. & Consolazio, F. C. (1944) Work in the heat as affected by intake of water, salt and glucose. *Amer. J. Physiol.* **142**, 253.

Rowell, L. B., Blackmon, J. R. & Bruce, R. A. (1964) Indocyanine green clearance and estimated hepatic blood flow during mild exercise to maximal exercise in upright man. *J. Clin. Invest.* **43**, 1677.

Seiple, R. S., Vivian, V. M., Fox, E. L. & Bartels, R. L. (1983) Gastric-emptying characteristics of two glucose polymer-electrolyte solutions. *Med. Sci. Sports Exerc.* **15**, 366.

Sherman, W. M., Costill, D. L., Fink, W. J. & Miller, J. M. (1981) Effect of exercise-diet manipulation on muscle glycogen and its subsequent utilization during performance. *Int. J. Sports Med.* **2**, 114.

Sjøgaard, G., Nielsen, B., Mikkelsen, F., Saltin, B. & Burke, E. (1986) *Physiology in Bicycling.* Movement Publications, Ithaca, NY.

Wahlqvist, M. L., Wilmshurst, E. G., Murton, C. R. & Richardson, E. N. (1978) The effect of chain length on glucose absorption and the related metabolic response. *Am. J. Clin. Nutr.* **31**, 1998.

Wahren, J. (1966) Quantitative aspects of blood flow and oxygen uptake in the human forearm during rhythmic exercise. *Acta Physiol. Scand.* (Suppl. 269) **67**, 1.

Wahren, J., Felig, P., Ahlborg, G. *et al.* (1971) Glucose metabolism during exercise in man. *J. Clin. Invest.* **50**, 2715.

Williams, J. H., Mager, M. & Jacobson, E. D. (1964) Relationship of mesenteric blood flow to intestinal absorption of carbohydrates. *J. Lab. Clin. Med* **63**, 853.

Further reading

Blom, P., Vollestad, N. K. & Costill, D. L. (1986) Factors affecting changes in muscle glycogen concentration during and after prolonged exercise. *Acta Physiol. Scand.* (Suppl. 556) **128**, 67.

Segal, K., Nyman, A., Kral, J. G., Bjorntrop, P., Kotler, D. P. *et al.* (1985) Effects of glucose ingestion on submaximal intermittent exercise (Abstract). *Med. Sci. Sports Exerc.* **17**, 205.

Sherman, W. M., Plyley, M. J., Sharp, R. L., Van Handel, P. J., McAllister, R. M., Fink, W. J. & Costill, D. L. (1982) Muscle glycogen storage and its relationship with water. *Int. J. Sports Med.* **3**, 22.

Wahren, J. (1977) Glucose turnover during exercise in man. *Ann. NY Acad. Sci.* **301**, 45.

12.7 Overtraining and sports psychology

M. O'BRIEN

Overtraining

Overtraining has been a problem in sports for many years and was described by Archibald Maclaren in 1866 and by Thorleif Haug, a famous Norwegian cross-country skier in 1922 (Nilsson, 1987). It is the result of overstressing an athlete either physically or mentally and results in abnormal psychological and physiological performance responses. Everyone has a certain capacity to adapt to stress, but as Hans Seyle (1956) postulated, once you exceed this, adaptation fails and triggers the symptoms of overtraining, which may be a protective physiological response to too much stress. Overtraining tends to occur in highly motivated athletes, in those who are training themselves, or in those who are coached by enthusiastic amateurs with little understanding of basic physiological principles. It also occurs commonly in athletes who are competing frequently in races and matches without adequate rest intervals, with the added stress of environmental changes such as excess heat or humidity, cold, altitude, crossing of time zones associated with competitions in different continents, strange environments and unfamiliar food.

Physiological stress can precipitate the symptoms of overtraining as often as physical stress. The emotional demands of competition, fear of failure, unrealistically high goals and the high expectations of a coach, which the athlete wishes to comply with, may all increase the level of anxiety and precipitate the symptoms of overtraining.

Symptoms and signs The symptoms of overtraining may vary from one athlete to the next. The commonest symptoms are a feeling of fatigue, loss of motivation, and lack of a desire to train and compete. Overtrained athletes tire easily and do not feel any better even with a few days rest. They do not perform well in training or competition. There is usually weight loss, decreased appetite, and a disturbed sleep pattern, e.g. trouble getting to sleep or waking up in the middle of the night for no reason, as a result of which they are tired and irritable during the day. There is usually a difference between the symptoms of overtraining experienced by young inexperienced athletes and older experienced athletes. Younger athletes tend to have more sympathetic signs (Nilsson, 1987), with increased heart rate and blood pressure changes, while in the latter a parasympathetic form occurs, where decreased performance and disturbed coordination are the predominant symptoms. Other complaints are increased susceptibility to colds, headaches, depression, muscle tenderness and tightness, and an increased incidence of injuries. Female athletes may become amenorrhoeic.

Athletes who are not being monitored may not realize that they are in trouble, and many think that if a little work does you good, a lot more is even better. This is more likely to occur in training camps, where athletes usually train for much longer periods of time than normal, e.g. swimmers may increase their training from 3 to 6 h a day over a very short interval. An athlete who has been absent from training for a variety of reasons, who rejoins the squad without allowing for a gradual build-up is also more susceptible. The sudden introduction of a heavy weight training session into a training programme without adequate rest periods is also an added risk.

There are few warning signs, and unless the physician and the coach have worked closely with the athletes and monitored them over a period of time, they will miss the early signs of overtraining. A decrease in performance time during competition and training is highly suspicious. The athlete who is overtrained tends to feel depressed. He or she wants to train but when this is tried, the athlete is too tired and makes mistakes, and gets even more depressed. It becomes a vicious circle, with the athlete trying to work to please the coach. This cycle must be broken by a complete rest from training.

The most reliable and simple physiological indications of overtraining include an increase in resting heart rate, blood pressure and an increase in exercise heart rate and blood pressure associated with a slow recovery time after exercise. If athletes record their resting heart rates each morning in their training diary, an increase of 5 beats/min for no apparent cause necessitates a review of their training and competition programme and a reduction in both. The increase in exercise heart rate can be assessed in several ways depending on the equipment available. For example, heart rate response to a particular swimming distance, e.g. to test swimming speed of 20 m swim from a push off; a 100 m swim from a push-off to test aerobic time; or a 600–700 m swim to test the anaerobic time. Specific distances for cycling or for running can also be used (Houston, 1982).

Costill (1986) monitors runners physiological reactions during standard submaximal 6 min runs. This can be done simply by using telemetry alone to monitor the heart rate, or combined with direct measurements of oxygen and carbon dioxide using a metabolic cart or an Oxycon. A coach can perform some of these tests repeatedly and at relatively little cost to monitor the training performance of the athlete. Increases in exercise blood pressure and also in recovery time can easily be monitored without too much extra cost.

Investigations Fatigue is the commonest symptom that athletes complain of. In each case a medical cause for the fatigue must be excluded before a diagnosis of overtraining is made. Investigations should include full blood count, serum ferritin, ASO (antistreptolysin-O) titre and monospot to rule out anaemia haemolytic strep infection and glandular fever. Cardiac causes for fatigue, though rare, must be ruled out by clinical examination and echocardiography. Low haemoglobin and normal haematocrit levels may be a sign of inadequate iron intake. During training the plasma volume normally expands more than the red cell mass increases. As a result, there is normally a lower haematocrit.

Peaking is the state of perfect physical, psychological readiness which allows the athlete to perform at his or her very best (Montpettit & Hogg, 1982). If an athlete is peaking for a particular event, he or she normally reduces the workload, and the haemoglobin level should increase. If an athlete continues the workload level and is overtrained, the haemoglobin will fall (Falsetti, 1983). Haemoglobin and haematocrit levels are relatively easy and inexpensive to measure. If the haemoglobin levels are below normal, e.g. 13 g for a man, 10 g for a woman, despite adequate iron intake and absorption, and no abnormal loss, overtraining should be suspected.

Elevated resting blood lactate levels may be a sign of overstress but other factors such as diet or previous activity may be the cause (Maglischo, 1982). A higher level of lactate than normal for a particular workload may also be suggestive of overtraining although a lot more work must be done in this area before it can be used as an indication of overtraining. Levels of CPK, LDH and SGOT may also be increased. These muscle enzymes are normally found inside the cell, but their serum levels are often raised in the blood after a heavy training session, and particularly after a marathon, due to muscle damage. As a result they have not proved a reliable sign of overtraining (Maglischo, 1982; Hagerman et al., 1984).

Hormonal changes

Intense physical exercise leads to an increase in the levels of plasma cortisol, which is a catabolic hormone, and a decrease in plasma testosterone, which is anabolic. Prolonged exhaustive physical exercise in man results in a decrease in plasma testosterone, which may be down to female levels. There is an increase in the serum hormone binding gobulin which results in very low testosterone levels (Adlercreutz et al., 1986). There is an increase in the binding of cortisol in muscle tissue and this combined with the high level of cortisol may lead to greater protein catabolism (breakdown) than anabolism inside the muscle cells, which may explain some of the weight loss which occurs. Weight loss can be monitored by weighing the athletes each day at the same time.

Up to recently there was no single physiological measurement which was diagnostic of overtraining, but Adlercreutz et al. (1986) at the Department of Clinical Chemistry in the University of Helsinki found that if there was a decrease in the ratio of plasma-free testosterone to cortisone of more than 30% in overtraining, and if this is combined with a high level of sex hormone binding globulin capacity, it is a good diagnostic pointer and may be useful in monitoring overtraining. The level of serum carnitine is also depressed in overtraining, and at an international symposium in Prague in 1987 Adlercreutz suggested that the level of carnitine may be a useful diagnostic test of overtraining, but these tests are expensive and limited to a few special laboratories.

Female athletes with a history of amenorrhoea or stress fractures should always be investigated, and an adequate hormone profile should be done, in order to determine the oestrogen, progesterone and gonadotrophin-releasing hormone and prolactin levels.

Susceptibility to infection may be the result of reduced immunoglobulin, particularly IgA. If the athlete has had mononucleosis or a severe bout of influenza sometime previously, they may complain of fatigue or an inability to cope with training for some months afterwards. Their IgA may be in the region of 100 mg/100 ml. The normal range is 200 to 400 mg. It may take from 6 months to 2 years to return to normal. During this period they will complain of fatigue, and they are more susceptible to upper respiratory tract infections.

The overtrained athlete is often more accident prone and overuse injuries are common. Bicipital tendinitis is a common finding in swimmers and Achilles tendinitis in runners, particularly if the cause of the overtraining has been excessive work. There is often a history of shin splints or stress fractures.

Psychological factors   Psychological effects of overtraining, anxiety, depression and lack of concentration, are extremely important and should not be neglected. If possible, they should be assessed and treated by a sympathetic clinical sports psychologist. An example of the help possible from a clinical psychologist is the case of a young female swimmer who was amenorrhoeic and complained of feeling tired and had difficulty in training for several months. Medical examinations and investigations were all negative. Psychological tests showed a very high level of depression and anxiety on the neuroticism scale. Using a fatigue questionnaire, J. A. Connolly (personal communication, 1986) showed there was a very high level of physical, emotional and mental fatigue. She was advised to stop training. The coach was very cooperative, but it was very difficult to convince the parents of the necessity of stopping training completely. After a 4-week period she was re-assessed by the psychologist. The emotional and mental fatigue had returned to normal, but her physical fatigue was still above the normal level and she was still amenorrhoeic. It is important to talk to the coach, the athlete and in certain sports to the parents to emphasize the importance of complete rest.

Treatment   Treatment of overtraining is first to identify the cause of the condition and to see if any external factors may be aggravating it, e.g. problems at home or school, lack of sleep, poor nutrition. Time must be spent with the athlete to convince him or her of the necessity for rest, as they often feel guilty because they are not training. Overtrained athletes recover much faster when rest is complete, rather than by just reducing the level of training (Costill, 1986). Psychological counselling should include the coach, parents and athlete. Good nutrition with adequate sleep will aid in recovery. Any injuries, particularly overuse injuries, should be treated adequately and a correct training schedule should be devised. It is essential that after injury an athlete should only be allowed back very slowly to training, and to competition only when he/she is fully recovered. Educating the athlete, coach and physician on the correct physiological principles of training is the most effective way of preventing overtraining.

Sports psychology

Psychology has been used in sport for many generations. Sports psychology as a specific discipline has developed in the last few decades with its own international society and journal. However, its role in the training and preparation of athletes for competition is still often misunderstood by athletes, coaches and physicians.

The increasing demands of training and competition place an added stress on athletes, and it is the uninjured athlete, who keeps his or her head, that wins the medals. The sports psychologist can play an important part in teaching athletes the psychological skills that are essential to their development and performance. They include emotional control, attentional control, self esteem and interpersonal skills (Hoggs, 1982).

The sports psychologist should work as part of a team with the athlete, coach, physiotherapist, nutritionist and physician, who should all understand the demands of training and competition on the athlete and the demands on their time and the personal and social problems that are likely to occur. Athletes most at risk should be identified and counselled. The aim is to help the athlete to enjoy training and competition and to lead a full life.

Sports psychology should be done in a practical clinical area, that should be incorporated as part of the initial medical examination of the athlete and should be included into the monitoring programme of the athlete. It should not be relegated only to the time when the athlete runs into trouble. Athletes may develop the same problems as non-athletes, for example, anxiety states or depression.

Certain athletes perform well in training sessions but are afraid of competition, and an injury is often used as an excuse not to compete (Ride, 1965). Personality type may also play a role in the reaction to injury. The extrovert who is impulsive is generally insensitive to pain and usually returns to competition too early. The introvert tends to have a low tolerance to pain and will tend to over-react and make his or her injury appear more serious (Sands, 1981).

Different personality types tend to react in different ways to stress, and the personality of the athlete can be evaluated using a variety of questionnaires. Among these are the Catell 16 PF (16 personality factor) Questionnaire, which measures 16 basic personality dimensions (Catell et al., 1970), and the Minnesota Multiphasic Personality Inventory. If they are answered correctly, they can give valuable information on, for example, the tough-mindedness and emotional stability of the athlete. The Profile of Mood States (POMS) measures six dimensions of mood (McNair et al., 1981): tension, depression, anger, vigour, fatigue and confusion. The normal levels for mood scales varies from 10 to 15. The Olympic cyclists showed higher than normal levels of vigour and lower values on other scales (Johnson et al., 1985). This is the typical iceberg profile for élite athletes (Eysenck et al., 1982).

An example of the use of the POMS questionnaire is an athlete whose sport involved numerous matches, who prior to competition was found

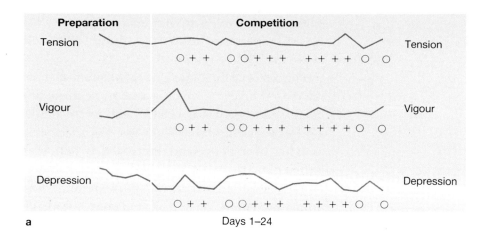

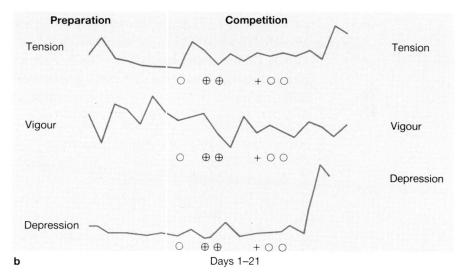

Fig. 12.7.1 POMS questionnaire (three dimensions of mood only shown). (a) Completed by a stable athlete showing a relatively constant mood profile. (b) Completed by a less stable athlete showing increasing tension and depression and reduced vigor. ○ = competition loss; + = competition win.

to have high levels of tension, depression and low vigour, with narrowed attention and a poor response to physiological testing. The management and the athlete were informed and she was advised not to travel, but due to the difficulty of obtaining a suitable replacement, she went. All the members of the squad were asked to complete the POMS questionnaire each day over a 3-week period. One member of the squad who was a mature, stable athlete, maintained a consistent mood profile, despite wins and losses (Fig. 12.7.1a). In contrast, the athlete with problems showed a profile with increasing levels of tension and depression, with reduced vigour, and had to be withdrawn from competition (Fig. 12.7.1b).

The two dimensions of neuroticism and extroversion can be measured by the Epipersonality Inventory (Eysenck, 1964). The introvert has a low pain threshold and tends to be more apprehensive and to over-react, while the neurotic extrovert tends to be more reckless and impatient and has a tendency to under-react, and with inadequate rehabilitation is more likely to be reinjured.

The Neuroticism Scale Questionnaire measures anxiety and depression. Increased levels of anxiety and hyperarousal will affect performance. Increased anxiety is associated with increased distractability, and strategy and tactics are ignored. There is a loss of drive and an aversion to the task that has to be performed. Increased anxiety is associated with increased sweating, a tendency to hyperventilation and a feeling of fatigue. There is increased tension in the muscles and diarrhoea is common. The unnecessary tension and wasted energy makes the athlete feel tired, and will have a marked adverse effect on skill performance.

Athletes need to know the correct level of arousal for optimum performance; too little or too much have an adverse effect on performance. In hyperarousal states attention involuntarily narrows, and information intake is restricted. Attention becomes internally focussed, and its manner varies with the potential styles of which there are a number of different types:

1 A broad external attention style tends to be found in team sports where the reading of complex situations and anticipating events is important. With loss of attention athletes tend to repeat mistakes.
2 A narrow external attention style is found in place kickers and in fencers. The attention is needed at the moment of response, which is narrowed but focussed externally. This may become too rigid.
3 A broad internal attention attitude analyses a game plan and is found often in 1500 m runners. With increasing fatigue or overarousal they tend to overanalyse and get tunnel vision.
4 The internal narrow attention style is found in jumping and shooting events where it is necessary for the athletes to be sensitive to their own bodies, to be calm and to be able to mentally rehearse their actions, if this breaks down they get overarousal.

Athletes need to be in control of themselves. If they are dominated by external factors, for example, by the coach or family, they are said to have an external locus of control and they are more likely to run into trouble, as their arousal levels tend to be higher. They have poor control and their performance in a competition situation tends to be more labile. Individuals with an internal locus of control, generally use their arousal levels under stress more effectively.

Athletes should have realistic goals that are specific, measurable and attainable. They should be flexible, not rigid, so that they offer a

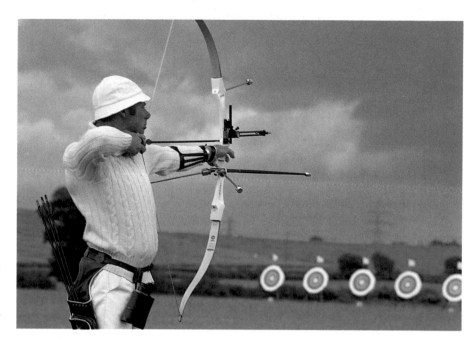

Fig. 12.7.2 Athletes need to be able to control their arousal and attention levels to achieve high performance standards. Activities such as archery demand high levels of internal, narrow attention. Courtesy of Ace Photo Agency, photo by G. Stuart-Turner.

challenge; they should be discussed with the coach. Athletes must have control of their goals. Within the final analysis it is the athlete who has to attain them.

There are many questions that can be asked by the psychologist: 'Are these goals realistic?' 'How is the level of expectation arrived at?' 'Is it based on the expectations or the needs of the coach, manager or parents?' 'How does it relate to previous performance, i.e. the level of skill and the basis of training?' 'Does the level of stress or motivation allow for a high level of performance?' Success is dictated by the goals you set.

Various techniques can be used to help the athlete attain his/her goal; these include relaxation techniques, mental imagery, and the control of arousal. Relaxation techniques include biofeedback and meditation. Mental imagery or mental rehearsal, can assist in the acquisition and retention of new skills (Sheedy, 1987). Mental imagery can also help the athlete to think about the techniques involved and plan before competition. When an athlete is injured, mental rehearsal can help to retain some of his/her skills.

Many athletes never reach their potential because of negative thoughts, e.g. in tennis they may think that they will double fault under pressure and they do. Coaches and athletes agree that negative thoughts are the single most devastating opponent an athlete can face. By realizing how often these thoughts occur and by changing them into a positive statement an athlete's performance can be improved. One basketball player reported an average of 56 negative thoughts for a day, despite the fact that he thought he had a very positive outlook (Ziegler, 1987).

Training experiences should be similar to competition setting. If athletes have to travel to competitions, they should arrive at least 2 days beforehand to allow them to visit the competition site and to discover the geography of the area. Before major competitions it is extremely helpful if videos of previous competitions held there with the noise and the crowd can be reproduced so that the athletes will get some idea of what to expect.

Biofeedback devices can help the athlete to relax along with other relaxation techniques. Biofeedback units provide the athlete with information about their body, e.g. their heart rate or muscle tension, so that they can learn how to control or correct it. Psychological testing combined with physiological monitoring of stress-related tasks can give valuable information (Johnson *et al.*, 1985). In this study the reaction time was measured and the heart rate and blood pressure was recorded while the athletes performed specific computerized tasks, e.g. to recognize specific letters on a screen. The response of an athlete to the mental and physical tasks vary. Athletes from sports that required high concentration, e.g. archery and fencing, tended to hold down their heart rate and blood pressure during the tasks, while athletes in the aerobic sports tended to have two peaks. Athletes who are unable to control their heart rate and blood pressure did not usually do so well in competition (Connolly, personal communication, 1984).

Psychological factors can play an important part in precipitating the overtrained syndrome, and the correct evaluation and treatment is essential to the rehabilitation of the athlete.

Successful athletes tend to be emotionally stable, tough-minded and relaxed. Important qualities in a successful athlete are their coachability, physical excellence, their openness to instruction, retention of critical power and the ability to integrate the new, the different and the innovative; also the ability to express aggression and drive without guilt. Psychology can help athletes in many ways to enjoy training and competition and to help them cope with failure and success.

References

Adlercreutz, H., Harkønen, M., Kuoppasalmi, K., Naveri, H., Huhtaniemi, I., Tikkanen, H., Remes, K., Dessypris, A. & Karvonen, J. (1986) Effect of training on plasma anabolic and catabolic steroid hormones and their response during physical exercise. *Int. J. Sports Med.* **7**, 27.

Catell, R., Eber, H. & Tatzucka, M. (1970) *Handbook of the Sixteen Personality Factor Questionnaire.* Institute for Personality & Ability Testing, Champaign.

Costill, D. L. (1986) Peaking for performance. In *Inside Running*, p. 123. Benchmark Press Inc.

Eysenck, H. J. (1964) *Personality Inventory. Manual of the Eysenck Personality Inventory.* Hodder & Stoughton, London.

Eysenck, H. J., Nias, D. B. K. & Cox, D. N. (1982) Sport and personality. *Adv. Behav. Res. Ther.* **4**, 1.

Falsetti, H. (1983) Overtraining of athletes. A round table. *Physician Sportsmed.* **11**, 93.

Hagerman, F. C., Hikide, S. R. S., Sherman, M. W. & Costill, D. L. (1984) Muscle damage in marathon runners. *Physician Sportsmed.* **12**, 39.

Hoggs, M. (1982) Psychological skills. In *Level 3. Coaching the Championship Swimmer*, p. 245–256. Canadian Swimming Association Congress Proceedings. Johannes Graphics, Waterloo, Ont.

Houston, M. E. (1982) Adaption and physiological stress. In *Level 3. Coaching the Championship Swimmer*, pp. 166–169. Canadian Swimming Association Congress Proceedings. Johannes Graphics, Waterloo, Ont.

Johnson, A., Collins, P., Higgins, I., Harrington, D., Conolly, J., Dolphin, C., McCreery, M., Brady, L. & O'Brien, M. (1985) Psychological, nutritional and physical status of Olympic road cyclists. *Br. J. Sports Med.* **19(1)**, 11.

McNair, D. M., Lorr, M. & Droppleman, L. F. (1981) *Manual for Profile of Mood States.* Educational & Industrial Testing Service, San Diego.

Maglicho, F. W. (1982) *Swimming Faster.* Mayfield Publishing, Palo Alto.

Montpetit, R. & Hogg, M. (1982). Tapering. In *Level 3. Coaching the Championship Swimmer*, pp. 143–156. Canadian Swimming Association Congress Proceedings. Johannes Graphics, Waterloo, Ont.

Nilsson, S. (1987) *Overtraining. Proceedings of the Advanced Conference in Sports Medicine, Oslo*, pp. 45–49.

Ride, L. (1965) Some psychological factors in sports injuries. *J. Sports Med. Phys. Fitness* **5**, 152.

Sands, F. H. (1981) Psychological implications of injury. In *Sports Fitness and Sports Injuries*, pp. 37–51.

Selye, H. (1956) *The Stress of Life.* McGraw Hill, New York.

Sheedy, J. (1987) Applied sports psychology. The sports trainer and athletic injuries. *Sport Health* **5(1)**, 21.

Ziegler, S. G. (1987) Negative thought stopping. *J. Phys. Educ. Rec. Dance* **58(4)**, 66.

Further reading

Costill, D. L., Bowers, R., Branam, G. & Sparks, K. (1971) Muscle glycogen utilization during prolonged exercise on successive days. *J. Appl. Physiol.* **31**, 834.

Gollnick, P. D., Armstrong, R. B., Sembrowich, W. L., Shephard, R. E. & Saltin, B. (1973) Glycogen depletion pattern in human skeletal muscle fibres after heavy exercise. *J. Appl. Physiol.* **34**, 615.

Sherman, M. W., Costill, D. L., Fink, W. J., Hagerman, F. C., Armstrong, L. E. *et al.* (1983) Effect of a 42.2 K footrace and subsequent rest or exercise on muscle glycogen and enzymes. *J. Appl. Physiol.* **55**, 1219.

12.8 Standardization of medical care during international sports events

D. HANNEMANN

International sports competitions—continental and world championships and in particular the Olympic Games—make particularly high demands on sports medical care. The basic ethical and medical attitude to do everything for the benefit of the athlete and for preserving and promoting health and physical powers is valid for any medical activities. If the well-being of the athlete is made the focus of the work of the sports physician and if the participation of the athlete in international championships and the Olympic Games is considered as the highest objectives of his/her sporting career, then it will be absolutely necessary to know that the quality of medical preconditions and care during the competitions/Games is of the same high standard for all athletes. The competitor has a right to medical care, to at least the standard received during the long period of preparation at home.

Responsibility of the team physician during the immediate preparation for international competitions

In a period of great physical and psychological strain confidence between the athlete and physician is very important. Therefore, the contact between the team physician and the sports team should be particularly continuous in the phase before a contest. In that phase the physician is faced with the following medical tasks:

1 Continuous check-up of the state of health, of general and special maximum stress, of fatigue, of the sleeping behaviour, as well as the search for indications of overstrain, functional disturbances or damages.
2 Ensuring general vaccine protection and the vaccine protection specially required for the region where the competition is taking place, according to WHO recommendations.
3 Completion of the athlete's bill of health (if one is kept) with important data for medical aid that might be needed in the place of the event (blood group including subgroups, existing allergies, inoculations, etc.).

4 Instructing the athlete in the medical rules and their meaning in the competition regulations of the international sports federations and of the Olympic Charter, respectively.

5 Educational influence and explanation on the danger of doping substances from an ethical and medical view. Making the athlete familiar with the doping regulations, in particular with doping controls, with the rights and duties of the athlete, and with the procedure of acceptance.

6 Instructions on the personal behaviour of the athlete in consideration of the climatic conditions existing or to be expected in the place of the event (temperature, relative humidity, wind flow, solar radiation, height above sea level).

7 Preparation of all medical documents for the sports team requested by the competition organizers.

8 Instruction and coordination of the entire medical staff (masseur, physiotherapists, further physicians) who will be involved in the preparation of the athletes for the international competition. As the person bearing the final responsibility of the health and well-being of the athlete the physician needs to have confidence in this team. He or she has to be informed on their work, on the methods and drugs used, and on special results of examinations.

Responsibility of the medical commissions of the international sports federations

The competition regulations of an international sports federation should ensure the protection of the health and life of all athletes participating in the competition. Taking into account the sports involved, the medical regulations have to contain general and special medical and hygienic demands on the competition conditions and on the athlete; their observance guarantees fair and equal participation for all athletes. The medical commission needs to continuously update the regulations in order to include essential new medical findings, particularly with regard to different kinds of sport. The following medical principles should be covered by the regulations:

1 Demands on the conditions in the place of training and competition (on sports equipment, etc.), for example:
(a) Water hygiene for swimming and show jumping.
(b) Hygiene of the mats for wrestling and judo.
(c) Temperature limits for winter sports.

(d) Wearing safety devices/guards of a suitable quality (safety helmets for bob-sleighing, racing, face guard for fencing, etc.).

(e) Demands on changing, warming and common rooms corresponding to the structure of the competition and the type of sports.

(f) Catering in longer competitions.

2 Demands on first aid stations, medical examination and control rooms, depending on the respective kind of sport, for example:

(a) Doping control station.

(b) Weighing room.

(c) First aid station, water rescue service, Alpine rescue service.

Here, the room conditions, the demands on equipment and material and also the usefulness of the places (start, finish, etc.) have to be demonstrated.

3 Rights of the team physicians and of the accompanying medical staff.

4 The doping regulations of the federation.

Sports medical rules in the frame of the Olympic Charter

In the interest of ensuring effective medical care of all Olympic teams participating in the Games, the Medical Commission of the IOC has been working intensively on the improvement of Rule 29 of the Olympic Charter over the past 4 years. Due to the continuous cooperation between the Olympic physicians of the National Olympic Committees (NOCs) and the Medical Commissions of the International Sports Federations, the *Guidelines of the Medical Commission of the IOC* was formulated and many important items resolved. The Medical Commission of the IOC, in line with the importance of the Olympic Games, is responsible for guaranteeing all required preconditions of the medical care of the Olympic competitors. The commission has to ensure that the demands made on medical facilities and their functions in these guidelines are met by the responsible sections of the organizing committee.

The organizing committee of the respective Games is responsible for creating all preconditions in personnel and organization, regarding rooms and medical facilities, to facilitate the unrestricted work of the medical staff of the Olympic teams, as laid down in the guidelines.

The National Olympic Committees have to ensure that the medical staff nominated by them for their Olympic teams on the basis of Rule 37 of the Olympic Charter possess the required qualifications for their functions. The medical staff will fulfil their tasks within the frame of the guidelines. The guidelines also cover the medical care of Olympic competitors and demands on medical facilities.

The following points are binding on all persons involved (Medical Commission of the IOC, organizing committee, NOC physicians).

Professional status of medical staff

Acknowledgement of the professional status of the medical staff of the Olympic teams: In accordance with its responsibility for the nomination of the medical staff, the NOC confirms the required qualifications of the physicians and other medical staff in the written nominal entry of the Olympic team. On the basis of this, the medical staff is entitled to care for and treat the athletes of their Olympic team, the officials and additional officials of their team and the members of the Olympic family of their country (IOC members, NOC representatives, guests and journalists). This right is effective on the whole Olympic territory and over the period of the official function of the Olympic Village (Rule 36).

As the NOCs bear the responsibility for the protection of the health of their athletes and of the members of the Olympic family of their countries, it has to be ensured that, in case of a treatment by medical staff or institutions of the host country, the consent of the management of the respective Olympic team will be procured. The accredited physicians of the Olympic team are entitled to accompany injured or ill members of their Olympic team to a hospital or other medical institution of the host country, to take the decision on necessary medical diagnosis and therapy in consultation with specialists, and to be present at possible treatments if desired.

Accrediting medical staff

Accrediting the medical staff of an Olympic team: The members of the medical staff receive an F-accreditation, including additional badges for medical staff, issued by the organizing committee. These badges entitle them to access to all accommodation of the athletes, members of the Olympic team and of the Olympic family of their country. They allow free admission to all venues and training places if athletes of their country are staying there for training or competition. The identified physicians have the right to any contacts with the athletes of their country, including the right to decide upon early breaking-off of participation in the competition for reasons of health. Close cooperation with the medical staff of the organizing committee is important, as are the possibility of entering medical facilities of the organizing committee, and the possible use of assistance of medical staff of the COJO (Comité d'Organisation de Jeux Olympiques) as well as the use of existing facilities including ambulance service.

Accredited medical staff have the right to accompany athletes of their country to possible doping controls and to be present at the time the sample is collected and sealed.

Medical staff quotas *Uniform quotas for medical staff of the Olympic teams*: According to the justified wish of athletes for medical advice and care by their own team physicians and medical staff, considerable changes have taken place at past Olympic Games. The following regulations are considered effective at present: five medical people for 25 athletes, and one further medical person for every extra 15 athletes.

The medical facilities appropriate for the number of medical staff, such as their accommodation, must not be at the expense of the athletes' accommodation.

Import of medical materials *Import and re-export of medical materials and drugs*: The medical staff of the Olympic teams may import (duty free) the equipment, materials, drugs and cosmetics required for their athletes and the members of the Olympic family. Corresponding lists of imports have to be provided by the NOC and to be presented to the controlling bodies upon entry and exit.

Working conditions of medical staff *Working conditions of the medical staff of an Olympic team in the Olympic Village*:

1 Physicians' rooms: the basic standard is one physician's room (15–20 m^2 of floor space) per 100 delegation members. Each team automatically gets their own physician room; with a maximum of three rooms per team.

2 Standard equipment: sufficient illumination of the room, hot water and cold water supply, air conditioning, electrical connections and hand basin.

3 Special equipment per room: one couch with adjustable head end, one desk with drawers, one work table (drug table), one medicine chest (lockable), one flexible lamp, one bin for medical wastes, one wastepaper basket, one desk chair, one examination chair, scales, a folding screen, one hallstand, one wall mirror, sheets for the couch, towels for daily use, two woollen blankets, and positioning rolls or cushions.

4 Equipment for sports medical working conditions as a whole: hot air sterilizer, one refrigerator (100–120 litre, lockable), one illuminator, one filing cabinet, and one typewriter.

5 Physiotherapeutical and massage rooms: basic standard is four broad massage couches per 100 athletes with a working space of 10 m^2 per couch, 15 couches per team at most.

6 General standard of equipment: sufficient illumination of the room, hot water and cold water supply, one or two instrument tables with trays, one to two stools, three folding screens per massage room, hand basin, wall mirror, electric connections, one wastepaper basket, one waste bin, two woollen blankets and one knee roll per couch, one positioning cushion, one cabinet for instruments, dressing material, etc., sheets for the massage couches, and towels.

7 Equipment in the entire physiotherapeutical complex as a whole: one cooking facility for preparing hot water, one hot water basin for the preparation of packs, one refrigerator for the preparation of cryopacks and for the storage of ointments and massage preparations, one foot basin, one forearm basin, a shower and a toilet.

8 Basic hygienic standards, daily cleaning and daily replacement of the used linen are required for all medical working places.

Standardization of examination *Uniform doping-control programme,* sex examinations and further medical examinations.

Medical care by the COJO

The health services required for the Olympic Games by the COJO cover three categories:

1 Medical services for all athletes, officials and people participating in the Olympic Games in the Olympic Village, in the training places and venues and at other institutions associated with the Olympic Games.

2 Medical examinations of the athletes (check-ups, doping controls).

3 Responsibility for providing hygiene and other prophylactic and protective measures in the sports sites, accommodation, catering facilities, and food hygiene including measures in case of severe accidents.

The outpatient's department at the Olympic Village and the health service at the training places and venues have to:

1 Ensure the sports medical care and medical basic care of athletes and officials.

2 Ensure the preparation of proper doping controls.

3 Carry out hygiene inspections and prophylactic medicine.

4 Provide ambulance service and medical emergency services for hospitalization.

5 Create facilities for mobile medical stand-by duty (marathon race, road cycle race).

The medical guide for the Olympic Games, which has to be confirmed by the Medical Commission of the IOC, contain details of the above regulations. These have to correspond to the Olympic Charter and its implementing regulations and to take into account the standards defined for the respective kind of sports in the rules of the federation.

Basic standards of living conditions in the Olympic Village

It is the responsibility of the Medical Commission of the IOC, the medical department of the organizing committee and the medical staff of the NOC to ensure that living conditions for the athletes are adequate to the high sports standard of the Olympic competitions.

There should be two-person bedrooms with the necessary furnishings, a common room per 15 to 20 athletes, and sufficient cloakrooms. Preset hygienic standards (one sanitary unit—toilet, shower, bath tub—for every five athletes) have to be met, and washing and cleaning facilities for clothes (including drying facilities) have to be provided. Depending on the peculiarities of each sport, sufficient and partly-specific changing facilities, as well as hygienic facilities (toilets, showers, hair dryers, cloakrooms) have to be provided.

A close cooperation between the organizing committee, the Medical Commission of the IOC and experienced Olympic physicians is recommended to draw up suitable menus. A particularly careful regulation is required for catering for athletes whose competitions may take place under extreme conditions, e.g. in certain winter sports, or who may be involved in long-lasting tournaments.

PART 13

DOPING AND DOPING CONTROL

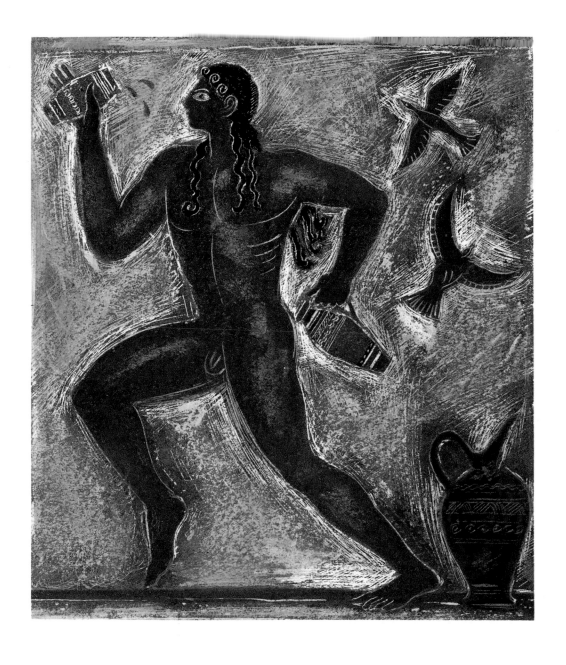

13.1 The doping problem

A. H. BECKETT

The dramatic increase in drug misuse in sport started in about 1960 as society as a whole came to believe increasingly that there were drugs available to deal with most ills, diseases and problems. Inevitably, sport, as part of society, became caught up with this drug culture and some competitors, coaches and doctors began to look upon drugs as aids in taking short cuts to success. Unfortunately, deaths in sport were necessary before leaders and legislators were shaken out of their complacency and mobilized a counterattack upon the cancer which had been established in the body of sport and was becoming increasingly invasive.

Appropriate action by international organizations required a firm basis of a coherent philosophy and the delineation of the borders between permissible use of drugs in medical treatments and inappropriate and obvious abuse. The IOC and the International Amateur Athletic Federation (IAAF) Medical Commissions, although recognizing that the misuse of drugs in attempts to alter performance in sport contravened the basic ethics of fair play and fair competition between competitors, concentrated their main emphasis on providing clear rules which could lead to action if contravened. It was recognized that not all doctors and coaches considered the welfare of competitors under their care to be their first priority. Pressures to succeed at all costs were in evidence in top class sports. If competitions in sport were allowed to degenerate into competitions between pharmacologists and physicians, with competitors being used as guinea pigs and receiving potent drugs for non-medical use, then inevitably this would lead to more deaths in sport.

It was decided to draw a firm line between permitted use and unacceptable use of drugs in sport by producing a list of banned classes of compounds, and giving sufficient examples in each class to demonstrate the purpose and the control envisaged. Any attempt to produce a definitive list of banned compounds would only have led to the use of related compounds with similar pharmacological actions and even to the use of compounds not marketed as drugs for medical use, as was already occurring in society. Thus the first list, and even the present ones, contain the phrase '. . . and related compounds'.

The first classes banned were psychomotor stimulants, sympathomimetic amines, miscellaneous central nervous system stimulants and narcotic analgesics. In April 1975 the class of anabolic steroids was included. The banning of the psychomotor stimulant drugs presented no problems since there is no medical justification for using such drugs in sport, and their abuse constitutes a potential danger to the user and to other competitors and spectators. Similarly, the use of narcotic analgesics for therapeutic reasons could not be accepted; the danger of addiction to the use of such compounds is well recognized.

The sympathomimetic amines represent a special problem, however, because some of the compounds are used to treat colds, allergies and asthma. However, to exclude compounds like ephedrine from any ban would have undermined the whole system of doping control, because much use has been made of these compounds in doping in sport after the amphetamines had been controlled. To allow the medical use would lead only to spurious statements of ailments by physicians, coaches or competitors. Some drugs have been developed to deal with these medical problems which have negligible stimulant effects on the central nervous system and are therefore not on the banned list.

The IOC Medical Commission also decided to only include the banned classes for which suitable analytical methods were available to determine the compounds unequivocally as being in that class and their metabolites unequivocally in urine. Thus, although it was well known that anabolic steroids were being misused in sport before 1960, the IOC did not ban the class until 1975, when suitable methods of analysis had been developed. The development of analytical methods alone is not sufficient to ensure good dope control. A knowledge of the application of the methods to the biological system is necessary and a knowledge of what happens to the drug in man under different conditions is also required.

It was decided not to use blood but to use urine as the biological fluid to be sampled, because there was resistance to taking 20 ml or more of blood and it was, and still is, impossible to determine most of the drugs of the banned classes in one drop of blood. Thus objective scientific information rather than subjective assessment was to be used to establish that contravention of the rules had occurred.

The taking of urine samples and the control of these samples and then transport and receipt in the laboratory and their treatment there, is just as important as the final analytical step. Thus clear guide lines about the procedures were established and published by the IOC Medical Commission. Duplicate samples are obtained from the competitor and if the results of analysis on the first sample establish the presence of a drug of the banned classes, then the rules allow for the analysis of the reserve sample in front of experts from the team and the competitor who might have contravened the rules. It is essential that the analytical result is not considered as 'positive' until the result of the second analysis has established the identification of the drug obtained in the analysis of the first sample. Analysis in itself does not constitute a case of 'doping' — all the facts must be reported to an appropriately constituted Medical Commission to come to a decision when all the facts are known. It is unacceptable for a case to be reported as positive simply on analytical results of the first sample — the laboratory function is to report results of analysis while the Committee function is to consider the 'doping' aspects.

The introduction of doping controls led to a dramatic reduction in drug misuse of the banned classes in those sports and competitions in which testing was carried out, but drug misuses escalated in sports not carrying out tests. The misuse of anabolic steroids became a major problem until tests were introduced, but tests at competitions alone can not control the situation because increasingly the drugs have been used outside competition periods and their use discontinued some time before competitions at which testing was expected. Because performance then falls, since depression often results from withdrawal of the drug, the 'gap' is covered by using the male hormone testosterone with the expectation that action can not be taken because of the difficulty of distinguishing

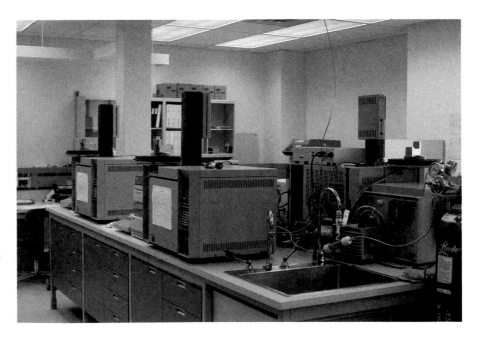

Fig. 13.1.1 The analyses of urine specimens from élite competitors involves sophisticated equipment and considerable expense. Courtesy of B. Challis.

between exogenous and endogenous material. An appropriate test was devised but, again, this in itself will not control anabolic steroid misuse — the only way is to have out-of-competition as well as at-competition testing. Some countries have now adopted this procedure and others are moving in that direction. It is important, however, that in such testing, control is for anabolic steroids and related drugs and stimulants such as amphetamines, but does not control sympathomimetic amines and narcotic drugs. Doping control 'out-of-competition' must recognize that therapeutic treatment for coughs and colds, etc. must be allowed without producing the problem of an athlete being considered as using a doping agent when he or she is not engaged in competition. Doping controls must command respect by being fair and realistic. We must never forget that their purpose is to deter drug misuse not cause problems in the correct therapeutic usage of drugs.

The problem of the easy accessibility of anabolic steroids throughout the world is causing great concern. Tighter regulations concerning internal distribution in countries and movement between countries are essential. Fortunately, policiticans are beginning to realize the impact of doping in sport on misuse of drugs in young people in society and are becoming receptive to the call for action.

The so-called 'blood doping' (see Chapter 13.3) represents a serious basic challenge. The costs of producing appropriate tests and ensuring that they do not class an innocent person as guilty because of individual differences in blood patterns, would be horrendously expensive. Despite the financial problem, the IOC Medical Commission has banned the procedure of blood doping but will rely upon the laws dealing with movement of biological specimens across national frontiers as one method to deal with the problem.

The IOC Medical Commission has attempted to adhere to its basic philosophy of preventing drug misuse in a realistic and fair manner without infringing the right of the medical practitioner to treat a competitor. However, when the use of drugs and procedures is carried out with the intent of altering performance rather than treating a medical problem, there can be no compromise. The recent information (1987) given by the Commission on classes of compounds and procedures banned and its statements about stimulants, narcotics, anabolic steroids, β-blockers, diuretics, blood doping, alcohol, local anaesthetics and corticosteroids, are illustrative of the attempt to draw this difficult line between correct drug use and drug misuse. This is essential if the true ethics of sport are to be preserved.

13.2 Clinical aspects of the doping classes

R. O. VOY

Beginning with the modern Olympic movement in 1863, athletes have devoted themselves to dedicated training and personal sacrifice in order to obtain their ultimate performances. However, in this decade dedicated training just does not seem to be enough for many athletes. The athletic community has turned towards use of chemical substances in order to maximize and enhance performance. This combination of athlete, scientist and physician has resulted in exposure to perceived performance-enhancing drugs. Athletes, who have worked so hard at preparing their bodies for health, are willing to take serious health risks by using chemical shortcuts to gain competitive edge. Striving for sports excellence through drug use has made doping of concern to sports officials and the public.

The word doping comes from the African Kaffirs who used a local liquor called 'dop' as a stimulant (Puffer, 1986). As far back as the third century BC, documents show that the Greek athletes ingested mushrooms to enhance their performance (Burks, 1981). With the 19th century there came widespread use of caffeine, alcohol, nitroglycerine, ethyl ether, strychnine and opium (Burks, 1981). It was at the 1960 Summer Olympic Games in Rome, that attention was really brought to drugs in athletics. The death of cyclist Kurt Enemar Jensen, which was linked to amphetamine use, opened the eyes of European sports-governing bodies. At the 1964 Olympic Games, there was an obvious increase in muscular appearance of the athletes. It was here in Tokyo, October 1964, that 'the definition of doping was adopted by the International Doping Conference of the Fédération Internationale de Médicine Sportive as well as the International (IOC) Olympic Committee' (Puffer, 1986). The IOC now defines doping as based on the banning of certain classes of pharmacological agents. The United States Olympic Committee (USOC), however, continues to use the following definition as previously defined by the IOC:

> The administration of or use by a competing athlete of any substance foreign to the body or of any physiological substance taken in abnormal quantity or taken by an abnormal route of entry into the body with the

sole intention of increasing in an artificial and unfair manner his/her performance in competition.

(MOA/USOC and the NGB, 1985)

Because athletes did not stop using drugs on their own, the IOC Medical Commission at the Olympiad of 1964 petitioned the IOC President to ban the use of drugs by Olympic athletes (Puffer, 1986). The end result was the establishment of a banned substances list and formal drug testing. According to the IOC Medical Commission, the most recent doping classes include five categories: stimulants, narcotics, anabolic steroids, β-blockers and diuretics (IOC Medical Commission, 1986).

Stimulants

Amphetamines, caffeine and cocaine are among the most common central nervous stimulants used by athletes. Clinically, stimulants give one a feeling of reduced fatigue, an increase in aggressiveness, hostility and, therefore, competitiveness. As a group, they produce a false sense of ability and may cause a loss of judgement. This may result in accidents to themselves and others within the sport (Puffer, 1986). Amphetamines are used by the athletes because they are believed to produce endurance and speed (Burks, 1981). Much publicity concerning this drug has revolved around football players; during the 1960s and 1970s, amphetamines appeared to be epidemic among professional football teams (Bell & Doege, 1986). With the National Football League drug control and monitoring system of 1975, the use seemed to decrease (Marshal, 1979). Taking its anorexic effects into consideration, wrestlers, jockeys and other weight-concerned sports people have used the drug to lose weight prior to competition.

The masking of pain, which may aggravate an already serious injury, the false sense of self confidence, the delay of fatigue, and increased aggressiveness are all factors leading athletes to this drug (Burks, 1981). Many studies have been done regarding the effects of amphetamines and most are controversial in nature. The only things which are agreed upon in the literature are that heart rates are significantly elevated by the drug and that totally fatigued subjects may be more alert with the ingestion of this drug (Chandler & Blair, 1980). Literature on this drug, relating to its use in sports, dates back to the 1950s. In the early 1950s, Smith and Beecher came up with results that showed a slight increase, of 1–4%, in performance in certain track and field events (Cooper, 1972).

They also claimed that athletes demonstrated feelings of being more alert and 'revved up' before competition (Puffer, 1986). Since then various studies have shown increases, decreases, and no change in physical activity. In the experiment of Chandler in 1981, it was documented that no significant increase occurred in athletic performance during the administration of amphetamines (Chandler & Blair, 1980). In 1981, Laties and Weiss found that, after taking this drug, performance usually improves by a few percent. They stated that in a competitive sport this increase can mean the difference between victory and defeat (Bell & Doege, 1986). Therefore, no definite conclusions regarding performance enhancement can be made regarding stimulants.

However, stimulants in general and amphetamines specifically produce many undesirable side effects. These include irregular heart rate, which may lead to cardiac arrest, the development of paranoid psychosis, a rise in body temperature that can lead to dehydration in warm weather, and the masking of fatigue that can lead to circulatory collapse, heat exhaustion and stroke (Bell & Doege, 1986).

Caffeine may be the world's most popular stimulant drug. It can be found in tea, coffee, cocoa, and products like diet pills and cold medicines. The effects of this drug are heavily dependent on dosage. The average amount of caffeine in one cup of coffee is approximately 100–150 mg, while instant coffee contains 80–100 mg. To the surprise of many, tea has anywhere from 30 to 75 mg of caffeine (Bell & Doege, 1986). When a person drinks two cups of coffee, effects begin within 15 to 30 min (National Institute on Drug Abuse, 1986). The person's metabolism, body temperature and blood pressure all increase. Caffeine also increases urine production, and results in higher blood sugar levels, hand tremors, decreased appetite and delayed sleep. Extremely high levels could cause nausea, diarrhoea, trembling, headache and nervousness (National Institute on Drug Abuse, 1986). Scientific studies have also shown there may be a tie between caffeine and its ability to burn blood fats for energy; the implication being that it may increase endurance. However, this may be negated since caffeine also acts as a diuretic, which can lead to fatigue and dehydration (USOC on Substance Abuse, 1987).

Caffeine seems to be most popular amongst runners and cyclists (Burks, 1981). During the 1976 Olympic Games in Montreal, high blood concentrations were found in some athletes (Puffer, 1986). Athletes and non-athletes were part of a controlled study done on cycle ergometers. It was demonstrated that it only took two and a half cups of coffee to start and increase the effects of maximal oxygen consumption and endurance

(Costill *et al.*, 1978). Costill and Fink also stated that 'at least part of the performance improvements were related to psychological effects'. A study by Ivy showed an increased work output from the administration of caffeine, but found it more important that it increased rates of lipid metabolism and increased mobilization of free fatty acids (Ivy *et al.*, 1978). Recent studies show ingestion of caffeine as a way to increase power output in skeletal muscle (Costill *et al.*, 1978). It is also suggested that too much caffeine does not show beneficial effects.

Because athletes generally use more of a substance than is therapeutically recommended, the IOC Medical Commission added a caffeine limit of 15 μg/ml in urine to the drug programme for the 1984 Olympic Games. In April of 1986, this was decreased to 12 μg/ml (Bell & Doege, 1986).

Cocaine, also a central nervous system stimulant, has gained popularity in professional athletics as well as with others. When cocaine is snorted, the effects begin within a few minutes, peak within 15–20 min, and disappear within an hour (National Institute on Drug Abuse, 1986). Injected cocaine takes about 15 s to reach the brain, while crack (smokable cocaine) takes 7 s (Cooper, 1986). Athletes use this drug because of its stimulant effect and its ability to mask pain, both of which may cause injury. Cocaine blocks the ability of one's own body to reabsorb adrenaline normally. This 'rush' makes the heart work twice as hard, but does not give it a chance to warm-up. This may result in incomplete and incorrect signals to the brain and heart, ending up in cardiac arrest (Cooper, 1986). The stimulating effect of cocaine can also cause destruction of nasal tissues, personality changes, and conflict in interpersonal relationships (Bell & Doege, 1986).

Particular attention needs to be paid to ephedrine and its derivatives—pseudoephedrine, phenylpropanolamine and phenylephrine, stimulants used as vasoconstrictors (decongestants) in over-the-counter cough, cold and sinus medicines. Inadvertent or innocent use of medications containing these substances can result in a positive test for banned substances.

Narcotics

As with the stimulants, the narcotic doping class acts in a way to give athletes a higher threshold of pain and a sudden rush of euphoria. Clinically, narcotics may be used as analgesics in treatment of mild to severe pain. However, as with the other classes, they carry many serious side effects along with them. Among these are physical and psychological dependence, and respiratory depression (USOC on Substance Abuse, 1987). Little evidence is found about the effects of these drugs on athletes. It has been said that the 'positive effects on performance would be far outweighed by the adverse health effects that may follow its use, including addiction' (Bell & Doege, 1986). Since evidence exists that these drugs have been and continue to be misused, the IOC Medical Commission has issued and maintains a ban on their use during Olympic Games

Anabolic steroids

The use and abuse of anabolic steroids is one of the most controversial topics in sport today. Athletes often refer to these drugs as the 'breakfast of champions', which shows how prevalent and innocent athletes feel is their use. First isolated in the 1930s, steroids were shown to have anabolic effects (muscle building) and were used to create positive nitrogen balances in starvation victims of World War II (Bergman & Leach, 1984). Anabolic steroids, which are derivations of testosterone (male hormone) were developed in the 1950s. Attempts have been made to separate the anabolic and androgenic effects of testosterone, maintaining the anabolic effects while decreasing the androgenic effects (Haupt & Rovere, 1984). This has not and might never be successfully accomplished.

Following these attempts, Zeigler worked to produce a less masculinizing anabolic steroid than testosterone; the result was Dianabol. The use of anabolic steroids, such as Dianabol, were included on the banned substance list for the 1976 Olympic Summer Games in Montreal (Bergman & Leach, 1984). In the case of testosterone (a naturally occurring hormone), it is difficult to distinguish from exogenous amounts, therefore, testosterone was not on the banned substance list before the 1984 Olympic Games (Puffer, 1986). Although drug testing has been done in the past, it is only recently, due to the addition of highly reliable gas chromotography and mass spectometry analysis, that anabolic steroid and testosterone detection has become reliable.

A common misconception is that 'anabolic steroids have been put on the banned substance list not because they enhance performance, but because they can be dangerous to the health of the user' (Bergman & Leach, 1984). The truth is that they were banned for both reasons. The key issue here is the perception by the athlete that the drug enhances performance since it has been shown that the drug increases protein synthesis and, therefore, an increase in muscle mass. The American College of Sports Medicine and the National Strength and Conditioning Association have stated that 'anabolic steroids can contribute to the increases of lean body weight often in the lean mass compartment, in the presence of an adequate diet and repetitive training' (American College of Sports Medicine, 1984). If, in fact, these drugs increase muscle mass and strength, their use in sport constitutes unfair competition and creates serious health risks to the athlete.

There are today only a few specific and uncommon medical uses for anabolic steroids in legitimate medical practice. These include stimulation of the bone marrow in certain patients with rare anaemia, stimulation of sexual development in hypogonadal males, treatment of certain types of breast cancer, and in treating a certain condition known as angioedema (Haupt & Rovere, 1984). These drugs, which may be taken orally or injected, have an abundance of dangerous side effects. They can cause premature fusion of the epiphysis (growth centre) of long bones in young children, liver disorders and tumours, testicular atrophy, lowered sperm count, enlargement of male breasts and nipples, and lowered high-density lipoprotein cholesterol levels which may result in cardiovascular disease. Women gain masculine features such as facial hair, baldness, deepening of the voice, shrinkage of breast size, enlargement of the clitoris, uterine atrophy, and irregularity of menstruation cycle (Lamb, 1984). Psychological effects may include aggressive behaviour, mood swings and increased libido (Bell & Doege, 1986). This list is, however, by no means complete; recently there have also been recorded cases of criminal behaviour while on anabolic steroids (*New York Times*, 1986).

Athletes take anabolic steroids with the intention of enhancing their athletic performance. They believe that if the steroids build muscle, it will benefit their strength and endurance. Even though it is accepted that anabolic steroids can increase muscle mass, the muscles produced contain a higher concentration of water and salt. This may result in making the muscles larger, but the muscles may be weaker due to the increased concentrations of salt and water; tendinitis and ruptured tendons may also be a problem (USOC on Substance Abuse, 1987). It is still not proven that the increase of muscle due to the use of anabolic steroids has any connection in increasing muscular strength. Every investigation points this out clearly. Athletes may also feel that these drugs shorten the recovery period after exercise, allowing them to exercise more frequently. The American College of Sports Medicine states that anabolic–androgenic steroids do not increase aerobic power or capacity for muscular exercise (American College of Sports Medicine, 1984). The psychological stance on this issue is that the athletes convince themselves they need these drugs in order to be competitive against those they think are doping (Bergman & Leach, 1984). The overall desire to win, along with peer pressure and team coercion lead to the taking of anabolic steroids.

β-Blockers

β-Adrenergic blockers are considered one of the doping classes. Clinically, these drugs are used to help reduce frequent migraines, to treat hypertension, to help control anxiety, and in treatment of movement tremors (US Pharmocopeial Convention, 1984). Some athletes have used these drugs in sports where physical activity is not stressed (IOC Medical Commission, 1986). Marksmen, golfers, archers and trap shooters have used β-blockers to achieve steadiness of the hands and to encourage sleep before competitions. Since the drug slows the heart down, skiers have also taken β-blockers to help decrease heart palpitations before their run (Goldman, 1984). Taking this information into consideration, the IOC Medical Committee has placed these drugs on the banned substance list. The IOC Medical Commission 'reserves the right to test those sports which it deems appropriate' (IOC Medical Commission, 1986). It is very unlikely that sports requiring vast amounts of physical activity and endurance, which these drugs decrease, would require testing as β-blockers would only prove to be a hindrance.

Diuretics

The newest addition to the banned substance list is diuretics. They were added in April of 1986, and will be considered a doping class for the 1988 Olympic Games (IOC Medical Commission, 1986). Diuretics do have important theraputic applications. Primarily they are used to treat high blood pressure and problems in fluid retention (Shangold & Mirkin, 1985).

Unfortunately, many athletes use these drugs to decrease weight in such sports as wrestling, boxing, judo and weight lifting. In addition, diuretics are used illegally to escape detection of banned substances by reducing their concentration in the urine. Since these drugs act on your kidneys to push potassium into urine, the low level of potassium in the blood causes fatigue, tired muscles and cramps. When taking diuretics, you are altering the balance between electrolytes and fluids (Goldman, 1984). These drugs cause weight loss by dehydrating fat that is 70% water; a significant weight loss in 24 h due to diuretics may cause leg and stomach muscle cramps. Diuretics may also cause an imbalance of the body's thermoregulatory system leading to exhaustion, irregular heart beats, and ultimately heart stoppage or death (USOC on Substance Abuse, 1987). In 1980, the International Federation of Body Builders (IFBB) Lightweight Mr Universe died of a heart attack due to diuretic use. A Swedish bodybuilder died a few weeks later, which was also attributed to a heart attack due to diuretic use (Goldman 1984).

Anabolic steroid users also use diuretics to rid their bodies of extra fluid build up (Goldman, 1984).

The IOC believes that 'deliberate attempts to reduce weight artificially in order to compete in lower weight classes or to dilute urine constitute clear manipulations which are unacceptable on ethical grounds' (IOC Medical Commission, 1986). For this reason as well as the serious health risks, diuretics are now included on the banned substance list.

Human growth hormone

The use of human growth hormone has gained popularity recently with athletes. It has been used clinically for the past 25 years to help treat children lacking sufficient amounts of growth hormone to reach normal height (Spilliotis *et al.*, 1984). It is also documented that injections of human growth hormone produce positive nitrogen balances in both man and experimental animals (Davidson & Passmore, 1986). Human growth hormone is considered a doping drug by the USOC and the IOC Committee.

Because drug testing for anabolic steroids and testosterone is so much more efficient, many athletes are turning to human growth hormone to enhance their performance. There is not yet an effective or reliable means of detecting exogenous amounts of this drug from normal body amounts (Puffer, 1986). Even though there is no scientific evidence to prove that the use of human growth hormone can improve muscular strength by inducing muscular hypertrophy, athletes still use it in spite of the negative side effects. In addition, growth hormone is used along with anabolic steroids to produce muscle growth (Strauss, 1984). The USOC drug control programme states that the side effects are well documented. They include growth in all tissues in the body, such as internal organs, bones, facial features and an increase in skin thickness (USOC on Substance Abuse, 1987). It also increases laxity of muscles and decreases the protective fat surrounding the abdominal organs. It can also cause the disease acromegaly, which includes overgrowth of the jaw and thickening of the fingers (Strauss, 1984). Now that synthetic growth hormone is processed with methods involving recumbent DNA, it will be more available to athletes and, unfortunately, acromegaly and other side effects will become more widespread.

Corticosteroids

In 1975 the IOC Medical Commission found out that corticosteroids were being used for reasons other than therapeutic ones. Some sports people were taking them orally, intravenously or intramuscularly. These drugs cause serious medical complications such as electrolyte imbalance, high blood pressure, oedema, ulcer disease and muscle weakness, to name just a few. Restrictions did not help cure the misuse, so the use of corticosteroids was ultimately banned. They are allowed in 'inhalation form, local or intra-articular injections, and topical use' (IOC Medical Commission, 1986). It is necessary for a team doctor to formally notify the IOC Medical Commission if this drug is to be administered to the athlete.

Corticosteroids are highly effective for anti-inflammatory purposes to relieve pain (IOC Medical Commission, 1986). They are also useful in preventing allergy attacks and in the treatment of acute ulcerative colitis (Davidson & Passmore, 1986). The sensitivity to insulin in Addison's disease and hypopituitarism are also correctable with the use of corti-costeroids. These drugs have also been known to cause a sense of euphoria (IOC Medical Commission, 1986). Anyone using this drug should be under direct medical supervision.

Conclusion

After reviewing the clinical aspects and dangerous side effects of the various doping classes, the question arises as to what should be done about the problem. Physicians, coaches, lay people and scientists should take every opportunity to educate athletes against drug abuse on every level and in every sport. Drug testing is also an important tool in this regard. Detection is part of the equation in stopping abuse; without detection, there is no real deterrent. Without a deterrent there is no opportunity to educate. Detection is an integral part of an educational programme. The main cure, however, lies within the athletes themselves. If they can realize that 'chemical shortcuts' are not a substitute for what we know works, such as dedicated training, good coaching and balanced nutrition, then there is hope for the present situation. Unless this is realized, and substance abuse is stopped, the true meaning of sport and fair play may be at risk, and hence the true meaning of sport lost.

References

American College of Sports Medicine (1984) *Position Stand on the Use of Anabolic Steroids in Sports.* American College of Sports Medicine, Indianapolis.

Bell, A. J. & Doege, C. T. (1986) *Athletes Use and Abuse of Drugs. Physician Sportsmed.* **15**, 99.

Bergman, R. & Leach, E. R. (1984) The use and abuse of anabolic steroids in Olympic-caliber athletes. *Clin. Orthop.* **198**, 170.

Burks, F. T. (1981) Drug use in athletics. *Federation Proceedings* **40**, 2679.

Chandler, V. J. & Blair, N. S. (1980) The effect of amphetamines on selected physiological components related to athletic success. *Med. Sci. Sports Exerc.* **12**, 65.

Cooper, L. D. (1972) Drugs and the athlete. *JAMA* **221**, 108.

Cooper, N. (1986) Cocaine is a loaded gun. *Newsweek*, **July 7.**

Costill, D. L., Palsky, G. P. & Fink, W. J. (1978) Effects of caffeine ingestion on metabolism and exercise performance. *Med. Sci. Sports* **10**, 155.

Davidson, S., Passmore, R., Brock, J. F. & Truswell, A. S. (1986) *Human Nutrition and Dietetics.* Churchill Livingstone, Edinburgh.

Goldman, B. (1984) *Death in the Locker Room.* Icarus Press, South Bend, Indiana.

Haupt, A. H. & Rovere, D. G. (1984) Anabolic steroids: a review of the literature. *Am. J. Sports Med.* **12(6)**, 470.

International Olympic Committee Medical Commission (1986) *List of Doping Classes and Methods of Doping.* IOC, Lausanne.

Ivy, J. L., Costill, D. L. & Fink, W. J. (1978) Role of caffeine and glucose ingestion on metabolism during exercise. *Med. Sci. Sports* **10**, 66.

Lamb, R. D. (1984) Anabolic steroids in athletics: how well do they work and how dangerous are they? *Am. J. Sports Med.* **12(1)**, 35.

Marshal, E. (1979) Drugging of football players cured by central monitoring plan, NFL claims. *Science* **203**, 626.

Memorandum of Agreement between the United States Olympic Committee and the NGB (1985). USOC, Colorado Springs.

National Institute on Drug Abuse (1986) *Stimulants and Cocaine.* Dept. of Health and Human Services, Rockville.

New York Times (1986) Prince George's County Court Judgment. *New York Times* **April 2.**

Puffer, C. J. (1986) The use of drugs in swimming. *Clinics Sports Med.* **5(1)**, 77.

Shangold, M. & Mirkin, G. (1985) *The Complete Sports Medicine Book for Women.* Simon & Schuster, New York.

Spilliotis, E. B., August, G. P., Hung, W., Sonis, W., Mendelson, W. & Bercu, B. (1984) Growth hormone neurosecretory dysfunction. *JAMA* **251**, 2223.

Strauss, H. R. (1984) Anabolic steroids. *Clin. Sports Med.* **3**, 746.

The United States Pharmocopeial Convention (1984) *1984 Drug Information for the Health Care Provider.* Medical Economics Books, Oradell, New Jersey.

United States Olympic Committee on Substance Abuse (1987) *Questions and Answers.* USOC, Colorado Springs.

13.3 Classes and methods

A. DIRIX

The practice of doping in modern-day sport has increased steadily over many years. In 1964 at the Olympic Games in Tokyo, with the assistance of Dr Dumas, a control was conducted of the cyclists participating in the 100 km timed team event. This task remained incomplete due to a boycott.

Following these events, Prince Alexandre de Merode, who had just been elected a member of the IOC, organized a meeting with Avery Brundage, then President of the IOC, resulting in the creation of a Medical Commission in 1966 and the subsequent organization of the first official dope controls during the Olympic Games in 1968 in Grenoble and Mexico.

A law against doping in sport was adopted in Belgium in 1965 and since that time, controls have been carried out during events of the Belgian Cyclist Union. The number of dope controls which took place during the Olympic Games in 1968 to 1984 amounted to 9235, of which 35 were positive. The number of controls carried out for the Belgian Cyclist Union from 1965 to 1986 amounts to 14 346 of which 489 were positive.

The experience acquired, along with controls carried out by other organizations, enabled the establishment of a list of banned classes of substances, which is regularly updated. The latter necessitates permanent study and a particular effort on behalf of the laboratories. The list is universally accepted and serves as a basis for the fight against doping carried out in liaison with the individual international sports federations, GAISF (General Association of International Sports Federations), FIMS, the National Olympic Committees and the governments.

The doping definition of the IOC Medical Commission is based on the banning of pharmacological classes of agents. The definition has the advantage that new drugs, some of which may be especially designed for doping purposes, are also banned.

The following lists represent examples of the different dope classes to illustrate the doping definition. Unless indicated, all substances belonging to the banned classes may not be used for medical treatment, even if they are not listed as examples. If substances of the banned classes are detected in the laboratory, the IOC Medical Commission will act. It should be noted that the presence of the drug in urine constitutes an offence, irrespective of the route of administration. The following classes and regulations for the 1988 Olympic Games are given in full in the *List of Doping Classes and Methods* drawn up by the IOC Medical Commission.

Doping classes

Stimulants

For example:

amfepramone
amfetaminil
amiphenazole
amphetamine
benzphetamine
caffeine*
cathine
chlorphentermine
clobenzorex
clorprenaline
cocaine
cropropamide (component of Micoren)
crothetamide (component of Micoren)
dimetamfetamine
ephedrine
etafedrine
ethamivan
etilamfetamine
fencamfamin
fenetylline

fenproporex
furfenorex
mefenorex
methamphetamine
methoxyphenamine
methylephedrine
methylphenidate
morazone
nikethamide
pemoline
pentetrazol
phendimetrazine
phenmetrazine
phentermine
phenylpropanolamine
pipradol
prolintane
propylhexedrine
pyrovalerone
strychnine
and related compounds.

Stimulants comprise various types of drugs which increase alertness, reduce fatigue and may increase competitiveness and hostility. Their use can also produce loss of judgement, which may lead to accidents in some sports. Amphetamines and related compounds have the most notorious reputation in producing problems in sport. Some deaths of sportspeople have resulted even when normal doses have been used under conditions of maximum physical activity. There is no medical justification for the use of amphetamines in sport.

Another group of stimulants are the sympathomimetic amines of

* For caffeine the definition of a positive depends upon the concentration in urine exceeding 12 µg/ml.

which ephedrine is an example. In high doses, this type of compound produces mental stimulation and increased blood flow. Adverse effects include elevated blood pressure and headache, increased and irregular heart beat, anxiety and tremor. In lower doses they (e.g. ephedrine, pseudoephedrine, phenylpropanolamine, norpseudoephedrine) are often present in cold and hay fever preparations which can be purchased in pharmacies and sometimes from other retail outlets without the need of a medical prescription.

Thus no product for use in colds, flu or hay fever purchased by a competitor or given to him or her should be used without first checking with a doctor or pharmacist that the product does not contain a drug of the banned stimulants class.

β-2 agonists

The choice of medication in the treatment of asthma and respiratory ailments has posed many problems. Some years ago, ephedrine and related substances were administered quite frequently. However, these substances are prohibited because they are classed in the category of sympathomimetic amines and therefore considered as stimulants.

Only the use of the following β-2 agonists is permitted, in aerosol form:

bitolterol	salbutamol
orciprenaline	terbutaline.
rimiterol	

Narcotics analgesics

For example:

alphaprodine	ethylmorphine
anileridine	levorphanol
buprenorphine	methadone
codeine	morphine
dextromoramide	nalbuphine
dextropropoxyphen	pentazocine
diamorphine (heroin)	pethidine
dihydrocodeine	phenazocine
dipipanone	trimeperidine
ethoheptazine	and related compounds.

The drugs belonging to this class, which are represented by morphine and its chemical and pharmacological analogues, act fairly specifically as analgesics for the management of moderate to severe pain. This description, however, by no means implies that their clinical effect is limited to the relief of trivial disabilities. Most of these drugs have major side effects, including dose-related respiratory depression, and carry a high risk of physical and psychological dependence. There exists evidence indicating that narcotic analgesics have been and are abused in sports, and therefore the IOC Medical Commission has issued and maintained a ban on their use during the Olympic Games. The ban is also justified by international restrictions affecting the movement of these compounds and is in line with the regulations and recommendations of the World Health Organization regarding narcotics.

Furthermore, it is felt that the treatment of slight to moderate pain can be effective using drugs—other than the narcotics—which have analgesic, anti-inflammatory and antipyretic actions. Such alternatives, which have been successfully used for the treatment of sports injuries, include anthranilic acid derivatives (such as mefenamic acid, floctafenine, glafenine, etc.), phenylalkanoic acid derivatives (such as diclofenac, ibuprofen, ketoprofen, naproxen, etc.) and compounds such as indomethacin and sulindac. The Medical Commission also reminds athletes and team doctors that aspirin and its newer derivatives (such as diflunisal) are not banned but cautions against some pharmaceutical preparations where aspirin is often associated to a banned drug such as codeine. The same precautions hold for cough and cold preparations which often contain drugs of the banned classes.

Note that dextromethorphan is not banned and may be used as an antitussive; diphenoxylate is also permitted.

Anabolic steroids   For example:

bolasterone	nandrolone
boldenone	norethandrolone
clostebol	oxandrolone
dehydrochlormethyltestosterone	oxymesterone
fluoxymesterone	oxymetholone
mesterolone	stanozolol
metandienone	testosterone*
metenolone	and related compounds.
methyltestosterone	

This class of drugs includes chemicals which are related in structure and activity to the male hormone testosterone, which is also included in this banned class. They have been misused in sport, not only to attempt to increase muscle bulk, strength and power when used with increased food intake, but also in lower doses and normal food intake to attempt to improve competitiveness.

* For testosterone, the definition of a positive depends upon the ratio in urine of testosterone : epitestosterone being above 6.

Their use in teenagers who have not fully developed can result in stunting growth by affecting growth at the ends of the long bones. Their use can produce psychological changes, liver damage and adversely affect the cardiovascular system. In males, their use can reduce testicular size and sperm production; in females, their use can produce masculinization, acne, development of male pattern hair growth and suppression of ovarian function and menstruation.

It is well known that the administration to males of human chorionic gonadotrophin and other compounds with related activity leads to an increased rate of production of androgenic steroids. The use of these substances is therefore also banned.

β-Blockers   For example:

acebutolol	nadolol
alprenolol	oxprenolol
atenolol	propranolol
labetalol	sotalol
metoprolol	and related compounds.

The IOC Medical Commission has reviewed the therapeutic indications for the use of β-blocking drugs and has noted that there is now a wide range of effective alternative preparations available in order to control hypertension, cardiac arrhythmias, angina pectoris and migraine. Due to the continued misuse of β-blockers in some sports where physical activity is of no or little importance, the IOC Medical Commission reserves the right to test those sports which it deems appropriate. These are unlikely to include endurance events which necessitate prolonged periods of high cardiac output and large stores of metabolic substrates in which β-blockers would severely decrease performance capacity.

Diuretics   For example:

acetazolamide	diclofenamide
amiloride	ethacrynic acid
bendroflumethiazide	furosemide
benzthiazide	hydrochlorothiazide
bumetanide	mersalyl
canrenone	spironolactone
chlormerodrin	triamterene
chlortalidone	and related compounds.

Diuretics have important therapeutic indications for the elimination of fluids from tissues in certain pathological conditions. However, strict medical control is required.

Diuretics are sometimes misused by competitors for two main reasons, namely, to reduce weight quickly in sports where weight categories are involved and to reduce the concentration of drugs in urine by producing a more rapid excretion of urine to attempt to minimize detection of drug misuse. Rapid reduction of weight in sport cannot be justified medically. Health risks are involved in such misuse because of serious side effects which might occur.

Furthermore, deliberate attempts to reduce weight artificially in order to compete in lower weight classes or to dilute urine constitute clear manipulations which are unacceptable on ethical grounds. Therefore, the IOC Medical Commission has decided to include diuretics on its list of banned classes of drugs.

Note that for sports involving weight classes, the IOC Medical Commission reserves the right to obtain urine samples from the competitor at the time of the weigh-in.

Doping methods

Blood doping Blood transfusion is the intravenous administration of blood, red blood cells or related blood products that contain red blood cells. Such products can be obtained from blood drawn from the same (autologous) or from a different (non-autologous) individual. The most common indications for red blood transfusion in conventional medical practice are acute blood loss and severe anaemia.

Blood doping is the administration of intravenous blood, red blood cells or related blood products to an athlete other than for legitimate medical treatment. This procedure may be preceded by withdrawal of blood from the athlete who continues to train in this blood-depleted state.

These procedures contravene the ethics of medicine and of sport. There are also risks involved in the transfusion of blood and related blood products. These include the development of allergic reactions (rash, fever, etc.) and acute haemolytic reaction with kidney damage if incorrectly typed blood is used, as well as delayed transfusion reaction resulting in fever and jaundice, transmission of infectious diseases (viral hepatitis and AIDS), overload of the circulation and metabolic shock.

Therefore the practice of blood doping in sport is banned by the IOC Medical Commission.

Pharmaco-logical, chemical and physical manipulation The IOC Medical Commission bans the use of substances and of methods which alter the integrity and validity of urine samples used in doping controls. Examples of banned methods are catheterization, urine substitution and/or tampering and inhibition of renal excretion, e.g. by probenecid and related compounds.

Classes of drugs subject to certain restrictions

Alcohol Alcohol is not prohibited. However breath or blood alcohol levels may be determined at the request of an international federation.

Local anaesthetics Injectable local anaesthetics are permitted under the following conditions:

1 That procaine, xylocaine, carbocaine, etc. are used, not cocaine.
2 Only local or intra-articular injections may be administered.
3 Only when medically justified (i.e. the details including diagnosis, dose and route of administration must be submitted immediately in writing to the IOC Medical Commission).

Corticosteroids Naturally occurring and synthetic corticosteroids are mainly used as anti-inflammatory drugs which also relieve pain. They influence circulating concentrations of natural corticosteroids in the body. They produce euphoria and side effects such that their medical use, except when used topically, requires medical control.

Since 1975, the IOC Medical Commission has attempted to restrict their use during the Olympic Games by requiring a declaration of use by the team doctors, because it was known that corticosteroids were being used non-therapeutically by oral, intramuscular and even intravenous routes in some sports. However, the problem was not solved by these restrictions and therefore stronger measures designed to not interfere with the appropriate medical use of these compounds became necessary.

The use of corticosteroids is banned except for topical use (aural, opthalmological and dermatological), inhalational therapy (asthma, allergic rhinitis) and local or intra-articular injections. Any team doctor wishing to administer corticosteroids intra-articularly or locally to a competitor must give written notification to the IOC Medical Commission.

13.4 Dope analysis

M. DONIKE

Introduction

Dope analysis is an integral part of the system of dope control. Its aim is to provide correct and defendable analytical results which are based on scientific data. Dope analysis is a very complex area and comprises not only the methods of modern analytical chemistry but also the know-how of many other scientific disciplines. For example, biochemistry explains the metabolism of dope agents, and pharmacokinetics describes the time course of the blood and urine concentrations of dope agents and their metabolites. In human sport, the biological liquid available for analysis is urine. It is worth mentioning that only very low concentrations of the dope agents will be present. For stimulants and narcotics the necessary detection limit is the lower ppm range (μg/ml $= 10^{-6}$ g/ml) and for anabolic steroids the lower ppb range (ng/ml $= 10^{-9}$ g/ml).

Comprehensive screening procedures

To fulfil the demands of national sports federations, international sports federations and of organizers of area games, world championships and the Olympic Games, a large number of samples must be tested for a variety of dope agents. The number of substances (or their metabolites) is determined by the dope definition of the IOC Medical Commission and other organizations.

The best approach to solve such an analytical problem is to screen the urine samples with comprehensive chromatographic methods using sensitive and selective/specific detectors. By using high-resolution capillary columns in one chromatographical run several hundred substances can be separated and preliminarily identified by their retention times. The first comprehensive screening procedure based on these principles was the screening procedure for volatile stimulants excreted

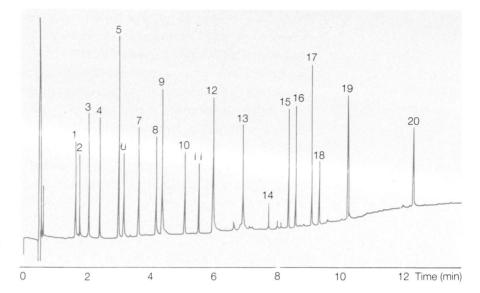

Fig. 13.4.1 Screening procedure for basic substances: fused silica capillary column, SE 54, cross-linked, length of column = 16 m, 0.2 mm i.d.; chromatogram of a calibration mixture containing 20 compounds.

free in urine (Donike *et al.*, 1970) (Fig. 13.4.1). The characteristic features of this approach are:

1   Alkaline ether extraction.
2   Injection of the extract on a gas chromatographic column without further steps such as concentration.
3   Temperature-programmed gas chromatography to shorten analysis and increase the detection limit for substances with long retention times.
4   Use of a nitrogen-specific detector to reduce the biological background and to increase the sensitivity for nitrogen organic compounds.
5   Registration of retention times and signal intensities by a computer.

The banned substances named as examples in the classes of dope agents defined by the IOC Medical Commission can be classified by their chemical and biochemical properties into five groups:

1   Nitrogen-containing compounds excreted free in the urine.
2   Nitrogen-containing compounds excreted as conjugates with sulphate or glucuronic acid and detectable by gas chromatography only after derivatization.
3   Stimulants with special chemical structures and properties.
4   Anabolic steroids.
5   Acidic compounds such as most of the diuretics.

Following the principles outlined earlier, special screening procedures for these chemical–biochemical classes of compounds were evaluated (Donike *et al.*, 1985). The substances classified under points 2 to 5 (above) bear polar functional groups which must be derivatized before gas chromatography. Derivatization increases the sensitivity of the applied analytical method, first by reducing the adsorption in the gas chromatographic system, and second leading to a higher response if a mass spectrometer is used as the gas chromatography detector.

To detect substances mentioned in points 3 and 5, it may be of advantage to use high-pressure liquid chromatography (Cartoni *et al.*, 1980).

Table 13.4.1 gives an overview of the analytical methods employed to detect different dope agents in urine samples.

Final identification

If initial urine analysis suggests the possibility of a banned drug, its metabolite or a related substance being present, the urine will be analysed by more sophisticated analytical methods. At this stage, with the information of the first analysis, the sample preparation may be modified

Table 13.4.1   Overview of the analytical methods used to detect dope agents in urine.

Chemical/biochemical classification	Sample preparation			Analytical methods		
	Hydrolysis	Extraction	Derivatization	Separation technique	Detection technique	Sensitivity (ng/ml)
Nitrogen-containing compounds excreted free in the urine, e.g. amphetamine, ephedrine	No	Ether	No	GLC	N–FID	100
Nitrogen-containing compounds excreted as conjugates with sulphate or glucuronic acid, e.g. phenolalkylamines, β-blockers, morphine	Yes	Ether + alcohol	Yes TMS/TFA TFA	GLC	N–FID/MS	10
Stimulants with special chemical structure and properties, e.g. pemoline, caffeine	No	Ethylacetate	No	HPLC	UV/VIS MS	100
Anabolic steroids (a) excreted free, e.g. metandienone, oxandrolone (b) excreted as conjugates, e.g. nandrolone, metenolone, testosterone	Yes No Yes	XAD$_2$/ ether XAD$_2$/ether	Yes TMS/HFB TMS	GLC GLC GLC	MS MS MS	1 1 1
Acidic compounds such as most of the diuretics, e.g. furosemide, etacrynic acid	No	Ether	Yes CH$_3$	GLC/HPLC	UV/VIS MS	10

CH$_3$, methyl group; GLC, gas liquid chromatography; HFB, heptafluorobutyryl group; HPLC, high-pressure liquid chromatography; MS, mass spectrometry; N–FID, nitrogen-specific detector; TFA, trifluoroacetyl group; TMS, trimethylsilyl group; UV/VIS, ultraviolet visible absorption spectroscopy; XAD$_2$, a polymeric adsorbent.

to increase sensitivity and/or specificity. The ultimate identification will be made by comparing the analytical data of the dope agent with those of authentic reference substances. These may be the pure agents or if the metabolites must be identified, urine of volunteers who have ingested the banned drugs. A positive result can only be accepted if the chromatographic and mass spectrometric data of the suspicious sample are in agreement with the reference.

IOC accredited laboratories

As dope analysis is a difficult type of biochemical analysis, related in some aspects to forensic–toxicological analysis, reports of false positive as well as false negative results have occurred. Both kinds of results will undermine the credibility of dope control—which is placed in a very sensitive area of sports, that of sport politics. The IOC Medical Commission followed in 1980 the proposal of the IAAF Medical Commission to create 'accredited laboratories'.

The requirements for accreditation were specified to check the competence of laboratories and to harmonize and standardize the quality of the analytical methods. It is a well-known fact that detection limits and coverage of banned substances may differ to a large extent between laboratories working in the same area. To receive comparable results, great efforts in terms of proficiency tests are necessary. Therefore the requirements specify:

1 The analytical equipment.
2 The analytical methods.
3 The proficiency tests to be performed to receive or to maintain accreditation.

Eighteen laboratories are accredited, most of them in Europe and North America. To create more laboratories in other areas is the common interest of the IOC Medical Commission, area authorities and international sports federations.

Anabolic steroids as problem drugs

In 1986 the 18 accredited laboratories performed 32 982 urine analyses. On 623 samples a positive result was reported (1.9%). In these positive samples 687 banned substances were identified (Table 13.4.2). In spite of the fact that anabolic steroids are mostly used in the training phase,

Table 13.4.2 Frequencies of detected substances, grouped in classes of dope agents.

Classes of dope agents	Number
Stimulants	177
Narcotics	23
Anabolic steroids	439
β-Blocker	31
Diuretics	2
Sedativa	15
Total	687

about two-thirds (63.9%) of the samples were found positive for anabolic steroids or their metabolites. This high percentage underlines the importance to not only screen for anabolic steroids at all competitions with tests of the highest possible sensitivity, but also to perform dope controls outside competitions, i.e. during the training period.

Conclusion

In the past, and in the present, dope analysis follows the challenges which are brought into sports by new developments on the pharmaceutical market as well as by the never-ending efforts to improve performance by chemistry.

The recent banning of diuretics and β-blockers is an example of the reaction of the responsible authorities. For these classes of compounds the analytical techniques—extraction, derivatization, combined gas chromatography/mass spectrometry or high-pressure liquid chromatography—are available. For blood doping, reliable analytical techniques do not yet exist. Another challenge—the application of pituitary and hypothalamic peptide hormones—has yet to be faced and the arguments for banning carefully weighed. In principle, the analytical techniques based on radioimmunassay are available as clinical tests, but the conditions under which these tests may be applied in dope analysis must be specified to avoid false positive and false negative results.

References

Cartoni, G. P., Ciardi, M., Giarrusso, A. & Rosati, F. (1980) Reverse-phase high-performance liquid chromatographic detection of pemoline in dope control. *J. Chromatogr.* **202**, 131.

Donike, M., Bärwald, K.-R., Christ, V., Opfermann, G., Sigmund, G., Zimmermann, J. & Schaenzer, W. (1985) Screening procedure in doping control. In A. Ljungqvist, P. Peltokallio & H. Tikkanen (eds) *Sports Medicine in Track and Field Athletics.* Lehtikanta Oy, Kouvola.

Donike, M., Jaenicke, L., Stratmann, D. & Hollmann, W. (1970) Gas-chromatographischer Nachweis von stickstoffhaltigen Pharmaka in wässrigen Lösungen mit dem Stickstoffdetektor. *J. Chromatogr.* **52**, 237.

Index

Page numbers in italic refer to tables and/or figures